HARVEY CUSHING

A Life in Surgery

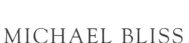

MICHAEL BLISS

UNIVERSITY OF TORONTO PRESS

Toronto Buffalo London

University of Toronto Press Incorporated
Toronto Buffalo London
Printed in Canada

ISBN 0-8020-8950-X

∞

Printed on acid-free paper

Library and Archives Canada Cataloguing in Publication

Bliss, Michael, 1941–
Harvey Cushing : a life in surgery / Michael Bliss.

Includes bibliographical references and index.
ISBN 0-8020-8950-X

1. Cushing, Harvey, 1869–1939.   2. Brain – Surgery – History.
3. Neurosurgeons – United States – Biography.   I. Title.

RD592.9.C87B5 2005   617.4'8'092   C2005-901941-7

University of Toronto Press acknowledges the financial assistance to its
publishing program of the Canada Council for the Arts and
the Ontario Arts Council.

University of Toronto Press acknowledges the financial support for
its publishing activities of the Government of Canada through
the Book Publishing Industry Development Program (BPIDP).

For my family

Contents

❧

Illustrations follow pages 180 and 372

Preface

~

Harvey Cushing (1869–1939) was one of the first American medical men to be the world leader in his field. He was one of the first great surgeons produced by the United States, and in the early years of the twentieth century he became the world's first successful brain surgeon. Cushing stands to neurosurgery as Sigmund Freud did to psychoanalysis – a comparison he would not have liked because he believed psychoanalysis was quackery. Better, perhaps, to call Cushing the Captain James Cook of neurosurgery, or the Babe Ruth of his game.

Cushing's life and work are splendidly documented, mostly because of his obsessive record keeping and letter writing, but also because so many others believed that his life should be recorded for posterity. The sources on which this book is based are extraordinarily rich and enable a biographer to describe Cushing's life and surgical times in immense detail. In an earlier time, when readers had more leisure, I might have written two or three volumes.

The documents make possible a rare re-creation of Cushing's private and public life and the interaction between his personal and professional values. Harvey Cushing operated on the brain the way he did because of the person he was – a doctors' descendant, conservative, ambitious, perfectionist, a Midwesterner, and a Republican. His life was an American epic, rooted in the nineteenth century and extending through the Gilded Age, the Progressive Era, the Jazz Age, and the Great Depression. It stretched 'from tallow dip to television' (as he entitled one of his essays). The American writer who in my view seems to have come closest to capturing many aspects of Cushing's world was F. Scott Fitzgerald. It would take a biographer of Fitzgeraldian sensibility and range to do full justice to Cushing and his family.

Cushing's friend and official biographer, John Farquhar Fulton, was to an uncanny degree the F. Scott Fitzgerald of American medicine. Unfortunately, by the time Fulton published the 754 pages of *Harvey Cushing: A Biography* in 1946, his talents had been so corroded by drink and other diversions that he was unable to do much more than let Cushing speak for himself in scissors-and-paste chapters. These were mostly assembled by two of Cushing's former secretaries, leading spirits of the group of talented women who worked for both Cushing and Fulton and more or less jokingly called themselves the 'harem.'

In 1950 a second-generation member of the harem, Elizabeth H. Thomson, published *Harvey Cushing: Surgeon, Author, Artist*. More intimate and readable and less chauvinist than the official biography, it was, like the secretaries themselves, discreet and, at bottom, deeply devotional. Thomson's understanding of Cushing's professional achievement and its context was limited. Both biographies, as well as the many article-length biographical portraits of Cushing written by his contemporaries and colleagues, were also constrained by the limits of their sources. I have had access to virtually all of the sources that previous Cushing biographers used and many more, including intimate diaries and family correspondence. The only constraint I must observe is to protect the privacy of some of his patients.

I began to get to know Harvey Cushing when I decided that his two-volume 1925 biography of his mentor, William Osler, which was long considered a medical classic, had become out of date and inaccessible to modern readers. I undertook to write a new biography of the Canadian-born physician who is widely regarded as one of the founders of modern medicine and one of history's great doctors. While working on

William Osler: A Life in Medicine, I had to immerse myself not only in Cushing's Osler records but also in the Osler-Cushing friendship as it developed during their years together at Johns Hopkins Hospital in Baltimore. My appreciation of the richness of the Cushing papers and of Cushing's own relationship to Osler's career grew. If William Osler, in the late nineteenth century, was the transmitter of crucial Old World innovations in research and medical education to the United States, via Canada and via Johns Hopkins, then Harvey Cushing became the first great American product of the vision held by Osler and some of his other colleagues at Johns Hopkins. Osler and his Hopkins surgical counterpart, William Stewart Halsted, went to Europe to learn from Old World masters and brought back to North America what they had learned. A few years later, Europeans began coming to America to learn surgery from Harvey Cushing.

By the time I finished the Osler biography I had realized that it required a sequel, a biography of Cushing. Each would stand alone, but together the two volumes would be a biographical study of the rise of North American medicine and surgery. They would also be unusually detailed portraits of two great figures in medical history. In Osler's case, the determination to present a balanced view of his life, stressing shortcomings as well as achievements, was made exceptionally difficult by the man's remarkable saintliness. Osler became something of a modern biographer's nightmare by living up to his reputation as mentor and icon. Cushing, I found, was very different. Mentor and icon, yes, but also at times hard-driving, egotistical, and mean. In those ways he was perhaps more human than Osler, perhaps more revealing of his time and place, perhaps more talented and more driven, certainly more American.

While this is a scholarly biography, complete with footnotes, I have tried to make it intelligible to any reader, lay or medical. Medical readers will have to pardon my occasional simplifications; non-medical readers will have to master a few technical terms, each one explained the first time it is used. My aim as a biographer is always to follow Walt Whitman, who wrote that the poet 'drags the dead out of their coffins and stands them again on their feet ... He says to the past, Rise and walk before me that I may realize you.' Harvey Cushing, who seems to have clung to a belief in some kind of spirit-life after death, would have liked that image.

Another image that influenced me in the writing of this biography comes from Fitzgerald's *The Great Gatsby*. It happens that I grew up in a little Ontario town on the shores of Lake Erie almost directly across the water from Cushing's hometown of Cleveland. This is my first book on a person or event that did not originate in Canada. Partly because many of us study American history in detail, partly because of our own culture and history, Canadians hope that they have the right balance of knowledge and detachment to write well about the United States. In my case, I would like to think that the lake and the border running through it created the distance a scholar needs to get the perspective right. The complication lies in all the connotations of the image of the flashing green light across the water.

MICHAEL BLISS
KINGSVILLE, ONTARIO
SPRINGFIELD, PRINCE EDWARD ISLAND
OCTOBER 2004

HARVEY CUSHING
A Life in Surgery

It was good to be hard, then; all nice people were hard on themselves.

F. SCOTT FITZGERALD, *TENDER IS THE NIGHT*

The Surgeon and the General

One day in 1898 General Leonard Wood, an American military governor of occupied Cuba, stood up abruptly from his desk and hit his head on a low-hanging chandelier. He was badly stunned for a few minutes and developed a large bump on his skull, but otherwise thought nothing of the incident.[1]

Wood was both a physical fitness fanatic and a trained physician. His personal approach to signs of illness or debility was to ignore them and just get on with his job of improving the health of the Cuban people. When his tour of duty in that country ended, he could take considerable credit for the anti-mosquito campaign that wiped out yellow fever on the island, a great American gift to Cuba. The bump on Wood's head subsided but never entirely disappeared.

Wood was a close personal friend of Theodore Roosevelt. They were completely kindred spirits, and Wood, who had earlier won the Congressional Medal of Honor in the campaign against Geronimo, had been the commanding officer of Roosevelt's Rough Riders in Cuba. After he became president in 1901, Roosevelt appointed Wood a military governor in the Philippines – the other islands taken over by the United States in its 'splendid little war' with Spain. Wood thus became America's first significant proconsul, a ruler of conquered provinces, as the United States began to strut and flex its muscles on the world stage and debate what kind of imperial power it would become.

About the time he began serving in the Philippines, in 1901–2, Wood began to have trouble controlling his left foot. It often felt as if it were asleep, and it dragged as he walked. He tried to ignore the problem. Feeling numbness also in his left hand, Wood began shaving and shooting left-handedly to force the limb into action. Then the cramping in his left leg began to spread to his arm and chest. Wood sensed that he might be on the verge of having some form of epileptic convulsions, and he took to carrying a vial of chloroform, one good whiff of which would forestall an attack. Once or twice he failed to take the precaution and did pass out. Hating to admit to infirmity and very busy suppressing native insurrections in the Philippines, Wood was finally driven to consult other doctors. They thought his problem must be neurological, somehow related to the bony and now-expanding lump on his head, just to the right of center.

In 1905 Wood placed himself in the hands of Arthur T. Cabot, a Boston surgeon of impeccable medical credentials and social lineage. Cabot operated on Wood's head, trephining, or drilling, through his cranium and removing the bony lump. It contained a small tumor studded with sandlike grains known as psammoma bodies. Cabot was careful not to go further. He did not pierce the dura, the tough membrane encasing the brain. Surgeons did not go there if they could possibly avoid it. When some tried, their patients usually did not come back.

Cabot's surgery gave Wood no relief. The general then consulted the British Empire's leading authority on surgical approaches to the brain, Victor Horsley of London. Horsley could not decide what was wrong with Wood and made no recommendation.[2] Cabot suggested that Wood try the one specialist in brain surgery in the United States, young Harvey Cushing at the Johns Hopkins Hospital in Baltimore.

Cushing examined Wood in the spring of 1909. Probably at Cushing's request, Wood was also seen by two of America's legendary physicians, Silas Weir Mitchell and William Osler, respectively the patriarch and the high priest of the country's medical profession. Cushing was very much their protégé.

The doctors were baffled. Part of their diagnostic problem was that they had no way of seeing what was happening inside Leonard Wood's head. The era's miracle technology, the x-ray, was not helpful because it could make pictures only of bone structures, not of the body's soft tissues, such as the brain. The external symptoms suggested that there must be some lesion affecting Wood's brain under the dura, which Cabot had not reached. Perhaps it was an old cyst or a broken-down clot, probably stemming from the chandelier incident. It could hardly be a tumor, somehow related to the one Cabot had removed, the doctors reasoned, because Wood was not showing any of the classic symptoms of brain tumor – headaches, dizziness, impaired vision.

Cushing raised but did not push the possibility of exploratory surgery, for it was risky even with the revolutionary techniques he had developed during the few years he had specialized in neurosurgery. He had never seen a case quite like this. Even on more familiar ground he was having a run of bad results, having lost several patients while trying to excise tumors. Truth to tell, his success at finding and removing brain tumors was pretty limited. General Wood's mental vigor was unimpaired and his physical capacities still excellent, so the doctors sensibly advised a wait-and-see approach. Cushing was relieved when Wood agreed. 'Glad that his operation has been postponed, for everyone dies that I touch,' the despondent surgeon told his wife that summer.[3]

By the beginning of 1910, America's ranking general, about to become army chief of staff, could no longer keep up with his men on an obstacle course, and when on horseback he was in danger of falling off. Wood telegraphed Cushing that he wanted an operation regardless of the risk. He was quietly admitted to the Johns Hopkins Hospital on February 4, and the next day, using a general anesthetic, Cushing opened his cranium.

He cut through the general's scalp, drilled and sawed through the skull, and with great difficulty, because of heavy bleeding, was able to open a flap of bone on the vault of the cranium, exposing the dura. Pressing the dura, Cushing found it unusually firm and concluded that there must be some kind of growth beneath it. He removed additional bone to try to estimate the area of the problem, cut through the dura, thought he glimpsed a growth, but had so much trouble with constantly oozing blood that he decided to withdraw. He sutured the dura, inserted drains to help deal with bleeding, then partially replaced the bone flap and sutured the scalp closed.

Wood had stood up well to the anesthetic and the loss of blood. Four days later Cushing tried again, at first using only local anesthetic because he already had his opening into the brain, which is an insensitive organ – literally lacking any feeling. As he folded the dura back on itself and the cortex of Wood's brain bulged into the opening, Cushing saw the edge of a tumor. He had to apply clamp after clamp to try to stop hemorrhage from the tiny vessels permeating the fringe of the brain, and realized he had better put the general under. 'It was evident that matters were going to be so desparate,' he wrote in his surgical notes, 'that it was thought best to have the patient anaesthetized and chloroform was again administered.'

Cushing had done several hundred craniotomies over a period of about eight years but had successfully removed only about ten tumors. As he studied Wood's growth, his first thought was that it was a glioma, the tissue of the brain itself running wild and so disrupting the organ that he might as well abandon the operation and leave the patient to his sad fate. Then Cushing realized that if he could not remove the growth, he could at least fall back on palliation, as he often did with his patients. He could ease the pressure inside Wood's head and make room for the tumor to grow for a few more months or years before it killed the general. 'With some hesitation, the exposure was persisted in with the expectation that the removal of dura and complete obliteration of the bony island which contained the primary growth might give the unquestionably large tumor chance to extrude itself and thus to postpone pressure symptoms that would unavoidably have to set in in time.'

Surprise: With the tumor tissue itself swelling into his operative field, Cushing found that he could work around its edges, now in one place, now in another, slowly carefully, isolating the tumor and separating it from the healthy tissue. Finally he was able to tilt the whole mass upward, reach in and cut its stalklike attachment deep against the longitudinal sinus of Wood's brain, and take it all out. The potato-shaped tumor weighed about 6.5 ounces (198 grams).

Cushing then patiently began to back out of the operative cavity, fighting residual bleeding all the way. He got it under control, filled the depression left by the tumor with saline solution, inserted drains, closed the dura, replaced the bone flap, and closed the scalp. The operation had lasted more than four hours, incredibly long for surgery in that era. It was later said, possibly apocryphally, that Arthur Cabot, observing the procedure, left the room at intervals to tell the relatives that the general had put up a marvelous fight and shown great courage – but said it all in the past tense.[4]

When Leonard Wood regained consciousness his left side was completely paralyzed and he showed symptoms of imminent convulsion. They soon passed. The wound healed without infection or incident. The tumor Cushing removed had not gone deep into the brain after all. It proved to be a rare form of slow-growing meningioma (a term that Cushing coined, some twelve years later). It was identical in appearance to the exterior tumor Cabot had removed; it had grown inward from the brain's intermediate lining and had infiltrated sinuses and cavities without poking through the innermost lining into the cerebral tissue itself. It was benign, would recur only if Cushing had failed to remove it completely, and at worst would not be a problem again for many years.

Harvey and his wife Kate were at home the evening after the operation. Their doorbell rang, and Harvey found another general of the U.S. Army, Hugh L. Scott, standing on his doorstep. Scott explained that he had been walking the streets all day and couldn't stand the uncertainty any longer – he simply had to know how his friend and mentor Wood was doing. The surgeon invited the general into his home, where to everyone's surprise it turned out that Scott and Kate Cushing knew each other from a western trip they had been on years before with William F. Cody, the frontier showman. General Scott stayed until nearly midnight, chatting about the Wild West, Buffalo Bill, General Wood, and brain surgery.

Leonard Wood, an impatient patient, was up and walking in a few days, was soon able to tie his shoelaces, was discharged from hospital one month to the day after his first operation, and, Cushing wrote, 'as though nothing had happened immediately resumed his work with accustomed vigor.' He had some residual lameness in his left foot, which in no way impeded his mission of trying to modernize the U.S. Army to be ready for major combat in a European war.[5]

Harvey and Kate Cushing were Major General Wood's guests at the 1911 Army-Navy football game. Then as now in the United States, the gift of good seats to a big game was a significant favor. Cushing hugely admired the military leader as an American who was changing the world for the better through service to his country and his fellow man, especially in bringing public health to backward countries.

The operation that saved Wood's life was one of Harvey Cushing's finest pieces of surgical service. In 1910 only a handful of surgeons in the world could have opened Wood's cranium without killing him. No one could have done the operation with as much chance of success as Cushing – slight though it appeared – because no one else could come and go into the heads of patients with Cushing's facility and success. In the half-dozen years leading up to the Wood operation, Harvey Cushing, working at Johns Hopkins, had developed the techniques that made him the father of twentieth-century neurosurgery.

Soon after the Wood operation, Cushing was offered an appointment as chief surgeon at Boston and Harvard's new showpiece medical institution, the Peter Bent Brigham Hospital. He and his family moved to Boston, where until his retirement he was the world's most prominent brain surgeon – the American whom the serious medical world came to see in the era of Woodrow Wilson, Charles Lindbergh, Babe Ruth, and Franklin D. Roosevelt. Cushing was fairly certain that Arthur T. Cabot, who had been amazed by the Leonard Wood operation, had a decisive say in inviting him to join the Boston medical establishment. 'He had never seen an operation of the kind,' Cushing remembered, adding, 'no more had I.'[6]

By the end of his Boston years, Cushing had attacked more than two thousand tumors inside the heads of rich and poor, black and white, male and female patients. Few of his patients were as prominent as Leonard Wood. He had also trained a generation of disciples who were establishing neurosurgical units in major hospitals across the United States, in Canada and Great Britain, and throughout Western Europe. At the peak of his career, after a grueling and crippling tour of duty as a surgeon during the First World War, Cushing found time to write a two-volume biography of his friend and role model, Sir William Osler. It won him a Pulitzer Prize in 1926 and became a classic of its genre. The Cushing touch, with scalpel and pen, in operating room, clinic, journals, monographs, and at the podium, had a major impact on the generation that founded modern American medicine and on the evolution of the specialty of neurosurgery around the world. The superlatives – a great pioneer, a giant, heroic, larger than life – really do apply in Cushing's case.

Cushing and Leonard Wood were both Americans whose work could be said to have helped shape the modern world. In the long run, Cushing's impact was greater than Wood's – and a bit less controversial if no less dramatic. (Wood, who eventually had to be disciplined for insubordination, seriously aspired to the presidency and was a role model for one of his protégés, General Douglas MacArthur.) It happened that Cushing and Wood and others of their era, including the Roosevelts, had much in common: ambition; boundless, driving energy; a fanatical work ethic; a penchant for self-promotion and ruthlessness; more than a soupçon of American prejudice and chauvinism; and an enormous appetite for life.

There was a price to be paid for surgical greatness – by Harvey Cushing himself, by Kate Cushing, and even by their daughters, Betsey, Mary, and Barbara – though few who followed the glittering careers of the fabulous Cushing sisters in the 1940s and 1950s would have thought they enjoyed anything but the ultimate in privilege, status, and wealth. There was also Leonard Wood and his parasagittal meningioma. Cushing's breakthrough operation bought Wood many good years as a military man and a politician. But the growth did recur. When Cushing again had Leonard Wood on his operating table, in 1927, the Boston surgeon had become one of the men who had helped make medical miracles an everyday occurrence, and he was far more confident at this trade. On this occasion, Cushing made one mistake and General Wood paid in full.

The following chapters explain how Harvey Cushing, a doctor's son from Cleveland, came to be the maker of epic medical events at a formative time in American history.

ONE

Western Reserve: The Cushings of Cleveland

~

Harvey Williams Cushing was born in the old Western Reserve, in the city of Cleveland, Ohio, on April 8, 1869. He was the tenth child of Henry Kirke Cushing, MD, and Betsey Maria Williams Cushing.

Like Nick Carraway, he was born with advantages not available to many other people in the world. His family was embedded in American history and the history of American medicine. Grandfathers Cushing and Williams had taken part in the epic journeys of New Englanders over the mountains to open the heart of the continent. Grandfather Cushing was the second generation of Cushing physicians. Harvey's father became the third, Harvey and one of his brothers would become the fourth.

The Cushings prospered while Cleveland grew from a frontier town into one of America's largest and most beautiful cities. As the son of affluent parents who retained their New England values, Harvey had as good and rich an upbringing by the shore of Lake Erie as America could provide – a carefree, cultured, and happy boyhood. He inherited his parents' temperaments, becoming much like them in later life, as well as inheriting some of the wealth that their enterprise and the growth of Cleveland created.

~

Both sides of Harvey Cushing's family had a strong sense of lineage and a pioneer tradition. The convention, of course, was to highlight the male line. The Cushings had come from Norfolk, England, during the great seventeenth century emigration of religious dissenters. The English family, whose name evolved from McOssian through Cusheyn, was undistinguished until it adopted the Puritan faith and set sail for America. Matthew Cushing and Nazareth Pitcher Cushing and their children arrived in Boston aboard the *Diligent* on August 10, 1638, eighteen years after the landing of the *Mayflower*. They settled in the village of Hingham in the Massachusetts Bay colony and began the Cushing line in the New World. Cushings joked about all of them having issued from 'Matthew's Pitcher.'[1]

Cushings became planters (farmers) and merchants and strong churchmen and prominent New England citizens. They became known as the 'family of judges.' Judge William Cushing of Massachusetts was one of the first justices of the Supreme Court and near the end of his career declined George Washington's request that he serve as chief justice. A maverick branch of the Cushings migrated to Canada as United Empire Loyalists. Harvey's ancestors were farmers at first, but they became medicalized towards the end of the 1700s when David Cushing Jr of Rehoboth, Massachusetts, studied physic with a noted local doctor, James Bliss, and decided he knew enough to enter practice.

David chose to move west, as many New Englanders were doing by that time. He found a promising stopping-point at Stafford Hill in the Berkshire region of western Massachusetts, where the local physician had recently died. He settled down, married the doctor's widow, Freelove Brown Jenckes, and developed a prosperous medical practice. Known as a 'forehanded' (straightforward) man, Cushing became a landowner and an investor in local industries. He owned an unusually large collection of medical books for his time and was remembered by his son as a sensible and highly esteemed member of the profession. David Cushing Jr died at the age of forty-seven in 1814 from typhus apparently con-tracted while he was treating prisoners captured during one of the battles of the war between the United States and England.

David's son Erastus, who was born in 1802 and lived to influence his grandson Harvey, followed his father's profession. He first studied medicine with a local doctor, then attended lectures at the College of Physicians and Surgeons in New York City, and finally took an MD degree in 1824 from a newly established local medical college in the Berkshires. For his thesis, Erastus wrote a reasonably learned two-thousand-word dissertation on medical aspects of *Conium maculatum*, or hemlock (the drug used to poison Socrates), which included his own observations on the utility of the plant in practice. He once saw the narcotic apparently have some good effect on a woman suffering from horrible facial pain, a condition his grandson might have diagnosed and treated surgically as tic douloureux.[2]

Erastus Cushing married Mary Ann Platt, also of Puritan descent, and began to raise a family and ply his trade in the Berkshire hills around the town of Lanesboro. But that hardscrabble region had had its moment, and the tide of settlers was moving on. Like many country doctors in that century and afterwards, Erastus found it exhausting to be on call twenty-four hours a day, struggling through snow and mud from patient to patient. He decided to protect his health and also to better himself.[3] He first toured some of the principal settlements farther west – the towns of Buffalo, Cleveland, Detroit, and Columbus – then upgraded his medical knowledge by attending lectures in Philadelphia at the United States' oldest and best medical school, the Medical Department of the University of Pennsylvania. In the autumn of 1835 Erastus, Mary Ann, and their three children moved west. As the family was leaving its hill-country home, an elder of their church met them on horseback, bid them farewell, bared his head, raised his eyes and hands to Heaven, and asked for God's blessing on their journey.

The doctor and his family traveled overland from the Berkshires to Albany, New York, where they boarded a canal boat for the week-long trip through the Erie Canal to its western terminus at Buffalo on the chain of inland seas known as the Great Lakes. A lake boat took them another hundred miles west along the south shore of Lake Erie. They embarked at the little town of Cleveland, Ohio, at the mouth of the Cuyahoga River. Family lore has it that as the Cushings walked up Superior Street from the landing into the town, one of their first sights was a white cat, surely a good omen.[4]

∽

The area around Cleveland was attracting many settlers from Connecticut because it was originally part of that state's territory. The Connecticut colony's charter included a grant of vast western lands, formalized after the Revolution as its Western Reserve. In the late 1790s the Connecticut Land Company surveyed the territory, and a town site at the mouth of the Cuyahoga was laid out by the chief surveyor, a graduate of Yale College named Moses Cleaveland. In the first decade of the nineteenth century the Western Reserve began to be settled by the descendants of Connecticut Puritans. Harvey Cushing would one day write a good account of the opening of the Western Reserve in which he quoted an unnamed source on the region's uniqueness as 'the last distinct footprint of Puritanism.'[5]

His mother's family – the Williams line – and the families of the Fitch and Mygatt women the Williams men married were among the Connecticut Puritans who migrated to the Western Reserve. Grandfather William Williams, born in 1803 into a family that had been in America since the 1660s, left a good autobiographical account of his father's 1811 decision to move from Windsor, Connecticut, to 'New Connecticut.' At that time there were neither canals nor practical steamboats. The Williamses went by ox-drawn covered wagon, rolling west on corduroy roads towards the setting sun, their slave boy Joel with them. They tried to sail west from Buffalo but were becalmed for weeks and then nearly shipwrecked in wild storms. Finally, they struggled in midwinter through the primeval Lake Erie wilderness to the settlement of Painesville in the Reserve, where they stopped. The slave boy, at that time said to be the only black in northern Ohio, was treated as just another member of the family, according to the Williamses. One day Joel sliced into his knee with an ax. The wound became infected, and a local surgeon eventually amputated the leg, but the boy died soon after. William Williams also told vivid stories about riders in the night who called the settlers to arms in 1812 with warnings that the British were coming to pillage and murder, having crossed over from Canada and captured Detroit. Fortunately for the Americans, the foreign forces stayed on the north side of the lake.

As a young man, William Williams backtracked to Buffalo – in those years very much a New England outpost – where he served an apprenticeship in banking and land speculation. He became one of the bustling city's most active real estate dealers, prospering in the orgy of speculation that bracketed 'the marriage of the two oceans' when the Erie Canal was opened in 1825. He married Lucy Fitch, daughter of a pioneer Reserve family in 1827; after she died giving birth to their second child, Williams married her sister Laura. In 1837, a year of severe financial distress, he decided to move with his family back up the lake to Cleveland.[6]

~

The Cushings, the Williamses, and their forebears were a product of the rough egalitarianism of early New England. Reminiscing in the 1870s, Erastus Cushing stressed 'how uniform the condition of life of our ancestors … has been. They have all apparently, as far as we can trace them, belonged to very much the same rank in society; all tolerably honorable men and women, neither quite rich nor very poor, but in a middle class.' To grandfather Cushing, being a successful physician was to be middle class, middle rank.[7]

Grandfather Williams, a businessman who had learned Latin and Greek at a private academy in the Western Reserve, saw social distinctions more finely. In his early years in Buffalo he had lived 'in close association … with the best and wisest material, mentally, intellectually and practically … a class of men of more than equal worth and ability.'

'It could scarcely be,' he remarked, 'that ... I could fail of appropriating or absorbing more or less of this element into my own forming character. The families of these men also stood at the head of all social order and influence in the community.' They were common folk with high aspirations, who had brought their Bibles and other books and their musical instruments with them through the wilderness, and they had no sooner settled than they began to think of schooling and getting ahead. One historian described the Western Reserve as being opened by 'common people exerting themselves ... for some form of ideal excellence,' a definition that exactly captured the image Harvey Cushing would imbibe of his family and its goals.[8] A birthmark, a footprint, the handiwork of Puritanism.

~

There were about five thousand Clevelanders when the Cushing and Williams families arrived in the mid-1830s. The town's prospects hinged on its location at the Lake Erie end of an old portage route to the Ohio-Mississippi river system. Just as the Erie Canal had been the making of Buffalo, so the Ohio and Erie Canal, linking Cleveland with the Ohio in 1825, became the key to Cleveland's early growth. In the 1830s Cleveland became the great transshipment point for agricultural produce pouring out of the American West, and for goods and people pouring in, a role that a few decades later would pass to Chicago.

Distances in the United States were immense, and Americans' identification with their home state or region was still very strong. Erastus Cushing's wife Mary, writing in 1836 after her first winter in Cleveland, saw herself in a 'western world' far removed from her 'native land' in the Berkshires. But she was not unhappy:

> Every thing seems to be stirring, buildings are going up – people moving, carmen have their carts in readiness – steamboats in port are being put in order, and everybody on tip toe for the opening of navigation ...
>
> Erastus' business is increasing, and is for the most part in the best families

– for the past four weeks his time has been constantly occupied in the practice of his profession, and with good success thus far ... Land purchase is much more of an object than we had any idea of.[9]

Erastus Cushing had developed an interest in obstetrics during his Philadelphia studies, and one of the instruments he brought with him over the mountains was a special pair of forceps for use in difficult deliveries. No one else in the Western Reserve had its equal, as Erastus apparently proved in one of his early services to a prominent Cleveland family. This became the making of his practice.[10] The Cushings bought town property fronting on the intersection of Euclid Street and Central Square (later known as Public Square), and Erastus settled into what a friend described as 'the silver door-bell practice' in Cleveland: he doctored the core families of old and affluent Cleveland, the ones who had silver bells on their doors. For a year or two, Erastus and a partner also ran a drug store.[11]

Erastus saw eight to twelve patients a day, usually charging seventy-five cents to a dollar for a 'visit and advice.' His patients were not only the well-to-do. A servant girl was seen and charged twelve cents. Harvey remembered Erastus's story of having gone out to deliver the child of a woodchopper one winter night; the town still stood on the edge of the forest (even when it grew up, Cleveland called itself the Forest City), and the doctor found himself being chased home by wolves.[12] In the yard of their home on Central Square, the Cushing children, Kirke, William, and Cornelia, kept pigs, chickens, ducks, and any number of smaller pets. When the William Williams family settled in Cleveland in 1837, they located nearby on Euclid Street.

The slender, sharp-featured, and kindly Dr Cushing became one of Cleveland's most respected physicians. Little is known about how he actually practiced except that he worked extremely hard, taking 'but little rest night or day.' He probably had the strength and weaknesses of most good doctors of his era – the strength being his ability to gain his patients' confidence and keep their confidences, the weaknesses stemming from the primitive state of medical knowledge and therapeutics.

In the 1830s Erastus Cushing's own children were regularly venesected, or 'bled,' in hope of relieving their spring fevers, which in the Western Reserve might still have included malaria. The only daughter, Cornelia, was sickly all her life. She suffered from what was first thought to be asthma, then diagnosed as inflammation of the lungs, and finally realized to be the dread scourge of the nineteenth century – 'consumption,' or tuberculosis. No physician's black bag contained an effective treatment for the wasting, racking, bloody cough of the consumptive. Erastus wrote that he wished he could give his daughter restorative relief, 'but in this case, as well as in many others, my ability falls far short of my desires.'[13]

During a crisis in her disease in 1856 Cornelia was treated with anodynes, 'light blistering,' and the application of leeches. Erastus himself had a chronic health problem diagnosed as 'inflammation of the liver,' which periodically flared up and immobilized him. In 1856, as Cornelia lay in her room near death, her father suddenly had a relapse: 'Doc was seized this morning with one of his attacks of neuralgia in the stomach and has been suffering prodigiously ever since. You may know what agony it must be that extorts continuous groans and drives him to run from room to room and to roll on the floor.' Erastus recovered quickly – he was probably having problems with gallstones – but Cornelia did not, dying in her twenty-fourth year.[14]

With his father working so hard and his mother looking after Cornelia and a sickly brother, Erastus's eldest son, Henry Kirke, born in 1827, grew up more or less on his own, 'without much stamina and of nervous tendencies,' he remembered. He was educated at private schools catering to the Reserve's transplanted New Englanders, and in 1845 went east to attend Union College in Schenectady, New York, graduating in 1848. He returned to Cleveland and learned medicine by working with his father and by taking lectures at the local medical school, the Cleveland Medical College, where Erastus moonlighted. All the 'professors' at this New World medical school were full-time practitioners making a bit of money from teaching on the side; the quality of the courses was probably not high. Like his father before him, Kirke went on from the local school to take a finishing year in medicine at the University of Pennsylvania. Erastus, whose letters to Kirke that year are filled with gentle wisdom and liberality – especially in urging him to buy all the books he wanted – hoped the boy would get a sounder medical training than he had had. Erastus felt that the shortcomings of his medical education had hampered his practice: 'May you profit by the errors of my experiences.'[15]

Erastus urged Kirke to investigate opportunities for further education, then make up his own mind about his future. Kirke decided to stay in Philadelphia for advanced training in one of its hospitals, but in the spring of 1851, when his father was prostrated with illness, he was suddenly called back and thrown into the family practice. Kirke, too, always regretted that he had not been better trained, though there is no direct evidence that he resisted going home to Cleveland to work with his father. Any such inclination would have dissolved in his sense of family duty.[16]

William Williams's eldest daughter, Betsey Maria ('Bessie'), born in 1828, had a similar sense of family obligation. After settling in Cleveland, her father and his second wife, Laura Fitch, had seven more children. Bessie's stepmother (who was also her aunt) needed help raising her brood at the best of times, and more so during her frequent illnesses. In her early teens, Bessie Williams added a repertoire of mothering and housekeeping skills to the classical language, literary, and musical training she received in school. A teacher called her one of the most remarkable children he ever saw, absorbing knowledge effortlessly, hardly ever making a mistake. At home Bessie was full of energy, apt to recite long poems from memory while performing marvels of knitting and crocheting. Her singing and cooking and her loving discipline convinced her stepbrothers and stepsisters that she was practically perfect. She was beautiful, too – black-haired, with large bright eyes and an erect 'carriage' that made her appear tall and slender. As she entered womanhood, Bessie Williams shone as a great prize for the man who could take her as his wife.

Kirke Cushing and Bessie attended school together, and the families often mingled. Kirke's mother once remarked that she knew of no one doing as much mothering as 'that dear girl,' Bessie Williams. 'She is a rich pattern for all for her untiring industry, patience and happy tact in household duties.' 'What a mother in Israel she was,' one of her step-brothers wrote (referring to Deborah, the dark-eyed prophetess who mothered the people of Israel and led them against the Canaanites).[17] Nothing is known of the courtship of Kirke Cushing and Betsey Maria Williams. They married on June 17, 1851, and went on a bridal tour to visit Massachusetts relatives.

∾

Bessie soon became a mother in her own right. During the sixteen years from 1853 to 1869 she gave birth to ten children. Sickness and death seemed to haunt the household. There was no problem with the first-born, William Erastus (1853), but Charlotte (1855), Julia (1856), and Cornelia (1857) all died in their first year. Alice (1859) was in her second year of life and Henry (1860) was still nursing when the outside world broke in on the family. In the aftermath of Abraham Lincoln's election to the presidency, the slave states seceded. The Cushings were immediately caught up in the Civil War.

Like many New Englanders, the Williams and Cushing families had supported the crusade to abolish slavery. They were ardent supporters of the radical antislavery party, the Republicans. When Lincoln issued his first call for volunteers, to serve for three months, Kirke Cushing immediately enlisted and received a commission as surgeon to the 7th Regiment Ohio Volunteer Militia. Leaving his wife and children at home, he went off for training and then to war.

Despite all her skills and her self-reliance and the comfort she took in knowing that she and Kirke were reading the same passages of Scripture each night, Bessie found her husband's absence almost unbearable.

She was frightened about what might happen to him, frightened to be alone, frightened for the children, and worried about how hard her father-in-law Erastus had to work to maintain the family's medical practice. She was a loving and passionate wife, and in long, almost daily letters, she pleaded for her husband's return:

> Oh! if I could see you to-night, my love! If I could have one good night kiss! One caressing touch of your hand! my husband! If you could only look in upon these dear, little sleeping ones, who are yours, God-given! How fervently I pray for the time when we may be reunited. It seems like a part of my life lost – this separation ...
>
> Oh Kirke! baby is such a treasure! You are losing his sweetest days ... Do you think you would forget sometimes that you have a home and family, if my letters did not come to remind you? ...
>
> How often I thought of the hours in which we have watched *together* over our sick little ones, when I walked the floor, with baby in my arms, or sat rocking him in the chair through the weary, *lonely* hours of last night! Don't you think I remember how many demands I have always made upon you in such emergencies? And how ready you always were to aid, and to relieve me of responsibility and care? I wonder sometimes that you have been so patient with my helplessness, and so willing to give up your time to your own great inconvenience. Dear Kirke, this is a great care and anxiety for me to have, without you, but perhaps it is what I need to make me less dependent.[18]

Bessie's worst fear was that her doctor-husband would not come home when his three months were up but would re-enlist for three years, as most of the volunteers had done. She was afraid that he might come to like the wild and free life of men in camps, afraid that he would give in to military ambition ('Do not let motives of honor and promotion influence you more than you are aware'), and she worried that his sense of duty might cause him to abandon his family.[19]

A fastidious and shy man who had had a fairly sheltered upbringing and neither drank nor smoked, Kirke found much of camp life 'unpleasant and unseemly,' yet he thrived on the food, the outdoor life, and, after a few weeks of training, the adventure of his regiment's advance into the hill country of western Virginia:

> My faith is still firm that slavery is to be ended by this revolution, but how is the question. I am now seeing a little of slavery for the first time. The slaves are quite black, civil, and apparently not aroused by our presence in any way. There are occasional exceptions however ...
>
>   The inhabitants are mostly clad in homespun and have a slouched, limpey, greasy look ... The women here knowing that we will not disturb them are insolent hateful & abusive ... In the main our boys have avoided offense in the way of pillage and abuse of power.[20]

The free-wheeling individualism and rude democracy of army life gradually began to grate on the young doctor. He formed no close friendships except with the chaplain. As a medical officer, dealing mostly with cases of measles and dysentery, he took a stern approach to the volunteers' health, including their lack of cleanliness and their malingering. 'He has not pandered to the whims of men who thought they were sick when they were not, or who pretended to be sick to shirk duty, or who were a little sick and wished to be petted,' the chaplain wrote home. 'This has made him seem to some cold severe and unsympathizing.'[21]

Despite his misgivings and his wife's pleadings, Kirke decided to re-enlist after the first three months. Knowing he was a good medical officer, he aspired to advance to brigade surgeon. But his unpopularity jeopardized even his current position. Learning of a plan to have him transferred to some other regiment, he chose to go home pending a decision on promotion. It was a lucky move; not long after he left, the 7th Ohio, which had enjoyed an unopposed advance deep into 'secesh' territory, was suddenly surrounded by Confederate troops. Most of the northerners surrendered and were taken prisoner.[22]

Kirke Cushing returned to Cleveland expecting to be called to further duty. The life had agreed with him to the extent that he now found it hard to sleep in a bed and considered setting up a tent in the yard.

When Bessie served him peach preserves, he wondered whether it was an extravagance better saved for visitors. Although he was asked to report to Washington for an interview, he never went. Bessie, it appears, was determined not to lose her man again. She made clear to him that his real duty was to stay at home. Kirke never talked about why he left the army, though one of his sons mused: 'I think I have heard mother say it was because he found her worn out, [baby] Harry quite ill, and his father also far from well and overburdened with family and professional cases, and he concluded it was his duty to stay here.'[23] The timing of the birth of their seventh child, Edward (1862), suggests that Kirke impregnated his wife immediately after getting back from the war.

Nor did his return ease her burden in other ways. As his father had done, Kirke lectured at the Cleveland Medical School. He fell on the steps of the school one day, probably in the autumn of 1861, and cut his knee through his trousers. The wound became infected, and he was immobilized for most of the next twelve months, eight of them in bed, with amputation a possibility. With the help of one servant, Bessie ran the household, minded the babies and baby illnesses, and lifted, bathed, and nursed her sick husband. 'Well she must have been made of iron,' Harvey told his own wife many years later.[24]

Kirke Cushing recovered from his domestic wound but dragged a stiff knee for the rest of his life, and three times during the Civil War he volunteered to work with wounded soldiers after great battles. When the North began drafting men for service in 1864, he paid $1,000 to have a substitute, a recent immigrant, take his place.[25] It was not an unusual or necessarily dishonorable practice. The eighth Cushing child, George, was born that year. Alleyne followed in 1867, and Harvey Williams on April 8, 1869.

~

Kirke Cushing was constantly busy. He worked unremittingly, never taking a holiday. During the 1860s, with the family living in a small house at 10 Euclid (which Street became Euclid Avenue in 1865 and evolved into one of America's most fashionable residential areas), he often worked late into the night at his office. Although Kirke had effectively taken over his father's high-class obstetrical practice and his was not an extravagant household, he felt under constant pressure to make ends meet. He was classically frugal: he spent little on himself, paid promptly and in cash, never borrowed. Like his father before him, Kirke never had a formal picture taken or painted; the Cushing doctors eschewed such vanities. A puritan in everything but religion, Kirke eventually stopped going to church. His ledgers show that by the early 1890s he was seeing patients seven days a week.

His practice eventually generated a very comfortable income for the late nineteenth century, some $8,000–12,000 annually (perhaps $300,000 in today's purchasing power).[26] The spectacular growth of Cleveland from small town to America's sixth largest city in less than half a century had pleasant real estate consequences for the Cushings. Both Erastus's original property (facing Public Square) and the site of Kirke's first home were redeveloped with the erection of multistory business 'blocks.' Rental income from these holdings would become very important in the life of his son Harvey. In 1873 the Cushing family moved 'uptown' into a fine rambling frame house at 786 Prospect Street, a block over from and parallel to the now-swanky Euclid Avenue.

∾

Harvey's first memories were of being read to by his mother at bedtime, of saying his prayers, and then having poetry recited to him before he fell asleep. As the youngest of Bessie's children, he may have been her special favorite – certainly he was not taken for granted, which was often the fate of double-digit offspring. One of the earliest references to Harvey is in a letter that his eldest brother, Will, a law student at Harvard in the mid-1870s, wrote to their mother: 'Why do you ring the "wonderful baby" in my ears each week? I have no respect for infants in general – but if he has done anything of mention and different from each baby, let us hear it.'[27]

All the Cushing babies were much loved and well provided for. Kirke's closeness with money was only to ensure that his family lived comfortably and could afford to take advantage of the opportunities opening to young Americans after the Civil War. Bessie's mother love was as boundless as her belief in reading, education, music, family loyalty, cleanliness, temperance, and regular attendance at the Presbyterians' Old Stone Church. One of her half-brothers commented that as a result of her surrogate mothering experience before marriage, Bessie made no mistakes with her own children.[28] None of the Cushing children ever recorded a word of criticism about their perfectly wonderful mother. Harvey recalled that she even did most of the family doctoring, doling out the paregoric, nux vomica, eye drops, and other potions from the medical cabinet. Not surprisingly, Harvey came to assume that a doctor's wife should know enough not to bother her husband with the children's little illnesses.

When he jotted down memories of his father, Harvey's first words were 'Severity – spanking.' Kirke used his open hand or the back of a hairbrush across bare buttocks. Bessie spanked too. 'I'm sure it was good for us and probably hurt them the most.' In the eyes of his family and the world, Dr Kirke Cushing was a reserved, stern man and a strict father. He hardly features in his sons' memories of their boyhood – obviously because he worked so hard and because he left most of the parenting to Bessie. He severely compartmentalized his life, so that the family, for example, knew almost nothing about his medical practice except that he believed in strict confidentiality and the most rigorous professional ethics.

After the Civil War crisis, Kirke was certainly not an absent father. There he was stoking the coal furnace every night – no one else was allowed to do it. There he was 'relaxing' at his carpenter's bench, making and mending furniture, and impressing his children with his handiness. He, of course, presided at meals and family prayers. But all remembered how remarkably silent their father could be. For a week or more at a time he would not say a word to anyone. He may have been angry for some domestic reason or troubled in his work, the children thought. Perhaps he suffered periods of mild depression as the daily grind and the years took their toll. Kirke Cushing had broad intellectual interests – he followed current events and the exploits of explorers and scientists and military men. He may have felt that in going back to Cleveland to take over Erastus's practice and then staying there with Bessie and the children he had not maximized his opportunities. In later years he never urged Harvey to come home.

What the world did not see of the elder Cushing was his dry sense of humor, his ambition for his sons, and, in conflicts with them, his flexibility and liberality. The fact that he tended to stay out of his boys' daily lives, letting the young colts have their head, was not necessarily a black mark. Unlike Ernest Hemingway, the boys did not have any 'Nick Adams' stories of watching their father deliver babies – Kirke would have considered such voyeurism shockingly unprofessional – but neither was any pressure put on them to follow in the family's medical footsteps.

Family rituals and duties were well understood. The children were expected to be punctual and to do their share of household chores. 'It was a house in which there was no loafing or sitting about,' Harvey remembered. Novel reading, especially dime Westerns, and card playing were mostly forbidden. Good reading was encouraged, but Harvey could not remember being influenced by any particular book, except perhaps the McGuffey series of school readers. Nor, to his later puzzlement, did he develop much sense of music: 'We always had two grand pianos in the house, and eight-hand duets were constantly being played. I never got nearer to it than as a child to find that if I hugged the leg of one of the pianos and pressed my youthful ear against it, the vibrations were considerably louder and quite enjoyable.'[29]

For many years there were morning prayers and grace at meals. Sunday was for churchgoing and Bible reading – no toys, no games, no other books. The family took the streetcar to the Old Stone Church in Central Square and sat in a row in the Cushing pew, little Harvey squirming in a corner at the end. Kindly Mr Parsons from the pew behind would slip the boy a peppermint candy while his mother smiled indulgently and his father paid no attention. Mr Parsons once said that he wouldn't feel at home in heaven unless his pew was behind Mrs Cushing's. Harvey never became deeply religious, was never steeped in the Bible or Presbyterian hymns, never seems to have worried about heaven or hell. His had been peppermint-flavored Presbyterianism.[30]

Harvey started his schooling at a small private school for neighborhood children. Just as he was about to transfer to a junior public school, at about age six, he had a bout of scarlet fever: 'I was quarantined in so far as to sleep on a cot alongside the double bed in which Father and Mother always slept, and it was characteristic of her that she not only did all the nursing and doctoring for me but saw to it that while convalescing I kept up with my lessons by games that were educational. It was made play that I should write out the menus for my meals, for example, and to my lasting chagrin the other children howled with delight at my spelling of "bananna."'

All his life he had trouble with spelling, despite his mother's insistence that he repeat his spelling lessons over and over during their noon-hour carriage rides when he was in public school (to be sure, spelling standards in nineteenth-century Cleveland were high; Cushing's schoolboy words included 'ichthyophagous'). When he was in high school she helped him with his Latin and Greek. His earliest surviving letter, written to brother Will when he was eight years old, shows both his spelling problem and his father's affectionate presence:

> I want you to come home. We have got a new hen ... we had two turkeys on Thanksgiving and one the day after. Papa made me a man and it was made of wishbon and it was made of a turkeys wishbon and it had a feather in its hat and it had wire arms and mama mad some clothes for it and I am going to hang it on the Christmas tree ... Ed broke a great piece of our bed ... and up in your room the window blew wright in and papa came up stares and fixed it up as well as he could.[31]

Cushing's boyhood was full of playmates: siblings, a horde of cousins, chums from other old and respectable Cleveland families. The Williams clan was especially close-knit and congenial. Over the years its social puritanism had been moderated by observing the *gemütlichkeit* of some of the city's early German immigrants. Christmas, for example, evolved from a minor holiday into a rich, family celebration. Music nights and amateur theatricals in the Williams circle occasionally even drew in Dr Kirke. The singing games verged on dancing, with rhythms and rhymes acted out in the fashion of the Shakers who had settled near Cleveland and believed in dancing before the Lord: 'I give my right hand a shake shake shake and I turn my body about / I give my ugly mug a shake shake shake and turn my body about.'[32]

The boys' favorite character was grandfather William Williams, a loose-collared, gray-haired, gruff old patriarch, neck bulging with what Harvey described as a 'Western Reserve goitre,' who loved to play the word game Verbarium with them. After the Puritan bans were lifted, W.W. enjoyed card games. He always played to win and was smart enough usually to win, but would be allowed to win anyway, and insisted that everyone in the game hop to it – exactly as Harvey did when playing tennis with young surgeons years later. Harvey remembered his grandfather's sense of humor: his epitaph was to read 'Here lies W.W. / Who never more will trouble you, trouble you.'[33]

The Cushing boys had barnfuls of pets: pigeons, chickens, doves, dogs (Harvey's 'Jack' became a famous trick dog in the neighborhood), cats, and more. Their attic was full of collections – birds' eggs, insects, butterflies, coins, stamps, postmarks – while the house overflowed with books and magazines. Harvey probably remembered little about early reading habits because he spent so much time out of doors. The boys played endless chasing and hiding games in their yard, in the Williamses' yard and in neighbors' yards. They raided everyone's fruit trees and spun tops, shot marbles, played croquet and a kind of vacant-lot football, and also pick-up baseball, which was becoming very fashionable. They let off firecrackers on the Fourth of July, hiked down to Lake Erie for summer swims, went on excursions to uncles' farms outside town, flew kites, coasted down Cobb's Hill in the winter, made outdoor ice rinks, and skated and played shinny.[34] Imagine the classic scenes of late-nineteenth century-childhood – they were Tom Sawyers and Huck Finns without the serious edge.

But they were not without their scraps. Harvey seems to have been quick-tempered from childhood. At a family party when he was about five years old, someone joked about him: 'Pepper Pot, Pepper Pot, when you were young / They tell me you had a most fiery tongue.' Yet there are no signs that Harvey needed more than the normal spankings at home or had any unusual troubles at school (unlike the man who became his mentor, William Osler, who during his Canadian boyhood chopped off the end of a sister's finger, was expelled from a local grammar school, and was taken to court for assaulting a school matron). He did occasionally fight with his fists. 'Harvey very properly called me a freckle-faced freshy, and I retaliated by calling him a stuck-up snob, and we went to it,' a distinguished doctor remembered about eighty years later. 'For forty minutes we punched and wrestled and sweated ... When we were winded we finally sat down on the ground and kicked at each other and, with our faces grotesque in sweat and dust ... we sheepishly grinned at each other and shook hands.'[35]

⌘

Harvey's oldest brother, Will, attended Western Reserve College, which was then in Hudson, Ohio, took a law degree at Harvard, and returned to Cleveland to settle down as a successful lawyer. The only surviving sister, Alice, never went to university, never married, and lived at home, occupied by books and poetry. Harry attended Cornell University, became a geologist, studied in Europe, eventually taught at Western Reserve (which relocated to Cleveland), and became a leading expert on the Adirondack mountain barrier that had played such a role in his family's history.[36] In 1883, just as Harvey entered high school, brother Edward ('Ned') finished a degree at Cornell and entered Harvard Medical School.

This was a record of high family achievement by any standards, more so when it was still rare for young men and women to attend, let alone graduate from, high school. With a population approaching 200,000, Cleveland still had only one high school, Central High School, a classic red-brick Victorian pile that had been the first free secondary school built west of the mountains.[37] The Cushing boys did not all measure up academically. If older brother George finished school, he certainly did not go to college; at age twenty he joined the U.S. Army and went farther west, taking part in at least one campaign against the Sioux.[38] Alleyne, closest in age to Harvey, was apparently often ill and not interested in school; he was to be a great worry to Kirke and Bessie.

By contrast, Harvey was a good scholar, socially popular, and athletically gifted. He developed into a wiry, dark-haired teenager, very fond of baseball and gymnastics. He played on an excellent Cleveland amateur ball team, and he and a couple of friends developed a tumbling routine – Harvey was number two in the pyramid – that once performed in a charity show. He liked to work out on the horizontal bars at the YMCA gym. His father must have been a little perturbed the day he was called to attend to his son who had broken his arm in a bad landing. Harvey was scared stiff to face his father, 'but he was kindness and tenderness itself, reduced the fracture and whittled out a splint ... no questions asked about what foolishness I had been up to.' A bit accident prone, as his own children would be, he suffered various other dislocations and sprains.[39]

Nothing about his formal schooling left any particular impression, not even the excitable Greek teacher who later went crazy. Nor did the piano and dancing lessons he took from an aunt or the French and drawing lessons from an uncle, except that he became an excellent dancer and began to show great talent at drawing. The 'Cushing lion,' a colored pencil drawing of a richly flowing lion's head ascribed to Harvey at age sixteen, still adorns a granddaughter's Manhattan apartment.

One mentor did stand out, a physics teacher named Newton Anderson, who was interested in craftsmanship and camping before there was much of either activity for American boys. Boy Scouts and summer camps had not yet been organized. In the summer of 1884 Anderson took Harvey and three of his cousins up the Great Lakes to Sault Ste Marie on a fishing expedition. That winter he began giving the local boys a manual training course in a neighborhood barn. Within a couple of years, this had evolved into the Cleveland Manual Training School, an adjunct to high school. Anderson bought a small island at the head of Lake Huron near the Sault and took his boys there for summers at what they called Camp Maskenoza, an embryonic boys' camp.

Anderson's activities gave the lads splendid opportunities to escape from scholarship, to escape from what had become an industrial city blanketed with oily soot from John D. Rockefeller's refineries. (The Rockefellers were Cleveland parvenus, a Baptist family that peddled quack medicines and then became fabulously wealthy after the Civil War by exploiting the gushing oilfields of Ohio and Pennsylvania. Kirke Cushing was doctor to a branch of the Rockefellers and for the first three years of its history was landlord to Standard Oil, which had its original offices in the Cushing Block on Euclid. There is no evidence of any social interaction between the families.) At Maskenoza the boys began to break loose from their family circles while developing their own self-discipline and leadership skills. The group built a substantial wooden schooner that some of them, Harvey included, sailed to and from their camp – a major adventure on Lakes Erie and Huron. On their wilderness island they spent high school summers hunting and fishing and improving the campsite, collecting flora and fauna, and dabbling in another of Anderson's interests, photography.

Harvey was one of the most enthusiastic collectors and photographers. All his life he was eager to see and record the world around him, and by high school he was already making deft sketches of various sights. The woodworking and blacksmithing and machining and mechanical drawing that he did in Anderson's classes were the beginning of his manual training with tools other than pen and pencil. A classmate who took second prize in one of Anderson's courses remembered that Cushing won the first prize, a complete set of machine-shop tools.

Oddly, the sources do not mention the instrument which, in that era, was as inspiring to future scientists as computers became to young boys a century later. We might expect that by about age thirteen Harvey Cushing would have taken as avidly to the microscope as young Willie Osler did on the northern shores of Lake Ontario two decades earlier. It appears, however, that there were no microscopes in his Cleveland circles for Cushing to take to. The Cushing doctors practiced with forceps, not microscopes. Neither the local medical school nor the high school appears to have yet discovered the microscope. One of Harvey's classmates remembered that in Anderson's metalworking classes they did design and build a microscope, 'complete with all the adjustments except the lenses.' If they managed to buy lenses, it was perhaps after Cushing had graduated.[40]

Harvey's vocation does not seem in any way to have been preordained or even thought about. At Central High School he took the classical course, which was heavy with Latin grammar, Greek, and literature. He was a good student, obtaining relatively high marks across the board, and in his final year stood eleventh in a class of eighty-three. He was also class president that year, though the only speech anyone remembered him giving was apparently a flop.[41]

Girls are almost as scarce as microscopes in the documentation of Cushing's Cleveland years. But no boy who danced as well as he did, wrote clever doggerel verse, and drew cute little pictures in friends' autograph books could have been totally without girlfriends. Happening to be without a girl at a party one night during high school, he managed to persuade a classmate's date to let him take her home. The classmate followed the couple and confronted Cushing on the sidewalk after he had dropped her off. 'They set to and had a grand battle, which Harvey won,' a friend remembered.[42] There is also a pictorial record: a photo in an old family album of a gang of Cleveland high school kids in which Harvey is sitting beside Kate Crowell, the girl he would eventually marry.

~

When the Connecticut families who had settled and prospered in the Western Reserve talked about colleges for their children, it seemed self-evident that Moses Cleaveland's alma mater, Yale College in New Haven, was the gold standard. Cleveland was known as a Yale town. Three of Harvey's cousins had attended, a second cousin was on the faculty, and six more cousins would eventually go there. Although Harvey's brothers' educational connections were mostly with New York institutions, something about their experiences at Cornell caused Kirke to sour on that college.[43] In the spring or summer of 1887 Harvey went west to Chicago to write the Yale entrance exam. He passed it, and when Yale received the formal testimonial to his character from Central High School he was admitted. In 1887, after another summer at Camp Maskenoza, eighteen-year-old Harvey boarded a train for the long trip east from Cleveland through the mountains and back to Connecticut to begin college in the heart of New England.

TWO

Making a Yale Man

Before Harvey left for Yale, there was an earnest father-son talk. Dr Kirke explained that they were going into a partnership, with mutual responsibilities and duties. The father would supply the money for the education, the son had to conduct himself to his father's 'approval while the partnership survived.' Harvey was not to smoke, drink, 'or be guilty of any immoral conduct or join a College ball club or boat crew.' At age eighteen, he agreed to be bound by his father's terms.[1]

Cushings had high expectations. They expected much from one another, from servants and institutions, and, ultimately, from themselves. They tended to hold everyone and everything to high standards and could be visibly and volubly unhappy – their favorite word to describe being upset was 'sore' – when their standards were not met. Especially within the family circle, Cushings watched over one another, warned, reproved, scolded, usually relented, and almost always supported.

Everyone had to stay in touch. Long-distance telephoning was not yet practical, and telegrams were expensive. The family lived by letter writing – newsy letters, at least one a week, often written on Sundays. Most of the hundreds of letters that Harvey wrote to his parents during their lifetime and many of Bessie's and Kirke's letters to him have survived. As Harvey's life broadened, and as he took up the family habit of making records of all of life's interesting experiences, his letters become the tip of a mountain of diaries, scrapbooks, notebooks, articles, reminiscences, and other sources, including, importantly, his patient records. Beginning with Cushing's Yale years, and moving through his medical education at Harvard and his apprenticeship in Baltimore, his writings document his struggles with his parents' expectations, the emergence of his own sense of values and priorities, the beginning of his single-minded desire to achieve, and much more.

At Yale College in the late 1880s Cushing tested and tempered himself and joined the American social and intellectual elite, and he was duly branded a Yale man for the rest of his life. He went on to Harvard Medical School in the early 1890s to absorb nearly the best medical training America could offer, and graduated into the brotherhood of physicians to follow in his brother's, father's, grandfather's, and great-grandfather's footsteps. During his education Harvey's family played the role of stern guardian angels, hovering to remind him of his commitments and duties, but also to shovel out money, books, food, holiday excursions, and advice on improving his health, improving his spelling, improving his manners, further improving his spelling, and keeping his temper. These hard-driving neo-Puritans could scold and get 'sore' at one another for being so prone to scold and get sore. Through it all, their partnership held solid.

~

Harvey's first reaction to a new place was usually to be disappointed. The small city of New Haven, Connecticut, in September 1887 seemed an odd jumble of old and new buildings. The room Cushing and his cousin, Perry ('Tot') Harvey, rented at 166 York Street was little more than a garret, reeking of calcimine. Their landlady was old, exceedingly fawning, and did not serve meals. Resolving to look for a better place as soon as possible, the boys' first priority was to check out Yale's athletic fields. By the next weekly letter, Harvey and Perry had fixed up their room, joined an eating club for meals, begun classes, survived

hazing and rushing, bought a 'frightful' amount of books, and spent so
much money that Harvey needed to ask his father for more.[2]

The institution had just formally changed its name to Yale University. The old Yale College had been founded some 185 years earlier
when Connecticut Puritans decided that Boston's Harvard College had
become theologically and morally decadent. In Cushing's day, the college was the liberal arts core of an institution also offering studies in
science, law, medicine, and divinity. It was not a very large university –
in 1887 all of the Yale schools enrolled a total of about a thousand
students and employed a hundred and twenty teachers. Yale's old campus across from the New Haven Green was three or four blocks of aged
lecture halls, chapels, dorms, and gymnasia, with the landmark Yale
rail fence still extant. Conservatism and respect for tradition were among
the institution's core values. Yale's governing body still consisted entirely of Connecticut Congregational ministers; compulsory morning
chapel for the undergraduates was to continue for another forty years.

The college curriculum heavily emphasized the classics, mathematics, and rhetoric in the first two years (Harvard dropped compulsory
Greek in 1887; Yale did not), and Cushing's sixteen weekly hours of
classes were still called 'recitations.' The students recited back to their
teachers work they had memorized. The quality of teaching at Yale was
not high by present standards. For example, Harvey's second cousin,
George Trumbull Ladd, the professor of moral philosophy, was a distinguished philosopher but a stupefyingly dull teacher, and there were few
classes in which the students were encouraged to think for themselves.
As one of the characters in Owen Johnson's famous novel, *Stover at
Yale*, puts it, 'Here if you ask a man if he's a Republican or a Democrat,
he writes home and asks his father.' In Harvey's early years at Yale, his
father would have expected no less.[3]

Despite basking in conformity and tradition, Yale by the mid-1880s
was quickening almost as swiftly as industrializing America itself was.
Under its new president, Timothy Dwight, Yale began to attract more
students than ever before, hired more professors, saw more of its graduates go into business, began receiving large donations and bequests

from affluent alumni and friends, and began to rebuild its campus. It dominated American college athletics to a degree never seen before or since. To be at Yale in the 1880s was to be near the pinnacle of American campus life – even if it meant being in relative darkness: the university's new buildings, unlike Harvard's, did not have electricity. Many Yale men, the true-blue sons of Eli, were destined for high achievement. In his four years there, Cushing became a proud, striving, perfect Yale man.

~

Like Dink Stover and most Elis of their generation and most undergraduates everywhere, Harvey at first regarded his courses mainly as a necessary evil. Some of the profs were good, others were 'stinkers.' When his father asked for more detail about his courses, Harvey could not see the point of talking about matters only of interest to others in the class: 'If you do want to know I can tell you they are mighty long and take a heap of studying.' Of course, his father responded with a pep talk about the lifelong benefits of hard study: 'Every victory gained over Latin Composition is a preparation for Success in the hard things of life wh. come to all. So work away at it and feel that after all it is a blessing in disguise. Difficulties squarely met and overcome by faithful work are the tests of character which show the reliable man from the fair weather crowd of sailors.'[4]

The freshman's real enthusiasm was not with the curriculum but with the extracurriculum – the recent explosion in college life of literary, musical, and social activities, and above all of athletic competitions. Beginning with rowing in the 1850s, then football in the 1870s, and then baseball, gymnastics, and track and field, American universities up and down the East Coast had begun to compete fiercely for athletic glory. Tremendous public interest in the college matches was a new phenomenon in American life, the first flourishing of spectator sport.

For Harvey Cushing, the most exciting event in his first few months of college was the Yale-Princeton football game played at the old Polo Grounds in New York on November 19, 1887. Three-quarters of the students and most of the professors took a special train into the city, warmed their stomachs with oyster stew, and shielded themselves with umbrellas: 'It was a fine sight I can tell you. On one side of the grounds were the stands and the other side was lined with coaches of the Yale blue and Princeton yellow trying to out yell each other. The boys all had flags and there were about as many yellow as blue. There were about five thousand people there and lots of them tony NY people out in fancy rigs of all kinds in spite of the rain.'[5]

Cushing was back in New York a week later to spend Thanksgiving at a classmate's home, do some 'gawping around' ('the Brooklyn bridge beats anything I ever saw'), and take in the biggest of all games, the Yale-Harvard contest, which brought out twenty thousand fans and was judged at the time to be the finest football game ever played in America, not least because the practice of 'slugging' opposing players with the closed fist had largely been eliminated. (Yale beat Princeton 12–0, beat Harvard 17–8, and won all the rest of its games that year.)[6]

Kirke Cushing had never sent a son so far away from home or so close to the temptations of a city as wicked as New York. His idea of college life was that boys would go to their classes and study. Gadding about in the big city and attending these sporting events, which were rife with drinking and gambling, seemed to him to verge on immoral student conduct. Harvey made an unfortunate slip that first autumn by suggesting that with football over and the baseball season far off, there was little to do but study. The father was alarmed and angry. The son, who would not be broken by parental silliness, stood up for himself:

Dear Father: I was very sorry to have received such a letter from you as I did last week. What I said about studying hard after Thanksgiving for examinations you seemed to apply to myself and said you thought it a rather sorry confession to come from me. If ... you thought I meant myself I am very sorry, but I don't know as you have any reason to think that I have not, and do not intend to study faithfully. I am sure you know I always did at home, and I don't see why you should suspect I have not here. As for repenting that you sent me here, I am sorry if I have been the cause but if you are afraid I won't study here then I don't see why you should suppose I would elsewhere.[7]

A good performance on his Christmas exams made everything right.

Even when most sore about his son's activities, Kirke did not deny his frequent financial appeals. Yes, Harvey should go ahead and buy two new pairs of shoes. Yes, he could pay a dollar more a week to get into a better, more sociable eating club. He had to be trusted to strike a balance: 'You have been told repeatedly that I hold myself ready to meet all expenses that can contribute to your comfort and advantage. But I must expect that you deny yourself as much as possible, superfluities, that are of no lasting return, and which I am told amount to a good deal in a term.'[8] Here Harvey did comply: he kept careful accounts, faithfully submitted them to his father, stayed out of debt, and took care to make his jackets and pants last until they shone from contact with the wooden seats of the lecture halls.

His parents kept him in touch with Cleveland news, sent along his *Harper's Weekly* and regular food parcels, and bombarded him with advice about looking after his health. Like most nineteenth-century students, Yale men were vulnerable to eyestrain, overwork, and winter-long colds: 'Have you forgotten the rubber cloth and strip of flannel which I put among your belongings when you went away last fall?' writes his mother. 'Will thinks there is nothing like it for a sore throat, and always puts his on at nights at the first symptom. So does your father, if his throat is sore. You need to wring out the flannel in hot water, put it around your neck as hot as you can, and put the rubber over it, securing them with safety pins. Then on taking it off in the morning, bathe the neck throughly with cold water, and rub it dry. You have lozenges of both kinds, have you not?'

His mother told him how to wash his socks so that he could save on washerwoman's charges, and he dutifully complied. Attending carefully to minor details would become one of his most pronounced, and sometimes most irritating, lifelong habits. Already as a freshman at Yale he expected the same from others: 'I gave the "bid" a blowing up one morning and told her she didn't know how to make a bed, she has since tucked in the clothes and they have remained on the bed during the night to my great comfort.' In her reply to this news Bessie gently scolded her son: 'You know that you have a propensity to scold. Watch against it, my dear.'[9]

Although Yale prided itself on being a democratic place, the student body was larded with sons of the rich and powerful, graduates of private schools, and exclusive secret societies. From his earliest days at Yale, Harvey managed to combine a sense of being an outsider – the Clevelanders thought of themselves as 'Western boys' – with a keen appreciation of the value of becoming an insider. Disliking the 'terrible chumps' at their first eating club, Cushing and Perry Harvey joined a higher-priced one with a more select crowd. By virtue of family connnections with the Ladds and others, the boys had an entré into some of New Haven's finest homes. When they took tea at the home of the widow of the founder of Yale's Sheffield Scientific School, Harvey told his mother that 'she is a big gun and we felt pretty stuck up to have dined with them.' Bessie explained that the invitation had probably come because the Cleveland Sheffields were patients of the Cushings, and warned Harvey about too-frequent indulgence in slang.[10]

'Cush' seems to have made friends easily at Yale, and towards the end of his first year both he and his cousin were sounded out about joining one of the sophomore societies – farm teams for Yale's already notorious senior societies. He explained to his father:

There are only two Sophomore societies ... They are very hard to get in as each only takes in 15 men which you see is pretty small out of a class of two hundred. Perry had received a pledge to one of them ... before Christmas. After Christmas some men in the other society came around to see me several times and finally offered me a pledge and as I liked them very much ... I finally accepted it, with your permission that is ... It was quite an honor to make either of them ... It is the only way one has of meeting upper class men ...

I don't want you to think that I am going with a crowd who expect to meet

once a week or so to carouse which I know more than a few do but I promised
you Christmas that I had not touched a drop since I had been here and I know
the first part of Freshman year is the hardest to keep from it so I think I am
pretty well out of it, for by this time most of them know just who don't drink,
though I am sorry to say they are pretty few.

His father saw both sides of the society question: it would be good to be
with a 'steady' set of men, disastrous to fall in with a 'fast' set, as some of
the Cleveland boys were rumored to have done.[11]

The parents tried to draw the line at intercollegiate sports. Fre-
quenting the gym, where he won a horizontal bars prize his first winter,
Harvey worked out regularly, and as spring approached he decided to
try out for the freshman baseball team. He had played a lot of ball in
Cleveland, was small – too small to try out for football (he weighed
130–150 lb in college, and his adult height was 5 ft 7½ in) – and he was
lithe and quick-handed. 'I haven't the ghost of a show to get on,' he
told his mother, but in a game between the frosh and Yale's varsity
'nine,' he found himself inserted at shortstop. 'I didn't feel so big about
it long, for I made an error on the first ball knocked.'[12] He somehow
made the team, thereby setting the stage for a major confrontation
with parental authority.

The trouble was that big-time intercollegiate sport in the United
States in the 1880s was already almost as fraught with semiprofessionalism
as big-time NCAA sports are today. Big money was being bet on big
games. Student athletic associations used admission revenues to fund
special training tables, had created freshman teams as feeders for the
varsity, and encouraged elaborate off-season training to improve performance (Yale baseball workouts began in the gym in February). Athletic scholarships had yet to be invented, but already there were charges
and countercharges that Yale, Harvard, Princeton, and the other big
schools had some pretty suspicious 'students' hanging around only for
the football and baseball seasons – or, in the case of Yale's great all-
round athlete Amos Alonzo Stagg, taking a suspiciously long time to
finish professional training.

At the best of times student athletes seemed to be skimping on their studies to go gallivanting from town to town. Yale's baseball team played not only against other colleges but often against professional teams. The collegians' superior training and discipline often made them competitive. Universities had no formal control over their student teams, which had developed totally extra to the curriculum. The defense of college sports was that it was a healthy, selfless sublimation of the old-time student propensity to rowdyism and riot, but on many occasions the big game triggered wild, drunken celebration. The moralists and their newspapers viewed with alarm; the families back in Cleveland worried about their boys being corrupted.[13]

Both parents objected to Harvey playing intercollegiate baseball. They suggested an apparently reasonable compromise, that he play ball in New Haven but not neglect his studies by making trips out of town. This posed the crucial problem of the freshman team's series against Harvard. At stake in the spring of 1888 was not only bragging rights and the greater glory of Yale but a far more important matter – the right of the whole freshman class to sit on the famous rail fence that enclosed the campus on three sides. Banned from the fence during their early months in New Haven, freshmen had traditionally seized it in a 'fence rush' (i.e., a brawl) with the sophomore class. To reduce rowdiness and property damage, it had been decided that the class of '91 would be able to sit on the fence if its baseball team could beat Harvard's. The matter assumed great urgency because the fence was doomed to be torn down that summer as part of Yale's building program. It was now or never for fence sitting.[14]

Harvey used every argument he could think of to persuade his parents to let him go to Boston for the Harvard game. His marks were good (unlike his cousin and many other athletes he stood in the first division of his class), the physical exercise was good for him, the food at training table was unusually wholesome, his uniforms and team blazer saved him money, and he had lived up to all the other terms of his bargain with his father ('I did smoke a very little last fall, but I am on a fair way to stop now'). The newspapers were falsely sensationalist, he argued. Sport was not corrupting Yale men; in fact, athletes like Stagg and Corbin, the captain of the football team, were looked up to and respected on campus. Freshman contests were not nearly as serious as regular ones, the training was not nearly as serious, but it was almost a duty to one's classmates to help win the right to sit on the fence. The team was depending on him.[15]

Harvey's father gave in, with bad grace: 'If you cannnot withdraw without hardship to others from the Harvard contest I shall say no more about it, but when that is through with, *that must be the end of that sort of thing absolutely* and for good ... I must have an explicit promise ... This matter has made me too nervous to write or do any work today.' His more understanding mother not only dropped her protests but suggested to Harvey that Kirke's harshness might be related to the boils that were plaguing him.[16]

The line on Cushing at shortstop was that he had good hands 'but often throws wildly, and loses his head.' He made two errors – had one hit in four tries and a stolen base – as Yale lost to Harvard in Cambridge, 9–6. The field was soaking wet for the return match in New Haven, but the Elis hung in and won the series with a run in the final inning. 'When we got back to the campus the class formed in line and marched around the corner, where each class was standing by their section of the fence and cheering us, as we went by them, till we came to our fence. The glee club came out and sang and some of the upper class men made speeches but I was so wet I didn't stay but got some supper and had a good shower bath in the gym and was tired Enough too go to bed.'[17]

'I suppose the end of your ambition is attained, if you can sit on the fence,' his mother teased. 'I have had more enjoyment out of our privalege to sit on the fence this last week than in anything, since I have been here, and I guess every one else in the class has,' the nineteen year old shot back. 'Every evening after supper for an hour or two before you have to study there is always a crowd there talking and singing. I have become acquainted with more boys there than in ten times that amount of time elsewhere and boys whom I had never seen before. ... You are always sure to find someone there you know and want to see. It makes me sick to think it will be gone next fall.'[18]

⟨∿⟩

Harvey's nostalgia for the passing of the fence was one sign that his college world might become larger than baseball and sports. On another occasion he thought a lecture by President Dwight on how to select and read books was unusually interesting. Dwight normally put students to sleep. When the Herodotus professor tried 'a new wrinkle' and had the boys find sources other than the textbook, Harvey went to the library and got out a 'great book' on an ancient battle. He forgot this when in later years he denied ever having used Yale's library as an undergraduate, and perhaps he also forgot telling his mother how every day he and a classmate noted the progress of construction on Yale's big new Chittenden library.[19]

It was too early in his Yale life for Cushing to think seriously about the future, but there were a few straws in the breeze. A classmate, Grosvenor Atterbury, tried to interest him in drawing for one of the campus newspapers. On the baseball trip to Boston he visited medical brother Ned, who was serving part of his internship in the operating room at the Massachusetts General Hospital. Ned showed Harvey around the hospital, introduced him to his friends, and allowed him to sit with the medical students and watch him operate. Harvey liked the hospital. Otherwise he had little use for Harvard's campus: 'I don't like the bull pup and pink shirt feeling.'[20]

The fence crisis helped make him a young believer in the importance of tradition. Yale's old fence was coming down, in the teeth of student and alumni protest, to please the donor of a new building. Harvey sided with the past, explaining to his skeptical mother, 'People think a fence especially an old thing like that one is, is a pretty small thing in comparison with a new building but it is the associations of that corner and everything about it that attaches one to it. One of the boys who was down here last commencement time to take his examinations said you would see old men who had come up to commencement and had graduated forty years ago sitting on the fence every morning.'

Cushing was one of a group of students who decided to stage a late-night protest at the desecration by altering the just laid cornerstone of the controversial new building, Osborn Hall. They removed the special copper box of memorabilia that had been cemented into the cornerstone and replaced it with a chamber pot. Most Yale students, including Harvey, eventually snagged a piece of the fence as a souvenir; they effectively tore down the fence in the spring of 1888 before the builders got a chance.[21]

❧

He was already so proudly Yale that he attended the annual Cleveland-Yale Christmas dinners before he graduated. About the beginning of his second year, Harvey's parents lightened up and began to trust him to get along at college without undue solicitude or scolding. Kirke Cushing's boils may have gone away, or he may simply have been satisfied with Harvey's decent grades. Harvey was always a solid B student, doing best in the subjects he liked, toughing out the others. His marks put him in the top third or quarter of the class, but he did not make Phi Beta Kappa.[22]

On the lingering sore point, baseball, the senior Cushings would have paid attention to their relative, Professor G.T. Ladd, who told the Yale dinner in Cleveland that Yale's supremacy 'with the oar the bat and the kick' reflected the students' application of the same discipline they gave to their studies and would carry through life. In the spring of his sophomore year, Harvey wrote an eloquent plea to his father to release him from his promise not to play ball outside New Haven. His whole social future at Yale, including his hope of being tapped for membership in a senior society, seemed to him to depend on doing his bit for the team and thus for the school. His parents quietly surrendered, and for the next three springs Cushing was a regular on the Yale nine. Some years later a faculty report observed how athletes at the school were perceived to be working for Yale, the scholars merely for themselves. 'Hard study,' it concluded, 'has become unfashionable at Yale.'[23]

Increasingly, though, Harvey wrote home about his courses and his response to them, including the time he 'got mad and sailed into the Prof' when he felt he wasn't being treated fairly in Latin recitations. When his horizons were allowed to expand beyond Greek, Latin, and mathematics, he became interested almost in spite of himself. His second-year course in 'rhetoric' was really a course in the English essay, with readings from Addison, Steele, Lamb, Macaulay, De Quincey, and others. The boys had to write essays, a terrifying prospect. So in November, with football season still on and Tot Harvey starting at halfback for the eleven, Harvey passed up a game on a rainy day to go to the library – and told his mother that he 'got so interested looking at other books and relics over in the library' that he 'forgot all about a composition till the librarian rang his bell for closing.' He wrote his first essay on 'The Study of Entomology,' told his mother he found it very difficult, and berated himself for not doing a better job. Here is a student who has fully absorbed family expectations:

> After burning much midnight oil I succeeded in finishing my composition in time to hand it in yesterday morning. With the exception of the former one which I wrote I think it is positively the worst piece of composition I ever read. Unless I take some rapid strides worthy of the seven league boots I will never make much success out of writing. I am sorry you took it so much to heart, my laughing at you for correcting my spelling. I know that is just what I need and wish you and father would always speak of it for I remember it that way better than any other.[24]

Third-year students could choose from a range of electives. Cushing found himself indifferent to William Graham Sumner's lectures in political economy, which touched too often on free trade ideas to suit his Republican tastes. His American history lecturer, on the other hand, was a staunch protectionist who liked scoring off Sumner. The intellectual sparring was good fun; Cushing found American history very interesting, and he did well in it. The next year he added European history and a good introduction to Shakespearean drama, along with a course in evolution from Sumner. 'I like all my courses very much,' he announced to his mother at the start of his senior year. [25]

At the end of sophomore year Harvey asked for his father's advice in choosing electives, because, he said, he still did not know what he wanted to do in life: 'I don't know whether you have any desire of what you want me to do after I leave college or not. I have thought about it a good deal and can't come to any determination at all." Kirke was careful not to try to dictate a profession for his son, possibly thinking that advice might be counterproductive. Despite his friendship with books and history, despite a passing interest in architecture stimulated by his chum Grove Atterbury, Cushing was drifting towards science and medicine. He was influenced by his interest in nature, by the medical gene in the family, and by brother Ned's example. It was also still common for a son to follow his father's profession. Even as Harvey told his father of his uncertainty, he suggested that the opportunity to study chemistry and physiology in third year should be seized 'if I am going to study medicine.' He was on the receiving end of a nearly disastrous explosion in his first chemistry lab and flunked his first recitation in physiology when he could not get a book in time, but liked both courses very much.[26] In senior year he signed up for an introductory course in physiological chemistry from Yale's most distinguished scientist, Russell Henry Chittenden.

The first presentation Harvey Cushing gave on the brain was in the senior course he took from G.T. Ladd on physiological psychology. Ladd asked him to go to the slaughterhouse and get a calf brain to show the class. Harvey instead found an old mongrel dog on campus, cut out its brain at the Sheffield Scientific School, and, hoping the organ would not smell bad, displayed it to the class of theologs and medical students.[27] Most of Ladd's course he found incomprehensible, remembering all his life how stupefying Ladd could be on such subjects as 'the thingness of the thing.' Abstract reasoning in another course was of little interest except to parody:

I don't know most of the time in class whether I am afoot or on horseback. It was with great difficulty at the last recitation that I got some syllogism about the moon and green cheese unraveled. I should hate now to have to tell why a cat can't have nine tails, if no cat has eight tails and one cat has one more tail than no cat, which remark you have probably heard many a time. And when it comes to applying negative conception to a proposition and then showing that the contrapositive of the convertend is inconsistent with something else, then I'm right out in the swim ... I suppose it cultivates the mind however, but I find that I have to plow pretty deep in mine as yet to get any fruits out of it.[28]

His reports home about his 'frog' course, by contrast, glow with interest as the boys dissect the nervous system, learn to use the microscope and micrometer, and experience a bad day in the lab: 'Such as Friday when I broke a large water bottle ... After that I couldn't break enough things, and fail in enough experiments, inwardly swearing at everything in the room, myself principally, during the rest of the afternoon. I could not get any decent crystals ... and stayed three quarters of an hour after the others till I finally succeeded in getting some very fine ones.' He was pleased to discover the value of his sketching ability in making a good set of notes in this course. They are the only notes he kept from his undergraduate studies, and it is a model notebook: principal points underlined, a rough index made for study purposes, and no gaps, doodles, or rude remarks.[29]

◅◅◅◅◅

When Harvey later reminisced about not having worked hard at Yale, it was because he chiefly remembered his extracurricular activities. The two scrapbooks he kept from Yale days consist mainly of clippings about athletics, including accounts of most of the baseball games he played. (He also saved a couple of baseballs, which are still with his memorabilia at Yale.) Whether or not he was actually the 'human sieve' he later joked about, he did make five of Yale's thirteen errors in one game at shortstop.

He was moved to the outfield as a sophomore and made his mark mostly with consistent hitting and good base running. Led by their perennial pitcher, divinity student Amos Alonzo Stagg, Yale was perennial overdog in intercollegiate matches during Cushing's years. In 1889, the year Yale won the College League title, Harvey tied for fifth in batting, averaging .286. It was tougher going in the frequent exhibition games Yale played against the Brooklyn, Philadelphia, Baltimore, and New York professional teams in the National League, but they did eke out occasional wins.

The traveling had its ups and downs. Harvey spent his twenty-first birthday (in 1890) in Baltimore, whose hilly, cobblestone streets he despised, and Yale lost the game. The year before, though, there had been an unexpected bonus when the college ballplayers were received in Washington at the executive mansion by President and Mrs Benjamin Harrison:

> Mrs Harrison had invited the Glee Club and when she heard the nine was also in Washington she invited us too. It made no difference about dress suits. So we went there after the concert and the President and his wife ... were brought in the big reception room, and we all lined up, about fifty of us counting the glee club and banjo club, and one by one were introduced to and shook hands with the Presidential couple.
>
> The glee club stayed quite late but we didn't feel much at home without dress suits and so only stayed a few minutes.
>
> It was quite an experience. He is the first President I have ever seen, I think. No, I heard exPresident Hayes one night at the Music Hall with you, but I don't know as they are any different from other people. The Pres. is very small, much to my surprise, and looks very tired and I guess it didn't rest him very much to shake hands with a crowd of young fellows, especially as his hand shake is very week.

The worst that Harvey had to show for his athletic career was a deformed knuckle as a result of breaking his left little finger during a game. Given the importance of his fingers in later life, it was just as well they moved him from shortstop.[30]

College ball never attracted the huge crowds that rowing and football brought out, but Cushing came to know what it was like to be adored by cheering blue-jacketed Yale men, violets in the buttonhole, and their blue-frocked ladies, violets at the bosom, on sunny spring days when no one had a worry in the world: 'Cushing's Great Sprinting for a Long Fly Starts 10,000 Persons Cheering.' His junior year at Yale ended in 1890 with the hard-fought championship game against Harvard, Amos Alonzo Stagg's last hurrah. Cushing had three hits and Stagg was 'tough as a hickory nut and wiry as a main-spring' as Yale eked out a 4–3 victory, champions again. Out with the flasks, and the 'Bingo' song:

> Here's to good old Yale
> Drink her down, drink her down
> For she's so hearty and so hale,
> Drink her down, down down!

Unlike his fans, and probably some of his teammates, Cushing seems not to have seriously experimented in college with drink, rowdyism, gambling, or easy women. He probably did not smoke regularly, at least during the baseball season. Nor is there any record of the ballplayer ever having lost his temper or been in a dispute with umpires. But baseball was a game to be played hard, and a clipping in his scrapbook about an incident in a game with Brown suggests that Cushing 'perforce' took every advantage he could:

Sexton's Vicious Blow: A Yale Ball Player Assaulted
Cushing had hit a ball hard towards left field, on which he made first easily, and then, seeing that the ball had been badly fumbled, started to add two more bases to his credit. Sexton stood squarely on second bag, and Cushing perforce brushed against him as he went by. He thought nothing of it, but kept on and made third on a slide. As he stood up on third base, brushing off the sand and dirt, he noticed Sexton coming quickly down towards him. In a moment later Cushing had received a vicious blow in the chest and Sexton

had turned to walk back to his position ... The 'muckism' of Sexton [contrasted with] Cushing's self-control, which tied his hands to his sides and kept him silent before Sexton's exasperating jeers.

It was said that everyone on the Brown team apologized to Cushing except Sexton, who was widely thought to be a professional.[31]

Harvey dabbled at gymnastics and rowing through sophomore year. Aside from studies, there were other diversions, including proms, where his dance cards, duly saved for the scrapbook, were agreeably full, with no one name dominating. He continued to be a popular man on campus, and as a junior was invited to join Delta Kappa Epsilon, one of the Greek letter societies beginning to sprout on American campuses. He was a member of the society's play committee that staged a Thanksgiving extravaganza, 'Pocohontas: A True Tale of Home Life in New England,' and he starred in it as 'that cute, coy coquette, Miss POCOHANTAS POWATAN, a Bar Harbor rosebud in her second session, and a terrible example of the effect of Fem. Seminaries.' In Act 2 Pocohontas entered with a double-back handspring, did a *pas de quatre* with Sir Walter Raleigh, and received 'Queen Lizzy's clemency and ... many fat offices of honor and boodle.'[32] There are no pictures of Cushing in drag, but someone did take a remarkable snap of him in the middle of a back somersault off a parapet at the entrance to the Yale gym.

Would he make one of Yale's elite senior societies, Skull and Bones, or Scroll and Key? Nothing much was known of their rituals, but the organizations had become well known for choosing the highest achievers on campus and helping their members keep on achieving throughout their lives. They were pretentiously high-toned male fraternal benefit clubs, the upper class's equivalent of Elks or Oddfellows. 'I don't know whether you or any one, except a Yale graduate, knows what it is to get an election to Skull and Bones or Scroll and Key,' Harvey told his father. 'It is the greatest honor a man can receive in college and is the one thing more than any other sought after by every one from the time of entering college to senior year.' Bones was said to do more for a man later in life and be easier to get into that year, but Harvey hoped

to go with the best men of his class into Keys. To his intense excitement
and delight, on Tap Day in 1890, a great public ceremony at Yale,
Cushing was tapped for Scroll and Key.[33]

~

During Yale terms, Cushing fought off sore eyes (probably conjunctivitis) and nagging winter colds. He escaped the typhoid fever that swept
through the college in the autumn of his junior year. It killed a classmate, and for thirty days the men of '91 wore black mourning badges.
There was equally profound mourning, some thought, when Princeton
ended Yale's five-year winning streak in the 1889 Thanksgiving Day
football game. Harvey's cousin, Tot Harvey, was a stalwart of the eleven,
its captain in his senior year. Cushing roomed by himself his last two
years. One day there was a small but revealing disaster when thirty
dollars was stolen from his wallet in his room in the Divinity dorm. He
attributed the theft to 'a little Jew whose looks I have never liked ... a
regular little fagin.' There was little ethnic diversity at Cushing's Yale,
and the racial stereotypes of the era were taken for granted. Yale seniors had a strange tradition of playing childish games: shooting marbles,
rolling hoops, spinning tops, and indulging in 'nigger baby' – a game,
Harvey told his parents, that was played only at Yale.[34]

Summer breaks were a time for resting from the grind rather than
taking paid work if one didn't need money. Harvey apparently did little
but relax and play sports, go camping, and travel. When the Cleveland
boys were back from college and the girls home from finishing school,
the Williamses, Boardmans, Harveys, Goodwillies, Crowells, MacBrides,
Garfields, Crehores, and Cushings would gather for 'porch parties' at
one of the rambling frame homes on Euclid or Prospect, play a little
ball or tennis, and sing the school songs. Or they would go out to one of
the rambling frame summer homes on the Lake Erie shore, Breezy Bluff
or Brightwood, where they would swim and picnic, light a beach fire,
and sing the school songs. Sociable, athletic, quick witted, and charming, Harvey was always near the center of the good times.[35]

As the circle of his friends expanded, he visited their houses and summer places up and down the eastern seaboard. Americans took trains as readily as they now fly. The Clevelanders liked to spend winter holidays at plantations in Georgia, summer heat waves on New Hampshire's Atlantic shore, and weeks or weekends back in Massachusetts or Connecticut seeing old friends and family. En route to New Haven for his senior year, Cushing visited Grosvenor Atterbury, Star Childs, and other well-to-do classmates at their elegant seaside homes. He found himself struggling to stay 'in the swim,' he told his father. 'I am afraid that being from the "wild and wooly west" I am not enlightened enough to appreciate all this formality,' particularly the balls, 'which begin about the time when a Christian should go to bed and end about as he should get up.' When a rich father insisted on showing him some old-time Yale fencing movements in the parlor, Cushing managed to knock a vase off the mantle.[36]

Visitors to New Haven at the time of Cushing's last winter prom included Kate Crowell from Cleveland and her widowed mother. The Crowells lived near the Cushings, and Kate's brother Ben was also at Yale. Harvey dined and danced with the Crowell women and went out of his way to show them the beautiful new Chittenden library. 'It was a part of the campus to which visitors don't often go as it probably never occurs to the men that they want to,' he told his mother, 'but I think it's the best place by far to take them and show them its not all play here. Besides the reading room in the main Library with the Tiffany windows is a remarkably handsome one ... The old library with its musty bookish odour and busts of old Profs & old-fashioned furniture which with its claw feet and carving attracted [Mrs Crowell] immediately.'[37]

Senior year was the time to begin thinking seriously about the future. While they were in New York for the big Thanksgiving football game (where Yale beat Princeton before 25,000 fans, and fifty people were maimed when part of the stands collapsed), Harvey and Grosvenor Atterbury were given a hospital tour by an Atterbury family doctor. Cushing was fascinated by the several surgical cases they saw; Grove, who planned to be an architect, was nauseated.[38]

Later, the Scroll and Key men had a series of Saturday-night talks about vocations from some of their senior brothers. Cushing was enthralled by Dr D. Bryson Delevan's talk about medicine:

> He told us a lot about the history & growth of the art or rather science of medicine, about the men who have done the most for it, of all of whom he had pictures and many of whom he seemed to know personally. Sir James Paget, Lord Lester, Pasteur, Virchow, and a lot more I don't at present remember. He told us about the Berlin Congress at which he was present, about Koch, his paper and how everything got so exaggerated, and then he went on to tell us about the schools and the study of surgery & medicine, recent advancement &c. It was mighty interesting and he must have talked about an hour and a half.

Harvey remembered the occasion all his life, sometimes claiming it saved him from being an architect like Atterbury. In fact, it only set him more firmly on the course he had never not been on. It may have helped him decide against Chittenden's and Ladd's suggestion that he postpone medical school to do a year of graduate work in science at Yale. Time to get on with becoming a doctor, like Cushings before him.[39]

The Yale nine lost the college championship to Princeton that June, ending a three-year streak. Harvey, who was putting his studies first, took the defeat lightly – he took his phys chem notebook with him to Princeton to study for Chittenden's final exam. After exams, there was a last out-of-town junket for an exhibition game. Harvey was mortified on return to find that his father had suddenly decided to attend his graduation and was in New Haven, the only visit he made during his son's years at Yale.

Harvey was able to introduce his father to Chittenden, and the Cushing men took in President Dwight's farewell sermon to the graduating class, 'in which he managed to tell us in sixty minutes that the past was behind and the future before us and not much more.' At Commencement Day ceremonies in Alumni Hall a voice from the past,

Effingham H. Nichols of the class of '41, warned that Yale was placing too much emphasis on athletic glory. The next day the class of '91, Yale's largest ever and the first to be decked out in caps and gowns, went through their presentation ceremony. Afterwards they paraded through New Haven behind a marching band, serenaded their professors, danced around the liberty pole, and enjoyed several days' more festivity. Eventually, Yale's blue-blooded class of '91 paid a bill of $210 for the damage their farewell celebrations had caused to a local restaurant. Harvey and his dad had left town the day before to go back west to Cleveland.[40]

THREE

Making a Harvard Doctor

September 1891. He was a lonely outsider in sweltering Boston, trudging the streets, checking his map at every corner, trying to find a place to stay. Brother Ned's old boarding house was already full. When he went to the not yet open Harvard Medical School for advice, all he got were a few recommendations from the caretaker. 'I must have walked about 10 miles and climbed 1000 feet of stairs ... I have not accomplished much more than to get a pretty good composite picture of a land lady whose name is legion and whom I do not admire. It seems to me I never saw so many people before who were all utter strangers & its most depressing.'

Out of the blue, Harvey bumped into a fellow Yale man, class of '89, who was attending the School of Technology (later MIT) and knew some lodging possibilities. By the time his classes began early in October, Harvey had found an acceptable boarding house at 32 Cedar Street and, in his twenty-third year, was ready to begin the grind of professional training.[1]

Grind it would be, a very different experience from his carefree, social, sporting time at Yale. The point of being at medical school was to get a professional education, not a liberal education. The Harvard Medical School was downtown on Boylston Street, near Boston's hospitals and far from Harvard's Cambridge campus. It offered courses, not collegiality. No ball teams (Harvey was technically eligible to try out for the Harvard nine but took no interest), no glee clubs, and instead of dormitories there were only dissecting rooms. Students were there to work at becoming doctors, to be trained to make a living at a difficult and competitive vocation. Cushing went to Harvard Medical School to work at becoming the best doctor he could, worthy to carry on the family trade.

As he began his medical studies, his father, who continued to pay all his expenses, inflicted on him a letter urging constant application as he entered 'the front entrance to the work of life.' He must stay away from the ruinous temptations, tippling, gambling, and immoral women: 'We hope a great deal from you.' Harvey expected much from himself and took his father's 'Lord Chesterfield letter' with a grain of salt. He put up pictures in his room of the three living Cushing doctors: his father, grandfather, and brother. The other medical symbol in his room was the skull he kept on his desk. This was relatively frugal; many medical students owned full skeletons.[2]

~

As a Yale graduate, Cushing was overqualified for Harvard Medical School, even though it was one of the four or five best in North America. The doctor factory dated from 1782, when it had been the third medical school founded in the colonies. Staffed by generations of prominent Boston doctors, the school had been reformed in the 1870s, rebuilt in the 1880s, and was now competitive with the University of Pennsylvania, Michigan, and Canada's McGill and Toronto medical schools. It offered state-of-the-art medical training that blended the old emphasis on clinical skills with the late nineteenth century's new interest in scientific medicine (characterized by an openness to evidence-based innovation, though not yet to systematic research). Harvard was in the process of extending its MD program from three years to four – Harvey's class could take an optional fourth year – but like all other medical schools, it still admitted students directly from high school as long as

they could pass its entrance exams. Having a Yale degree, Cushing was
required only to write a perfunctory test in chemistry.

Harvard's great names in medical education – the doctors Warren,
Bowditch, Holmes, Cheevers, Shattuck, and others – were well known
at the breakfast tables of medical America. Sons so often assumed a
father's profession, practice, and professorships that a dynastic tradition
dominated Harvard medicine (except in the Holmes family, where
Oliver Wendell Jr shifted fairly successfully to the law). This practice
was later eventually scoffed at as typical Boston inbreeding, but often
the sons and grandsons were at least as talented as their fathers, just as
young Cushing aspired to be worthy of his own family. Meanwhile,
competition in medical education and the high standards set by
Harvard's great reforming president, Charles W. Eliot, were forcing the
medical school to be reasonably open to innovation. By Cushing's day,
Harvard was even beginning to hire faculty who were neither Bostonians
nor its own graduates.

The professors' offerings amounted to a rigorous training in the academic bases of medicine as they were understood in the 1890s. Students mastered anatomy, biochemistry, knowledge of the physical manifestations of disease, and the theoretical practice of medicine (long on
diagnosis, prognosis, and sedation; short on specific therapies). They
nicely complemented their classwork by being able to study the variety
of patients at Boston's several hospitals, notably, the Massachusetts
General Hospital, founded and staffed since the 1820s by the same
medical families who controlled the medical school. Yale's benighted
medical school, by comparison, was crippled by its New Haven location, which offered neither a busy hospital nor great doctor dynasties.
At the end of the nineteenth century, Yale medicine remained, at best,
undistinguished. Cushing never seriously considered studying medicine
at the university he dearly loved.

Nor in 1891 was it feasible for him to become part of the controversial experiment in American medicine that was starting up in Baltimore, where the magnificent bequests of the merchant Johns Hopkins
had created a new university and a hospital, both aspiring to American

and world leadership. The richly endowed Johns Hopkins Hospital, its staff chosen from the best in North America, had opened for business in 1889. But financial setbacks caused Hopkins to postpone opening its medical school, which was intended to have the highest admission standard in North America – a full college degree. Johns Hopkins might be the coming place, but it wasn't just yet. Harvey had seen Harvard and the MGH on his baseball visits; they were good enough for his brother Ned, and good enough for him.

~

Cushing's courses at Yale with R.H. Chittenden had given him a big lead over most of his classmates, about 140 of them, the majority fresh out of high school. A handful had university training, though very few with a background as good as Harvey's. Elliott Joslin, Yale '90, another ambitious neo-puritan, had done a full extra year with Chittenden in New Haven before enrolling at Harvard. Keeping up with Joslin was to become one of Cushing's self-imposed goals.

Most of his class wondered how they could possibly keep up with Cushing. Studying cells and tissue under the microscope early in first year, Harvey made beautiful pen and ink drawings, remarkable works of medical art. His father soon bought him an expensive German-made microscope. Cushing recollected that he was urged to skip further preliminary courses and begin serious work in the dissecting room, where medical students really got to know the human body.[3]

Experienced only at eviscerating chickens, fish, squirrels, and deer, many of the students would still have been struggling to overcome awe and squeamishness in their first days with human cadavers. A classmate remembered the immediate impression Cushing made with his scalpel:

His first 'part' was a right 'upper extremity,' and before a day was passed, all the students as well as the teachers were watching the progress of Cushing's dissection. Dr. Mixter had placed him near a window, which in the old gas-lighted room, was important and by groups of twos and threes often came for a few minutes at a time to watch. Cushing himself talked little. First he sharpened his scalpel carefully and frequently, then he raised his skin flaps so as to keep as many of the cutaneous endings of the nerves as possible intact. At the end of three weeks, he had not only his intercost-humeral intact, but a multitude of anatomoses from the clavicle to the finger tips. He took the same care of the tissues to avoid drying as he afterwards took in his cranial operations ... He showed his professional pre-eminence from the start.

After the early weeks, he began to talk freely to his fellow workers – but first he stated his intentions. 'Be a leper,' he said, 'that is what I have decided to do,' and with that phrase he refused practically all social invitations that would have wasted his evenings.[4]

He had a special advantage entering Boston medicine as Edward Cushing's younger brother. Ned had been a good and popular student at Harvard and an intern at the Massachusetts General Hospital before studying abroad and then going home to practice in Cleveland. Well liked and well connected, he supplied letters of introduction, which their father urged Harvey to use to his advantage. Harvard's professor of surgery, Maurice H. Richardson, was so busy the day young Cushing introduced himself that he had little to say, but afterwards he made a point of writing Ned, a former assistant, to say that he would do all he could to help Harvey: 'He seems already to take hold with a great deal of interest. His dissections are spoken very highly of.'[5]

Cushing dutifully attended Richardson's surgical demonstrations to the anatomy students, but they were so crowded there was little to see. Students never could see much surgical detail from the benches in amphitheaters. Charles Scudder, a Yale man and a friend of Ned's, who had junior appointments at the medical school and the MGH, arranged better opportunities: one month into his first year Harvey was an ac-tive worker, giving anesthetics. 'Have been etherising twice thanks to Dr. Scudder,' he wrote Ned. 'Once with Dr. Cabot when he removed some pieces of ribs and once with Dr. Harrington in a Excision of knee. Enjoyed it immensely. Am in an advanced Practical Physiology course with Dr. Bowditch. Friday we operated on a dog and removed section of intestine.'[6]

He first formally observed surgery at the MGH in February 1892, viewing the action with a pair of opera glasses. In two hours he saw 'an amputation, excision of the knee, removal of an enlarged testicle, a perineal section, a breast & especially interesting was the removal of a plate of teeth from a woman's aesophagus without ether, the same having been swallowed six weeks ago.' 'Enjoyed them immensely,' he told his father.[7]

⁓

The men of Yale '91 had scattered to the four winds, but were keeping in touch, of course. Harvey's rich friend Grosvenor Atterbury was in Cairo that winter to study Moorish architecture. Perry Harvey had gone back to Cleveland, where he was enjoying the social whirl with the old gang while starting to make his way in business. He was one of the first of Cushing's friends to comment on the new ethnic group that certain aspiring Americans were beginning to notice: 'You ought to see me sell dry goods. I really believe I've found my hole – except where those damn stinking lousy Jews come in.'[8]

Jewish dry goods men in Cleveland scrambled and drove hard bargains, reinforcing a crude stereotype of their culture in an age of stereotypes and ethnic consciousness. During Harvey's early days in Boston when he sought company it was with the group of his classmates who had enrolled at Harvard's law school. If any of them was Jewish, Harvey did not notice. When brother Will had attended Harvard Law School more than a decade earlier, he had mentioned to their parents that the star student, Louis Brandeis, 'is currently believed to have some Jew blood in him, though you would not suppose it from his appearance.'[9] Old America was just beginning to feel the presence of the intensely striving and upwardly mobile group of newcomers.

Harvey and twenty-one-year-old Kate Crowell, who had known each other all their lives, had become sweethearts by the end of the summer vacation. We know this through a letter that Kate's mother, a longtime friend of the family who signed herself 'Aunt Ca'line,' wrote to Harvey on Kate's behalf just after he went to Boston. Kate was in bed with neuralgia: 'She thinks it will do her good if I write to you; she is partaking of a few concords before the next attack of face-ache ... To say that we miss you, Harvey, is simply a farce. It only shows what a big place you have made for yourself. *How* you have made it, I don't quite understand – or I haven't realized.'

Kate sent him her picture, they began to correspond, and he saw her when she came to Boston to visit Mary Goodwillie and other close friends from Miss Hersey's School, where she had finished her education. But his work came first – during Kate's spring 1892 visit, Harvey dropped in only to say 'how de,' he told his mother. 'Not having Energy to dress up ... I go looking more or less like a tramp and beat a hasty retreat before other callers may come. As my mind is occupied with non conversational subjects these days I fear I am not a very entertaining caller.'[10]

He was dissecting a head that season, was not satisfied with his progress or with the school for prohibiting night dissecting, and hoped he would be able to keep the noggin to work on during Easter vacation. 'Now look here,' Perry Harvey wrote him, 'make it *vacation* and leave your old hours alone for a while. Take a rest and for heaven's sake don't get run down, Cush. Somehow or other doctors seem to take good enough care of other people's health but damn poor of their own. Take a pill or two for luck.'[11] All the rest of his life, friends would urge him not to work so hard.

He became good friends in first year with a classmate, E. Amory Codman, scion of an old New England family, an outstanding student, amateur baseball player, and would-be surgeon. Both were elected to the medical students' elite Boylston Society. As exams approached, they exchanged lecture notes and sometimes went on study outings together. Like most medical students of their era, they took private 'quiz' classes offered by demonstrators such as Scudder. Cushing thought

Codman had better working and learning capacity than he did. The class was not ranked at the end of the year, but Harvey clearly did well, earning two As (anatomy and medical chemistry) and a B (physiology).[12] The opportunity to do a few days' work at the M.G.H. substituting for one of the interns caused him to delay going home to Cleveland to his family and his girl.

~

Dr Scudder arranged for him to spend September 1892 as a clerk in the hospital's outpatient department. So he cut his vacation short and went back to Boston, leaving Kate at a resort in the Shinnecock Hills of Long Island. They joked about being in a Kipling story of the hill stations in India where the Raj's females lived in cool idleness while their husbands worked in the unlivably hot cities. Kate bemoaned her fate and tried to lure him back with nautical double-entendre:

> You cant think how horrid it was after you left ... The inn is full of lone women. We counted 24 women to six men in the dining room last night. Regular old *spinsters*. In the evening they sit around with *knitting* and look you over from top to toe and *gossip* ... Oh I wish you were here to sail with us ...
>
> You could go down to New London (only two hours), take the boat from there ... we could sail all day Sunday and I would show you how well I can steer and luff and do all kinds of tricks.

Harvey couldn't get away. At his desk after work, he wrote her about his early experiences with the human side of medicine:

> Most always some poor devil hangs around and pours a woeful tale into any sympathetic ear he can find. Yesterday I found a young Irishman out in the dressing room ... The poor man was weeping, which he tried to conceal, and I found out by a question or two that he came over to Phila to marry a girl he had known in Dublin – she threw him over – he shot himself ... no money – no surgical relief possible &c &c ... I cheered him up as well as I could and

got him away from the hospital ... I expect he'll be brought in some day after a more successful attempt ... Excuse this melancholy story but my thoughts are full of them most of the time and this is only one of a dozen as sad.[13]

That autumn, Professor Richardson offered Harvey a job as one of his assistants. It mainly involved preparing patients for Richardson's demonstrations, including etherizing them. Harvey worried to Kate about the high expectations the doctors in the hospital had for Edward Cushing's little brother. He put hospital work before his morning lectures, copying friends' notes to keep up.[14] Whether at first or second hand, his note taking was a model: Cushing's medical school notebooks are complete and detailed, beautifully illustrated with sketches sometimes done in several colours. He underlined salient points, inserted marginal subheadings, and indexed his notebooks' contents.

Here is an earnest student burning real midnight oil, sometimes putting work aside to write late-night letters, his only companion the dim light on his desk:

> I have been pretty busy all this week – have worked all the time but have not done much work – a distinction without a difference you'll say, but not so – The hospital work is still exceedingly interesting and consequently distracting and my triple row of books are pointing the finger of scorn at me for their accumulated dust. So you see that you need have no fear for the lamp's being over-worked.
>
> I have been the lamp's milliner ... aided by a pair of scissors and a large piece of wrapping paper and she now beams benignly down upon me from under a sun bonnet and responsively gurgles to the name of 'Sister.' Sister has a bad habit of smoking which though companionable I don't aprove of in her sex. She is allowed to go out nights however and as I have no time for such luxuries I insist on doing all the smoking to even up.[15]

He cut back on holiday observance, forgoing the Thanksgiving football match in New York (though finding time for the Yale-Harvard game). Columbus Day in Boston led only to more work – dealing

with 'the broken heads and black eyes which appeared the next morning at the hospital.' He lived to the rhythms of the week: 'The periods
of seven days are marked off about as regularly as the big hall clock
checks off the seconds, and in much the same way for there is a rush
in the middle and a gradual slowing up toward Sunday where there is
a breathing spell, a little time to think about something except pills
and then a rapid descent to the middle of the week when the "fur
flies" and one hopes the momentum gained will carry him to the next
stop.'[16]

Normally working late, Harvey took an occasional evening off for a
concert or a play (Joseph Jefferson in *Rip Van Winkle* had him bowling
ten pins with Henrick Hudson all night, he wrote home). He might
dine out on Saturday night, and on Sundays he caught up on socializing, letter writing, excursions, light reading, and leftover work. One
Sunday he happened to pick up a copy of *The Scarlet Letter* and was
'held under a spell by the magic pen of Nathanial Hawthorn all this
afternoon ... It's a powerful book.' This was the third time he had read
the book – not bad literary taste in a twenty-three-year-old medical
student. Despite his busyness, he usually had some nonmedical reading
on the go, often shared with or inspired by Kate. He was versed in
Kipling, Robert Louis Stevenson, and other popular authors. He liked
the heft and feel of books of all kinds, spent freely on medical texts,
and had a hard time dragging himself away from bookstores and the
splendid new Boston Public Library. 'Tuesday afternoon I went down to
the Post office to get some money from father and stopped in a book
store on the way back for a moment which turned out to have been
over an hour when I came to myself.'[17]

A powerful literary bent and no small writing ability emerge in letters home that are much more than duty notes. One Sunday, as he
described it to his mother, was

> a day to sit by the fire and spin. No cross patch has been here though the fire
> has and much spinning has been done in the way of yarns while the wind
> whistled and rattled at the windows at will. Painter and Dolliver, medici,

were here this morning and we read papers & bandaged imaginary injuries & tied ligatures till noon. They were supplanted by Childs and Hitchcock, legici, we talked football, read poetry and I listened while they discussed the political situation ... After lunch Dr. Sears and Arthur Clement of 89 Charles Street dropped in to digest and soon one Howland, legicus, also appeared, on whose departure I arrayed myself in all my glory and a clean collar and made a call on the Misses Ward which I have owed since last February – had a pleasant time, though only stayed half an hour.[18]

Harvey decided to stay in Boston over Christmas 1892 to get extra hospital work (Kate held a 'spinster dinner' in Cleveland to commemorate his absence). He made a point of getting out on winter excursions, such as skating on the Charles River, and writing them up nicely for the home folks:

The river presents quite a gala day appearance in the afternoons – parties of young people – an occasional crowd of youngsters playing hockey – corpulent old gentlemen who must have seen twenty winters before that cold one of '49 ... and who would much better have left such sport to the grandchildren – lots of people riding bicycles on the ice – wealthy pappa's dragging their children about on sleds – Eminent doctors like Cabot and Shattuck cavorting about and so on without end. I should not have been surprised to have seen Grover Cleveland and baby Ruth, Phillips Brooks or any one else so many notables were pointed out to me ... 'My tallow dip is almost done' so I must to bed.

Over the New Year there was an excursion to a classmate's place up the coast in the fishing town of Gloucester, where they spent a day 'gadding about' on the waterfront. Harvey was interested in everything:

I still have a feeling as though my hair was full of sea weed and my mouth of salt halibut, for they have a custom in the smoke houses of offering the visitors appetising pieces to chew which must be done with as much good grace as possible. I consider the habit on a par with that of the good German

Anatomist – his name I forget now – who is said to chew connective tissue while dissecting ...

I was surprised to see the varieties of fish and to learn of the out of the way places they are gathered from. The best Mackerel come way from Norway or Iceland. They had quantities of salmon from the Oregon River sent way east in bulk to be prepared & distributed here abouts after the manner of a post office station. We saw a boat ... just in from a six weeks trip to the Western Banks with 14,000 lbs of Halibut – Enormous fellows some perhaps 200 lbs. It was a very small haul. 'In ye olden time' trips sometimes 'fetched' 150,000 pounds of Halibut. Then there were Cod Haddock &c &c in all grades of 'being made' which means being saturated with salt – I was presented with some 'xtry fine' boneless cod which I shall send home to mother.[19]

Returning from Christmas celebrations with family friends, Harvey came across a snow slide that a group of street children had built along a hilly street. He gave in to temptation, and for a few moments the medical student far from home at Christmas was king of the sliding hill: 'I haven't had such a slide for ten years and found I could stand up with the best of them and might have been there yet but for a miserable small brat who yelled out much to my embarrassment just as I was starting out for about the tenth time – "Look out for the dude doctor with the cane." I recognized a small mick who used to come into the surgical room last summer to have his finger dressed and that was my last slide.'[20]

⁓

The lectures and textbooks he studied from were only a part, often a small part, of his early years in medicine. He was constantly taking on work in the hospital. Much of it was routine, as he wrote amusingly to his father after the Christmas 1892 stint in the outpatient department: 'I don't know how much I have learned there except to ask people with more or less grace – "How are your bowels?" One good old creature told me his were in Ireland. I presume he didn't quite catch the drift of

my question. I hope it has made me a little more at home with a stethoscope in my ears though I still feel a good deal like a great big mosquito
with a formidable proboscis buzzing about and prodding an innocent
creature here and there. I also hope Materia Medica will seem less dry.'[21]

The operating room assistance he was required to perform most often, 'etherizing,' was much trickier than it sounds. By the 1890s surgery
everywhere had been changed by the impact of the coming of anesthesia. Just a few decades earlier, surgeons had found that ether or chloroform could put patients into a sleep so deep that they did not feel pain.
One of two preconditions for an enormous advance in the history of
medicine was at hand. The other condition, still being worked out in
Cushing's student days, was the use of antiseptic and aseptic procedures to forestall infection. Using anesthetics and keeping wounds clean,
surgeons could begin to take their time. They could begin to operate
on organs and on conditions, and inside bodily cavities, which they
had never before dared to touch.

No institution in the world celebrated the anesthesia revolution more
enthusiastically than the Massachusetts General Hospital. This was the
place where, on October 16, 1846, John Collins Warren had performed
the first surgical procedure on a patient under ether inhalation. The
ether was administered by a Boston dentist, William T.G. Morton. Many
supposed the whole idea reeked of quackery. At the end of the operation, Warren is said to have proclaimed, 'Gentlemen, this is no hum-
bug.' Oliver Wendell Holmes coined 'anaesthesia' to describe the loss
of *aiesthesis* (sensation). No matter that controversy would rage forever
about the MGH's priority in the 'discovery' of anesthesia (because there
turned out to have been many predecessors). Every MGH surgeon,
intern, and medical student took pride in the story of the great events
that had taken place under Bulfinch's beautiful hospital dome, the 'ether
dome.' Throughout the twentieth century the story would be told and
retold in annual Ether Day addresses, including that given in 1921 by
the world-famous Harvey Cushing.[22]

In 1892–3 he was just another clever medical student, and the procedure he followed was little changed from the 1840s. The etherizer's

job was to hold an ether-soaked sea sponge to the patient's face until he or she passed out, check to see breathing stayed normal while the surgeon cut, and be particularly careful that the patient not swallow the tongue or choke on vomit. Most of the time there were no problems. Etherization was routine enough that first-year medical students did it. Midway through his second year, on New Year's Day 1893, Harvey was called on to etherize while J. Collins Warren, grandson of the great initiator, excised a breast tumor. Nothing went wrong.

The next week one of the interns, a graduate physician named Frank Lynam, asked Cushing to sub for him as etherizer during regular hospital surgery. Harvey was a little anxious about assuming so much formal responsibility – what if they lost a patient under his care? – but agreed to start under Lynam's supervision. On January 10 they had to etherize a woman who was about to be operated on for a strangulated hernia, and whose chance of surviving was slight. Lying etherized upon the table, the patient died before the beginning of the operation, which was to be witnessed by students.

The death made Harvey 'pretty low in mind,' he noted in a pocket diary for that day. When Lynam asked him to carry on, he tried to beg off, suggesting that he might drop out of medicine. Lynam berated him as 'one damned fool' for being so upset, bucked him up, and Cushing finally agreed to continue. He gave two anesthetics on the twelfth: 'A pretty poor etherizer I. Lynam a good fellow.' On the sixteenth: 'Etherized 3–4 times and pretty poorly.' The nineteenth: 'Hard luck again etherizing ... Ovariotomy ... and a cervix ... who behaved bad – had to put string in tongue. Dr. P[orter] must think I'm a clumsy dunce.' He always remembered the woman who died, reminiscing thirty years later about how he had 'burned with chagrin and remorse,' walked the streets of Boston, and planned to go into some other business.[23] All his medical life he was prone to depression or anger or both when patients were lost.

As well as teaching him about anesthesia and the hard lives of the house officers ('about as hard worked men as I have ever seen'), these hospital experiences were a marvelous window for observing surgeons at work. Cushing saw 'beautiful' operations, he saw them handling rare conditions, he saw surgeons failing in routine situations, and he noted the death of a surgeon from raging septicemia caught from a patient. He exulted when things went well in the operating room, he dissected amputated body parts, and when things did not go well he did his first autopsies. He also had his first experience of begging grieving relatives to permit autopsy. When he asked permission in the middle of a wake, the widow screamed at him and the mourners chased him away.[24]

Harvey learned to get on with the house men and became well known to Boston's prominent surgeons, Richardson, C.B. Porter, A.T. Cabot, J. Collins Warren, and others. When he later wrote of MGH's 'aristo-cratic aloofness and indifference to all students except a favored few,' he must have counted himself among the few. His pocket diary records what was probably his first bit of active work with scalpel or suture: on April 15, 1893, during his second year of medicine and yet to take any course in surgery, Cushing 'assisted Dr. Warren at a Breast amputation' and was 'clumsy at it.'[25]

More interested in the hospital than his courses, he continued to cut classes, especially in therapeutics. He admitted to his father that he was sadly neglecting his course in materia medica. He hated studying poi-sons for an examination; 'contemplate taking some myself,' he jotted in his diary. On occasional breaks, usually initiated by classmates, he real-ized how narrow he was becoming: 'I have done more social mingling today than for a very long time. Joslin invited three or four medical embryos to dinner at his house where were three or four unmarried women of the genus spinster which as you know abounds in this New England region. They were very pleasant however and I actually found myself talking two or three times, though I can't for the life of me imag-ine now what I had to say.'[26]

In the spring of 1893 the eldest Dr Cushing, grandfather Erastus, died quietly in Cleveland at the age of ninety-one, and the embryo doctor, Harvey Cushing in Boston, gave his first paper on a medical subject. It was on anthrax and read to the Boylston Society. Anthrax was not a very practical subject, Harvey had realized, because it so rarely afflicted humans, but it was of great historical interest because of the role the anthrax bacillus had played in the birth of bacteriology a generation earlier. Harvey's dissatisfaction with his performance ('Not very successful. Headache all day') set the mold for his anxiety about practically every talk he ever gave. In the same month, while visiting Grove Atterbury in New York over Easter, Cushing had his first encounter with the famous textbook writer and chief physician at Johns Hopkins Hospital, William Osler. Of the occasion he only noted, 'To Dr. Weir's Clinic w. Osler & Howell.' He owned a copy of the first edition of Osler's text, *The Principles and Practice of Medicine*.[27]

As term ended and second-year examinations loomed, he was run down and had frequent headaches and occasional short bouts of depression. A spring visit from Kate not only failed to cheer him up but appears to have reminded him that he could not afford to be seriously in love while still a student. 'Shes a fine girl,' he told his diary, 'but its best methinks for me not to see much of her.' A bad time: 'Am seriously worried about myself. I have been able to do no studying for some time. Sit and stare at my book – So stupid I can't read words or say anything. Suicide about only alternative – Don't wonder that people turn to it.'[28]

It was a rare and transient moment of despair. Most former students know the mood. What he turned to when he felt mentally befogged was the volume of Sherlock Holmes stories Kate had given him. He was particularly taken by 'The Speckled Band.' His other stimulant was nicotine, for he had become a heavy cigarette smoker. In those days, cigarettes were the 'light' alternative to cigars. His diary that spring shows several short-lived attempts to break the habit: 'Couldn't stand it and smoked again after about 10 days ... Hate myself these days.' A classmate remembered Harvey scorning smokers who did not inhale and telling the boys that 'when he drew the smoke deep into his lungs, he felt every nerve tingle to the ends of his fingers and toes.'[29]

He pulled himself together, joined a rowing club for exercise, and spent a week by the sea with Amory Codman 'to season our grinding with salt air.' The out-of-town time was refreshing, he later thought, but he wanted to put in longer hours of study than Codman seemed to want or need. So he went back to Boston, gave himself an hour a day at the boat club, and spent the rest of his time at his desk in his underwear. The last few days of his second year:

> *June 12*: ... Grind at Materia Medica. Hopeless ...
> *June 13*: Grind all day till I couldn't tell Opium from Alcohol ... Read some Sherlock Holmes in evening in despair.
> *June 14*: 9.30 Anguish. Will go to Materia Med. Exam. w. despair depicted on my face & shame in my soul. I am not sufficiently bright or well memoried to take such subjects & know anything about them.
> *June 15*: Materia Med. Exam. this A.M. Did poorly. No memory ... Pops concert in evening.[30]

'It has not been a very satisfying year,' Cushing told his father. 'We are just on the border line of practical work and have reached in theory the stage where things are no longer definate and assured and as I am not much of a theorist its been pretty hard. Then the year has been broken up a lot by the out patient work I did – the hospital substituting and Dr. Richardsons work for which we had to cut all the Therapeutics lectures ... Its over with now and I hope I have gotten as much out of it as I ought. It certainly has been long hours.'

Cushing scraped through materia medica and therapeutics with a C. But he got another A for his work in advanced anatomy, and in pathology he received the first perfect grade ever given in that subject at Harvard. Yet he would not let up on himself. The June 28 entry in his diary reads: 'Joslin told me I got the first 100 ever given in Pathology. Ashamed of knowing so little & having such luck.'

The beginning of summer work at the hospital had been postponed, so Harvey was able to go over to New Haven for a week and help the Yale nine prepare for the Harvard game. A struggling fielder remembered his tough advice: 'Speer, if you can't stop them with your body or legs stop them with your face.'[31]

⟳

When the medical world got him down and sports were not therapeutic enough, Cushing liked to look at paintings and drawings. He sometimes imagined developing his own skills or fleeing into architecture. His visual sense was very strong, as was his interest in using drawings, photographs, and words to preserve what he saw. He was interested in nature – leaves, trees, flowers, vistas – and he was interested in exotica, from circus performers to famous explorers, such as Robert Peary and his company, who were spending a few days in Boston before leaving in quest of the North Pole. Cushing spent a July afternoon inspecting Peary's *Falcon* in the harbor and many late nights at his boarding house talking with Langdon Gibson, a veteran of Peary's first expedition.

> Most everything was packed away so that we could not see the sledges the house &c nor sniff at the pemmican or other provisions. The dogs however were well worth seeing lying around panting on the deck with their four or more inches of coarse yellowish hair ... The spirit of adventure must be a dangerous one to handle when once well rooted. Did you know that those men during the winter months used to go out to relieve themselves naked, the thermometer 56 below or theirabouts? ... Gibson says he never had the suggestion of a cold while there & does not remember that anyone else had. One night they got up a foot race of 100 yards on the ice to be run without clothes which resulted in nothing worse than a frozen toe – a mere nothing.[32]

There were other adventurers around the Boston boarding-house table that summer of 1893, men who had been to India, Latin America, and the American West. Harvey, who had not even crossed the Atlantic, felt conversationally crippled.[33] He would even be one of the last of his family to visit the great world's fair in Chicago, the Columbian Exposition, at which the architectural and technological marvels of the age – many of the American frontiers – were on display.

He got back to Cleveland for a few weeks in August. Aside from 'making a fool of myself' in some unspecified way over Kate, he picked up a little more work at the city's Lakeside Hospital. He experienced medical frontiers, old and new, when he was asked to assist a local surgeon on a call into the countryside. As American surgeons had been doing since the 1600s, Cushing and Dr Dudley Allen operated in a farm home, probably on the kitchen table. But the operation they performed was new and still daring. It was an appendectomy, invented only about four years earlier to eliminate a condition, appendicitis, which had been described only in 1886 by one of Cushing's Harvard professors, Reginald Fitz. As well as assisting at such advanced surgery, Cushing had a chance to do routine work on his own: 'Opened (too wide) an abscess in neck in little Etsansburger girl – darn clumsy fool – rattled.'[34]

He finally took a week in September to go to the world's fair in Chicago, traveling with brother Ned and keeping a special illustrated journal, the first of many travel diaries. The brothers took in all the wonders of America's great 'White City' – the Dahomey village, Cairo, the mammoth redwood plank, Nuremberg, the ostrich farm, Buffalo Bill's Wild West show (but they missed Custer's last stand), the Bedouin village and Turkish 'bizarre,' the wonderful Bell telephone exhibit, the Illinois building, the cliff dwellers' homes, and much more. Like many Americans, Harvey was most impressed with the Japanese exhibits, especially the art and design. He was most disappointed by the Eskimo village – 'miserable unhealthy looking Esquimaux in white dirty clothes w. conjunctivitis and other disfiguring ailments' paddling around a pond in their kayaks.

Ned and Harvey drank good beer, Harvey bought Japanese pictures and rode in an elevator (but apparently not on the world's first Ferris wheel), and they ran into 'all the Clevelanders we ever knew.' He spent hours in the fair's art gallery but made his most detailed notes on the English nurses' exhibit in the Woman's Building. He observed the special labels these daughters of Florence Nightingale used for various dishes and pans, their color-coded glassware, their thermometer holders, and the special operating clothes recommended for both patients and physicians. He seldom went anywhere without finding out what there was to see on the frontiers of medicine, and he always took nursing very seriously.[35]

∾

As a third-year student, Cushing was finally taught in courses and hospital clinics about treating patients. The first medical case he was given to report on, at the Boston City Hospital, baffled him because he could find nothing much wrong with the patient: 'The lad's history pointed to some cardiac trouble but I could hear nothing in the way of murmurs except those which issued from my lips.' This was the correct diagnosis. His second patient, suffering delerium tremens and early pneumonia, was more obvious. His notes from surgery lectures that year are routine. The course was a once-over-lightly given by Drs Warren and Richardson, with much attention to amputations, excisions, and problems of anesthetizing, and almost nothing about work in the abdomen or the head. At exam time Cushing commented to his father that the course had 'been so wretchedly presented to us that no one seems to care particularly about the outcome.'[36]

Nothing on the curriculum seems to have excited Cushing at this stage. 'What a drone this all is to be sure,' he told Grove Atterbury. He later remembered that what must have been some excellent neurological or endocrine clinics – he saw acromegaly, cretinism, exophthalmic goiter, and other conditions – left him uninterested in what seemed to be medical backwaters. His letters are conspicuously free from positive comment about any of his professors. Neither then or later did Cushing write of having had great mentors or models at medical school, roles actually filled by his brother, father, and grandfather.

Judging from his correspondence, his most interesting conversations in third year were around the table at his boarding house at 89 Charles Street. He talked a lot of architecture with a fellow Clevelander, Abe Garfield, took a great interest in one of the boarders' work with long-distance telephone lines (Harvey got through all the way to Chicago and Cleveland), and enjoyed discussing whether an airtight box with a goose in it weighs less if the goose is flying (it does, but the goose soon suffocates). He was fairly even-tempered about the daily routine, though to Kate he admitted falling back on bad habits: 'Since I got away from your good influence I've been getting critical again and have made a compact with Abe whenever either says anything derogatory of anyone, the other has the privilage & in fact is compelled to kick him.'[37]

He did less at the hospital, only to load himself with so much extra work at the medical school that even his father – in retirement a recovered workaholic – suggested that he not attempt too much. On weekend mornings he did advanced dissection under the direction of William T. Councilman, the pathology professor who had awarded him the perfect grade (and had offered him a cash fellowship, which he declined, suggesting it ought to go to a more needy student). He spent still more time in the dissecting room working with a younger student, a Yale man who was trying to carry on with his medical education despite a series of epileptic seizures.[38]

The winter of 1893–4 was a time of severe cyclical depression in the United States. Harvey was often accosted by beggars on the streets of Boston and witnessed a demonstration of curiously well-dressed and well-fed unemployed on Boston Common. There were also unusually severe epidemics of infectious disease. While there was protection against the dreaded smallpox – Cushing vaccinated Elliott Joslin – as yet there was no good shield against influenza, a disease making its first major appearance in the eastern United States. Cushing fended off what he thought was an early attack – 'Prodromal symptoms of ye Grippe put off by whiskey & phenacetine' – but after Christmas succumbed and had a long bout that apparently left him tired and depressed. The family decided that he needed a holiday, and Ned booked a trip to Havana, Cuba, for the two of them.[39]

∼

They had a happy and interesting two weeks in the old Spanish colony. Harvey recorded and sketched their sightseeing, siesta-ing, stamp collecting, cigar smoking, picture taking, and medical tourism. This last included inspecting a foundling hospital, which had a box in the wall where mothers could leave their unwanted newborns, and seeing exotic forms of leprosy at the municipal lazaretto. Harvey gushed to Kate:

> Eddie and I have just been flitting about every where and what he can't tell about this town and this 'gem of the ocean, Pearl of the Antilles' or what ever you want to call Cuba is not worth the knowing ... and you should just see me Katy – I'm yards round and brown as a real dark Cuban and instead of my being an invalid the tables were turned and I have had to nurse Ed who was awful sea sick for a little while at which I had to roar ... Americans are pretty plentiful hereabouts ... but they don't seem to appreciate these skies blue beyond belief, and the water equally so ... the curious little narrow streets ... the plaster houses of all imaginable colors, old ruined fortresses & prisons, chain gangs, slaves, lepers, and oh such fruits, beyond measure in amount and variety ... What I mean is they don't seem to get hold of that old 'Local Color' which perhaps too much is said about. The fish markets, plantations, 'niggers' (the best looking people here as far as physique goes – for the Cubans proper are merely puny little weasened creatures on the end of a cigar) and the flowers and oh its an endless wonderland.

After the trip, he was soon back at the grind in his Boston room, munching crackers and smoking: 'I come back to earth with a dull thud and found myself sitting here alone at an uncanny hour with only the purr of my tired lamp, the ticking of the clock and the sound of rain outside to break the stillness.'[40]

He still had trouble concentrating, which he blamed on the effects of the flu, but it may also have been related to uncertainty about the immediate future. He could take his degree at the end of his third year, as most of his class would do, or he could stay on for Harvard's optional fourth year. In either case, he would probably take a further year's training as a house officer in Boston and perhaps finish off, like Ned and many of his classmates, with a year's study in Europe. He turned twenty-five in April 1894 and would have to wait several years before he could settle down and marry. It was almost universally assumed that the young

American male on the frontiers of life – geographic, business, or professional – had little or no time for romance. Harvey thought his long-
term future lay in Cleveland, and he was becoming impatient: 'I suppose the three years before I finally drive my tent pegs into Cleveland
soil will seem brief in the retrospect but Lord: they do seem long from
this end.'[41]

Another possibility suddenly opened up when a medical friend passed
on news about a position available in Baltimore at the Johns Hopkins
Hospital. It might be an unusual opportunity, Cushing thought, but he
had no strong feeling and asked his father for advice: 'I suppose if the
applicant is wanted it means work under Osler. I submit the same to
you and Ed.' Whatever they suggested, there was no follow-up. A later
Cushing anecdote about having applied to work with Osler seems to
have been a trick of memory.[42] Harvey decided to take a fourth year in
Boston, combining classes with hospital work.

Third-year exams were the usual grind, and the stress upset his stomach: 'All my spare moments were taken up in hating myself as I seem to
be on the royal road to chronic dyspepticism which is not cheerful in
contemplation nor predisposing to any decent mental work. Having
experimented with the usual drugs in vain I am reduced to living on a
starvation diet and *chewing gum*, think of it.' He compared himself variously to a clam and a hermit, and played on Oliver Wendell Holmes's
definition of social events as 'gabble, gobble, git' – all he could do was
git. His friend Codman, who had blithely spent most of the academic
year roaming around Europe, was now cramming for the exams using
Harvey's surgery notes, working fourteen-hour stints while Harvey flagged
after three.[43]

He planned to begin hospital work immediately after exams, but a
crisis developed at home when Ned came down with a bout of typhoid
fever. The physician treated himself badly – he would not stop going
into work – but pulled through and finally agreed to take a holiday. It
was Harvey's turn to be the healthy companion on a voyage of convalescence, this time to England. Their father, who had continued to finance Harvey through medical school, paid his fare. Just as the

Cephalonia was leaving Boston harbor, Harvey learned that he had received A's in all his principal subjects.[44] Codman, who had also passed, came down to see them off.

~

'The sea – the sunset – the dinner and the tobacco are delicious,' Harvey wrote in the ubiquitous diary their first day out. They were traveling with their Uncle Edward and Aunt Louise Williams, whom they soon learned to avoid (he was 'a tactless stinker,' Harvey decided; she spent most of her time in her cabin). Instead, the brothers made friends with the ship's physician, who asked Harvey to stitch up a third-class passenger who had cut himself in a fall. Landing in England, they overspent on first-class train tickets to London: 'Don't know whether they take us for fools or Americans.' They were good American literary tourists, spending their first night drinking Cheshire punch in Dr Johnson's famous old haunt, the Cheshire Cheese pub. 'Ride home in a cab very merry after Half & Half punch & stewed cheese and Uncle Ed says it's the finest hour he's spent in months.'

The Cushing brothers left uncle and aunt far behind as they took in various London sights, including slums and slum workers in the East End, and then journeyed north for walking tours in Derbyshire's Peak District. They tramped in knickerbockers, plaid socks, and golf caps, marveling at the foliage, the flowers, picturesque country houses, literary landmarks, and Anglo-Saxon tombstones. At one of their London hotels they wrote their letters with quill pens. They also spent a couple of days wandering around Oxford colleges. Towards the end of their trip they were back in London, where they made several visits to the Great Ormond Street Children's Hospital, hoping to observe its leading clinicians and surgeons.

Cushing would always love the English countryside and British literary culture, but he had mixed feelings about the English people. His first comment about medicine in the United Kingdom, on inspecting cases of chronic rheumatoid arthritis in children at Great Ormond Street,

was 'English indifference.' He and Ned saw some unusual and interesting cases on a visit to the chambers of the prominent consulting surgeon, Jonathan Hutchinson, and were thrilled at Great Ormond Street
to meet Edmund Owen: 'A *dandy* – spoke to me & had me try to
diagnose some cases. I was not very keen … Saw him open a big abscess
– & he invited us to dinner at the Saville Club.' Embarrassed by too
much friendliness, the American tourists begged off.

Harvey saw England in 1894 on six dollars a day, as recorded in the
careful accounts he sent his father. With his father's concurrence, there
was also upwards of a hundred dollars for tailored suits in London – still
the sartorial capital of America. Cushing eventually became tired of
tailors and tired of other American tourists. He sometimes got tired of
his brother, too, noting that sightseeing was best done by the individual
at his own pace. He seemed not to tire of dining at the Cheshire Cheese.[45]

~

Before fourth-year courses started in 1894, Harvey worked as an outpatient physician at the Massachusetts General Hospital, saw some patients at the Boston Children's Hospital, and took obstetrical training
among the Jewish population of Boston's North End. Clinical obstetrics
generated his lowest fourth-year grade, a C. To Kate he described a day
of outreach rounds:

> With Joslin I visited Italians Poles Portugese & 'Chews' in various tenements
> of all grades of squalor. One young one we tore from his parents arms midst
> wailings and gnashings of teeth and packed him off to the City Hospital else
> the other four children who slept in the same bed with him would in all
> probability have been down with diphtheria as well in a few days, if they will
> not be anyway. Not even the good District nurse, who is of necessity more of
> a linguist than we, could make them understand that our intentions were of
> the kindest. I should not like to go there after dark.
>
> Then we saw ten or twelve more sick families, fathers, mothers, meager
> infants & what not with various ills urgent & otherwise. The ones we did

most for were least grateful and those for which we could do nothing or perhaps could not recognise the trouble would overwhelm us with 'God blessings' as is usually the case even with more intelligent parties in different grades of society. In one room about half as large as mine here there were living a father largely boosy and nationality unknown, an Italian mother and six children the oldest being so many years of age & the most recent arrivals twins. In that room was combined kitchen bedroom – one bed & one cradle & a box or two – sitting room & I guess that's all the variety they needed.

Thus we wandered up & down dark stair ways in and out of courts pretty extensively throughout 'Little Italy' and the Portugese quarters till half past seven. Joslin & I then repaired to Youngs & ate enough for all day and here I am and that's more about charity medical work than I've told anyone for a long time.[46]

He had never had strong religious feelings, had attended chapel at Yale as a duty, and only occasionally went to church in Boston to hear an outstanding preacher. Most of his Sunday mornings this year he spent working in the biological lab at the medical school, 'nature's church – a much more inspiring and instructive lesson can be learned there than from most preachers.' Otherwise, he coasted a bit, taking a variety of clinical courses, an introduction to biology, and a course in legal medicine. He did not think he learned much from a course in operative surgery using human cadavers – experience gained assisting at real surgery was far more important.[47] In March 1895 he wrote the examination to qualify for a house appointment at the MGH.

The trips with Ed had been so pleasant that in this final spring they junketed off from New York for a couple of weeks of sightseeing and socializing in Bermuda, just coming into its own as a quaint, picturesque tourist paradise. They were shown about by various 'darkies' and 'niggers,' rode a donkey, marveled at Bermuda's natural beauty, sent onions to the folks at home, were invited to the governor's tennis party, and, in formal dress, danced at least one night away with some of the 'gay damsels' they met. Many years later, one of these women remembered the gay time being tempered by Harvey telling her that he couldn't possibly see her in Boston as he was much too busy at his studies.[48]

His relationship with Kate Crowell had cooled after some kind of crisis a year or so earlier, when he had urged her to get over him – perhaps because it would be such a long wait until he would be ready for marriage. They exchanged only a few cordial letters and seldom saw each other while Cushing was finishing at Harvard and embarking on his new apprenticeship. When Kate and her mother visited Boston in the spring of 1895, Cushing showed them the hospital where he would be working, and could not understand their lack of enthusiasm: 'I am always a little surprised to find people depressed by a hospital. I suppose familiarity makes one callow but the Massachusetts is essentially a bright place. There are hospitals and hospitals.'[49]

He began work at the Massachusetts General as a replacement house man in April 1895, two months before graduation and before his formal appointment. Amory Codman, who had not opted for fourth year, was just finishing up as a house officer. They were both interested in the need to improve anesthetics, Cushing because he remembered his difficult second-year experiences, Codman after losing a patient through inattention, which he (later and probably facetiously) blamed on Cushing's hijinks. Codman's supervisor suggested that it would focus the etherizer's attention during an operation if he regularly monitored the patient's pulse, recording the findings on a chart. Codman began to keep 'ether charts' during surgery; Cushing picked up the habit from him that spring and made the charts more elaborate. It was hardly the earth-shattering contribution to 'the technique of surgery' claimed by Cushing's first biographer, but it was a starting-point, the beginning of Cushing's creative obsession with improving everything about the surgical experience.[50]

He finally took a set of exams in stride, though he felt the usual sense of relief when they were over. 'Yesterday I finished my last examination in the Harvard Medical School,' he wrote his mother on June 16, 1895, 'and glad I am. If I had known what a struggle it was to be I don't believe I should ever have had the soul to begin.'[51] He cleared out his boarding-house room, shipping the detritus of his four student years back to Cleveland, and moved into the MGH to begin his year as an intern. On duty at the hospital, he missed his graduation ceremony at Harvard on the twenty-sixth. 'I hope I have not entirely wasted the years spent in pursuit of these sheepskins,' he told his father. He was now Harvey Cushing, MD, and had graduated *cum laude*.

FOUR

Making an American Surgeon

~

Where did you start after medical school? Newly minted doctors needed first jobs and clinical experience to complete their training. Hospitals needed staff. By the end of the nineteenth century, the hiring of recent graduates to do stints as hospital house physicians had become systematized. They worked for very low or no wages either as 'externs,' living outside the hospital and usually treating outpatients, or as 'interns,' or 'residents,' who lived in the institutions and were on call to treat the patients on the wards. Thus, Dr Harvey Cushing began his career by living and working at the Massachusetts General Hospital in 1895 as an intern.

Hospitals varied widely in the experience they offered interns. The MGH, a big and busy urban hospital, doing much more surgery than medicine, had a large staff of house men (few if any house women), assistants, and students. These 'house pups' or house pupils, organized in a complex hierarchy, were always coming and going, invariably working long hours. The interns did not rotate through different services – medical, surgical, obstetrical – but stayed with one specialty throughout their year. Cushing's appointment was on the South Surgical Service.

After a year or so of internship (extended a bit by those who wanted to sharpen special skills or interests), the best and most advantaged of the medics would go abroad to tour and study at great hospitals, universities, and clinics. Throughout the nineteenth century, Europe had been the professional finishing school for thousands of American doctors, most of them graduates of the elite schools and hospitals in Boston, Philadelphia, and New York. 'There is much foreign talk here at the M.G.H.,' Harvey reported to his mother as he settled in at the hospital. 'Five men go out August 3 and several of them go abroad immediately.'[1] He and his father expected that he would do the same after his intern year and before settling down in Cleveland.

There was never a time when Harvey Cushing's main medical interest was not surgical. He seems to have intended to do surgery from the day he entered medical school. It was a natural choice, not only because of his obvious manual dexterity but because there had never been a better time in America to focus on the surgical side of doctoring.

By the 1890s surgery and surgeons had come into their own in the United States. They had always been the frontiersmen of American medicine, but mostly as the dead-end, last-resort crowd. When all else failed, the surgeon with his knives and saws and blood-stained frock coat was called in to strap down the patient, give everyone whisky, take some himself, and go to it. Now, though, the surgeons came armed not only with anesthesia but with the ability to limit infection through the anti- and aseptical procedures, riffs on cleanliness, first pioneered by Britain's Joseph Lister in the late 1860s. As surgery became relatively painless and germ free, it was transformed in one generation from a cut, run, and pray business, stinking of pus and gangrene, into an almost routine 'medical' procedure. Surgeons quickly began to extend their range from the surfaces of the body and its major orifices into its previously sacred cavities. Surgery worked – not just in the crude way that, say, amputation worked, but in more conservative, less heroic ways: to repair broken and ruptured organs and to save limbs and tissue that would otherwise be lost.

Surgery also worked in more radical ways: to remove diseased organs, such as ovaries or appendixes, that might have killed their host.

In general, surgeons could deal with disease and its consequences more effectively and safely than ever before. Arguably, they could deal with many kinds of disease more effectively than mere physicians, who still had almost no curative drugs – only bags full of narcotics, sedatives, stimulants, and placebos. Sometimes, as with the terrible abdominal pains that had carried off thousands before Fitz had delineated appendicitis in 1886, almost one's first resort by the 1890s was an operation by someone capable of doing the new surgery.

In America, most doctors had always done a certain amount of surgery, and those who specialized in it had not been looked down on as tradesmen and butchers, as was often the case in the Old World. As fin-de-siècle demand for their services soared, surgeons went from strength to strength – becoming better trained, more specialized, busier, ever more successful and inventive, and able to command and collect high fees for life-saving services. Members of the surgical elite, such as Cushing's Boston teachers, were medical gentlemen, who in the last few years had exchanged their old work clothes for white jackets and trousers. They washed their hands vigorously, sterilized their instruments, and worked in spotless operating theaters assisted by tough-minded and very professional female nurses. In 1889 the MGH opened Ward E, an operating pavilion meant to be completely aseptic, lit by skylights and electricity, with asphalt floors and rounded interior corners to minimize dust. Two years later, antiseptic procedures were extended throughout the hospital.[2]

Boston's finest belonged to the fledgling American Surgical Association, founded in 1880, membership by invitation only. They published articles in specialized journals such as the *Annals of Surgery* or in the venerable *Boston Medical and Surgical Journal* (later the *New England Journal of Medicine*). Surgeons typically submitted details of their unique or interesting cases and reported on their innovations in technique. In surgery as in medicine, though, it was still felt in America that the masters and models were to be found in the Old World.

Yet there was talk of exciting new developments at home. In July 1895 Edward Cushing told Harvey about a colleague who had recently

finished training in Baltimore. 'I have seen much of [Hunter] Robb in
the past three weeks and have been interested by what he has to say of
Halsted & the Johns Hopkins Hospital,' Ned wrote. 'He says that to his
mind there is no surgeon like him in the land, that his aseptic technique is perfect, and that the scientific manner of his work keeping at it
from the laboratory side simultaneously with his clinical & operation
work is a revelation to a man ... He says strongly that if a place is
available after you finish your M.G.H. service take it by all means –
that a year there would be worth five abroad &c &c. Think it over.'[3]

Harvey liked the challenge of being a house surgeon at the MGH, one
of the busiest hospitals in America. 'It's a great place here with a constant succession of curious and interesting cases,' he told his father.
Much of his time was in the 'accident room,' sewing up lacerations,
setting broken and dislocated bones, and sometimes amputating. 'The
unexpected always turns up in this place.' He normally worked under
the supervision of four of the hospital's principal surgeons – John
Homans, Charles B. Porter, J.W. Elliott, and W.M. Conant – assisting
and etherizing, taking histories, and keeping the careful patient records
for which the hospital was noted. There was hernia and hemorrhoid
work on men, mastectomies and ovariotomies on women, and the occasional appendectomy and gallbladder removal. The surgeons were
even doing investigative openings of the abdomen, sometimes on very
young patients. 'A laparotomy on a child 48 hours old is not so common,' Harvey told his mother, 'but the child does not seem much disturbed.'[4]

He scarcely left the hospital. Working very hard, constantly on call,
he seldom got more than five or six hours' sleep a night and paid no
attention to the day of the week or the weather. 'Had a great 24 hours,'
Cushing enthused towards the end of his tenure:

Started the morning with usual dressings – had a bad cut wrist with tendon sutures in Acc. room followed by a subglenoid disloc of humerus. Several operations by Dr. Conant – till 3 p.m. – an emergency extra uterine pregnancy. Lunch. Two histories in afternoon – one case a cancer of caecum probably – A gunshot wound of abdomen at 7.15 p.m. – operations 3 hours long – intestinal resection &c –

Raft of small things in Acc. room the rest of night it being June 17th [Bunker Hill Day] – lacerated common cracker hands – gunshot wound of thigh – fractured leg et cetera.

Stayed up with gunshot belly man till he died at 7.45 a.m. [He] picked up above 4 a.m. after an intravenous infusion remarkably but no use. Just about to take a bath before breakfast when in piled a crush foot – from a trolly car – Choparts amputation [by] HWC. Breakfast. No time for ward visit. Hysterectomy for fibroid – Hydrocele of canal of neck – Exterpation of rectum for cancer. Put a fracture up in plaster in PM and I am now very feeble – several operations tomorrow. No place in the country does the work the M.G.H. does. I am only one of thirteen.[5]

Early in Cushing's tenure one of his mentors, J.W. Elliott, tried to help several patients suffering from brain tumor. Cushing anesthetized at operations that involved guessing where a tumor might be found and then hopefully drilling into (trephining) the skull to get at it. They missed one patient's tumor and tried to remove another's by shelling it out with the bare fingers ('leaving pieces here and there adherent,' according to the case report). Both patients died soon after the surgery; a third survived in misery.[6] Other surgeons in other centers were attempting to work on the brain in those years, with similarly disappointing results.

Cushing did an autopsy on one of the sufferers and found the body riddled with tumors. He kept a picture of another patient and a fragment of skullcap as souvenirs of these unusual experiences. A friend wrote up the two fatal cases, which had some interesting features, for publication in the *Boston Medical and Surgical Journal*. Inserting Cushing's autopsy report in the text, he offered to put Harvey's name on the paper too. 'Not on your life,' Harvey was later said to have replied.

Why would he want his first article to be a description of failure?[7]

Despite later speculation, there is no evidence that Cushing had any unusual interest in these patients. He valued working with Elliott because of the latter's skill in the abdomen, but when he first met William Williams Keen of Philadelphia, a giant of American surgery who had actually succeeded in removing a brain tumor, he was not inclined to genuflect. Keen, he wrote, 'left rather a poor impression. Windy about his own cases and work. Everyone knows its good, without having it forced down ones throat.'[8]

The truly fascinating breakthrough while Cushing was an intern – one of the great discoveries in the history of technology – was the announcement in December 1895 by the German physicist Wilhelm Conrad Röntgen that a form of radiation could penetrate solid objects and produce outline images of their interiors. News of the discovery of what Röntgen called 'X-rays' and their possible medical application raced through the medical world. 'Everyone is much excited over the new photographic discovery ...' Harvey told his mother in February 1896. 'Imagine taking photographs of gall stones in situ – stone in the bladder – foreign bodies anywhere – fracture etc etc ... Its fearfully uncanny. We won't be able to have any secrets if people can take photographs through stone walls etc. Some letters have come from the men abroad, letters of the wonderful things they are doing in Vienna with the X-Rays.'[9]

Within three more months Cushing had helped secure the apparatus for his hospital's outpatient service: 'We have at last succeeded in having an X-ray machine put in for which I have subscribed largely and hope the conservative staff will ultimately remunerate us for it. It is great sport, very useful in the out Patient to locate needles &c. We could look through the chest readily this morning – count the ribs – see the heart beat – the edge of the liver etc. It is positively uncanny.'[10] Cushing's friend Amory Codman, who was specializing in orthopedic surgery and was particularly enthusiastic about the breakthrough, suffered serious radiation burns from the time he spent with the primitive equipment.

Cushing was remembered by a student serving under him that year as an ambitious and demanding intern who was hard to work with – traits that would later be remarked upon many times over.[11] His prickly behavior was accompanied and partly driven by a deep concern for patients. One of the hundreds of 'grateful patient' letters that Cushing came to accumulate refers to an incident of surgical conservatism, in which he disdained his elders' fatalistic desire to amputate:

> I was your first Patient to go under your knife when you became House Doctor – and you in one operation saved the leg that all the other Doctors wanted to take off.
>
> That operation Doctor seems to me to be one of the greatest of your many many big things in your great life. The leg to day [1930] is as sound and strong as a twenty dollar gold Piece – after giving it the hardest of abuse in hard labor.

The patient was a professional ballplayer. Cushing had found that careful drainage of the infected areas of his tubercular leg made amputation unnecessary.[12]

Like all surgeons, Cushing still had much to learn about effective asepsis. Neither masks nor rubber gloves were as yet worn in operating rooms. Many of the procedures at the sometimes hidebound MGH, such as the use of sea sponges rather than cones to give ether, were out-of-date. The surgeons still put a premium on getting in and out as fast as possible. 'We operated too much by the clock,' Cushing recalled. There was inadequate preoperative study of cases, inadequate postoperative attention, and 'no encouragement to follow up a bad result, whether to its home or to the deadhouse.' In the forgiving glow of nostalgia, he thought that his generation of MGH juniors had not been aware of their faults. In fact, as the leg case showed, young Cushing already had a constructively critical streak. 'Considerable sepsis in the house,' he told his brother Ned in April 1896. 'No wonder when these men operate about the way a commercial traveller grabs breakfast at a lunch counter.'[13]

~

What would he do after his internship? In November 1895 Harvey and Ned took a 'hospital trip' to New York, Philadelphia, and Baltimore, picking up pointers and checking out the stories about W.S. Halsted's magnificent work. Harvey later recalled that his first encounter with Johns Hopkins made him immediately 'enamoured of the place ... even a short visit was enough to show an outsider something of the spirit which permeated the early group of workers there.' We do not know whether the Cushings saw Halsted operate or how much they learned about his background (Harvey would have been further impressed to learn that Halsted was a Yale man and had been captain of its football team). They did see the camaraderie of the Johns Hopkins men, seniors and juniors alike, with their belief that the future of medicine lay in the work that they were doing. Back in Boston, Harvey promptly wrote to Halsted, Surgeon-in-Chief at Johns Hopkins, saying he aspired to become his house surgeon.[14]

Halsted discouraged the outsider, telling him that several men on the spot wanted the job. He advised him to 'go to Europe as soon as you can, and to remain as long as possible before coming to us ... You probably know that there is little if any scientific work done in this country in medicine, and that most of it is done in Germany ... Six months or a year in Europe just now for the purpose of learning German thoroughly would be of great benefit to you.' The Cushings thought the advice was sound, and in the spring of 1896 Harvey booked steamer passage with a fellow intern, C. Allen Porter, and also began studying German: 'I am already making some plans about Germany – courses their times of beginning and desirability – men to see, and places to go for the first German grind. Many of the men who are now abroad and beginning to turn their faces homeward will be anxiously looked to for advice ... I have four places under consideration to settle in, Bonn, Goettingen, Stuttgart and Freiburg.'[15]

But then Halsted, who had a habit of changing his mind, suggested to Cushing that he might work at Hopkins for a year or more and then go to Europe. Harvey happily agreed, sending in a formal application endorsed by all of his leading Harvard and MGH teachers. 'I hope I may not prove unworthy of their commendation,' he told his father. Scheduled to begin in Baltimore in October 1896, he still hoped to spend the summer in Germany with Ned, but they decided to take a shorter holiday in Canada instead. Harvey had thoroughly enjoyed his year's internship and dreaded a letdown after working at such high pressure. He would have liked six more months of it.[16]

He unwound with several weeks of touring through Nova Scotia, Prince Edward Island, and Quebec. This travel diary has disappeared, leaving us only the excerpts quoted by earlier biographers and accounts in his letters. It appears that on his short sojourn on Prince Edward Island, Cushing might have passed the Victorian farmhouse where, more than a century later in an unchanged countryside, I am writing these chapters: 'Great fields of waving wheat – white acres of potatoes – woods of spruce and hemlock, groves of large beech – balm of Gilead – silver-barked birch shining against the dark evergreens – fertile country, looking as though every farmhouse was full of milk, butter, eggs, and mutton chops 2" thick.'

The Americans canoed in northern Quebec and were thrilled with the romantic picturesqueness of old Quebec City. They were saddened to see the beautiful young women who, while helping with the nursing at the city's Hôtel-Dieu, were committed to spending the rest of their days wearing black veils. 'Though I suppose,' noted Harvey, 'their lives are very useful ones compared to many ... The novices learn nursing by "observation" alone; there is no instruction.' Ned told Harvey that the hospital was like the ones he had seen in Europe – 'clean but small rooms and the air of an old monastery and candle snuffings.' At the Grey Nuns' orphanage in Montreal, Harvey was disheartened by 'pathetic sights of bastard children deserted – turned over to soulless creatures who in an English land teach them a foreign language. The poor peaked children – everything done in unison – automatons in life.' The city's new English hospital, the Royal Victoria, struck the visitors as complete and interesting, but they said nothing more about it.[17]

That summer Allie Porter and other friends left for Europe, warning Harvey not to unlearn at Hopkins the good things the MGH had taught him. Halsted's reputation for being a slow and meticulous operator might be good science, but it wasn't good use of time if you took twice as long as you really needed: 'So please combine their methods & scientific spirit with some of our Boston "*Gimp*."'[18]

~

The culture shock of becoming an assistant resident in surgery at the Johns Hopkins Hospital in the southern city of Baltimore, Maryland, was intense. All his life Cushing had moved in fairly familiar circles, surrounded by like-minded New Englanders and their Ohio descendants. At Yale, he had been invited to join the right clubs. At Harvard and the Massachusetts General, he had followed in his brother's footsteps and been introduced to the people who mattered. He had many friends and relatives in Boston, the cultural hub of America.

Now he found himself in a bare room in the staff quarters of a new and traditionless hospital on a hilltop overlooking a sprawling, alien city: 'My sole adornment consists of an old time discolored photograph of Neddie on the mantel. My few books look very lonesome in the corner of a huge book case ... There is a small iron bedstead in one corner covered with mosquito netting.' He knew no one at Johns Hopkins, and no one knew him. After all his years of education, he was starting over again. 'I am a very humble member of a large staff here. I have been given a part of a ward with a few patients as a start and have not as much to do as is salutary. Everyone is very kind however and I expect soon to feel more at home.'[19]

He found everything strange: the people, the hospital, a city full of row houses 'as alike as streptococci.' His letters were a litany of complaint: 'Am not having a very good time as yet ... Baltimore is fearful ... a curious place – slow hardly expresses it ... The house staff are a new sort of men to me, all but one or two, southernors ... I miss my books very much. The library here is rather inaccessible ... Am much dissapointed to find the Hospital a very sloppy place and the work of everyone most unsystematic, i.e. on the surgical side ... Hope things will clear up or I can't stand it.'[20]

The idea that house staff had to work hard in the early years at Johns Hopkins is quite wrong. Cushing had little to do in the way of surgical work and little else to do other than offer routine patient care for one of the colored wards (the wards were segregated) and the children's ward. Nor did it look as if he would be able to learn very much from his chief, Halsted, who seemed a chronic absentee: 'Dr. Halsted has only operated once this month and rarely appears.' When Halsted did appear, Cushing found the experience perplexing:

> It was most disconcerting to me, after the hurley-burley of the M.G.H., to have my new chief come, as it were apologetically, some day into Ward G; ask if he might be allowed to examine a particular patient; to have him spend an hour fiddling over a patient with a cancer of the breast who had recently been admitted; and then to have him depart saying he was tired and would be able to do nothing more that day.
>
> If he were sufficiently interested, he might ask that he be permitted to do the operation; and if he came and did operate, as soon as the breast was removed, leaving the huge closure and skin graft for Bloodgood [the resident], he would depart with the tissues. These he would study and ruminate over for an interminable time, meanwhile tagging innumerable areas which he wished to have sectioned – a duty which devolved upon the house officer [Cushing].[21]

When Cushing did get to watch Halsted operate, he found he could see very little because Halsted had a way of smothering the view with his shoulders. He was exasperatingly slow, lacked both showmanship and easy dexterity, made no helpful comments to observers, and constantly nagged his assistant, Joe Bloodgood. A joint research project on dogs that Halsted proposed to Cushing turned into an embarrassment when Halsted, having incorporated the session into his teaching, failed to turn up. Harvey found himself trying to show medical students canine parathyroids, which he had trouble locating and were too small to see clearly anyway.[22]

Not much about the surgery at Hopkins impressed Cushing. Joseph Bloodgood seemed unsystematic. The hospital had been designed before the great rise in demand for surgery: its operating room was a tiny, wooden-floored, ill–lit space with an old wooden army table which Halsted had brought back from Germany. Aseptic surgery was only gradually replacing older antiseptic methods, and the operating room still ran 'wet' with the disinfecting solutions that were applied to patients, instruments, and operators. The floor was littered with discarded sponges. Halsted and his staff still wore rubber aprons and rubber boots to protect themselves from the harsh disinfectants and other loose fluids. To protect their hands, Halsted's team was just beginning to use the rubber gloves that became their most famous invention; the early gloves were heavy and cumbersome, and Cushing scoffed at the practice.[23]

He considered quitting. 'You will have to make the best of it, hopefully, until fair trial has been made,' his father advised. 'This I have no doubt is also your own judgment and intention.' Ned urged him to talk things over with the two Harvard men they knew at Hopkins, William S. Thayer and John M.T. Finney, and to see the possibilities for professional growth:

> Isn't the surgical pathology and the rubbings up against a new set of men going to pay? Cant you take too some of their post graduate courses? The bacteriological and pathological work I don't believe you'd get anywhere so satisfactorily, and their operative techniques down there must be worth studying even if their methods seem to you rather backward.
>
> Indeed if you had more responsibility and more to do in the way of operations and bed-side work would you have time for the other things you want to do? The M.G.H. has given you good clinical and operative training – and taught you how to handle patients, and that sort of knowledge stays with one; and I can't help feeling that your work at Baltimore will be very valuable just for being rather different.

If all else failed, he could work on his German.[24]

Grumbling, he settled in: 'Curious to be with so many men with whom one has absolutely no association or mutual acquaintances.' But he began to get to know them and their ways. 'It's a good experience – and that's what we look for, experience. Medicine of course is an all sufficient bond.' As Ned had suggested, he played to Hopkins's scientific strength and began spending long hours with his microscope in the laboratory: 'The talk was of pathology and bacteriology of which I knew so little that much of my time the first few months was passed alone at night ... in the old pathological building looking at specimens with a German text book at hand.' As well, he had brought to Baltimore the x-ray apparatus, an early fluoroscope, which he had helped pay for at the MGH (and presumably had not been reimbursed), and began to tinker with it. By the end of November he was beginning to get used to the place 'and though not wildly enthusiastic hope I am making it pay.'[25]

He even began to appreciate the splendid parks and trees and flowers of Baltimore and its rolling countryside, as well as the strange Maryland cuisine. 'These Baltimoreans have more ingenious ways of serving up viscera than I imagined possible. Good muscle is a rarity. Oysters we never see. It's most curious. The Marylander serves his chicken fried. Sunday mornings we have griddle cakes and sausage served together – a general custom and an insult to good digestion the equal of beans and fish balls.' Family friends from Cleveland, the Goodwillies, lived in Baltimore and provided a home away from home. Getting to know the city, Harvey sent his mother a fine description of its famous market:

> Lexington market is immense ... I never saw so many things worth taking home in one. The butcher the baker and the broom-stick maker sleek and ruddy stand in their stalls and slice off great bologna sausages or four Maryland fresh biscuits or anything you like into the gaping basket ... Candy; all sorts of bread stuff; flowers; vegetables; meat – miles of it. Can you imagine a hundred yards of skinny, skinned rabbits, hanging on a rope with a row of

grinning darkies behind them? It's the sort of market one only expects to read about. I wandered about and munched and acted the Northern Spy [and bought Northern Spy apples] for about an hour till my 'abide' got sore from countless encounters with the corners of heavy laden baskets. When you go to the Lexington market don't ride home in a jerky electric car or you may step into a basket of eggs. [26]

Baltimore had a white Christmas in 1896, and young Dr Cushing made sure that the children on his ward at Johns Hopkins had stockings well stuffed. Ned came to visit, bringing their cousin Melanie Harvey with him, and surprised Harvey with the announcement that he and Melanie were engaged to be married next June. Harvey was at once delighted at the match and sad to lose his traveling companion. He had already decided he would stay at Hopkins for at least another year, 1897–8, if he were promoted to be senior resident. Otherwise he would go to Europe.

He took in the New Year's Day dance at the Hopkins nurses' residence, writing to Kate Crowell, with whom he still exchanged the occasional letter, that in this part of the world it would be considered a breach of etiquette not to go. 'I've been used to treating nurses with great hauteur and dignity. This social business kills me ... We are very frolicsome creatures here ... They don't work so hard down here as they used to in Boston – a good and a bad thing.'[27]

'I am getting more used to Baltimore,' he told his father in February. 'Don't mind their carelessness and slowness and unreliability now that I expect it. I wouldn't choose to dwell here however.' In March, not long after he took a day off to run over to Washington to see the inauguration of the new president, Ohio's own William McKinley, he learned he would be staying in the region for at least a little while. Halsted had come through with the much-sought-after residency appointment, pitchforking him over several contenders to succeed Bloodgood. It was typical of Halsted that Cushing first heard the news from others. 'I hope I will prove worthy of his Confidence,' he told his father.[28]

~

In the next few years Cushing proved himself spectacularly worthy, not only of Halsted's confidence but of the great experiment in American medicine that was Johns Hopkins Hospital and Medical School. Baltimore's millionaire merchant and financier, Johns Hopkins, had left the then huge sum of $3.5 million on his death in 1873 to finance 'a hospital which shall in construction and arrangement compare favorably with any other institution of like character in this country or in Europe.' It was to share a medical school with the new university that Hopkins equally endowed. Hopkins's trustees and the administrators they hired, notably Daniel Coit Gilman and John Shaw Billings, aspired to create great institutions for advanced care, education, and research – the fullest possible utilization of knowledge for human betterment.

They took all the time they needed to do the job well and within the estate's means. The hospital did not formally open until 1889, and the medical school required an extra endowment from a group of philanthropic, feminist women to open its doors in 1893. But from their earliest stirrings, the Johns Hopkins institutions attracted first-rate people, funded them generously, and assumed the leadership roles in higher education and medicine that their benefactor had envisaged.

The hospital, built on a hilltop in what is now East Baltimore with a stunning view of Chesapeake Bay, was smallish by later standards, only about three hundred beds. Surgical shortcomings aside, Hopkins was lavishly equipped with laboratory facilities and support staff. Its chiefs and department heads – William Welch in pathology, Howard Kelly in gynecology, William Osler in medicine, and William Stewart Halsted – were given authority comparable to executives in German institutions or American corporations, and had an almost open mandate to find the best possible ways of delivering their services. There was a very heavy emphasis on research to create new knowledge. The pathological and physiological laboratories had been up and running for six years before the hospital officially opened. Much staff time was spent on pilgrimages back to the great European centers. There was also a major in-house commitment to colloquia and other occasions for the presentation of advanced work. Never inclined to hide their lights, the Johns Hopkins institutions founded their own journals to spread the news of their research achievements.

Osler and Halsted, both familiar with the best continental practice, decided that graduate doctors would not just pass through Hopkins on short internships, as they did at the MGH and other American hospitals. Instead, Hopkins would have a hierarchical residential system, in which appointments were open-ended. Men might be around for five or ten years, learning their specialty while working their way up to being the senior resident in medicine or surgery, contributing to research, and becoming superbly qualified to move into a top position at another institution. During this high-level apprenticeship, the residents would do original research and would aim at achieving state-of-the-art care for the patients in the hospital, most of whom were charity cases, though there was a small private ward.

Most of the staff eventually became involved in teaching medical students. But the Johns Hopkins School of Medicine was almost an afterthought and at first a bit of a bastard child, as the researchers and clinicians concentrated on their primary interests. Anyway, the best way to teach students was by example, the Hopkins chiefs believed. The trick was to set very high admission standards – Johns Hopkins was the first North American medical school to require a previous undergraduate degree – so as to attract only first-rate students. Put these first-rate students in the same wards, labs, and dissecting rooms as first-rate researchers and clinicians and the osmotic outcome would surely be first-rate doctors.

The key was the quality of Hopkins's senior people. The trustees did a superb job of staffing the hospital. Ignoring the local favoritism that still governed appointments at most of America's older medical schools and hospitals, the Hopkins trustees scoured the English-speaking world for the best talent they could find. H. Newell Martin, an Englishman, got Hopkins off to a good start in physiology before descending into alcoholism and early death. William Welch, a Connecticut-born Yale graduate, trained in New York and Europe as a pathologist, was lured away from the highest medical circles in New York by the promise of almost unlimited research opportunities. 'Popsy' Welch and his labs became a magnet for European-trained Americans such as Franklin Mall and John J. Abel, who could now live the research dream in their homeland. William Osler, an energetic Canadian with impressive service at McGill and the University of Pennsylvania, became the master clinician of Johns Hopkins, author of the textbook that became the holy writ of modern medicine, and the teaching star of the medical school. The gynecological surgeon, young Howard Kelly from Philadelphia, dazzled everyone with his remarkable technical skills and boundless energy (which spilled over into a quirky and only occasionally offensive Christian evangelism).

Surgery, however, was a serious, ongoing problem. After a failed attempt to hire Sir William Macewen, who had been Lister's successor in Glasgow, the trustees agreed to give Welch's friend and protégé, W.S. Halsted, a chance. Halsted, who came from a well-to-do New York family and had done extensive graduate training in Germany, had been a surgical wunderkind in New York circles in the early 1880s, a dynamic operator and teacher and a prolific publisher. His research led him to be a pioneer in the use of cocaine as a local anesthetic. Halsted and most of his staff became addicted, his career collapsed, he had to be institutionalized, and he was just getting back on his feet in Baltimore, under Welch's patronage, when the Hopkins opportunity arose. The cautious trustees at first made him only acting head surgeon.

They firmed up Halsted's appointment as word spread of his excitingly innovative approach to surgical problems. Oddly, it may have been related to a major personality change caused by his cocaine habit. Halsted had morphed into an introverted, ruminative man, reluctant to operate, most interested in probing the physiological and pathological underpinnings of the discipline through animal experimentation. He had begun to address the fundamental problem of facilitating healing during and after the trauma of surgery. While so many of his colleagues in the 1880s and 1890s were obsessed with improving healing by aseptically keeping germs away from wounds, Halsted reasoned that despite every effort, the bacteria would probably get through and make contact. The best step forward would be to support the wound's, and therefore the body's, capacity for resistance and self-healing.

The key was to interfere with tissue as little as possible during surgery. 'It was, essentially, to operate with the utmost respect for the integrity and nutrition of the tissues,' Halsted's first biographer put it, 'to be extremely careful to stop haemorrhage from all the tiny severed blood-vessels, to bring together separated tissues in their natural relations if possible, and to leave no vacant spaces where stagnant fluid might collect and form a soil defenseless against the growth of bacteria, except when a bloodclot was deliberately allowed to fill an unavoidable vacant space. And that was all, but enough to make his operations procedures of mathematical precision, with healing almost as precisely ensured.'[29] It was also enough to make Halsted's operations notoriously long. His obsession with hemostasis led to seemingly endless clamping or ligating of every possible bleeding point. He closed with the neatest possible suturing, eschewing catgut to use layers of silver wire and fine black silk, the aim being to bring the tissues to fit perfectly for healing.

What came to be Halsted's trademark operation, the radical mastectomy for breast cancer, was lengthier still because of his determination to excise all tissue that might possibly have been invaded by tumor. Whereas others simply cut out the tumor or the breast, the Halsted mastectomy involved removing the pectoral muscles as well as the lymph nodes and adjacent loose tissue, well up into the neck. Halsted and his disciples, especially Bloodgood, his first long-serving resident, knew that the procedure often failed, for tumors recurred. Consequently, they made histological study of the tumors themselves a part of their continuing work.[30]

Halsted was so slow that colleagues joked about patients healing before he had finished operating on them. The mastectomies involved removing so much tissue that an orderly was said to have once asked him which half was to be returned to the ward.[31] In later life, Cushing spun a tale of waiting through his first Halsted mastectomy: As what the MGH considered a twenty-five-minute procedure dragged on hour after hour, Cushing gave up on the patient and prepared an arsenal of heroic restoratives, only to be astonished when the woman was returned to the ward in good condition.[32]

Halsted's good results could not be argued with, however. Cushing was often severely critical of fellow workers, but he did not clash with superiors whom he thought he should respect. On the other hand, he was not inclined to hero worship or to be overgenerous in giving credit. He never spelled out in print exactly what he learned from Halsted, though in his maturity he admitted to friends that Halsted had a revolutionary impact on him.[33] At the time in Baltimore, he settled down after the dismay of his early months and cultivated his own set of garden plots – as a technician, as a researcher, as a tough senior resident trained in a demanding school, and, most important, as an operating surgeon.

~

The first case that particularly interested Cushing was a young woman brought in with a gunshot wound in her neck. She had an unusually complicated pattern of sensory disturbance and paralysis from damage to her spinal column, the body's main nerve canal. During her six-month stay, Cushing made an elaborate study of her puzzling condition. (Yes, six months. Some patients stayed at Johns Hopkins for years. Part of the glory of the place was opportunity for prolonged, detailed study. Patient stays in most nineteenth-century hospitals were amazingly long by current standards). Cushing used his x-ray apparatus to take pictures of her neck, which showed the location of the bullet, made an exhaustive study of the literature of spinal cord injuries, prepared charts and diagrams, and offered the case as his maiden performance at the Johns Hopkins Medical Society in May 1897. In a tour de force of observation, scholarship, reasoning, and wonderful new visual evidence, Cushing concluded that the patient suffered from hematomyelia (hemorrhage into her spinal cord) and that in this and similar cases – here is the conservative in him – surgical intervention was *not* indicated.

His presentation, his first piece of sustained medical writing (which by a quirk of timing became his second publication) was remembered by a colleague, Hugh Young, as 'exhaustive ... beautiful ... remarkable ... splendid.' With it Cushing began to make his mark at Johns Hopkins. Later suggestions that the case also led him to neurological surgery are not supported by evidence. There was no follow-up with either patient or subject – in fact, Cushing seems to have lost interest in both – though he continued to use the x-ray apparatus for a few months as the hospital's unofficial radiologist until new equipment and staff took over. He was lucky, he remembered, to escape radiation burns.[34]

Most of his research time in the first year or two was spent in the drudgery of bacteriology, trying to puzzle out the etiology of the infections that ravaged so many patients. Circumstances: (1) Johns Hopkins had many typhoid fever victims; (2) its surgeons were increasingly operating to remove gallstones. Consequence: Cushing's actual debut publication, 'Typhoidal Cholecystitis and Cholelithiasis,' in the May 1898 issue of the *Johns Hopkins Hospital Bulletin*. He correlated his studies of bile duct bacteria with work by Welch and Osler and drew elaborate hypothetical connections between the typhoid bacillus and the creation of gallstones. This article seemed of more general interest than his unusual surgical case and was prominently discussed in an editorial in the *Journal of the American Medical Association*. Its conclusions did not stand up in the long run.

Cushing spent more long hours exploring the impact of the typhoid bacillus and related microbes. Could you create gallstones in rabbits by infecting the animals? What about the other exotic bacteria infesting the intestines of typhoid patients? There were so many bugs to be identified, he later reminisced, that every Hopkins worker claimed his own. His was a 'Bacteria O,' which had something to do with hog cholera; Hugh Young's, he joked, was Adam, the father of all bacilli.[35]

He probably studied the bacterial contents of his own feces. It was a

common laboratory exercise for Hopkins students, and it became important for Cushing when, after observing patients with abdominal gunshot wounds, he wondered about the possibility of reducing dangerous
microbes in the intestinal tract before surgery. Perhaps the bacterial
flora of the alimentary canal varied significantly with intake. Perhaps
the risk of infection from intestinal surgery could be reduced by eating
the right food, followed by the fasting already prescribed before etherization. Thus, the meticulous young surgeon, steeped in external asepsis, tried to move on to internal sanitation. For a time he became obsessed with making all patients' ingesta 'amicrobic.'[36]

~

As Halsted's senior resident, Cushing immediately pushed for improvement in the hospital's surgical procedures. He was determined to put
an end to carelessness and disorder in both operating and patient care.
He bombarded Halsted with suggestions for change, generating a remarkable letter of apology from the chief surgeon of what was supposed to be America's finest hospital:

> I need hardly tell you that I am in hearty sympathy with your efforts to correct
> some of our many bad habits. We have never had a man on the staff who
> understood the management of his assistants or, indeed, who had served in a
> well conducted hospital. It is a discouraging fact that good precedents are so
> often forgotten & bad ones seem to take such deep root. During the 1st 2 years
> of the Hospital I spent many hours in the Wards trying to stimulate or de-
> velop in the internes a taste for neat dressings.

Perhaps making a virtue of necessity, Halsted told Cushing of his 'hope
that you will never hesitate to criticize freely what you consider existing evils.'[37]

Cushing expected high performance from everyone who worked with
him, and he did not hesitate to scold anyone – interns, orderlies, nurses,
or colleagues – who failed to live up to his standards. His outspoken-

ness sometimes sparked resentment to the point of rebellion. Having apparently rid Hopkins of a German intern who had challenged a male operating-room nurse to a duel, Cushing found himself in a similar situation. An older southern physician, one Walker, who had come back to Hopkins for further training, was not going to have his work slandered by a northern hotshot. According to J.M.T. Finney,

> One day after Cushing had been particularly severe in his criticism of Walker, and unjustly so in Walker's opinion, the latter waited in the dressing room until after the others had gone. He then called Cushing into the room, closed the door, turned the key, took it out and put it in his pocket. He then told Cushing that he had stood all of the criticism in public that he intended to stand, and demanded an apology for what had been said to him that day and Cushing's promise that it would not be repeated in the future. Failing to secure this, he said that one or the other of them would get the worst licking that he had ever had in his life before leaving the room. Cushing tried to pacify Walker, but his hot Southern blood was up, and nothing short of an apology and a promise would satisfy him. When these were forthcoming, they shook hands and left the room.

Although Finney said they became 'good friends thereafter,' Walker soon left the hospital and Cushing took over his ward.[38]

Cushing himself was not beyond criticism; he was once chewed out by the hospital's vigilant superintendent, Henry Hurd, for leaving his wards surgically unattended while working in the lab. They exchanged 'warm words' about the incident, and then apologized. There are no reminiscences of Cushing in the operating room this early in his career, only his own observation that the kind of biting sarcasm Halsted was noted for hurt 'much more than a good cursing.'[39]

Throughout his career he had excellent relations with patients. He was all kindness and charm and sympathy. If young Dr Cushing happened to be tough on the nurses, determined that everything should be done just right, well, that was good for patient morale too. He worried about his patients, sacrificed free time to care for them, mourned those he lost, and, like most doctors of the era, continually risked infection to care for the living. A nurse never forgot the time a child who had been tracheotomized for diphtheria had his tube accidently withdrawn and rushed into the hallway choking. Cushing took hold of the boy, put his mouth to the wound, sucked out the mucus, blood, and dis-ease-membrane, then reinserted the tube.[40]

A sudden reversal: Kirke and Bessie Cushing get a telegram from Osler saying that Harvey is a patient on his own wards. His problems had begun with severe abdominal cramps and vomiting. The doctors were uncertain, perhaps partly because the food at the hospital was notoriously bad. Their first decision was to rely on morphine and not to operate. Harvey, who had just lost a patient from the effects of a rup-tured appendix, persuaded a medical student to do a second leukocyte count. When it revealed infection, he was rushed to the operating room. Instead of taking in the Baltimore Orioles' championship game on the afternoon of September 28, 1897, the Hopkins team took out Cushing's appendix.

They had done only a handful of appendectomies. Halsted preferred not to work in the abdomen. 'Halsted, Finney and Bloodgood did the operation and they had all six hands inside of me at once – big hands at that. Hugh Young gave me chloroform ... They used a mid-rectus inci-sion from ensiform to pubis and got mixed up in the epigastric artery which they had to tie twenty times with heavy black silk ligatures.' Cushing had left instructions for disposition of his possessions if he did not pull through, but all seemed well. Eight days after surgery he wrote Kate: 'I'm having a beautiful time ... am perfectly well literally living in a bed of roses ... American Beauties. Then there are great baskets of fruit outside of each window – a lot of rare old wine in the wardrobe – Everything one could wish to read on this table here – delicious viands brought in by a wonderful cook and the best of nurses ... Friends drop-ping in constantly ... What more could one wish. I have been com-pletely spoiled and am no fit subject for compassion.'[41]

The operation would have been an advertisement for the benefits of modern surgery, except that a few days later his abdominal wound broke down, minor infection developed, and the suturing had to be redone. Recovery was slow and painful. 'We have been bragging of our summer record of 200 cases or more without suppuration. I have broken the series.' Halsted had used heavy silver wire sutures subcutaneously to close Cushing's abdomen; for years, Harvey could feel his chief's handiwork under his skin.[42]

~

After recovering from his appendectomy – he took a couple of months off – Cushing threw himself into his job as day-to-day head of surgery at Johns Hopkins, and he began to blossom. 'Here I am, a youth, doing surgical work that not one of my school confreres will hope to do for years. It frightens me sometimes. The Chief rarely operates. Today I did all of his private cases ... I've been so fortunate lately that I hardly dare to speak of it lest some day may come a fall ... I am high cockalorum in the house ... I am thriving under it and never felt better.' He later acknowledged that Halsted's lax supervision – no rules and juniors being given all the responsibility they could handle – was the ideal way to teach men to think for themselves.[43]

His early publications, some fifteen articles in about a twenty-four-month period, contain lovely nuggets about the discovery of his powers. Doing a radical mastectomy, for example, which he must have learned from Halsted, Cushing accidently nicked the thoracic duct, which was then thought to be beyond surgical treatment. He found that he could use one of the delicate curved needles that Halsted imported from France to close the wound with a fine black-silk suture. In writing this up, he could not resist adding a footnote describing other minor triumphs he had accomplished with the wonderful needles.[44]

Then there was the remarkable case of the patient with the severed jejunum (small intestine) that had formed a fistula with the abdominal wall, out of which his nourishment poured almost undigested. The case was important for Cushing's studies of the progress of intestinal bacteria, and for a time the poor man became a guinea pig as the doctor fed

him oysters on strings and tried other experiments. Cushing finally resisted the temptation to think of himself as a latter-day Beaumont with
a new Alexis St Martin. He closed the fistula, resected the bowel, and
enabled the patient to return to life and sanity.[45]

He was proud when his contrarian diagnosis on an influential private patient in the hospital proved accurate – 'and I am such a kid.'
Proud when he saved one of Halsted's private patients, 'a swell from
Washington,' whom Halsted had said would die. And proud when he
did the first splenectomy at the Johns Hopkins Hospital. It was for a
case of Banti's disease that had been diagnosed by Osler, who had a
high appreciation of surgical work (which may have been misplaced in
this case, for though the patient lived many years, the operation did
him no discernable good). Osler was almost immediately impressed by
Cushing. 'Halsted and all of us have the most unbounded confidence
in him,' Osler wrote to Ned Cushing early in 1899, 'and within five
years he ought to have the reputation of one of the best operators and
most successful surgeons in the country.'[46]

Building that reputation involved getting everything right in his
operating room. A key starting point was just where it had been back
in Boston, the anesthetic. As Cushing knew from experience, anesthetizing ill and fragile patients with ether required considerable powers of
judgment and concentration, and the occasional application of brute
force, even as it imposed serious, sometimes disastrous side effects on
the patient, both during and after the operation. Cushing implemented
his Boston 'ether charts' at Hopkins, and one of his first suggestions to
Halsted was to set aside space adjoining the operating room as an ether
recovery room. Still, there was a major problem: the house men at
Hopkins served only four-month stints on surgery and Cushing decided
he had no one he could rely on to give anesthetics in prolonged mastectomies or complicated hernia repairs.[47]

Hernia cases, a staple of Hopkins surgery, often involved serious
intestinal strangulation in older patients, who also tended to respond
badly to anesthetics. The Hopkins working rule that it was not safe to
anesthetize anyone over sixty made many such cases inoperable. Early

in his residency, Cushing had a patient with a strangulated hernia die under ether on his table. Inhalation anesthesia also tended to create complications during goiter work in the neck; Cushing saw both experimental animals and patients die when respiration was blocked and desperate, bloody struggles at resuscitation failed.

He began experimenting with cocaine as a local anesthetic. Paralyzing nerves with injections of cocaine seemed in many cases less hazardous to the patient than inducing unconsciousness with ether. The surgeon was his own anesthetist. 'The author was driven into these cases by poor anesthetizers,' he scribbled on his first publication describing this work. He knew nothing at that time of Halsted's earlier experience with cocaine, and Halsted apparently neither told him of it nor took an interest in this work. The results of hernia surgery under cocaine anesthetic were so impressive that by late 1899 it had become the procedure of choice at Johns Hopkins.[48]

Cushing expanded his use of cocaine as part of an interest in the phenomenon of intestinal perforation caused by typhoid fever. The condition seemed unpreventable and untreatable. Perforation of the bowel as a result of necrosis and ulceration in typhoid cases led to acute peritonitis, indeed was often only recognized by the peritonitis, a state Osler labeled 'a rough draft of death.'[49] Even if the problems of anesthetizing and operating on a patient suffering from severe typhoid fever could be surmounted, surgical intervention would be too late.

Osler and his medical staff made typhoid fever a major area of study. The barriers between medicine and surgery at Hopkins barely existed, and in 1898 Osler's resident, Thomas McCrae, introduced Cushing to the 'autumnal crop' of typhoid cases. Examining the patients, Cushing thought he felt lesions that the medical men were ignoring as insignificant. He wondered if close observation might lead to the detection of intestinal perforation at the moment of occurrence, perhaps even in advance as 'preperforation.' Prompt laparotomy and repair of the bowel might be possible.

Cushing achieved remarkable results on a nine-year-old boy, saving his life by going in three times to repair and clean up the consequences

of perforation. Europeans hardly ever tried to operate even once in
such cases, and the Nestor of American surgeons, William W. Keen,
was on record as suggesting caution and warning that a second operation almost never worked. 'The boy is doing unexpectedly well though
I mustn't boast yet,' Harvey wrote Kate after his first operation on the
child. 'The game is young but we must win.'[50]

Proud of his success in saving even one of the three perforation cases
that he had worked on – and proud, surely, of Osler's comment that a
surgical treatment that saved one in three was better than the physicians' results ('they all die with us')[51] – Cushing made typhoid perforation another of his special interests. Here he was working on the frontiers of surgery, an American ahead of Europeans, or certainly bolder
than them. These were important early experiences at reconfiguring
the risk-benefit calculation as confidence in the safety of exploratory
laparotomy increased. There were parallels with the recent development of the appendectomy as a radical intervention to avoid the emergency of rupture.

Nor would Cushing hesitate to try a second operation for perforated
intestine. Where Keen counseled giving up, Cushing countered, 'It is
hard to agree with the statement that a patient should be left to his
fate, no matter how desperate the condition, provided surgical intervention offers any chance of relief, forlorn though it may be.'[52] Working with these cases, he was also absorbing lessons about the crucial
importance of 'fraternity' between surgeons and physicians on the wards,
and he was forming a lifelong belief that the surgeon should have a
major role in diagnosis.

Cushing found he could better manage his sometimes very long perforation operations when the patient was under cocaine anesthetic. He
was working entirely with Osler's staff on a procedure the boldness of
which was foreign to Halsted's surgical temperament. How proud
Cushing must have been in the summer of 1899 to receive a letter from
his former colleague at MGH, Allie Porter, describing how he had been
reading Cushing's first paper on perforation when word came from his
own wards of a patient with exactly the same symptoms, prompting

Porter immediately to undertake what proved to be a successful operation.[53]

An appreciative comment on Cushing's perforation work in the *Boston Medical and Surgical Journal* included a warning that such operations were without risk only in the hands of surgeons whose technique was so good that error was almost impossible. All of Cushing's early papers were sprinkled with comments on the importance of technique. In his cocaine studies he repeatedly drew attention to the importance of the surgeon having mastered the anatomy of nerves, a subject many of them neglected in the age of the general anesthetic.

He was still frustrated by the difficulty of monitoring patients during surgery. It was particularly important to know when they seemed to be slipping into the condition known as shock. It happened that George Washington Crile, who was making a name for himself in Cleveland surgery, was deeply interested in the subject and, both in Europe and America, had carried out a major program of animal research. In 1898 Cushing reviewed Crile's prize-winning monograph, *An Experimental Research into Surgical Shock*, which advocated preventing shock with surgical approaches similar to those being used at Hopkins, including careful control of bleeding, gentle handling of tissues, and greater use of cocaine anesthetic. Cushing hoped that the innovation of monitoring blood pressure, which Crile and others could do with laboratory animals, would soon become clinically feasible. Something better than a finger on the pulse was needed to warn of impending shock.[54] Meanwhile, he would keep on trying to perfect the preperforation operation and would continue to explore anesthesia through nerve blocking with cocaine.

~

In Baltimore, Cushing worked with men who became his good friends and whose careers touched his for several decades. The seniors at Johns Hopkins, including Welch, Osler, and Superintendent Hurd, entertained him in their comfortable homes or at the posh Maryland Club. After work the young residents and researchers might gather in their rooms in the hospital's administration building or perhaps go over to the 'Hopkins Chapel,' Hanselmann's saloon. The gang included Simon Flexner, a brilliant and ambitious pathologist working under Welch; Lewellys Barker, one of the many Canadians drawn to Hopkins in Osler's wake; and Tom McCrae, another Canadian, solid and unusually hard-working, who had risen to be Osler's resident. Cushing also knew all the middle rank, including William S. Thayer and John M.T. Finney, who had helped lure him to Baltimore in the first place and were becoming fixtures in the city.

The Hopkins family welcomed talented newcomers, such as the brilliant German medical artist Max Brödel. With their common interest in drawing, Cushing and Brödel became particularly good friends, and Max helped Harvey with his German. Oddly, Brödel's patron and Hopkins's most technically accomplished and productive surgeon, Howard Kelly, who did gynecological work, was never close to Cushing. Kelly, a human dynamo, seldom had time for anyone he was not trying to convert to his brand of Christian fundamentalism. When he did once notice Cushing, Harvey remarked to Kate, 'Dr. Kelly looks as effulgent as an Xray tube. He is distinctly phosphorescing. Its a privilege to be seen by him who does not hide it under a bushel.'[55]

The Johns Hopkins Medical School, which had been gathering strength since its 1893 opening, was little more than the hospital staff wearing professorial caps and gowns. 'Instructor in Surgery' since 1897, Cushing also taught occasional postgraduate courses to earn a few dollars, help out, and get some experience. He worked constantly with medical students on the wards; during the students' clinical clerkships – an Osler innovation – they did much useful work with patients. But Harvey did not have a major teaching commitment or interest. In fact, he did not approve of one of the most innovative features of the Johns Hopkins Medical School, its admission of women on equal terms with men. This had come at the insistence of the rich Baltimore women, led by railroad heiress Mary Garrett, who had raised the extra endowment money that enabled the medical school to open. In the seventy-member incoming medical class in Cushing's second year at Hopkins, there were twelve women. There had not been any women in Cushing's classes at Yale or Harvard. 'Bad luck to "em" and their patron saint Mrs [*sic*] Garrett,' he wrote to Kate. 'I believe in it but little.'[56]

He finally gave in, more or less, to his own need for female companionship. Convalescing in Cleveland from his appendectomy, and taking in a series of weddings in the winter of 1897–8, he renewed his romance with 'my dear little Katy.' When he returned to Baltimore, their desultory correspondence suddenly heated up. Harvey wondered whether he had been right to put her off for so long: 'It worries me a great deal sometimes when I think that perhaps I am treating you very badly after all, despite my endeavor to do what I thought was *fairest* to you. When you are everything in the world to me why should I be willing to run the risk of losing you?' By early 1898 she was 'beloved Katy,' they were reading Shakespeare sonnets together, and Harvey was scoffing at her fears, undoubtedly learned from him, that she might hinder him. '"Ruining my career!" What a funny idea … Whenever I used to accomplish anything I used to be pleased for the home people first … but I'm afraid that's all changed now and that everything will be for you first and always. By afraid I mean glad.'[57]

In February 1898, Kate visited Baltimore, staying with the Goodwillies. Harvey introduced her to the Halsteds, Oslers, and other Hopkinsites, who must have known she was his chosen. 'Dr. McCrae must have been blind as a bat and stupid as an owl if he hadn't some suspicion about me that afternoon after Mr Hurd's tea,' Kate wrote later. In the moonlight, on the Goodwillies' steps, he proposed to her and she accepted.[58]

The wedding would have to wait several years, until he finished his training. They were deeply in love and they would have a rich and busy epistolary romance, exchanging love letters almost daily, but even the fact of their engagement was still a secret. They told only Kate's mother, who completely approved of the match, told Harvey not to be so modest about himself and his prospects, and joked that he might be getting mother along with daughter. Kate, a healthy and athletic young woman, full faced, and slightly taller than Harvey and more full figured than he would ever be, lived at home in Cleveland, where she filled her days with golfing and other activities at a new social institution for active well-to-do Americans, the country club. She received letter after letter from her fiancé, dedicating and re-dedicating his life and work to her, pouring out details about his life and plans. 'I never felt my strength so before – never so confident of my ability to surmount obstacles. I've done more good work since I had you to help me than ever before.'[59]

Kate was deliriously happy with their engagement – 'I think this is the best time of my life' – and totally committed. 'Oh Harvey dear, I love you so much – I never thought that I was capable of it, & no one ever sees it but you & some times I'm half afraid to let you see it – It is very deep & all tangled up & twisted round & if anybody should try to pull it up I should die.' She settled in to wait: 'How is separation to grow easier every day if I will persist in dreaming about you every night? ... I cannot get through the day without a letter, or without writing. I shall have to write just a line every day ... it will be so many years, that we shall have to live on letters ... I should like to kiss you just once – *Please* don't miss a day. Your loving, KC.'[60]

So he worked harder than ever and wrote more letters than ever, describing his life and painting remarkable word pictures, sometimes with sketches:

> I have been submerged most of the time – Operating – trying to break in a new surgical staff – writing a medical paper – getting up lectures and clinics for the next symester et cetera. Last night however I went to the ball – the nurses New Years ball. The first time I've danced since just a year ago at the same function ... had some bully dances which made me think of you ... My legs seem to stay younger than my gray matter. I am reading Schaupenhauer's Essays – enough to make anyone morbid you will say ...
>
> I was asked to go to a Chafing dish party tonight at the Hurds ... but could not go ... Life seems to be spent in going to bed so as to get up early and get to

work in order to get through in time to go to bed and be able to get up – and not be behind the next morning.[61]

Early in 1898 he was finally invited to dine at the Halsted residence, a rare event for anyone in the Hopkins community. The Halsteds, a mid-life marriage between the surgeon and one of his operating-room nurses, Caroline Hampton, were notoriously reclusive. When they did entertain, theirs was complete hospitality. It was 'truly Chesapeake,' Harvey told Kate, listing dishes he could barely spell:

I. Caviare and thin slices of dry toast as a Hor d'eouvre.

II. Boulion.

III. Roast oysters – huge ones – brought in on a great dish of silver, an old hunting prize won by Mrs H's grandfather in the palmy days of the south. We were supposed to help ourselves and had to open the oysters instead of having the madschen do it. They *were* good (The big dish was planted right in the centre of the table).

IV. A terrapin stew made in a chafing dish from the real $50.00 bird picked out of a lot by the Professor himself and boiled and skinned and picked by him before the dinner.

V(a). An asparagus course – I forget

V. A wonderful quail arrangement with a whole bird in the middle of a block of a salty quail jelly. Also a slice of pate de fois gras.

VI. Omellette souffle I believe. Very delicious at all events.

VII. An ice served in most curious and quaint dishes.

VIII. Crackers and Camabere chese

IX. Fruit, candy et cetera

   Many rare wines at intervals appeared. Some old Madeira 60 years old, think of it. Also from Grandfather Hamptons cellar.

   Lastly coffee made in the library. The berries were picked out and roasted that afternoon. Ground in the quaint old brass arrangement before us – and the coffee made in an old brass pot with a long handle and brought to a boil over the fire. I never tasted Coffee before.

   I wish you could have been there.[62]

When Kate was there and they called on the Halsteds in their home
it became clear to Harvey that his chief's domestic fastidiousness was
not just the other side of his professional carefulness. The Halsteds, he
told his mother, were truly odd:

> A great magnificent old stone house full of rare old furniture, clocks pictures
> and what not in topsy turvy condition, cold as a stone and most unlivable.
> The dog room upstairs and the Cheifs library alone have fires in them ... Mrs
> H. met us or received us in the dog room in a large dirty butchers apron. Such
> a blunt outspoken plain creature you never saw. They are so peculiar, Eccen-
> tric, so unlike other people yet so interesting doubtless partly because of
> their oddities that one is inclined to shelve his thoughts about them along-
> side of those of people from fiction – Dickens perhaps ... The Professor
> himself is doubtless the best man in his specialty in this Country which of
> course makes being his slave a most valuable experience. I am very fond of
> and admire him immensely.

Having experienced Halsted's considerable charm – 'when the bars were
down ... as delightful as anyone I have ever known' – Cushing told
Kate that when they were married they would become great friends of
the couple and visit them in their summer retreat in the Carolina hills.[63]

Fat chance. The more he got to know of the Halsteds, the more
eccentric and trying he found their ways. They were almost invisible in
Baltimore and Hopkins society. When Cushing tried to visit unannounced, the maid lied to him, saying no one was home. Worse, Halsted
was often not in the hospital when he should have been. The more
Cushing took charge as resident, the less he saw of his chief, whose
excuses for absenteeism were as chronic as his confusion about the
state of his patients. Halsted would have a cold, a headache; famously,
he once excused his lateness by saying that he and his wife had been
catching rats. He encouraged his staff to begin operations without him
if he wasn't on time. He told Cushing to operate on any patients who
couldn't wait for him, and he offered to operate on cases that Cushing
had handled days earlier. At other times, he decided to do follow-up

studies on patients who turned out to have been discharged. Some of his excuses seemed to Cushing to be outright fabrications. For several weeks in the spring of 1900, Cushing annotated Halsted's notes to him as though preparing a case against a chief whose lack of professionalism was, at a minimum, deeply exasperating. 'He spent his medical life avoiding patients,' Cushing wrote in a published obituary of Halsted.[64]

What Cushing did not know and apparently never knew, though he might have suspected (only Osler knew the truth and he did not tell until a secret manuscript he wrote was published fifty years after his death), was that Halsted still had a serious drug problem. He had broken his addiction to cocaine only by switching to morphine. Through the 1890s, the Surgeon-in-Chief and Professor of Surgery at Johns Hopkins took three grains of morphia a day, which is nine to twenty times a normal dose. His addiction probably explains his chronic absenteeism, which Hopkins records indicate had nearly cost him his job even before Cushing's residency. He was a horrible teacher, feared and disliked by the medical students. The morphine habit surely contributed to his introverted personality. His world may have been further complicated in that the evidence – including his marriage to the mannish Caroline Hampton, who lived in separate quarters in their house – suggests that he may have been homosexual (as also, perhaps, was his friend and patron Welch). Sexual 'inversion,' as a few alleged experts were starting to call it, was a condition that even to physicians hardly had a name, let alone tolerance, a century ago.[65]

In all of these circumstances, Cushing's ability to take charge of the surgical wards at Johns Hopkins was a godsend for Halsted. Halsted certainly thought so. 'If you should break down,' he wrote Cushing in 1899, 'I would be in my grave in a month.' A year earlier Cushing had helped Caroline Halsted avoid an early grave when a horse ran away with her carriage and she was badly battered. Her husband was away at a medical meeting. In the Halsted home, Cushing operated on her for a fractured pelvis and other injuries. He was amused to find himself serving immediately afterwards as a kind of high-class doorman, greeting solicitous colleagues – the Oslers, President Gilman, and others –

all of whom, he suspected, were entering the Halsted residence for the first time.[66]

Halsted's generation of surgeons often operated in patients' homes – it was often more convenient and private and less septic than in hospital – and Cushing had already done other home operations. He would not have been surprised in July 1898 when he was asked to come on a Halsted expedition to the mansion of a very rich Irishman in Providence, Rhode Island, and to remain behind after the surgery, probably a hernia repair. He told Kate he was not comfortable in the haunts of the ultra rich: 'All this magnificence ... disturbs me. There are flunkies at every corner and I believe a steam yacht at my bidding and three nurses who as is quite usual, know it all. The carpets are about a foot thick and there are paintings from the last "Salon" on the walls – behind glimmering Electric lights ... Providence is cool and pretty though I refuse to ride through it in a victoria. I am afraid I am a very proud Child of the Public.'

Some kind of disagreement about patient care between Cushing and the local doctors caused them to insist that Halsted return to take over the case. Despite Halsted's support, Harvey felt he had no choice but to leave. Halsted's apology for the whole incident notwithstanding, Cushing found it 'a humiliating experience' and worried to Kate about whether his own sharp edge might have been partly responsible: 'Oh! I do hope I am not going to grow up tactless among my own people. Perhaps I have been too successful.' The 'Child of the Public' fled Providence for Boston, where he stayed at private clubs, saw old Harvard friends, and decided that he and Kate should live there.[67] He went on to Long Island to stay with the Atterburys, then back to Cleveland for a two-week junket up the Lakes with his family and Kate. He seldom again operated in anyone's house. Even Halsted soon stopped making high-fee surgical pilgrimages to patients; they had to come to the hospital instead.

There was also a war going on in the otherwise idyllic summer of 1898 as the United States fought Spain, mainly over Cuba. The main threat to American soldiers in the campaign was infectious disease, including the typhoid fever that ran through the 5th Maryland (Baltimore) Regiment at its base in Florida. On the outbreak of war, Harvey had volunteered to serve on an ambulance ship but was not needed. He wanted to go to Florida to tend the sick men: 'I do hate to be a stay at home.' Instead, he had to receive cases shipped back to Baltimore. He wrote to Kate about meeting the first trainload of sick volunteers:

I never have, nor expect to see 150 such emaciated, wan, forlorn, ragged, dirty creatures as were carted in on that train of six old disreputable sleepers. It was enough to make a strong man weep. As one of them told me 'We are and have been rotting.'

Perhaps a hundred of them, so called convalescents, were furloughed and one by one tottered off from the train with their packs, gaunt, haggard, feeble. It would have wrung your heart ... And then the sick ones big heavy fellows, their skins hot as a live coal, not sick long enough to have lost flesh and make carrying easy. There were about 20 ... hospital stewards with green Chevrons and red Crosses who knew no more how to pick up a sick man than how to keep him clean. We saw it was useless, so Finney turned them out and he and I carried out I think about 40 of them in all, one at a time and put them in the ambulances. It took us two hours, but it was one of the greatest privileges I have ever been granted. We could have done it all day and General Grigg thanked us with tears in his eyes.

The train was foul beyond description. Imagine an old Pullman sleeper, with shabbiest of fittings crowded with sick, many lower berths with two people, dirty clothes & equipment scattered about everywhere, no thought whatever of keeping the patients clean, and pans & cups & old hats & shoes and dirt and haggard bearded young faces, stupidly turning their eyes at you, who felt guiltily strong and well and vigorous and army blankets & pullman blankets & dirty sheets & pillows & bad odors and I don't know what was absent to complete a scene of extreme disgust & pity.

'If we'd only been at Santiago we wouldn't have minded so much, 'cause we a' had some reason to get well & get back to the front – but to rot like dogs down at Tampa with nothin' to look forward to – it was hell, sure enough.'[68]

He got as far as Huntsville, Alabama, to bring back more sick soldiers, some of whom were raw material in his typhoid perforation studies, and he exchanged views with his father on whether America had been properly prepared for the war. Otherwise, the Spanish-American conflict passed him by.

In 1899 he was again a stay-at-home when Johns Hopkins Hospital was invited to send a medical expedition to study tropical disease in the formerly Spanish Philippine Islands. He envied his friends, Simon Flexner and Lewellys Barker, for having the opportunity:

> Is it not *splendid* ... They are going to take a complete laboratory along ... Flexner told me last night that I was in the original plan but it did not seem feasable to take me nor necessary for a surgical man to go ... Such letters as they have to nabobs and giving them right of way – government service &c ... Lady Curzon is a personal friend of Garretts etc ... Mrs Garrett offered them her private car to Vancouver ... Isn't it simply good? Flexner says he will be willing to die if they accomplish a part even of what they anticipate. How hollow it seems to set around at home.[69]

Harvey's professional expeditions were to nearby cities to give presentations at medical gatherings. The first of these, a session at a southern medical society meeting in Birmingham in the autumn of 1898, was both more and less than the learned discussion of typhoid perforation he had expected. The youngsters from Johns Hopkins found themselves

> buttonholed on all sides and asked to discuss the relative value of some anti deluvian Brazilian drug we never heard of, by old 'Kentucky colonel' doctors full of corn whiskey and with whiskers all over their heads – gray heads, mostly. It is perfectly killing, but interesting too and a great treat. I have got to change my whole paper; subject perhaps. They (most of them) wouldn't understand a word of it, I fear ... Probably most of them never saw a microscope.
>
> Interesting old fellows from way up in the mountains of Tennessee and

Georgia, young apprentice sprigs, in town for the first time all enthusiastic but with mediaeval ideas. Poor fellows. I'm sorry for them. All with fine qualities and sacraficing health to exposure and work of which we City breeds little dream. So it has its pathetic side too.

I brought my frock to wear ... We are going to operate tomorrow. I wish I had a great beard for the occasion and my few gray hairs showed better.[70]

Mostly he was on duty in Baltimore, night and day, seven days a week, in charge of the surgical wards and staff, ready to operate any time in an emergency. 'Morning rounds, operations daily, laboratory work in the afternoon, library work when I can, German lesson every night with Brödel, more rounds, reading and literary work till midnight and a Chapter in Thackeray before my light goes out ... and let us hope no emergencies during the night.' The days sometimes faded together until he became 'woozy' with fatigue 'and prone to get cross with people on little provocation,' he told Kate, 'until I remember you when I become very sweet and amiable to everyone, which I am most of the time.'[71]

Lack of sleep could make him euphoric, intoxicated, exhilarated: 'I've been oh so chatty and feel active and vigorous, as though I had a grasp on life and work as never at other times. Everything has a rosy hue at these periods and whatever I touch seems to succeed. I suppose that's only a part of the mental state and so partly imaginary.' He knew he worked too hard and occasionally worried about it: 'I'm afraid you think me a dreadful digging old worm who never sees the light of day and is not capable of loving any body but is simply miserly over his work.' After they were married, he promised her, 'I shall never be very busy and Sunday will always be your day and no office hours.'[72]

He never suggested that fatigue might affect his surgical judgment or skills, but did allow that he could be overcome with 'hospitalismus': 'For a week I have looked a little white and yellow and a few green spots under the angle of each joint. These things have begun to get commented upon and I cant stand personal criticisms except from you.' He would take a few days in the Carolina or Virginia countryside to recover, half envying the person taking his place, and then throw himself back into the fray:

> We did not operate as I thought the staff was rather tired so the morning early
> was occupied with a sort of round up of the wards and then there were a
> thousand little details to see to, the floor varnished and parafined in our
> laboratory, some new shelves put up, the instrument man to consult, a lot of
> patients to see ... a new plaster room to be fitted up under one of the wards,
> the 'diener' to lecture because he did not keep up some operating room
> supplies, etcetera. This continual drumming and pushing and scolding to
> keep other people up to their work is dreadful wearing especially as you
> have to keep their respect and liking at the same time. And these southerners
> are the happy go luckiest lot you ever saw ...
>
> This afternoon I spent in the laboratory across the street ... played tennis
> for 3/4 of an hour before dinner. Unusually good dinner. Had a smoke with
> McCrea and have been in the wards the rest of the evening. Most of the time
> spent in trying to straighten out a forlorn family. A very nice boy whom we
> are very fond of is dying and his mother is here and his sweetheart, poor girl,
> came this afternoon – she's a good soldier too – and his father tonight. The
> latter is all gone – lost another boy at Santiago of fever and has proceeded to
> get most intoxicated. I've got him away from the rest on some pretext and
> asleep down stairs. Isn't it sad ...
>
> A woman said to me this morning in ward C 'Why are you Dr. Cushing?
> How young you are!' – this always pleases me mightily and I have got so used
> to it that it embarrasses me no longer. I must look young and why should I not.
> I'm happy. So many of the younger men in the house look older than I do ...
>
> Poor Davis, one of the men in the house, has gone home with a fatal afflic-
> tion. Too bad. He was one of our best men. Three of the 4th year class have
> consumption – developed the last year. A medical Course is a rough one
> certainly. What a lot of sickness. And you and I are so well and happy and have
> the whole world laid out at our feet. Why should fortune pick us out?[73]

The good luck almost ran out that Thanksgiving Day. Harvey operated in the morning, showed Kate's mother around the hospital in the

afternoon – also showed her her bones via x-rays – and went to President Gilman's for dinner:

> A very enjoyable affair except that I began to feel sick and heady and to realize that I had infected my finger with a needle prick in the morning. I stopped in at the Goodwillies on my way home, saw a sick darkie when I got back so that it was midnight before I could have anything done and everyone else had gone to bed so I tried to but found it no use ... I had to get up at six to see the same 'dark' and ordered him for immediate operation, got the operating room ready, called Bloodgood up to do it for me as I was incapacitated by that time.
>
> The darkie flatly refused to have anything done so I volunteered – took my old friend Chloroform, which I'm afraid makes me dreadful chatty and had my hand opened up – since then I have been better but one handed. The man from whom I got infected died – also the darkie. What serious things we dabble in at times.[74]

The best part about his month's convalescence from the infection was that he was able to spend most of it in Cleveland.

∽

He wanted to get abroad, marry Kate, write articles and make a name for himself, and he still did not know how or in what order these things might happen. A common view, that Cushing must have burned with focused ambition from his college days on, is a distorted retrospective reading based on his later achievement. During most of his training he took life a day at a time. In the summer of 1899, for example, he told Kate, 'I have no plans and do not think beyond the present day only hoping it will end in bed, which is hardly likely. I wonder why I keep at it. Ambition? And also how I stand it so well – Physique? I am aware of neither though I recognize in others that ambition brings work and a sturdy constitution prevents "Hospitalismus" from which so many around here are suffering more than I.'[75] There were other times when he weighed his options, sometimes with Kate, sometimes with his father and brother, sometimes with friends at the hospital. Where would his interests and talents take him?

There was little false modesty about ambition at Johns Hopkins. Seniors and juniors alike aspired to be and be recognized as the best. There seemed no limit to the medical greatness that a super-achiever like William Osler would attain. Cushing thought Osler would surely accept one of the offers coming to him from Great Britain and end his days as Sir William. Other Hopkinsites were content to stay in Baltimore and become nationally and internationally famous. The younger generation at Hopkins soon found themselves in demand for top positions in prestigious American medical schools.

Lewellys Barker, who took a chair at the University of Chicago in 1902, was a particularly interesting case of idealistic ambition. At Hopkins he caught the vision of the possibility of putting research work before private practice and sordid money grubbing, at least for a little while. Cushing often listened to Barker philosophizing about careerism – and once prophetically suggested that Barker would eventually succeed Osler at Hopkins. The problem for all the young medics was to figure out how long 'a little while' might be. Could it be stretched into a lifetime of teaching and research? How long would Harvey Cushing stay at Hopkins? How long would it be before he had that year in Europe? When he came home, would he be able to find that perfect position in a major hospital or medical school where he could break new surgical ground, train a few students, and live happily ever after?[76]

He hoped to go abroad in 1899 after his second year as senior resident. Halsted cajoled him into staying. McCrae passed on news that Osler, himself in Europe for the summer, 'said all kinds of splendid things about your work and thought very decidedly that you ought to stay on for some time yet. He seemed to think it would be a great loss to the place for you to go and a pity for yourself.' Still, Cushing's restlessness increased. It came to a head that winter with the possibility of taking a position in Cleveland at Lakeside Hospital and Western Reserve University. Here was the opportunity finally to go home and get married.

He had already half made up his mind when he wrote Kate in December: 'Will you be awfully disappointed if I don't come? Do you think I am too ambitious and that I have become a slave to Barkerism? If I should let go now I would become an old fat good for nothing money making operator. I could give you a home right away but you would hate me in a year – I know and I would myself. Its pitiful to think that I may be doing good work only because of my environment. No one can tell however.' But the Cleveland offer was a good one and the whole family was drawn into weighing pros and cons, with his aged parents making a special visit to Baltimore. The Cushings had long conversations among themselves and with some of the seniors at Hopkins, including Osler. Hopkins wanted Cushing to stay but had no significant promotion available to offer him. Harvey's mother urged him to decide his future on the basis of where he could best serve and how he could best repay his father, who had footed the bills for his education.

Kirke Cushing, who had returned to Cleveland in his youth to practice with his father, and perhaps had felt confined there, seems to have been unwavering in his belief in his son's destiny. Any doubts he might have would have vanished as Harvey told his dad about the sensational, still unpublished results he was getting operating on certain previously hopeless cases. Kirke advised his son to stay in Baltimore:

> My conviction is that you are much better off where you are than you could be with anything offered here.
>
> Every year you stay in Baltimore will add increasingly to the advantages of your opportunities. To this time, largely, you have been establishing a foundation, the superstructure is now in the making, and will be recognized as the earlier work would not have been.
>
> It does not matter so much what your title is, or what our relative rank is: the great thing is the opportunity to do good work and have it recognized ...
>
> The increased repute of 2 or 3 years more work, where you are, will tell powerfully on any opening there, here, or elsewhere that will eventuate. That something most Desirable will show up is hardly to be doubted.[77]

Harvey parlayed the Cleveland option into a vague arrangement with Halsted that he would go to Europe for a year in the summer of 1900. Kate would continue to wait patiently at home. 'You are ambitious but not too ambitious,' she told him. 'You are only bringing out the best that is in you, and that is your duty.'[78]

⁓

Cushing's 'superstructure' began to take clear shape in 1899–1900. He was supplementing his abdominal and intestinal repair work with a growing interest in the nervous system. By the time he left for Europe in June 1900 he had developed a bold and delicate new operation that took him literally to the edge of brain surgery. 'Your friend, Harvey Cushing, has opened the book of surgery in a new place,' Osler told a mutual acquaintance early in 1901.[79]

It evolved from his interest in local anesthesia. He anesthetized or blocked peripheral nerves, usually by injecting them with cocaine. In addition to the patients whose nerves Cushing temporarily deadened to prevent pain during surgery, there were some who came to Hopkins seeking relief from pain they felt as a result of diseased or damaged nerves. Often the pain was in or around the face. Could the doctors deaden nerves to stop pain?

Well, you could try to remove the offenders by doing a neurectomy. In August 1897 Cushing tore away five centimeters of the infraorbital nerve from the floor of the eye socket in a fifty-seven-year-old woman. In March 1899 he evulsed an inch or two of the inferior dental and infraorbital nerves in a thirty-seven-year-old shoemaker. He probably also tried cocainization in some of his facial cases (which at least was an advance on the hemlock that Erastus Cushing may have seen prescribed). Whatever he tried, he soon learned, if he did not already know, that such procedures gave temporary relief at best to those patients who suffered from the horrible, literally maddening pain spasms known as trigeminal neuralgia, or tic douloureux.[80]

Trigeminal neuralgia is a disorder of the largest facial nerve. Its cause is still obscure. 'Tic' refers to twitching grimaces caused by agonizing jolts of nerve pain. Cushing soon became familiar, for example, with the case of James Walker, a former sea captain very near the end of his rope after years of seeking relief from the malady. In the early stages of a spasm, Walker would feel 'a devil twisting a red-hot corkscrew into the corner of the mouth,' and then the pain would spread. The slightest movement of his face or beard could set off an attack. Drugs were useless. His teeth had long since been extracted. He could barely eat or talk, and in the summer of 1899 he appeared at Johns Hopkins threatening suicide if the surgeons couldn't help him. Walker was emaciated and shrunken, unwashed and red-eyed from sleeplessness, drooling and writhing and crying out in pain. Two previous operations for his nerve trouble had given him only short-term relief. Now he did not much care if he died on the table.

A few bold surgeons in Europe and America had recently attempted heroic intervention to deaden the trigeminal nerve by severing its juncture with the brain. Cushing had observed some of these operations, assisted at others, and had found the experience 'disheartening.' The procedure of drilling into the side of the skull and cutting through the dura, or lining of the brain, to reach the key area was often impossibly bloody. Cushing had seen at least one death from hemorrhage on the table; bleeding and other operative problems often caused surgeons to retreat in disarray without achieving anything. Mortality from the operation was an unacceptable 20 percent. At Hopkins they had lost two of the four patients on whom the procedure had been attempted.

On August 4, 1899, using chloroform anesthetic, Cushing trephined James Walker's cranium in the lower right temporal fossa, using a hammer and chisel, and opened a small operative well. He pushed aside the middle meningeal artery, pried up the dura, and with a blunt dissector worked free (or as he put it, 'liberated') the whole gasserian ganglion – the bundle of nerve cells connecting the brain with the trigeminal nerve. The next night Walker slept soundly for the first time in years. With the pain gone, he began to eat ravenously, putting on forty pounds in the next nine months. He lived normally, dying in his mid-seventies twelve years later.

The isolated cases of brain damage and tumor that Cushing had seen in his early training had not inspired him to do any brain work, even on animals, in his early years at Hopkins. His real trail towards neurosurgery led from problems of anesthetizing, then to cocaine work with the peripheral nerves in the abdomen, and then to the face and to cases like Walker's. The problem of trigeminal neuralgia led Cushing to develop his ganglionectomy, a delicate neurectomy at the very edge of the brain.

The exact timing cannot be nailed down, but before the Walker operation and probably after it as well, Cushing had built on his observations by studying the literature of gasserian ganglion removal and by practicing on cadavers. The method he developed was a modification of a procedure that others (Frank Hartley and Fedor Krause) had pioneered seven years earlier, differing 'only in its details,' he reported in his first article about the operation. 'It is, however, upon detail,' he added, 'that the success of this, supposedly one of the most delicate of surgical procedures, depends.' He was entering the skull lower than others had done, lifting rather than cutting the dura, and by coming in lower he could more easily retract the troublesome middle meningeal artery.

Cushing prepared himself in the company of the dead. He did about thirty operations on cadavers, finding that only fresh bodies were suitable for his purpose (the professor of anatomy and the medical students were surprised that all their specimens had had ganglionectomies).[81] In a long footnote in his first paper on the extirpation, Cushing described how he sensitized himself to the level of delicacy required:

> Only after a great number of operations at the autopsy table can one satisfactorily train his reflexes to appreciate the degree or force which it is necessary to apply at the edge of the ganglionic dural sheath in order that it may be split and the ganglion exposed by lifting away its superior covering ... Only after repeated operations on fresh cadavers possessing skulls of various indices did the writer feel justified in dealing with the ganglion at the operating-table and confident of removing it in toto. To satisfactorily free the entire ganglion is a delicate procedure and familiarity with the crackling sensations imparted to the hand while liberating it from its dural envelope can not be overvalued. I know of no operation which could be undertaken without such preliminary experience with equal rashness. I have found the experi-

ence gained from practice on ordinary anatomic material to be unsatisfactory. The toughening of the dried dura and altered consistency of the ganglion and brain imparts, through the dissecting instruments, sensations markedly different from those which are given by fresh tissues.

Cushing did a second ganglionectomy in December 1899, on a St Louis businessman who had lost everything and become maniacal with pain. He had a splendid outcome, the patient writing him a few years later about having been 'resurrected.'[82] In January 1900 he operated on the sufferers he had partially treated years before, getting good results despite problems with bleeding. These were the exciting results he described to his father when they talked over his future that month. Kirke Cushing would certainly have been impressed. In all his years of practice, he had seen only two cases of trigeminal neuralgia; both patients had committed suicide.[83]

Other surgeons were interested in the problem, including W.W. Keen, who had done trigeminal work himself and was already familiar with Cushing's work on typhoid perforation. Keen organized a symposium on trigeminal surgery at the College of Physicians in Philadelphia on April 20, 1900, and invited Cushing to present his results. Cushing did not think the seminar was very interesting, except for some remarks by Barker, who was already working with him on these nerve problems. The *Journal of the American Medical Association*, in its issue dated only eight days later, published Cushing's paper, 'A Method of Total Extirpation of the Gasserian Ganglion for Trigeminal Neuralgia: By a Route through the Temporal Fossa and beneath the Middle Meningeal Artery.' It was accompanied by beautiful drawings of the operation made by the author. Here was a major surgical triumph, the opening of the new page.

∽

Cushing already had his passage to Europe booked. Just before he left there was a strange burst of publicity, about which he had mixed feelings. The New York *Journal American*, one of William Randolph Hearst's newspapers, immediately sensationalized Cushing's JAMA report in a Sunday feature story entitled 'How Toothache and Neuralgia Are Cured.' It called Cushing's innovation 'probably the most daring operative procedure ever attempted by a surgeon.' Coincidently, other newspapers published a sensational story about the distinguished Canadian-born astronomer and professor at Johns Hopkins, Simon Newcomb, whose crippling pain in the leg had disappeared after Cushing and Barker, working with cocaine anesthetic, had removed part of a diseased nerve from his thigh. Suddenly able to walk miles again without his crutches, and bursting with gratitude to his doctors, Newcomb raved to reporters about the miracle. 'Cured after Years of Pain,' trumpeted the story, which read almost like a testimonial for a patent medicine or a faith healer: 'Prof. Newcomb believes himself to be entirely cured and leaves his crutches at Johns Hopkins as a souvenir just as the poor cripples who are cured by miracles leave theirs at Lourdes and at the shrine of St Ann De Beaupre.'

Notoriety like this deeply embarrassed doctors, who were forbidden by all their codes of ethics from advertising their skills. On the other hand, it was almost certainly effective advertising that would attract more cases. But not for Cushing. Having finally completed his American apprenticeship, he was going to see what more he could learn from the European masters.

He cleaned up his work in Baltimore, had a long visit from Kate, thanked his father for the beautiful steamer trunks and generous letter of credit he provided, began to cultivate a mustache to look older or more European or more like Osler, and sailed for the Old World at high noon on June 23, 1900.

He did not have very definite plans, either for his *wanderjahr* abroad or for his return. It was not clear what he would do if he went back to Johns Hopkins or even if he would go back there at all. 'I feel like a person who is just about to jump from a precipice,' he told Kate. 'I hope I will land easy and be able to climb back again.'[84]

FIVE

A *Window on the Brain*

The Atlantic crossing afforded Cushing a week off, time to relax, recover, get some sea legs, eat, drink, write, reflect, and socialize. As soon as he boarded the old Cunard liner *Servia*, he began his travel diary: 'I shall apparently be alone with a few books, some tobacco, my thoughts, and some pretty keen regrets at throwing up the J.H.H.' Then the first of his notes and letters to Kate: 'These Cunarder people are so nice and courtly and have such nice voices and never get annoyed like the Americans.'[1]

The energy went out of him like a deflating tire, and he spent the voyage with his mind a blank, reading Edith Wharton's *The Touchstone* and making the usual steamer friendships, including chats with his old Yale baseball teammate, Amos Alonzo Stagg. He traveled 'incognito' as Mr rather than Dr Cushing, so was left alone by the medically inclined. Most of the passengers were American pilgrims to Rome or Thomas Cook tourists, many of them 'English people who have been spending two weeks in the "States" and who think we are queer I doubt not.'

It was a crossing for putting on weight, with good weather and only a few hours of gastric queasiness. At landfall on the Irish coast, vendors came aboard with newspapers and boxes of fresh strawberries. On their last night out, a sudden shower gave way to a rainbow coming out of the water and arching over England. It was Great Britain's welcome to its American cousins, a courtly Britisher told Harvey.[2]

Then a prolonged social interlude, featuring several rounds of intense medical sightseeing and fraternizing in a climate of professional bonhomie during the summer of 1900. American doctors were thick on the ground in London and Paris that season: many of Harvey's colleagues had come over for the Centenary Festival of the Royal College of Surgeons of England, and even more for the Thirteenth International Medical Congress in Paris.

It was only Harvey's second trip abroad. Despite his thirty-one years and his Yale, Harvard, and Hopkins background, he was a gawky American, adjusting to customs he often found strange and irksome. London, the capital of the world at the height of the glory and power of the British Empire, seemed overwhelming. His first few days there felt like months, he told his mother: 'I do not remember to have been so impressed with the *bigness* of things when Neddie and I were here together. It gives one vertigo for a few days: the incessant motion of traffic – the constant roar, much tempered of course by asphalt pavements and rubber tires, but still a roar – the overpowering number of people – the concentration of interesting things all worthy of days of study.' On hot summer days he sweated in the obligatory dress for medical visiting, a frock coat and tall hat, feeling each day as though he were going to a wedding.[3]

Osler was also over for the summer, and he took Cushing and other Hopkins men, Thomas McCrae and Henry Barton Jacobs, under his wing. Being Canadian, Osler was as British as he was American. He knew British medicine intimately and happily introduced his young protégés to its highest circles. Cushing, whose acquaintance with Osler was still mostly professional, was very impressed. 'Dr O. is a big man here – even bigger than in his own country and just as nice,' he told his diary:

His name is passport anywhere. He gave a stirring address at the 'Polyclinic,' Jonathan Hutchinson's post graduate hospital the other night. I met Sir Wil-

liam Broadbent, Malcolm Morris, Ewert the heart man, and some other nabobs there. Dr O, Jacobs and I were down to Guy's Hospital this afternoon
and had a profitable visit. Its a fine place, less old foggyism than in our
comparatively young institutions, as the MGH for instance. The old Guy's
Museum is remarkable, second only to the Hunterian which surpasseth my
highest expectations ... Its a treat to go about with Dr Osler. He gets at the
meat of things in an extraordinary way. At Guy's we looked over some of
Addisons Brights Hodgkins old pathological and clinical reports – very interesting they were.

It was not Osler's doing, but there was even a viewing of Queen Victoria
passing by on the street: 'Nice old lady. There must have been 10,000
people along the way to see her and such a mass of swell equipages as I
never saw.'[4]

The young doctors made follow-up visits to the medical nabobs they
had met through Osler, had a marvelous picnic on the Thames with the
Oslers and their son Revere, and were invited to lunch in one of London's
higher social circles: 'Rather formal occasion, ladies smoke cigarettes
... many flunkies about, menu written on an ivory card & shown to you
– delicious frenchy things.' At a medical dinner in honor of Osler a few
days later, Harvey, who was not an abstainer, was still surprised by English drinking habits: 'Elaborate & delicious long course dinner with
much wine of which they all drank heavily. I was astonished. The amount
of alcohol consumed here is extraordinary anyway. Working men never
pass a "pub" without a peg and their betters are really no better.'[5]

He was spiritually intoxicated by a weekend with the Oslers in a
sleepy seaside resort, Swanage. They had tea at the ruins of Corfe Castle,
strolled on the Dorset downs, dipped and swam in the ocean, ate about
five meals a day, and sank into great feather beds at night. He felt he
was in a Thomas Hardy novel and wished he could spend a month
there.[6]

Back in London he took in the conversazione and other ceremonies
at the surgical centenary so he could see the 'big men' of Anglo-American surgery. He was proud that a number of his American colleagues –

W.W. Keen, J. Collins Warren, and Halsted himself – were being honored by the British. He paid an obligatory call on Halsted in London but saw nothing more of him socially. His penchant for schmoozing waxed and waned – his favorite hours at the Royal College of Surgeons were spent studying the marvelous collection of anatomical and pathological specimens in its Hunterian Museum. He also found time to see the great paintings of Europe, beginning with the National Gallery in London, and to have dinner at the Cheshire Cheese.

'Paris is beautiful beyond words.' The playing of 'The Marseillaise' at the opening and closing ceremonies of the Thirteenth International Medical Congress, an olympian gathering of some seven thousand physicians, sent chills down his spine. The congress featured endless grand receptions and famous people to size up, more hours in formal evening dress than Cushing thought he could stand, and, also in evening dress, a 'swell variety show' at the Casino de Paris. Like many Americans he felt more at home in Paris than in London: 'I like the Parisian medical people immensely. They are much more like Americans than are the English curious as it may seem, in appearance and manner. Such a hospitable lot I have never encountered.'[7]

He eventually tired of ceremonies and papers in foreign languages (German was still the language of science; French, of international conversation). One afternoon he sat by the Seine with Will Mayo from Rochester, Minnesota, and another colleague, and they talked about how the real highlight of the congress had been the spectacular surgical demonstrations offered by the famous (and in their view appallingly bad) Parisian master, Eugene Doyen. The young turks most liked to watch other surgeons at work, if only to see their true colors.[8] After the congress, Harvey moved to cheap digs on the Left Bank and prepared to see what the French could teach him.

~

The little he had seen of English surgery was not impressive. Of several general surgeons he had visited, one, Mayo Robson of Leeds, seemed pretty good. A surgeon at St Thomas's Hospital in London had made him 'shudder' as the man bungled a bile duct operation. Cushing saw the venerable surgical immortal, Lord Lister, at a meeting one day and then, to his astonishment, saw the head surgeon at Guy's Hospital operate using an old Listerian carbolic acid spray, as though nothing had changed since Lister's heyday thirty years earlier. 'The technique of all of these men is execrable from our standpoint and they must have many septic wounds,' Harvey told his father.[9]

Nor did he exclude the much-honored and highly specialized British surgeon, Victor Horsley, who had pioneered a number of neurosurgical procedures, including one of the first gasserian ganglionectomies. The only letter of introduction Harvey took to Europe was to Horsley (supplied by William Welch), and Horsley invited Cushing to breakfast with him and his family. On July 4, 1900 – perfect symbolism – the up-and-coming young American watched the English master enter a cranium, breaking open the bone with a huge pair of forceps. Cushing saw Horsley do a couple of other procedures, including a ganglionectomy in a private home, and judged that Horsley was a 'little disappointing,' a better laboratory worker than an operator. Any plan Cushing might have had for spending more time with Horsley was abandoned.[10]

He told brother Ned that the surgeons he saw in Paris were 'far and away above the Londoners I think.' Doyen's demonstrations apparently included a brain tumor removal, and Cushing praised the beautiful intestinal work of Henri Hartmann at the Hôpital de la Pitié. Still, in France he was disappointed too, telling his father that the surgical work was not very stimulating. His journal entries were often scathing, especially in describing the work of one Fauvre at the Hôpital Laennac:

A stumpy little man who ... slapped a patient and did not seem to know his business. He explored a deeply icteric [jaundiced] woman who did not seem to have had her history taken and closed her up ... most carelessly. Their technique is good though they have too many whiskers, espec. the assistants, one of whom would have made a good Pan. The visit 'au lit des malades' was distressing as usual – poor, old, dirty, over-crowded wards perhaps the best they can do under the circums. – women examined publicly – men bared promiscuously – no histories to be seen – careless examinations – ragged looking temperature charts and so ad infinitum. Fauvre wore gloves (rubber) during his visit and the usual linen butchers costume and apron. An acute appendix case was discussed and allowed to wait.[11]

Disrespect for the patient by European doctors bothered Cushing constantly, as it did many American physicians who came both before and after him. While one of the attractions of Europe was the willingness of doctors to put their patients on display for teaching purposes (especially women in obstetrical and gynecological clinics), many Americans were disgusted by doctors' treatment of their subjects as second- or third-class humans. This attitude came naturally in the hierarchical societies of the Old World but was deeply suspect in democratic, egalitarian America. In Cushing's day, German surgeons had been known for brilliance and innovation – Halsted was a proud disciple of German surgical training – but had also become notorious for their callousness. J.M.T. Finney of Hopkins had visited Berlin only a few years before Cushing's trip to Europe and vividly remembered a day in the clinic of one of the well-known figures:

The patient was a young woman about twenty. She was wheeled into the operating room on a stretcher, then stripped of all her clothing, lifted to the operating table and tied there by the orderlies with bandages binding her legs together and her arms to her sides, with her head pulled back over the end of the table and tied fast there in a most uncomfortable position. Thus she could not move her head, arms or legs, but could only cry. The whole procedure was brutal. There was no nurse present, only a maid, and the surgical amphitheater was full of doctors and medical students. When she cried from fright and from the rough handling, one of the orderlies would smack her on the side of the face and roughly tell her to shut up. When the surgeon himself came in, she was crying loudly and begging for mercy. He walked over and gave her a resounding smack on the cheek and in turn told her to be quiet. He then proceeded to do the operation, a most painful one, without a drop of anesthetic of any kind, believe it or not. The poor girl screamed and cried until she stopped from sheer exhaustion. The details of the operation are too horrible to relate. I waited until after it was over, just long enough to go up and ask the operator – I won't call him a surgeon – why he hadn't given the poor girl an anesthetic. With a shrug of the shoulders he replied, 'It wasn't necessary. We could hold her' …

It was at once obvious that one of the reasons why German surgery had advanced as it had at that time beyond the surgery done in most other countries, resulted largely from the apparent disregard for human life and suffering. They would attempt things that in most other countries would be considered unjustifiable … The patient was something to work on, interesting experimental material, but little more.[12]

Finney had probably briefed Cushing on what he would find in Europe, perhaps steering him away from Germany. Instead, Cushing traversed the south of France, observing every willing surgeon he could find, at least once politely declining to do guest surgery: 'One can always play better ball in his own back yard when he has his own bat &c.' He had congenial times with fellow physicians, who often took him into their homes for meals and drinks ('I was forced to make an intimate acquaintance with absinthe and other beverages which get under ones hat rapidly') and who swapped stories and showed him their rare books.[13] But he found few operators he could respect.

In Lyon, a major regional center, where he was initially interested:

My illusions were shattered this a.m. at the Hotel Dieu. Poncet's assistant did a very bad exploration of a case of cranial traumatism (recent) with right hemiplegia. He used Doyen's burr & after a chisel with which to enlarge the small opening he made in the temporal region. Cut the meningeal artery. Much hemorrhage. Tried to secure it with their outrageous Riverdin needles without success … Did not open dura for supposed underlying clot. The worst of the performance was that he tried to explain himself at the black board afterward … absolutely hopeless … I excused myself as soon as politeness would allow.

Then he saw appallingly careless abdominal work on a ruptured appendix. 'Abscess smeared everywhere (no cultures of course).'

As one after another of the established surgeons disappointed Cushing, he began to worry that he was hypercritical: 'I wonder if I am trying to find a perfect surgeon ... Have seen noone who has regard for tissues.' The most pathetic case was one Leopold Ollier, a pioneer in plastic and osseous surgery, who when Cushing visited was taking a photo of a patient whose elbow he had excised and who could now hold up a dumbbell. When Ollier left the room briefly, Cushing, thinking the patient looked tired, offered to hold the dumbbell, and found it was made of wood.[14]

Surgery was still so young. No two surgeons had the same technique, it seemed, no two operating rooms the same procedure. Cushing took exhaustive notes – how surgeons washed their hands, their use of nurses and assistants, their temperaments, their drinking and smoking habits. César Roux, chief surgeon in the medical school in Lausanne, Switzerland, looked like Rudyard Kipling, 'similarly intelligent & boorish je croix at the same time'; on first examination Cushing found him 'nearer to being the kind of man I am looking for than anyone I have seen.' Roux was a showman, ingenious, fast, a wizard at suturing. Cushing was a little bothered by his habit of smoking in the operating room and was then appalled at his barbaric operation on a girl with a goiter: 'Girl brought into op. room about naked – prepared on table before remainder of class – shivering with cold. Covered with wet cloths and operated with *no anaesthetic*, not even a little morphine. She cried out once or twice – not at skin incision however. R. did the extirp. beautifully.'[15]

The next day he watched Roux operate for inguinal hernia on an old man, again without anesthetic. 'A brutal performance and very badly done.' When Cushing told Roux about their use of cocaine as a local anesthetic in operations on the aged, Roux laughed and said he wouldn't have time to do that. 'Rather inconsiderate of patients but that is charac. of all,' Cushing noted in his diary. 'Patients enter op. room during preceeding op. climb on tables and are cleaned up amidst "bloody rags."'

The pièce de résistance with Roux, as it were, came the day he showed Cushing one of his famous gastroenterectomies. He somehow got his patient's bowel completely twisted, swore audibly, backtracked, swore some more, and became confused: 'I was dreadfully embarrassed my-self. Roux's vaso-motors began to dilate and it was pretty bad all round.' In his diary, Cushing again noted how badly the patient had been treated before the operation. 'It always shocks me the lack of regard they have for feelings of patients. Possibly we are too finicy.'[16]

Three or four years earlier, while researching his paper on spinal cord injuries, Cushing had come across impressive articles by Theodor Kocher of Berne, a general surgeon with a high reputation across Eu-rope, especially for his innovative work excising the goiters that were so common among the Swiss. Cushing told Halsted about Kocher, and in 1899 Halsted visited Berne and became very enthusiastic, partly because Kocher's methods were similar to his own (and very different from those of Roux who, when Halsted visited him, left a clamp in a patient's abdomen).[17] Cushing finally arrived in Berne to spend time with Kocher early in November.

On his first day he watched Kocher's son, Albert, operate and was bowled over: 'The operating!! – the JHH out done. Its easily seen why "the Professor" thought so highly of their work. Detailed technique – tedious operation – absolute hemostasis – intervals between op's ... Strange contrast to yesterday a.m. Roux did six operations in 2 hours – Kocher fils did two operations in six hours.' The Kochers ran their clinic much like those at Johns Hopkins. Cushing immediately felt comfort-able there and also with Theodor Kocher, a cadaverous little man with a nervous smile and Halsted-like habits with his nurses: 'He is kindly sarcastic in his impatience – His "Schwester, Schwester" long drawn with the usual *stupid* at the end must be hard to bear.'[18]

When Cushing finally got to see the great man operate, he was again disappointed:

Disillusionizing morning ... Patient very badly handled – uncovered most of time. I never saw such careless exposure of patients. An assistant operated 2 hours in cold amphitheatre on a mastoid ... the patient being half covered with a single sheet all of the time.

Arndt meanwhile operating on some hernias – very badly – finger dissections – Kocher then did a horrible operation for an impossible stricture ... He dallies over work to extraordinary degree – 3 1/2 hours over his two cases which for a busy man is too much. His inhibition relaxed this morning and he was needlessly sarcastic to the poor head nurse who does most of the assisting – the kind of Halsted sarcasm which hurts much more than a good cursing and makes people get red. The operating room too looked like the JHH in 1897 – wet to the ankles of the guests – the staff wear rubber boots – and bloody sponges knee deep.

Some of the things I liked about operating room technique – Method of covering head in neck operations. Hair is done up in bandage ... Also applic. of sheets to protect neck.[19]

Cushing later acknowledged a great debt to Kocher, but only small parts of it related to operating technique. Although he picked up bits and pieces of ideas from Kocher and others, Cushing failed to find 'the perfect surgeon' in Europe. Europe was in fact a laggard rather than a leader, especially in patient care. The Old World had almost nothing to teach Cushing about surgery. The approaches to perfection they had developed in Baltimore were the state of the art.

∾

He had to spend serious time somewhere during this year and had earlier arranged with Kocher to work in his lab at the University of Berne. He took a room at a medical students' boarding house, worked on his German, and waited to be assigned a problem. For several weeks nothing happened. Kocher, pushing to complete a series of some two thousand goiter extirpations (for which in 1909 he became the first surgeon to win a Nobel Prize) had little time for the American. Harvey considered moving on: 'I don't like Berne and am disappointed in Kocher.'[20]

To kill time, he sat in on lectures at the university and, as he was preparing to leave town, paid a courtesy call on Hugo Kronecker, the distinguished professor of physiology, who among other achievements had been a pioneer in blood pressure studies. 'Lovely old gentleman – enthusiastic about Welch Bowditch Chittenden &c,' Cushing noted. He decided to stay around a bit longer. He went to Kronecker's lectures, 'with the 20 Prussian females who constitute the bulk of the 3rd semestre class – mostly dirty fingered unkempt haired females,' and hung around the underused physiological research institute at the Berne Hochschule.[21] Finally, probably at Kronecker's prodding, Kocher presented Cushing with an *arbeit*, a problem he wanted elucidated to help with his study of cerebral circulation. There were several parts to it, but the essence was 'to decide the question, if in compression of the brain the small veins and capillary vessels are dilated by stasis or compressed?' For Cushing's future career, this proved to be a momentous question.

He wondered if he was doing the right thing in returning to the laboratory like a first-year medical student. 'It's wicked in me to have made you wait these long years,' he wrote Kate. He told his father that even if nothing came of the work he would still benefit from the collateral reading. He settled down to the task with his usual intensity and concentration, stayed in Berne through the winter of 1900–1, and returned there from a stint of similar research in Turin, Italy, to finish up in the spring. The Kochers and Kroneckers took him into their community and their homes, he made friends with other Anglo-American researchers in Berne and soon was complaining to his father of all his social obligations: 'Now that I have something serious to do its difficult to manage the social duties which seems to be expected on all sides. In Baltimore I could refuse to go anywhere.'[22]

Baltimore friends, who were keeping him up to date with Hopkins news, joked that he would catch the 'geist' of the dedicated German research worker, growing ever more unkempt until he reached the final stage of sleeping in his lab in his underwear. Notwithstanding his tendencies in exactly that direction – one day he virtually ordered Kocher and his assistant out of his lab so he could get on with his research – Cushing relished his Swiss socializing. He enjoyed elaborate meals and

musical evenings at the homes of the Kochers and Kroneckers, hiked
and climbed in the Alps, skated and learned to ski, and took up dancing again.

He charmed the maidens of Berne, and the young folk had particularly memorable sledding parties over the New Year's holiday. Cushing
named his Grundelwald sled the Gee Whizz, and by the time he left
town he had formed lifelong friendships with Lotte Kronecker and Jeanne
Michaud. Back in Cleveland, the faithful Kate must have wept at reading about the good times Harvey had enjoyed ushering in the twentieth century without her (in one letter he apologizes for hurting her
feelings and berates himself for having been 'dirt mean'; her letters from
this year have not survived). But there is no evidence that his social
dalliances were anything more than casual. In Berne, as everywhere he
had been since Yale, Cushing was wedded to his work and his career.[23]

His research problem was to find ways of putting the brain under
pressure, and then study the effects of that pressure on its blood vessels.
This was his first sustained piece of animal research, using dogs and
occasionally monkeys. (He also did a minor project for Kronecker on
the effects of the saline solutions used to irrigate the nerves and muscles
of frogs.) Cushing found that European workers were as hard on experimental animals as they were on humans – 'I have never seen less compassion for animals' – and insisted on anesthetizing his dogs before surgery. Long before he became involved in battles with antivivisectionists
about the handling of animals in research, Cushing wrote to his father
about the monkeys they were using: 'Nice little fellows they are, though
they do bite on occasion as my left thumb would show you, and though
they take ether apparently gladly their last blinks at us and the light of
day are rather pitiful. I wish I could explain to them the occasion of our
seemingly heartless treatment or could make up to them in some other
way for the shortening of their allotted time.'[24]

How does intracranial circulation respond to increased pressure? It
could be seen as both an abstract question in physiology and a real
issue in the surgeon's world of hemorrhages, abscesses, tumors, and other
cerebral events. As in most research, Cushing's final publications sim-

plified a story that his barely legible Berne notebook shows was complicated by the usual false starts and twists and turns.

To manipulate pressure on local areas of the brain, Cushing inserted an expandable rubber bag through the skull that he could inflate with mercury. To increase general pressure, he injected saline solution into the cranial vault. He could measure the pressure he was applying, and with apparatus physiologists had been using for some years he could also chart levels of arterial tension, or blood pressure, as the circulation in the brain responded. 'Busy every day with pressure observations,' he wrote in his diary. 'I can see many exciting things through a mist – which prevents me from defining their worth or newness with any exactitude ... I hope it will come to a good end.'[25]

To help clear away part of the mist, to study circulation in the tiny capillaries and veins on the brain's surface, he resorted to a technique others had used, though never in this kind of study, of building a glass window into dogs' skulls. He covered a trephine opening in the skull with a circular glass window, fixed it in place with a couple of bent screws, and found that through it he could observe the impact of his injections. With the help of a magnifying glass, he made elaborate, multicolored drawings of the exposed area of the cortex 'in order to fix in the mind's eye the minutiae of the smaller vessels and the ground-color of the brain ... to carry a mental picture of the topography of the fine radicles, and consequently to observe accurately the time of their appearance and disappearance from the field of vision.'

The scientific prose of the published descriptions of his experiments fails to mask his pride in the technical achievement or his excitement at literally having a window on a new world. His notebook is even more revealing: '*Astonishing to see how easily brain can be washed out. Much easier than organs in general ... Most interesting observations were on dislocation of brain and cord w slightest pressure medulla ... Saw* with astonishment variation in size of cerebral vessels during exposure of brain.'[26] 'We were the first that ever burst into that silent sea,' said Coleridge's ancient mariner, and all the pioneer brain researchers would have understood.

After a while it became clear to Cushing that the brain does not immediately buckle under pressure. The body fights back. Circulation at first seems impaired, and local areas of the brain become anemic, but the blood flow then surges back as the body works to maintain blood pressure at a level higher than the pressure being applied by compression. Cushing saw that this conservative response mechanism could continue until extremely high levels of blood pressure were reached. Eventually, of course, relentless foreign pressure would overwhelm the circulation, blood pressure would collapse as the system went into something like a state of shock, and then respiration and heartbeat would cease.

These observations seemed immensely exciting to the young American, who thought he had discovered an important new physiological principle:

> It is ordinarily stated ... that fatal symptoms originate when the intracranial pressure approaches or reaches the height of the arterial tension. The fact that the arterial tension is a varying quantity which regulates itself so as to overcome the effects of the increased intracranial pressure seems never to have received attention ... A simple and definite law may be established, namely that *an increase of intracranial tension occasions a rise of blood pressure which tends to find a level slightly above that of the pressure exerted against the medulla.*[27]

He first set out his conclusions in a paper given in Italy and later published in the United States. He had made his crucial observations in the Turin laboratory of one of Kronecker's former students, Angelo Mosso, in May 1901. (He did not like Mosso, claimed he only worked effectively when Mosso was absent, and punned about rolling stones gathering no Mosso.)[28] The group in Berne were all deeply impressed. Kocher and Kronecker shepherded a longer paper in German to publication. Working under high pressure and seriously fatigued, Cushing almost had a blow-up with Kronecker when, in Teutonic fashion, the senior professor tried to write the paper for him: 'This I told him was not my way and we had some pretty serious words fortunately avoiding rocks.'[29]

Cushing's findings were not as simple, brilliant, or important as they first seemed. His thinking about blood pressure, deeply influenced by George Crile's studies of surgical shock, rested on assumptions involving control of the venous circulation by the vasomoter nerves. On this foundation he spun out ideas of vasomoter defenses against compression, vasomoter exhaustion, shock, low blood pressure, and eventual collapse. Most of this theorizing would soon be challenged by physiologists and eventually discarded. Even his basic principle, which friendly commentators tried to immortalize as 'Cushing's law' or 'Cushing's response,' was not particularly original; many others had noticed that compression of the brain induces an increase in blood pressure. In fact, the distinguished German clinician, Bernard Naunyn, who edited the German journal to which Kocher submitted Cushing's paper, appended a note indicating his surprise that Cushing was, without attribution, confirming his own findings of twenty years earlier.[30]

Ambitious enthusiasts often overclaim and undercredit, and Cushing and some of his rivals were prone to this. His solid achievement in this research was to delineate the brain's reaction to compression more carefully than previous researchers. He paid more attention to timing, stages, detail, and local variation, realizing by observation that the brain was tougher, more resilient under pressure, than others had thought. His real windows on the brain focused his gaze more closely than others' views. He fixed his images of the brain's responses in his mind's eye and then on paper, while doing precise measurements of changing blood pressure. Previously a general surgeon with a special interest in the nervous system, he had seized this opportunity to use his remarkable technical skill and become a close observer of neuropathological functions. In simple words, he was really getting to know the brain.

In other ways too. One day he took careful notes of a lecture on cerebral localization given by a young physiologist friend. It was evidently the first time he had pondered the vitally important story of attempts to map the central nervous system. The clinical relevance of this experimental work also undoubtedly crossed his mind. In Italy, for example, he saw many patients with brain disorders, and he began to apply some of his laboratory observations to humans. More to the point, during medical sightseeing in that country, he happened on a hospital in Pavia where the doctors were measuring the blood pressure of patients in the clinic with a homemade, inflatable cuff, invented by Scipione Riva-Rocci. Everyone else's attempts to read blood pressure had been frustrated by cumbersome, impractical equipment. Cushing, now very familiar with the subject, sketched the Riva-Rocci instrument in his travel diary and arranged to take one home with him. Perhaps it might be useful in the operating room.[31]

Back in Berne, where he had often watched Kocher operate, he became particularly interested in the problem of brain tumors. One day in May 1901, both he and Kocher concluded that a patient whose brain had been exposed in the expectation of finding a local epileptic lesion was probably actually suffering from a tumor. They never found the tumor because bleeding forced Kocher to retreat and close.[32]

Only a few days after that operation a letter arrived from Halsted in Baltimore offering Cushing the 'surgery of the nervous system' at Johns Hopkins when he returned. If he took up Halsted's offer, this was the area of surgery in which he would specialize. It was certainly the area into which the main currents of his interests, first the ganglion work in America, now the neurological studies in Europe, had merged. Halsted may have known or guessed this, or he may have just taken a shot in the dark – we will see him have second thoughts. In any case, Cushing had already decided to spend his final months in Europe doing more neurological work.[33]

~

Cushing crammed his eleven months on the Continent with what Osler would have called nonmedicated sightseeing. In Paris he did the Louvre and the architectural sights and the 1900 International Exposition in company with his architect friend Grove Atterbury. They also made a four-day excursion to 'Le Plus Pittoresque Endroit du Monde,' which an article in *Century* magazine had identified as the village of Le Puys, in Auvergne. They went with kodak and sketchbook in search of the picturesque and had long discussions about which scenes contained the mix most pleasing to the eye. Did sycamore maples have more 'artistic foliage' than poplars, for example, perhaps because of their unusual 'pale green nakedness' in the spring? Even in the most picturesque spot in the world, Harvey made a point of calling on the local surgeon and toured the curious old hospital, 'all angles and passageways and unexpected steps and gardens and also bad smells.'[34]

The year before he went abroad, Harvey and his father had engaged in elaborate ruminations about the details of a Cushing family bookplate they had commissioned. A growing passion for old books, especially medical, quickened to fever pitch in the bookshops of Europe. So did Harvey's interest in medical history. He was an awestruck pilgrim in the old university towns of Bologna and Padua. In Padua, seeing the amphitheater in which Vesalius had done his great anatomical work justified his whole trip to Italy. He was thrilled to stand where William Harvey, Marcello Malpighi, 'and others without end' had watched the medical awakening of the seventeenth century.[35]

He toured hospitals and churches and museums in Italy. His first biographer diplomatically maintained that Cushing 'was impressed with the extraordinary service rendered by the Church to the ailing poor of various communities.' In fact, this American Protestant was appalled by the backwardness of practically all the institutions he saw in Italy, disliked Italian laboratory laziness, and was offended by the ignorance and superstition fostered by Roman Catholicism. The worst example was at La Consolata, the old church that housed the famous Shroud of Turin:

What a terrible thing for Italy is this Kingdom of the church within the Kingdom of the state ... Every Catholic goes once a week to La consolata – here miracles are performed – the 'idols' are seen to open their eyes – one half witted old woman sees it and all believe – a child is believed by its mother to be able to converse with the virgin – the child believes or makes believe and people crowd from all Piedmont to ask blessings through the infant ... It was dreadful to see the crowd of hogs and children fairly licking a dirty figure of Christ in the doorway ... Here also is the only shroud of Christ's body – shown once in 25 years ... There is a strange story about the imprint of Christs body on it ... wicked trickery ... The priests know all ... A most all-powerful wonderful organization which keeps Italy in the superstition of the middle ages.[36]

Despite the fruitfulness of his research, Cushing begrudged all the time he had to spend in Turin, complaining to Kate: 'I can tell you more about macaroni and poor wine than would fill a book ... This Chace after scientific facts is exciting but hard work and demoralizing.'[37]

He much preferred the rhythms of work and life in Berne, where in his spare time he became interested in the life of Albrecht von Haller, the eighteenth-century physiologist and botanist and the city's greatest name in medicine. Cushing looked up Haller's diaries and publications and made him the subject of a long essay, 'Haller and his Native Town,' which he sent to an American journal. It was the ritual letter from a wandering student, prepared at Osler's instigation and published anonymously, telling the folk a bit about this interesting community and its traditions. Cushing already showed the easy narrative style that makes his historical essays flow unusually smoothly. The essay ends with the dying Haller, fingers at his wrist, trying to feel his last pulsation.[38]

Cushing almost raced through Germany en route back to England in the summer of 1901. Although he planned to learn more neurology before going home, he did not bother to look up the pioneering continental experts, even those whose work he knew about. He completely skipped Vienna and Berlin, the traditional centers for American medical studies abroad. He spent only a few days in Heidelberg and Bonn, briefly meeting 'all the big medical people' and seeing German students at their ritual dueling, which he thought barbaric. His trip down the romantic Rhine, he told his mother, was made 'less interesting from my being alone and feeling some national responsibility on account of a swarm of gorgeous loud mouthed Chicago jews.'[39] In his Haller essay

he summed up his disinterest in the American infatuation with graduate courses in Germany:

> Nothing seems to me so unprofitable as the usual semester spent in Vienna by
> the concourse of American students, the signatures on whose diplomas still
> remember the blotter ... No opportunities better than those at home could be
> offered and it seems to me that the only excuse which today can be given for
> foreign study is a shocking need of modern languages and days too full of
> Kleinigkeiten [busy work] to allow of time for laboratory work. Presumably
> there is but one factor which will retard the realization of Dr Osler's prophecy
> made last summer in London that the great international postgraduate schools
> of medicine will ere long be transferred to America; that is the expense of
> living there.

The medical future belonged in North America.

∾

Back in London, he met up with Osler who was over for another summer, but he did not feel at ease: 'Its curious how deadly England seems
after bracing old Switzerland ... If I hadn't made this arrangement to
stay here during July I should have taken the next steamer home.'[40]

Victor Horsley had offered him some work in his lab, but Harvey
had been advised to look up the physiologist and neurologist Charles
Sherrington in Liverpool. Only eleven years older than Cushing,
Sherrington was a prolific publisher (Harvey was familiar with much of
his work) and was already launched on a career that would be capped
with a Nobel Prize and scientific immortality as one of the greatest of
all neurophysiologists. He was doing elaborate studies of cerebral localization among primates and welcomed Cushing – apparently, the
first American to visit his lab – for a few weeks' work and socializing.[41]

There was not enough time for him to undertake a new project, and
Sherrington did not have anything to suggest, so Cushing hung around,
offering to help where he could, and learned a bit about Sherrington's

studies of the brain's motor and sensory functions. He decided that 'an English laboratory may be in worse shape than an Italian one' and found Sherrington himself a puzzle:

> He operates well for a 'physiolog' but it seems to me much too much. I do not see how he can carry with any accuracy the great amount of experimental material he has under way ... He is not quite as big a man as I had expected. As far as I can see, the reason why he is so much quoted is not that he has done especially big things but that his predecessors have done them all so poorly before ...
>
> Experimental neurology much to my surprise is still in a most crude condition. The problems offered are immense. S. goes at them too fast. Few notes are taken during the observations, which is bad. S. says himself he has a bad memory – putters around his laboratory till after 7 in the evening trying to catch up on things & then is used up and doesn't begin till ten or eleven the next day.[42]

Sherrington asked for Cushing's help trephining some of his thick-skulled primates, first an orangutan and then a 250-pound gorilla. In a long letter to his father, Cushing blended compassion with vulgar stereotyping:

> I'm glad ... that I do not have to take the responsibility of sacaraficing these poor hairy *ape-like-men* for such they seem ... Pretty expensive research is it not? The gorilla cost over $1000 and was a fine big specimen from the West coast. He was ill however and apparently had pneumonia and I doubt if he would have lived more than a day or two. Its very difficult to keep them long alive here and this poor little man had only been in the country twenty-four hours. The bacterial flora of city air can hardly be endured by any who has spent his days in a mangrove swamp. Had you any idea that a gorilla is a negro – an orang a Chinaman or rather Mongol? It was most startlingly striking. The gorilla of yesterday was Coal black – I don't believe you could have distinguished his ear from a darkies. He smelled just like a dirty Negro – behaved like one. The orang came from Borneo – was yellow – a Mongol

even to his whiskers – It's a most suggestive Darwinian thing ... There are lots
of monkeys in the 'ménagerie' ... A dog faced monkey ('Fannie') very tame
and friendly – a Bonnett, whose salaams and salutes at command are most
comical, also friendly – a Jew and some others ... Ah they are a fine race More
human really than we are.[43]

In his three weeks with Sherrington, Cushing improved his approach
to doing craniotomies, made some careful drawings of the primate cortex, studied Sherrington's novel techniques of localization through cortical stimulation, and made a few notes on what must have been stimulating discussions with Sherrington about the brain and its functions
and where research should be going. For Cushing, the experience was a
window on other kinds of brains: the primates' and Sherrington's.
Sherrington used some of Cushing's drawings in some of his publications. Other legacies of his time in Liverpool were a lifelong friendship
with another visitor, Alfred Fröhlich from Germany, and a memorable
excursion to the Isle of Man on the trail of tailless cats. His European
companions on that junket, Cushing noted, were surprised by the
assertiveness of their American friend, 'who sends for tea when he does
not like his coffee instead of drinking it and who objects to being over
charged for cabs.'[44]

Cushing and Tom McCrae went to Scotland for the final two weeks
of what had been a fourteen-month surgical pilgrimage. His last professional visit was to the legendary Sir William Macewen in Glasgow, Lister's
successor and an even earlier pioneer than Horsley in brain surgery. It
was a final letdown. Macewen, Cushing noted, was 'disappointing except in his appearance.' The Scotsman was a humorless loner. In his
operating amphitheater he had set up a system of mirrors for observers,
and they found it impossible to see anything. Everything was clean, but
nothing else was impressive. Cushing later wrote that it would have
been 'an assured calamity' if Macewen, years before, had taken the
offer from Johns Hopkins that had then reverted to Halsted.[45]

A last holiday with the Oslers in the Highlands. Preparing finally to
return to the United States in mid-August, he was still unsure what he

would do next. The problem was that nothing had really been settled about his status at Johns Hopkins.

~

They had missed him in Baltimore – on the wards, in the operating room, among his circle of friends. Following his lead, the surgeons had been on the *qui vive* to catch typhoid perforations before they happened, and they had practiced the ganglionectomy operation on practically every fresh cadaver. But they told him it wasn't the same without his yodeling in the shower, his battles with nurses, his enthusiasm and driving energy. 'The surgical side has swamped Mitchell,' Tom McCrae had written to Harvey back in February, referring to his successor. 'They are bossing him I fear. I wish you could be here for about four hours to clean out the wards. "G" is awful. About 28 surgical patients most of whom are up & about – outpatients do not get proper care and there is soon going to be hell to pay.' McCrae had also kept him abreast of Halsted's vexing inability to plan for the future. One day Osler had asked McCrae about Cushing's situation: 'I said that I thought you were uncertain and that you had no very clear idea of what Dr Halsted thought. "No" said the Chief "nor has anyone else." He spoke about your importance to the surgical side as the man who had more "geist" and go than anyone they had. I hope you are not worrying over the future. Things will shape themselves and you are sure of a good high niche somewhere.'[46]

No one was able to pin Halsted down about what he intended to do for Cushing. Osler and perhaps others pressed Halsted to make up his mind, which he finally began to do in his letter offering the neurosurgical work to Cushing. But on what terms? Would Cushing be a resident? A professor? Salaried? An outsider with hospital privileges? No one knew, least of all Cushing. When he asked Superintendent Hurd for advice, the answer was that everyone was away for the summer and Cushing should come for a conference when they got back. Hurd, Welch, and Osler all wanted him, Hurd said, not least because of

Halsted's 'extremely unsatisfactory' handling of the surgical instruction for the medical students. They had all heard very favorable reports of Cushing's work abroad.[47]

Cushing's mustache did not survive re-entry to America, probably because Kate announced that he would have to choose between it and her. He remained clean-shaven and sharp-faced for the rest of his life. He probably eschewed facial hair for aseptic and comfort reasons too, especially in the summertime when Baltimore was, as Cole Porter put to music in 'Kiss Me Kate,' 'Too Darned Hot.' 'The very walls of the hospital today were wringing wet like an ice-pitcher on a summers day,' Harvey wrote to his father after arriving in town at the end of September, hoping to get his status clarified. Everyone welcomed him back; Osler had him over for dinner, and two of his friends, Henry Barton Jacobs and Thomas Futcher, suggested that he should live with them in the house they had rented at 3 West Franklin Street, next door to the Oslers. As he would probably go into private practice to supplement his Hopkins work, he could have an office there and hang out his shingle.[48]

So much was done on a remarkably casual and personal basis in Johns Hopkins's early years. Until the seniors made up their minds, Cushing was in a strange limbo without any surgical work to do and without any kind of appointment. When he finally had an interview with Halsted, who met him at home in dressing gown and bedroom slippers, the professor hemmed and hawed through his new gold false teeth. The problem, as Halsted saw it, seems to have been twofold. First, Cushing was not really qualified to do all the medical work involved in being a neurologist. Second, there would never be enough work at Hopkins to keep a neurosurgeon busy. No one in the world, not even the great Horsley, was doing neurosurgery only. Halsted suggested that orthopedics included practically all the neurological maladies with surgical implications, so why not take charge of this broader field?

Cushing balked. He was set on doing neurosurgery and thought the orthopedics proposal, which involved trenching on others' fields, absurd. 'I told him I didn't want it and in fact got rather mad,' he told

Kate. He pointed out to Halsted that on his impossibly flexible defini-
tions, neurosurgery might include the thyroid and goiter work that
Halsted himself was doing. 'I came very near writing him a letter that
night telling him that he and his people could go to __ that I was going
to Cleveland. Then I thought of you and didn't ... The days are spent
over here at the JHH doing some desultory work in the laboratory and
telling people I am not on duty.' A day later he added, 'I feel as tho' I
was a perfect idiot not to stay home with you and make some money
for us – instead of chasing a bubble which the Professor would prick if it
were not for the other people who continue to blow it for me a little
out of his reach. He's unique, interesting, but almost too queer to be
close to and be comfortable.'[49]

Kate was furious at Halsted's apparent spurning of Harvey and urged
him to come home. She had once warned him that they were both
temperamentally peppery, and proved it in passionate letters responding to his:

> Why must we be separated for so long you not quite settled in your mind
> down there, and I leading half a life up here? For the first time since we have
> been engaged, I am tempted to say 'come home' – where every one awaits
> you with open arms, and shake the dust of that damnable Johns Hopkins
> from your feet. Yes I am at the swearing point! ... And *everybody* is crazy to
> have you here! I don't see why you cant wait around here for things to turn
> up, and do a little business on the side, and you need not think you are settled
> here for a life time ... I want you to be satisfied – and contented. It really does
> not matter an atom to me where you are if I'm there too ... You never talk
> 'business' to me. I wish you would. Its all very vague in my mind, but I do wish
> you had told Dr Halsted to go to. The thought of him makes me furious. Why
> won't you let me come down for a few days? ... Do you suppose it would really
> make you take your eyes off the ball if I came down for a few days?

She tried to sleep on the matter, but

> the more I think of it, the more I feel that you have not a friend in Dr Halsted,

and that he will take pleasure in thwarting you, right along, if you stay in Baltimore ...

I begin to think it's your duty to come back. You know perfectly well that Dr Osler does just blow along your bubble, but what can he really do? Turn your back on it, come back here, begin to work, and your ship will come sailing in – *our* ship ...

We can go to Baltimore later on. There are no enemies here. Everybody – it goes with out saying – is wild to have you ... If you pursue a bubble it flies before you – if you ignore it and turn your mind to something else – it comes your way – then grasp it. I am actually shedding tears ... Oh write quickly and comfort me and say you will come. I love you so.[50]

Before Kate's letters reached him, Cushing had had a second meeting with Halsted and had set out his terms, which included holding him to the neurosurgical commitment. To Cushing's surprise, Halsted gave in on everything. Harvey now had to calm down his fiancée:

Dont be too hard on the Professor. I think he's really all right at bottom but he doesn't know how; and I am a good bit too sensative and easily hurt. I wont run up against him any more. I told him finally I didn't want the things he offered and told him what I did want and they have come my way. All I've got to do now is to show that I can do them. Can I? Heavens I can try.

If you had written me like this a week ago, dear, I would have been in Cleveland with all my belongings. Yesterday I sealed my arrangements ... To go away mad really would have been to sever associations that we would have regretted much in the end. Isn't it an anomalous condition: my sticking this out for your sake because I was too proud to have you think I'd failed: your anxiety to have me throw it all up. I'm glad I didn't now sweetheart because I'm sure it's going to be all right.[51]

Halsted had agreed that Cushing would become an 'Associate' in surgery, working with a local neurologist on the ward cases and having one day a week for neurological surgery. He would teach a course in surgical anatomy to the third-year medical students in the autumn and a course in operative surgery in the spring. His pay from Johns Hopkins for his undergraduate teaching would be $100. For the rest of his earned income he would have to rely on private practice, private teaching, writing, and speaking. Because Hopkins had only limited accommodation for private patients, Cushing, like the other young surgeons, would do any private operating in one of the other Baltimore hospitals. 'I knew I could have everything I asked for,' Harvey told his father. 'What I disliked was the asking. I wanted offers. Everything, however, has come about satisfactorily ... and all that is left is for me to come up to the scratch. I hope I will be able to.'[52]

He accepted the offer of Jacobs and Futcher to share quarters at 3 West Franklin, had a shiny brass plate engraved with his name, bought stationery announcing that his office hours were from 2:00 to 3:00 daily, and moved in at the end of October 1901. The three young doctors, Jacobs, Futcher, and Cushing, were greeted with a case of wine and boxes of cigars, courtesy of 'Professor Hopkins' – their neighbor, Osler.

~

Within a few days of settling his appointment, Cushing did another ganglionectomy for trigeminal neuralgia, his fifth. The operation was almost a disaster because of bleeding; he was about to give up when a sudden reprieve enabled him to finish. It was only a moderate success, since the patient could not shake off an opium addiction and accused the hospital of improperly experimenting on him.[53] Unfazed, Cushing did more ganglion operations. In this and all his surgery he was now experimenting with measuring blood pressure, using his Riva-Rocci sphygmomanometer. Its inflatable cuff was similar in principle to today's monitors and had many possibilities. In thinking about where to go with blood pressure, Cushing paid close attention to the research of his fellow Clevelander, George Crile.

His return to Hopkins coincided with the publication in American journals of his articles about his work abroad – more evidence that he was a coming man in Stateside surgery. This was underlined in December 1901 when Cushing gave the prestigious Mütter Lecture at the College of Physicians of Philadelphia, once again at the instigation of the talent-spotting W.W. Keen. He slaved over his talk to the point of neurasthenia, he told Kate from 3 West Franklin: 'I've done little the past few days but sit up here and swear and tear up papers and smoke cigarettes.' The final product was a tour-de-force presentation of his studies in cranial compression and blood pressure. His main theme was that these observations ought to have major clinical application in situations of intracranial compression.

He had already begun studies of patients with compression problems, trying to clarify what he called the 'clinical indications of intracranial mischief.' The course of things to come in Cushing's surgery was forecast in his Mütter conclusion: 'Prompt surgical relief, with a wide opening of the calvarium [skull cap], may save life even in desperate cases with pronounced medullary involvement. Thus an extensive craniectomy may completely, though temporarily, ward off the serious attacks which accompany the increasing tension of an intracranial growth.'

Philadelphia's medical elite toasted the young man of the hour at a glittering reception. 'I was pretty tired and would have courted a railroad accident, a fire, or typhoid fever to have escaped the ordeal – rallied fortunately after I got up and saw it through well. Largest crowd they ever had at a Mütter lecture.'[54]

There were no crowds of patients coming to Dr Cushing's private office in the afternoons, and he began to fret about making ends meet – even though, or perhaps because, his father still routinely underwrote his expenses. 'I'm "right smart" hard up,' he told Kate. 'Baltimore is a kind of foozle all round and I want to go home where my girl lives at.' He appreciated the $200 honorarium he got for the Mütter Lecture, cultivated other speaking opportunities, and made $50 dashing off a 'pot-boiler' article for a textbook on saline infusions. He collected his first two fees from practice in January 1902, three months after hanging out his bronze shingle.[55]

The Oslers welcomed the young doctors next door into their daily lives. William Osler had always been encouraging, friendly, and hospitable to Cushing and had probably done more than anyone else at Hopkins to advance his career. Now Harvey was exposed to Grace Revere Osler's enchanting blend of Boston graciousness and good-humored informality. She would yell out of the window for her neighbors to come and join a party, appear on their doorstep with her sewing to escape from her husband's student nights, offer to superintend their house cleaning, introduce them to visiting Osler cousins and nieces, and in a way that never happened with the Halsteds, make the young men feel instantly and always at home. The Oslers gave Jacobs, Futcher, and Cushing keys to their house – latchkeys – so they could come in and use the library whenever they wanted. Harvey often capped a long day's work with a game of tiddlywinks with Osler's second cousin and namesake, medical student Willie Francis.

Cushing soon tired of the winter round of Hopkins luncheons, teas, dinners, receptions, skating parties, concerts. Separation was no longer bearable for either Harvey or Kate, and over Christmas 1901 they decided to marry the next summer. If nothing else developed, they would set up house in Baltimore.

There was talk of other possibilities. Full of enthusiasm for the future of academic medicine in America, Lewellys Barker had moved to the University of Chicago, which had great plans for expansion, and he was urging Cushing to join him. There were very discreet murmurs from the highest circles in Boston, up to and including Harvard's President Eliot, about the possibility of an appointment there – if not right away, certainly in the near future. Everyone knew that Harvey Cushing was a man to watch.[56]

When the Crowell-Cushing engagement was formally announced, Kate received many letters telling her of Harvey's glittering prospects. From a former classmate of Harvey's: 'I admire "Cush" as we all call him more than any one I have ever studied with and I consider him by far the ablest man of his time ... Now that he is going to have a wife to help him I don't believe there will be many years elapse before his name stands way above the men of this New and those of the Old

World.' From George Crile: 'His work has always been masterly and has been favored with a recognition that has been rarely the good fortune of an American surgeon to receive, and he is destined for a most distinguished place in modern surgery.' 'Well, you are a lucky girl,' William Osler told her. Grace Osler phrased it slightly differently: 'I am glad that you have the *privilege* of becoming Dr Cushing's wife.'

Feeling very important, Kate wished that her mother could hear the nice things they all said about Harvey. Harvey passed on to her the not so nice but very prescient comment made by his friend Amory Codman: 'Tell your new wife not to be discouraged because you get sourbellied now and then for it is only your ambition running away with your soul and your heart is all right.' Harvey also told her of William Welch's curt comment: 'Glad it wasn't a nurse, Cushing.'[57]

Many doctors did marry nurses because their lives constantly mingled. Cushing's engagement gossip and marriage planning mingled during any given day with long, tense hours in the operating room, most of them in the shadow of death. He had never been an easy doctor for nurses to get along with, which helps explain Welch's comment. His manner with fellow workers, up to and including Halsted, was often preemptory. Occasionally he regretted it. 'I was very rude to the Professor yesterday,' he told Kate. 'Sorry, but couldn't help it. Some day I will tell him I don't like him and then pack up my duds and go home and bury my head in your lap.'[58]

That spring he so often openly criticized associates that Osler, in what for him was a rare rebuke to anyone, decided to draw the matter to Harvey's attention: 'You will not mind a reference to one point – the statement is current that you do not get on well with your surgical subordinates and colleagues. I heard of it last year & it was referred to by a strong admirer of yours in N.Y. The statement is also made that you have criticized before the students the modes of dressings, operations, etc. of members of the staff. This, I need scarcely say would be absolutely fatal to your success here. The arrangement of the Hospital staff is so peculiar that loyalty to each other, even in the minutest particulars is an essential. I know you will not mind this from me as I have your interests at heart.' This letter, tantamount to Jesus chastising Peter, must have shamed and humiliated Cushing, raising the specter that his career at Johns Hopkins was a miserable failure. He may have told Osler that he, Cushing, felt he should go away. Thus, another Osler note: 'Do nothing of the Kind! Who is free from faults & failings! It is a simple matter – "Keep your mouth" (as the Psalmist says).'[59]

Cushing's commitment to his kind of work meant that even at the happiest times of his life he could be haunted by a sense of faults and failings. He did his eighth ganglionectomy on March 24, 1902, on a forty-seven-year-old photographer who had come to the hospital moaning and crying in pain, the right side of his face a dirty, suppurating mess, too sensitive to be touched. Full of confidence, Cushing thought the operation was going so well that he paid little attention when told that the patient's blood pressure was falling. He suddenly found himself desperately trying to stimulate the patient, then giving artificial respiration, and, hours later, asking permission from the relatives to do an autopsy. They refused. Writing about the case two years later, Cushing was more critical of himself than Osler had ever been or any surgeon could be in today's litigious world: 'It is difficult to record fatalities due to operations, which ordinarily have a successful termination, without attempting on some grounds or another to excuse the unhappy outcome. There is none to offer in this case ... Whatever may have been the underlying condition, the operation was the immediate cause of death and should have been abandoned at the time of the patient's beginning failure.'[60]

The whole Baltimore medical community, indeed all of Baltimore, was flabbergasted that Easter to learn of the sudden marriage of the leader of the city's high society, Mary Frick Garrett, widow of Robert Garrett, former president of the Baltimore and Ohio Railroad, to her younger doctor, Henry Barton Jacobs of 3 West Franklin. No one was more surprised than Cushing, who was in Cleveland finalizing his own wedding plans. These had hit an unfortunate snag when Kate and Harvey's desire to marry on Kirke and Bessie's golden wedding anniversary, June 17, conflicted with a cousin's wedding plans. Both Harvey and Kate were furious, and Harvey wrote an intemperate letter to a mutual relative, who rebuked him sharply: 'Do not write to anyone else as you did to me. You would be a very unwise old blackface to use any of a good many expressions in your letter ... I have destroyed your letter as a dangerous document.' Kate had been even more intemperate, telling the innocent offender to her face, 'You can't have that day. It's ours!' – only to learn that her future mother-in-law had made the original suggestion. [61]

Harvey and Kate calmed down and advanced their date to June 10. Their letters were richer than ever in expressions of love. Kate to Harvey: 'I can't possibly live without you, and everybody might just as well know it.' Harvey to Kate: 'As long as I have you ... I feel so absolutely independent of everything else in the world – my family even (isn't it wicked?), my profession, everything. Its quite wrong I know to love you so much that I am willing to sacrafice the very things necessary to make us happy but I feel that way.' When he was not upset about the change of date, Harvey was full of good sense, urging Kate that their wedding shouldn't smack of an 'Arbeit' for their guests. 'Don't lets have any "glad its all over" feelings. I want people to wish they could go to another like it every week.' [62]

Abrupt, wrenching transitions were normal in his life, as they are for most physicians. On April 21 a Baltimore man shot his eighteen-year-old pregnant wife in the head. She was rushed to Johns Hopkins in a coma, sinking fast. They gave her artificial respiration and did a tracheotomy while Cushing managed to do a craniotomy, opening the skull in twelve minutes to try and relieve the pressure from her hemorrhage. 'With three lives at stake – that of the assailant, his victim, and a child – the moments consumed during this partial hemicraniotomy under artificial respiration were exciting enough,' he later wrote in a scientific paper, 'and we were rewarded, after the final opening of skull and dura, by the patient's taking, for the first time, a few spontaneous gasping inspirations. The hemisphere bulged under considerable tension from the opening, and a large amount of blood clot was evacuated. To our great disappointment, the voluntary efforts at respiration did not long continue.' Under artificial respiration the woman's heart continued to beat for twenty-three hours, but an obstetrician said there was no hope of saving the baby. All three lives were lost.[63]

Cushing found hope in thinking that by entering the brain in the emergency they had come close to success. A week later a sixteen-year-old girl he had operated on three times for a tumor he could not locate or alleviate (it proved to be deep in the brain, affecting the pituitary gland) died of starvation and pneumonia. In despair about this, his first attempt at tumor removal – or perhaps about some other case or about grim results in so many of his cases – Cushing went to Halsted's home to ask him if he really thought it was worth his staying on at Hopkins. Perhaps fortunately, Halsted was away. Cushing released the tension by writing to Kate instead.[64]

His professional life was a constant emotional roller coaster. Two weeks later, when operating on a patient whose face was paralyzed from a bullet wound, he ingeniously connected a totally severed nerve to a working one. As the patient's functions gradually returned, Harvey was able to claim one of the few successful nerve anastamoses anyone had yet performed. 'Done a *great* lot of work,' he wrote to Kate in mid-May. 'Been showing off for a New York doctor. Made his eyes stand out.' His first graduate teaching course at Johns Hopkins, on operative surgery, had been a great success, and for the next year he planned to raise the fee for it from ten to fifty dollars.[65]

The Oslers had a hole cut in the fence in their yard, big enough for two to get through, just so that the Cushings could come and visit and use their garden house. 'It makes life in Balto even, worth while to be next door to these people,' Harvey wrote Kate. The Oslers gave the Cushings two decanters as a wedding present, and their son Revere gave a pair of sugar tongs. Halsted gave them an etching. The Cushing parents gave a thousand dollars, Kate's mother six hundred. Kate's accounts contain a complete list of the 246 wedding presents the charmed couple received.

The wedding ceremony was held outdoors at the Crowell home, Breezy Bluff, on a summer day glittering with blue sky and the blue Lake Erie water. Mary Goodwillie was the maid of honor, Perry Harvey the best man, and Grosvenor Atterbury, Starling Childs, Lewellys Barker, and Simon Flexner also attended the groom. After the wedding several hundred guests came to the reception. The newlyweds went to Niagara Falls on their honeymoon and then to Ontario's Muskoka Lakes for a week of 'habitant days,' fishing and watching the sun set.[66]

They took over the house at 3 West Franklin, with its door to the Oslers through the fence. As so many told her, Kate had married the most promising surgeon in America. Although Harvey still fretted about having to find work to make his living – the need to earn John Hunter's 'damned guinea' – everyone else expected great things from his scalpel and pen.

At age thirty-three he still seemed amazingly young to have attained such eminence in the surgical world. In fact, the long bachelor apprenticeship having finally ended, his most creative period was only now at hand. Having looked at the brain, Cushing in the next few years learned how to gain access to it, relieve it, and let it heal. In doing this he founded neurosurgery.

SIX

Opening the Closed Box:
The Birth of Neurosurgery

~

'If it's to be a bad summer I'll send Kate home. I've got work to do.'
Thus Harvey had written his father before his wedding. By a 'bad
summer' he meant the heat of Baltimore which drove out everyone
who could possibly leave the city. The Cushings coped with the heat
that first summer by wearing very few clothes at home. 'I think we
rather enjoyed it, tho' we didn't know each other very well, did we
Peaches, then?' Harvey reminisced a few years later, 'And you tho't I
had no sense of humor – which I hadn't.' They called each other Peaches
after their favorite fruit. Kate was also his kitten, Harvey sometimes her
cat.[1]

Harvey had told Kate that he believed married people should have
long vacations from each other and that he would send her home often. By September she was back in Cleveland, visiting her family while
he worked in Baltimore. Neither of them much enjoyed this first separation, and Kate longed desperately for him. 'How glad glad *glad* I shall
be to see you – and to darn your socks again! ... I feel so idle and good
for nothing – no marketing no socks – no dressing to make – and no
peaches to cut up ... I feel so useful with you. I can't bear to think that
you do just as well without me ... Your letters are the only thing I live
for until I get back to you again. Darling I love you so much – and if I
once see you I shall never be able to leave you again. Don't ask me to.'[2]

Kate was not medical. She was neither a nurse nor a medical wife like Grace Osler, who had been widowed from one doctor before marrying another. Nor was she educated beyond her very good Boston finishing school. While Harvey had often used Kate as an emotional sounding board during their courtship, he did not really share the details of his professional life with her. The Dr Cushings never had done so with their women, nor did most men at the turn of the century.

Just how separate their spheres were became clear to Kate one day in Cleveland when her new brother-in-law, Ned, showed her Harvey's just-published Mütter lecture. He was about to give it to his father. When Kate asked to see it, Ned told her she wouldn't be able to understand it. 'He might have let me read it even if I can't understand,' she wrote Harvey. Then she had a more disturbing conversation with the former Grace MacBride, one of the old Cleveland gang whose education had included some training in science and who had married the other nationally prominent Cleveland surgeon, George Crile.

> She said she had just finished your article in Annals of Surgery, and found it intensely interesting, and didn't I think so? I'm afraid I looked a little bewildered, and asked to gain time, which one it was, and she explained that it was about the use of something or other in something or other, and I had to say I hadn't seen it. What? You haven't read it? Aren't you *interested* in such things? My dear Grace I shouldn't understand it if I did read it and Harvey can't be bothered explaining things.
>
> An expression of intense pity for us both. She said she spent much time in the laboratory and at *operations!!* Imagine! ...
>
> She's not so bad. For just a few moments, though, I wished that I had been Mrs [Doctor] Porter to throw some long words at her ... Made a perfectly *grand* cake yesterday – wish I had thought to show it to Grace. She can probably make cake and darn socks better than I can, because she's very capable.[3]

Kate never did spend time in the laboratory or at operations, and she probably never read any of Harvey's technical articles. In the early years of their marriage she gradually found her place as a housewife and hostess, albeit always with servants and caterers. Soon she would also be a mother. Harvey got on with his career.

We have only glimpses of the Cushings as a Baltimore couple, such as a servant's comment: 'She's a lovely lady: she's plain as a pipe stem but she's not a bit proud.'[4] In front of the servants she would have been a model of equanimity. The correspondence of husband and wife, much of which survives, reveals that Kate's insecurities and her independent spirit clashed early and fairly often with Harvey's insecurities, independent spirit, and love of work and travel. It was not easy to establish the terms for the compartmentalization of their marriage. There was never as much harmony for Harvey and Kate as his parents or the Oslers enjoyed. Harvey always loved Kate, after his fashion, and she, in her fashion, loved him. But he loved his work more and nearly always found a way to give it priority.

Usually she went along with this. The bond of their marriage was very strong. Much of the time, Kate was happy with the terms of their lives together. She also knew that Harvey was doing great work.

~

In the first decade of the twentieth century, Harvey Cushing became the father of effective neurosurgery. Ineffective neurosurgery had many fathers. Cushing became the first surgeon in history who could open what he referred to as 'the closed box' of the skull of living patients with a reasonable certainty that his operations would do more good than harm. His deliberate concentration on brain surgery marked the founding of a new surgical specialty, of which he became America's and then the world's leading enthusiast and guiding star.

It happened very quickly after Cushing's return to Hopkins in 1901. By 1904, when he penned a major but still tentative 'apologia' for 'the special field of neurological surgery,' Cushing was already devising the operative procedures that became the basis of his fame. Two years later he began publishing what were virtually how-to manuals for brain work. When he gave a magisterial address in 1910 on 'The Special Field of

Neurological Surgery: Five Years Later,' he was receiving brain tumor cases from all over America, was beginning to train students in the specialty, and could perform near-miracles in the operating room. The next month, February 1910, he operated on General Leonard Wood.

He had started in 1898 or 1899 with those first experiments severing the gasserian ganglion in fresh human cadavers. Less than ten years later, in March 1908, he removed a tumor from the cerebral cortex of a completely conscious patient, who endured neither anesthetic nor pain during the operation. Surgeon and patient talked about the situation as the operation proceeded. If working on the brain was surgery's equivalent of the Northwest Passage, as he once put it,[5] by 1908 the hand of Cushing had reached the Beaufort Sea. Einstein had published the theory of relativity three years earlier; in 1908 Henry Ford introduced his Model T.

Of course, there were important and high-achieving predecessors. Cushing stood to the confused, tentative early workers in neurosurgery as Cook did to Magellan, Champlain to Cartier, Lindbergh to the Wright brothers.

~

So much can go wrong with the closed box of the human skull and its contents: fractures, punctures, ruptures, obstructions, infections, growths of every shape and size, dislocations and terrible compressions – causing the literal destruction of the central nervous system, of motor and sensory function, sight, touch, taste, hearing, smell, of self-control and consciousness and personality itself. Terrible, unendurable pain in the head – demons? evil spirits? – had to be relieved. The box had to be opened. Hippocratic writings mentioned the already-ancient practice of trephining or trepanning, opening the skull. Skulls from around the world, from thousands of years ago, bear the marks of the blades, gouges, chisels, saws, and drills used to break in – processes that must have caused unbearable pain in the hope of easing even worse agony. Death was the trephiner's normal and often merciful handmaiden. In a few

cases – when you cut away some benign growth or managed to pick out
or reset the fragments of broken head bones, or were just unaccountably lucky – the good results might have been astonishing. Mostly, the
skull was attacked in desperation and with dismal outcomes.[6]

By the early nineteenth century, surgeons in the advanced countries
of Europe tended towards conservatism in approaching the head. Except in dire emergencies, such as massive fractures or hemorrhaging
gunshot wounds, it seemed better to hope for natural healing, or at
least let nature take its course, than to intervene and hasten death.
Even in the American Civil War of the early 1860s, military surgeons
were advised that most trephinations of wounded soldiers were more
dangerous than the wounds they were intended to treat.[7] Nearly always
when the cranium was opened – especially when the brain's outer lining, the dura, was pierced – a raging, fatal infection developed.

In the meantime, neurologists had begun to understand the gross
structure of the central nervous system and were embarking on a very
long journey to try to map its functions. Which areas of the brain controlled which physical and intellectual activities? If neurology could
develop a clear picture of where things were happening in the brain –
that is, if the quest for cerebral localization succeeded – then it might
also be possible to understand exactly where, inside that closed box,
the lesions might be found that disrupted any given activity. If a patient loses the function X – say, control of the right arm and leg – then
there must be something wrong in the X-controlling region of the brain.
Suppose it is a blood clot or an adhesion, an abscess, or a tumor. Once
the surgeons figure out how to open the box safely, perhaps they will be
able to go to the X-controlling region, find the lesion, treat it, and close
up. The old phrenologists were crude and silly, but mostly in believing
that brain functions could be mapped from the *outside* of the cranium.
The early enthusiasts of cerebral localization, such as Pierre Paul Broca,
David Ferrier, Hughlings Jackson, and Charles S. Sherrington, knew it
had to be an inside job.

With the coming of anesthesia and the antisepsis revolution, surgeons who were bold or foolish, or both, began to venture into the

forbidding territory. German, French, and, above all, British surgeons were the most daring. In 1876, for example, William Macewen in Glasgow, a former student and admirer of Joseph Lister, wanted to operate on an eleven-year-old boy for what he was certain was a brain abscess that he thought he could locate. Denied permission, Macewen concluded at autopsy that he could have found the abscess and saved the patient's life. Three years later he obtained consent and succeeded in removing a tumor, whose protrusion he could see, from a fourteen-year-old girl; she recovered completely. That same year, 1879, he drained a clot under the dura of a nine-year-old boy who had developed epilepticlike seizures after a fall. Macewen continued to operate on the cranium from time to time, mostly to relieve abscesses in the mastoid region. His success rate was fairly high – though case selection and many other variables make the statistics very subjective. Although Macewen enjoyed great fame as a general surgeon, his neurosurgical pioneering was somewhat underappreciated in his own lifetime; snafus such as those Cushing experienced when trying to watch him in 1901 did not help.[8]

The British claimed that a wonderful milestone in medicine was reached in 1884 at the Regent's Park Hospital in London. A physician, Alexander Hughes Bennett, concluded that a twenty-five-year-old man suffering seizures and left-side hemiparesis (paralysis) must have a tumor in the right cortical motor area. Under Bennett's persuasion, a surgeon, Rickman Godlee, trephined the patient's skull in three places, used a mallet and chisel to remove a portion of the bone, found a tumor exactly where it had been predicted, removed it, and managed to control bleeding by cauterizing the blood vessels with an electrode. The patient survived and seemed to do well. The Godlee-Bennett case – the location and successful removal of a brain tumor – was deemed a sensational achievement even when the patient developed an infection and died a month afterwards.[9]

Within months other surgeons were reporting similar feats, leading to the usual confusion over exactly who should get credit for exactly what procedure.[10] One of the most prominent British newcomers to

the field was Victor Horsley at London's neurological centre, the National Hospital for Nervous and Mental Diseases in Queen Square.
William Williams Keen of Philadelphia, whose surgical experience
stretched back to the Civil War, managed some of America's first successful tumor removals and, as we have seen, had an eye for talent-
spotting in the field.

In 1888 David Ferrier and Horsley told enthusiasts at a medical
congress in Washington, DC, of the bright future of brain surgery. Many
surgeons took the experts at their word and gave it a try – more than
five hundred general surgeons in the United States reported performing operations on the brain between 1886 and 1896. In 1893 Moses
Allen Starr, a New York neurologist, published the first American text
on brain tumors. Two years later the French surgeon M.J.N. Chipault
required 1,540 pages to survey the state of the field in his two-volume
Chirurgie opératoire du système nerveux. It included a 325-page section
on the surgical treatment of trigeminal neuralgia, the operation that
still had a 20 percent mortality rate when Cushing perfected it at the
end of the decade.

The mortality rate was the dark side of the early enthusiasm for brain
operations. As in the Godlee-Bennett case, many 'successful' operations resulted in dead patients. They may have died months afterwards
from an infection which the surgeon thought could have been pre-
vented or controlled, but they were just as dead as if they had expired
on the table. In 1889 the Berlin surgeon Ernst von Bergmann, concluded that reports of brain surgery showed an operative mortality rate
upwards of 50 percent. Studies in the early twentieth century were
almost as pessimistic: Harvey's friend E.A. Codman analysed the brain
tumor cases at the Massachusetts General Hospital between 1895 and
1904, and found that half the patients died.

Many of the surgeons who had tried their hand at brain operations
found the experience more than sobering and never did it again. In the
ten years after 1896, far fewer American and other surgeons attacked
sick brains than in the decade before. Almost no brain work was done
at Johns Hopkins before Cushing entered the field. The only two at-

tempted tumor removals, he learned from studying the hospital records, had ended disastrously.[11] Around the world a very few determined souls, beginning with Macewen and Horsley in Britain and Fedor Krause in Germany, stayed in the dangerous field which so many of their colleagues had tried to enter prematurely. A profession temperamentally inclined to exploration and pioneering had been defeated by an exotic, harsh, forbidding climate.

The two major problems were bleeding and bulging. From the moment a surgeon cut into a patient's shaved scalp he had to deal with highly and delicately vascularized regions of the body. It got worse when he got through the skull (even the bone can ooze blood) and opened the meninges, the three membranes – dura, arachnoid, and pia mater – that envelop the brain. The vessels saturating the meninges, surface, and tissues of the brain bleed easily and often. As in the pre-Cushing ganglion operation, and in the tumor case Cushing saw defeat Kocher, surgeons often had to retreat from a bloody mess without achieving anything. They would be lucky to get out without causing the patient to bleed to death.

Sometimes when you first broke into the box and its linings, releasing the intracranial tension or pressure, your drill or scalpel would trigger a shower of blood, not unlike an oil gusher. More commonly, the release of pressure would cause portions of the brain to bulge or herniate through your opening, and you could not get them back in again. Sometimes you could not close the dura after an operation. After 1890 most of the best operators followed Wilhelm Wagner in making a bone 'flap' by connecting their drill or trephine holes, which they would fold back using the scalp as a hinge. But with bulging they could not close the flap. When brain tissue herniated, it soon became infected, creating a dreaded 'fungus cerebri,' and the patient soon died, as in the Godlee-Bennett case.

Bennett and other surgeons were able to console themselves that they had at least located and removed tumors that would have killed the patient anyway. Occasionally the brain did not herniate or the hernia did not become infected and the patient survived. But there was yet another level of frustration. Suppose you expose the brain, keep the hemorrhaging and release of pressure under control, and then can't find the source of the trouble? Perhaps you've missed your diagnosis completely and there is no tumor; perhaps the tumor is buried deep in the brain; perhaps you're just in the wrong region.

It was largely a matter of guesswork – informed but very imprecise – to deduce what was happening inside the closed box. Even the x-rays had many limits. They might be able to help locate bullets in the brain, and illuminate certain skull fractures, but they could not show distinctions among soft tissues – say, the difference between tumor and regular brain. If a surgeon chose to go into the cranium and found he was in the wrong place, there was nothing he do, it seemed, but close and go home – and hope that his sutures did not break open, that the drain he had installed would help remove pus, that the suffering would not be too great, and that someone might pay the bill for an operation that had achieved nothing.

⁓

Cushing brought to the dismal field of brain surgery a highly developed set of techniques to control bleeding, crucial knowledge of and sensitivity to the problem of intracranial pressure, his awesome dexterity, and his equally awesome combination of enthusiasm and a determination to succeed. Without quite realizing it, he also drew on the relatively awesome resources of the Johns Hopkins Hospital and Medical School – and on the financial resources generated by the Cushing Cleveland properties, which made him independently wealthy.

The early experience with the gasserian ganglion operation had been a triumphant demonstration of his potential. Cushing had not understood problems of intracranial and vascular tension until he did his work in Europe, but he came back doubly enlightened: he had seen through his window how the brain responded to compression, and with the Riva-Rocci cuff he had brought to America the crucial instrument for measuring blood pressure during all kinds of surgery. What luck to be the first American surgeon with a device almost as important as the stethoscope or the thermometer! No wonder Cushing believed in the possibilities of his new specialty and of surgery in general.

His early work owed more to his enthusiasm than to immediate results. So far as blood pressure monitoring was concerned, it was a diffuse enthusiasm. Cushing believed that all surgeons should adopt the new device, especially to forewarn against shock. From 1901, blood-pressure monitoring was used in his, and soon in others', operations at Johns Hopkins. 'One barely knows what cases to select, what ones to pass by,' he gushed in the *Boston Medical and Surgical Journal*. 'New facts of interest from a purely physiological point of view, or, what is to us more essential, of prognostic, diagnostic or therapeutic value to the clinician, are constantly being brought to light.' He explored the usefulness of blood pressure in differential diagnosis, to test traditional drugs and procedures, as a tool in patient management, and above all in the operating room. Cushing's 'ether' charts now also recorded blood pressure.

Of course the device would be overused, Cushing wrote in 1902: 'Many a long chart will be plotted seemingly to no purpose before there is a final selection of conditions wherein it will be considered negligent to omit these observations.' The users would be bound to make their share of mistakes: a story was told of the student operating-room nurse at Hopkins who, when told by Dr Cushing to take a blood pressure reading, began applying the cuff to his leg. Samuel Greenblatt has unearthed from an obscure Cushing footnote an occasion on which Harvey decided to apply the cuff to his own neck, he and a colleague observing the results as he strangled himself to the brink of faintness and nausea.[12]

Cushing had probably known George Crile, the noted researcher into blood pressure and surgical shock, both professionally and socially in Cleveland. They definitely met after Cushing's return from Europe, and Cushing apparently introduced Crile to the Riva-Rocci cuff during his Christmas 1901 visit. Crile immediately saw its value. Cushing's former Harvard professor, W.T. Councilman, overheard some of their

discussion, was intrigued by surgeons talking about physiology and research, and invited them to give a presentation in Boston in January
1903. That talk convinced Harvard's Department of Surgery to have
its research committee investigate further: Were the devices accurate
and could they play a valuable role in surgery?

Cushing and Crile could hardly believe the committee's 1904 finding: 'The adoption of blood-pressure observations in surgical patients
does not at present appear to be necessary as a routine measure.' In
later years, when everyone was routinely measuring blood pressure, he
poked fun at this study as an example of medical obscurantism, reminiscent of opposition to the introduction of the stethoscope. In fact,
the young surgeons in their enthusiasm oversold their story. The Harvard
study was thorough and honest, and built a strong case for using traditional forms of patient assessment – respiration, pulse, appearance – in
preference to single-index measurement by imperfect technology, however promising it might be in specialized cases and for the future. It
probably had not helped when Crile displayed a cumbersome pneumatic suit he intended to have patients wear during surgery to control
their blood pressure. The surgeons' theoretical view that it ought to be
possible to stop blood pressure from falling by cocainizing local
vasomotor nerves was also suspect. Cushing, who also experimented
with inflatable tourniquets, wrote two of his least enduring papers on
aspects of this subject.[13]

That the establishment clung to its conservative approach to monitoring patients did not really surprise Cushing and his friends. The young
turks considered the American Surgical Association, with its limited
membership elected by seniority, clogged with deadwood. Following
up on his 1900 discussion with his friends beside the Seine in Paris,
Cushing was enthusiastic about Crile's idea of forming a new club of
younger surgeons to watch one another operate. An energetic friend at
the Massachusetts General Hospital, Jim Mumford, joined their discussions, and they decided to expand a little Boston group into a new
national organization. The Society of Clinical Surgery held its first
meeting in Baltimore in November 1903. All the Hopkins surgeons

showed off their skills, with Cushing putting some of his head patients on display.[14]

The society allowed Cushing, who would always be of two minds about specialization, to keep up with the latest in general surgery. He occasionally did general work after coming back from Europe (but soon stopped holding office hours at 3 West Franklin), though by 1904 he was complaining to his father that everyone assumed he did only neurosurgery.[15] He taught the fundamentals of surgery at Hopkins, and he never forgot that both his surgical and medical roots were general; he never lost his respect for the generalist or his general interest in the future of surgery and medicine.

His cultivation of 'the special field of neurosurgery,' he explained in his 1904 address, was based on the desire to open up a neglected field in which surgeons had too often been handmaids to neurologists, who themselves were poor guides to the mysteries of the closed box. With enough study and laboratory work and practical experience, it ought to be possible to do many new things in neurosurgery: 'I shall keep away, so far as possible, from beaten paths: for that a cerebral abscess should be evacuated, a ruptured meningeal vessel tied, the spinal cord relieved from pressure, and a severed nerve sutured, has long needed no comment.' What he most wanted to do was perfect a technique that would give neurological patients surgical relief from their most common complaint, the effects of severe intracranial pressure, most often caused by tumors.

Neurologists were well aware of a common symptom complex: headaches, vomiting, and the impairment of vision associated with 'choked disc' or apparent edema of the optimic nerve. These, Cushing argued, were indications for exploratory surgery. Unfortunately, 'the dread of the operating room, which many doctors share with their patients, together with the supposed uncertainties of an exploration, has led and still leads to one invariable course of treatment, large doses of the iodids being given with the vague hope that lues venerea [syphilis] may be at the bottom of the trouble.'[16] Although Cushing was ostensibly working in partnership with Hopkins's consulting neurologist, H.M. Thomas, he appears to have done his own examinations and diagnosis virtually from the beginning, almost certainly because Osler, who had unbounded confidence in him, allowed him to.

By 1904 he was well on his way to making exploration for and palliation of intracranial problems routine procedures. He had already worked out some of his basic methods of opening the cranium. The pneumatic tourniquet that he modeled on the blood-pressure cuff, for example, was used to compress the blood supply to the scalp before the first incisions. He used a hand trephine (even today they look like hardware store products) to drill his holes in the skull, being particularly careful not to break through and pierce the dura. To connect the drill holes he used the Gigli wire saw, which he passed through the holes and cut upward through the bone. The bone would be folded back or perhaps removed. He advocated making relatively large openings in the skull to reduce the problem of herniation through a small space. Bone wax, as introduced by Horsley, along with a supply of cotton pledgets, were at the ready to control oozing blood. At the end of the operation, when he sutured the dura and then closed the scalp, Cushing used the fine black silk sutures and curved French needles introduced to Hopkins by Halsted. He carefully sutured in layers, first the inner scalp, or galea, then the outer.

He could do these craniectomies and craniotomies without causing infection or herniation. In the early years, Cushing had only two cases of fungus cerebri, one caused by a bad decision to install a drain through the primary wound. Usually he was so sure of himself that he no longer provided for drainage; there would not be any pus. But he hardly ever hurried either. A common theme of all his neurosurgical papers was the need to abandon the fetish for haste. These need not be hazardous procedures. Be careful enough, Cushing wrote in his first published discussion of his technique, and you will find that 'no cases, when handled properly, are technically so simple, nor have such an uneventful convalescence as these very cases of exploratory craniotomy – for unlike similar abdominal operations a period of recumbancy after the operation is not essential.'[17]

Knowing he could enter and exit the cranium at will, his enthusiasm led Cushing to attempt to relieve head trauma by relieving the effects of hemorrhage. He thought he could save some stroke victims – the results were not very good, though the old practice of 'bleeding' for apoplexy was probably worse – and he was almost certain that newborns who had suffered cerebral hemorrhage could be helped.[18] His surgery on infants led to remarkable experiences, including an operation in March 1904 on the convulsing seven-day-old daughter of a Cleveland friend, brought to him on the advice of Ned Cushing and George Crile. Harvey removed blood clots, and the child convalesced without incident and developed into a 'a fine specimen of wholesome babyhood.' An eight-day-old baby's life was despaired of when Cushing was called in, and he too doubted that the misshapen, convulsing child could survive. Operating in a private home, he cleaned up clots on one side of the baby's brain and had to go in again on the other side. After the operation, 'the child, contrary to our expectations, and almost against our desires, immediately began to improve.' While Cushing worked, a woman, a professed Christian Scientist, had waited outside the room. When he told her that the operation seemed to have gone well, she said, 'Ah, I had the right thought.'

His own thought, in the paper he published about these procedures, was ambivalent, for he knew that much permanent damage had been done to that baby. He continued to do these operations, but with only about a 50 percent survival rate and with some uncertainty about whether mere survival was a worthwhile outcome. Operating on stroke victims raised similar issues. 'From a therapeutic side this neurological business is not very bright,' he told his father in 1906 apropos of yet another hopeless case. Even when he was not responsible, the infant deaths depressed him, and he wondered if his father had felt the same way about losing patients. Halsted is said to have commented during these years that he didn't know whether to refer to 'poor Cushing's patients' or 'Cushing's poor patients.'[19]

In these years Cushing saw many cases of Jacksonian, or focal, epilepsy in which cleaning up adhesions on the surfaces of the brain might reduce convulsive seizures. Cushing thought he had some success, but the pattern of outcomes – only about half the cases seemed to benefit – was inconsistent and baffling, though perhaps better than medical treatment afforded. Sometimes operations seemed to have what are now called placebo effects, making the patient feel better even though the attacks continued.[20]

~

The cases of suspected tumor that Cushing saw steadily increased. In his 1904 survey of neurological surgery he was moderately optimistic about the possibilities of tumor removal, noting that reports of successful extirpations were increasing, and even venturing to predict in a footnote that some day a diseased pituitary body might be successfully attacked. He said nothing in this paper about his own results with tumor, which were not impressive despite occasional spectacular success. In November 1903 he removed an intradural tumor at the upper end of the spinal cord, with full restoration of function, only the tenth reported case in history. Osler had recommended surgery to the patient, since it could hardly make his condition worse. 'It's the first case of the kind hereabouts,' Harvey told his father, 'and really only happens about once in an operator's lifetime.'[21]

In a way the situation got worse before it got better. The more Cushing saw of tumors in these early years, the less sanguine he was about surgery's ability to deal with them. Despite the high hopes of the cerebral localizers, most suspected tumors could not be found, and many of those that could be found could not be removed. Many tumors were locatable only because they had done irreparable damage, causing irreversible blindness, mental derangement, and other disorders. The outlook for 'cure' by removal was not good.

Cushing fell back on palliation as the only alternative, and a respectable one: Give the patient relief; buy time. To do this, he developed a subtemporal decompression as his basic intracranial operation, his signature craniectomy. Between 1905 and 1910, it was his all-purpose response to the standard symptomology. Subtemporal de-compression was usually beneficial, almost never harmful, and it could serve as a platform for going in a second or third time to try and find the tumor.

Cushing was not the first brain surgeon to understand the value of decompression. Whenever a surgeon opened the cranium he released some of the pressure and gave the poor soul a bit of relief, whether or not he found the tumor. Often the operator would not try to push the tissue back in under pressure and replace the bone; he might simply close the scalp over the hole in the head (thus doing a craniectomy rather than a craniotomy). The trouble was that the relief often came in the form of so much herniation that fungation and infection could not be stopped. One of Cushing's 1904 patients developed a hernia as big as the remainder of her head, from which liters of fluid were drained before she died.

He reasoned that if he was going to leave a decompressive opening in the cranium, he should do it deliberately and in an area where the scalp had the strength, through its fascia and muscles, to contain the brain matter. So he focused his decompressive approach – an opera-tion of choice rather than a fallback – low on the side of the cranium, under the temporal muscle. He first described the operation in 1905 and by December 1906 had a series of about thirty cases, most of which had been given immediate and striking relief. He had come to believe, he wrote, 'that every patient should be operated upon in some such way as this as soon as the diagnosis of intracranial tumor has been made.' He criticized surgeons who advocated operating only on and over lo-calizable tumors:

Contrary to the opinion held by many, that only those cases of cerebral tumor should be operated upon in which there are localizing symptoms, I feel that the cases which are *most favourable* for operation are those in which there are no localizing symptoms whatsoever. For in these cases it is possible to relieve the underlying symptoms, and inasmuch as the tumor is implicating some silent area of the brain, it may, in case it is a slow growing tumor, continue to enlarge for months or perhaps years without damaging in any way the more important centers. On the other hand, if the growth has already so damaged centers as to enable us by our as yet gross methods of diagnosis to determine its situation, it has incapacited the patient to such an extent that decompression merely for the relief of subjective symptoms is much less satisfactory than it would be under these other circumstances. Furthermore, operation and removal in such cases of cerebral tumor as indicate their presence by irritative or paralytic symptoms means, usually, a persistence, if not an increase, of these same symptoms.[22]

By 1908, with well over three hundred craniotomies and craniectomies under his belt, Cushing had routinized his procedures. He described them in great detail in a major address in St Louis entitled 'Technical Methods of Performing Certain Cranial Operations,' as well as in a massive 259-page chapter on 'Surgery of the Head' that he contributed to a multivolume textbook edited by W.W. Keen. His discussions of methods of drilling, sawing, and sewing included pros and cons about burrs, forceps, and dissectors and about the need to bevel the brain flap and why he had abandoned the pneumatic tourniquet (it would not withstand repeated sterilization). He was already conservative in some respects. He trephined by hand, for example. Some surgeons had adopted motorized drills from dentistry – what an awful mess in the operating room when they sawed through skull, dura, and into the brain itself!

Cushing always underlined the need to perfect every detail of the surgical experience. Perfection included the preoperative ritual (to minimize infection, the head was not to be shaved until the patient was on the table and then was preferably done by the surgeon himself); perfection included the placing of the patient on the table (before anesthetization and using a special extender to position the head), the need for an expert anesthetizer (Cushing used a specialist for all his neurosurgical work), the need to have a bellows ready for artificial respiration, and above all the imperative of being careful: 'An operator who persists in taking dangerous corners at high speed will be the cause of a

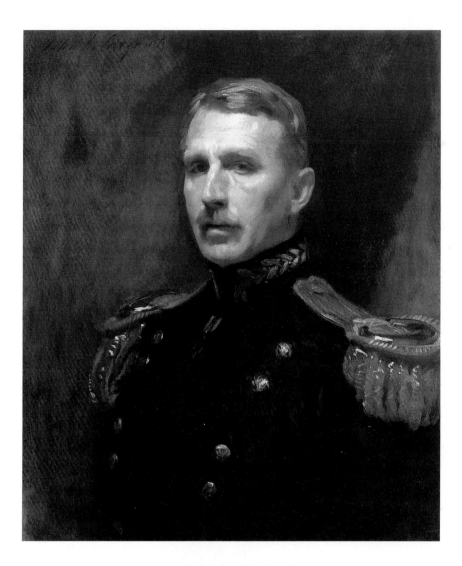

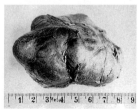

General Leonard Wood, 1903, by John Singer Sargent, and the tumor
Cushing removed in 1910.

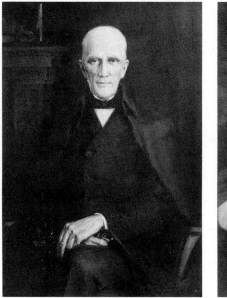

Erastus Cushing, grandfather.

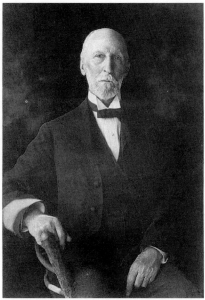

Henry Kirke Cushing, father.

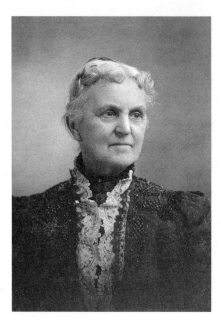

Betsey Williams Cushing, mother.

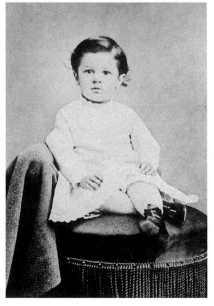

Harvey Cushing, age two,
youngest of ten children.

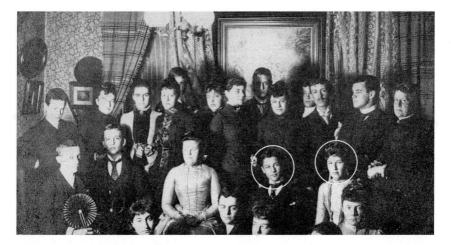

Cleveland cousins and friends. Harvey with Kate Crowell.

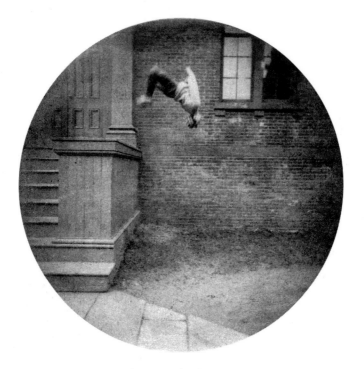

Cushing at Yale, about 1889.

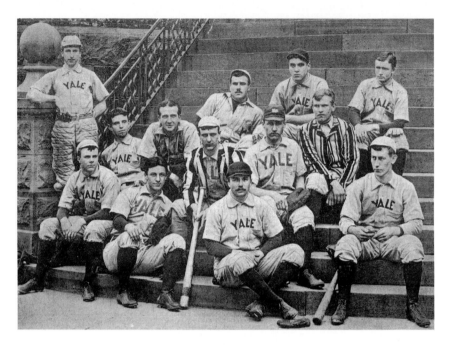

With bandaged finger, the Yale Nine, 1891 (bottom row, 2nd from left).

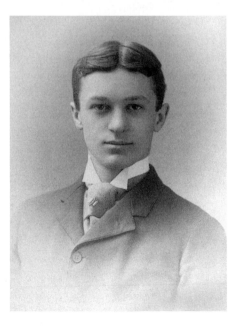

Harvey Cushing, Yale '91.

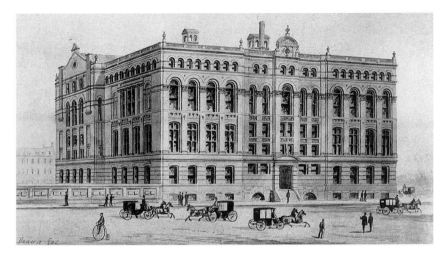

Harvard Medical School when Cushing was a student. A tough professional grind.

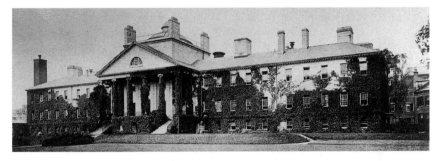

The Massachusetts General Hospital. Hard work under the Ether Dome.

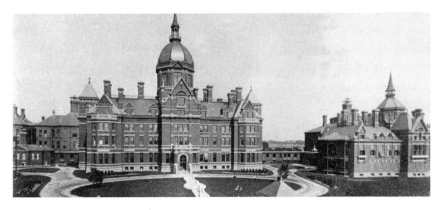

Johns Hopkins Hospital, Baltimore. Time to cultivate excellence.

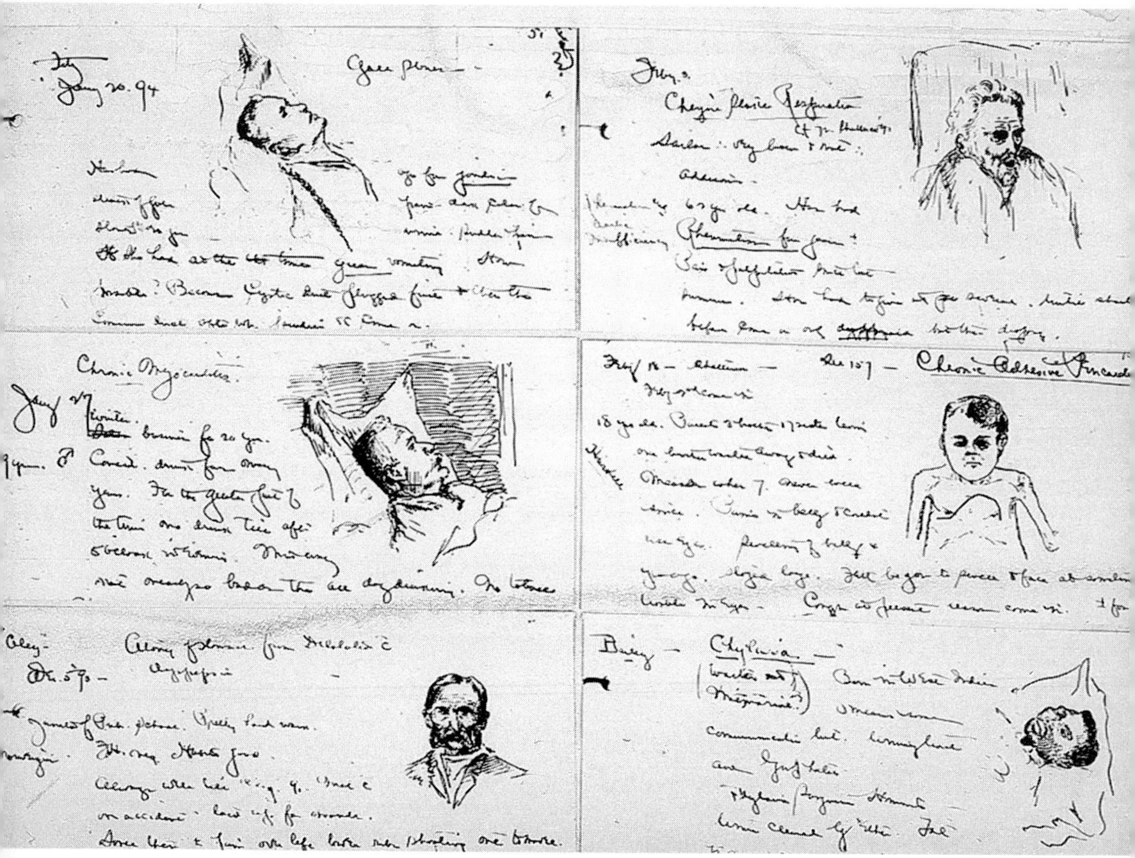

Cushing's sketches of patients seen as a medical student.

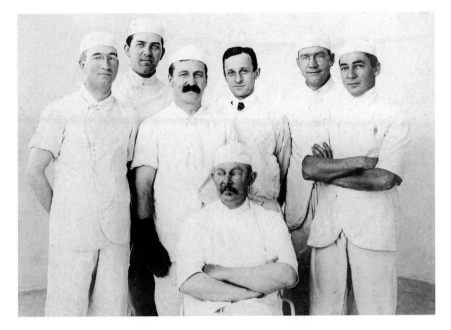

All-star surgeons, Baltimore, 1904. Hugh Young, R.H. Follis, John Finney, Harvey Cushing, Joe Bloodgood, Jim Mitchell. Seated: W.S. Halsted.

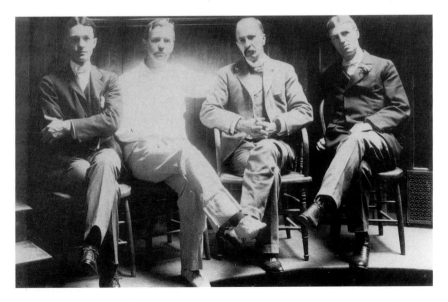

Latch-keyers. Harvey Cushing, Thomas Futcher, William Osler, Thomas McCrae.

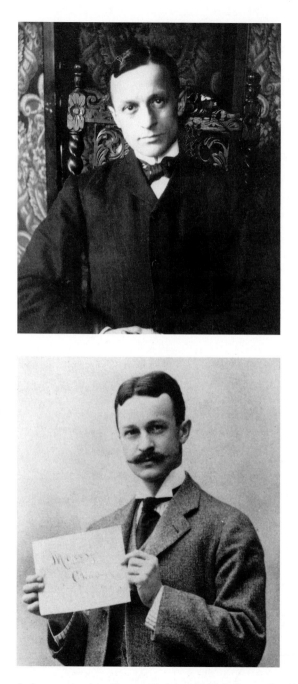

The end of apprenticeship. Harvey Cushing, 1900, before and with his traveling mustache.

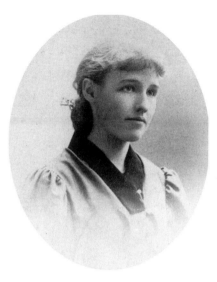

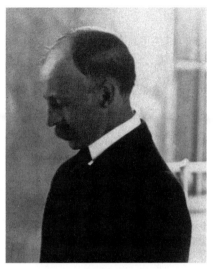

Kate Crowell, 1894.

Ned Cushing. Almost indistinguishable
from William Osler.

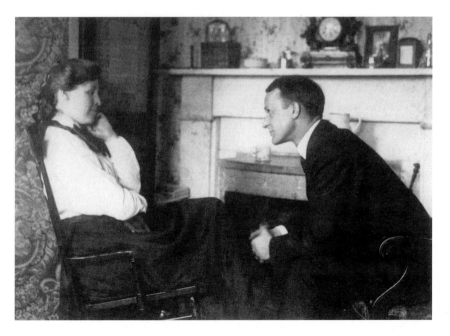

Harvey wooing Kate. They married in 1902.

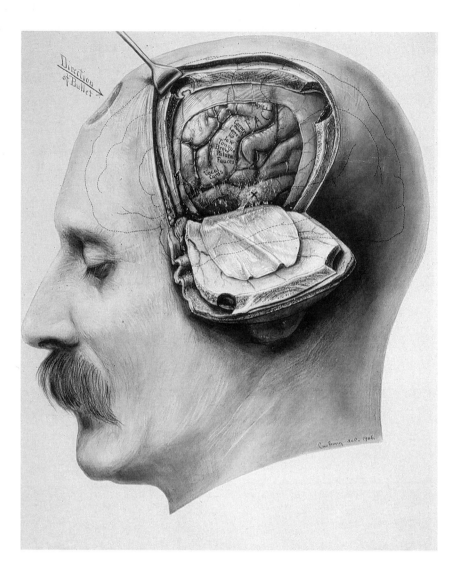

Harvey's sketch of the motor area of the brain, 1906. The patient probably has
Ned Cushing's features, not Osler's.

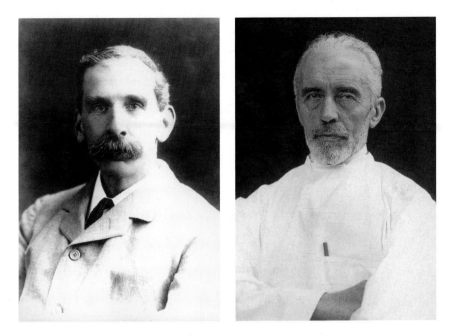

Victor Horsley.   Theodor Kocher.

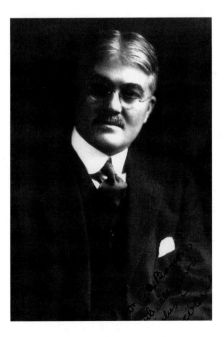

George Washington Crile.

THE JOHNS HOPKINS HOSPITAL.

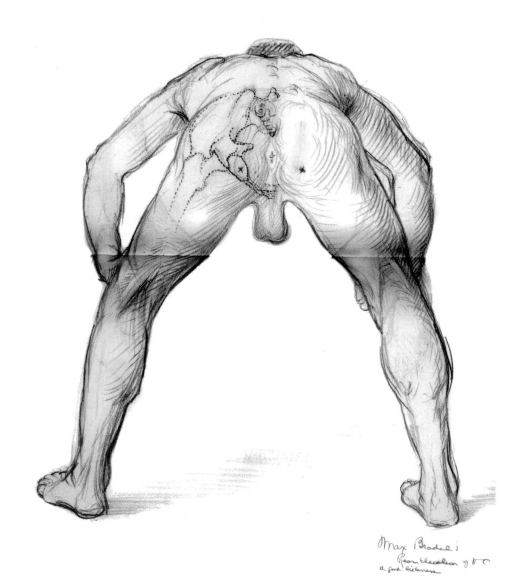

Anything for research. A hitherto unknown sketch of Cushing by Max Brödel, 1903,
to delineate a sacral nerve.

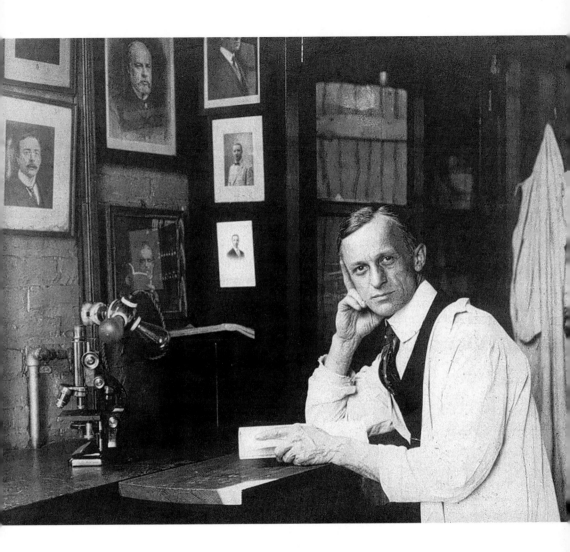

The research pose. Harvey Cushing, 1907, with pictures of his mentors.

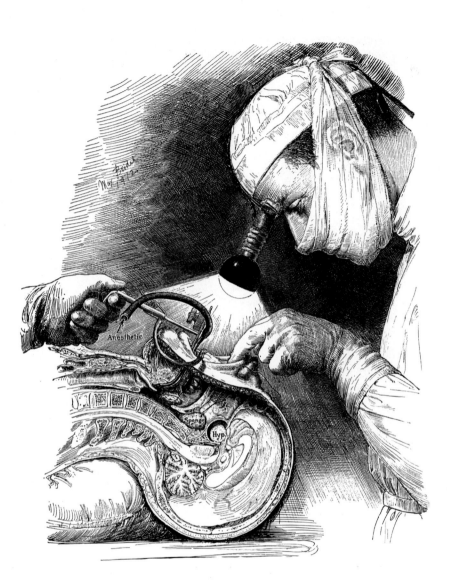

The transphenoidal approach to the pituitary. Cushing sketched by Max Brödel, 1914.

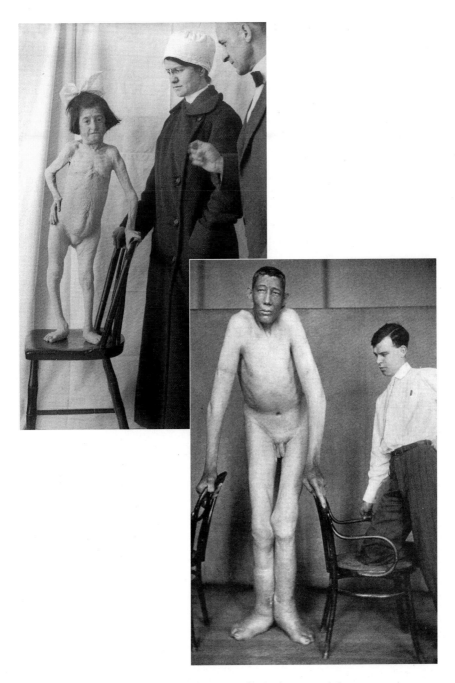

Pituitary disorders: dwarfism and acromegaly. Cushing is with his tiny patient;
Samuel Crowe with the giant.

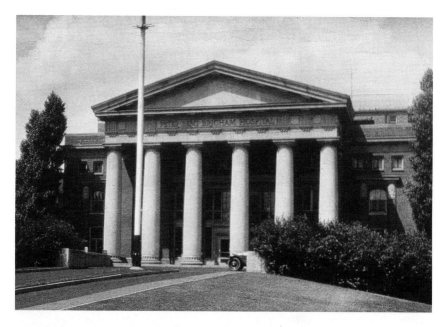

The Peter Bent Brigham Hospital, Boston.

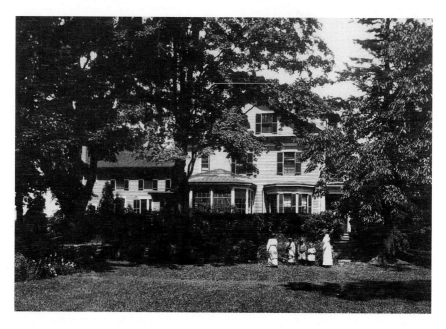

The Cushing home, 305 Walnut St., Brookline.

serious or fatal accident some day, whether he is driving an automobile or opening a skull.'[23]

He emphasized the need to learn from mistakes, explaining how on several occasions where they had pairs of similar cases in which resort to surgery was debatable, they had operated on the least serious case and used the other as a 'therapeutic control.' He knew that he seemed obsessed with trivia. He probably sensed that he was already known for being impossibly perfectionist and almost impossible to work for, but he would make no concessions:

> I earnestly believe that, in operative work upon the brain more than anywhere else on the body, the surgeon must follow his patient through every detail of preparation, position on the table, anesthetization, etc., if he will avoid the surgical calamities which sometimes come to these cases out of a clear sky; for there can be no doubt that in many respects it is the most difficult and at the same time most delicate field of operative endeavor.
>
> Some of the principles of technique which I have laid down heretofore and in this place may seem finicky to many surgeons, but our excessive precautions must receive consideration in view of our results if for no other reason, for we have never had an infection, deep or superficial, in our long series of craniotomies, and our immediate operative accidents have been practically nill.[24]

Even as he was publishing his techniques, Cushing was pressing further, improving on them, honing his diagnostic skills, preparing to move from decompression to exploration, wondering about how to study the circulation of the cerebrospinal fluid in and around the brain. Learning how to open and close the skull and give the patient some relief was the *sine qua non*, but it was only the beginning.

❧

He also worked on the peripheral nervous system, experimenting with nerve suturing, and continuing to perfect and write about his bread-

and-butter operation, the ganglionectomy for trigeminal neuralgia. In his first five years back at Hopkins he published almost as much about the trigeminal and related nerves as he did on intracranial matters. In Montreal in early 1904, for example, he presented a study of his first nineteen trigeminal patients, a tour-de-force exploration of the terrible disease and his method of curing it. A Montreal friend of Osler's wrote that it was quite the most finished presentation ever given in the city. 'This, of course, is rather talky talk,' Kate told her father-in-law, 'but comforting as Harvey has worked so hard on this paper.'[25]

He spun out other papers on these patients and the effect of his operation on their facial nerves, contributing neurophysiological observations about sensory nerves and the independence of taste fibers from the trigeminal system. He continued to perfect his operation, taking great pride when he learned how to avoid severing the twig of a nerve that controlled the raising of the eyebrow, and in the appearance of patients who showed only what he called an 'invisible scar.'[26] The perfect surgeon also aimed at the best possible cosmetic outcome.

He engaged in a running debate with Philadelphia competitors, the team of William G. Spiller, neurologist, and Charles H. Frazier, surgeon, who had been present at the symposium when Cushing first described his operation. A year later they announced a major improvement on it. Their method was not to try to sever or remove the whole gasserian ganglion, as Cushing did, but only to detach the nerve's sensory root at the base of the brain. It was a simpler and often safer procedure, one that Cushing himself, after much conservative hesitation, grudgingly adopted. At the time and later, Spiller and Frazier were credited with an important innovative advance in trigeminal surgery, and this disconcerted Cushing because they relied on what he considered to be his more important innovative (infra-arterial) approach to the ganglion. Everyone knew that polite and careful references to one another's work by these intense competitors masked a tense struggle for credit, glory, and prominence in the eyes of referring physicians and their patients. Who were the most significant innovaters? Who had contributed only minor modifications? Who should garner most of the trigeminal glory? And in consequence – although no one ever spelled this out – who should be the surgeon to whom the profession referred most of the trigeminal cases? Was the biggest man in the field Cushing at Hopkins or that team in Philadelphia?[27]

Cushing was not too proud to make the most of his mistakes and to stoop to conquer in the oddest, most literal way. In 1903 a fifty-three-year-old man developed a case of herpes zoster (shingles) on his buttocks after a Cushing ganglionectomy. Harvey realized that he had inadvertently damaged the man's fifth sacral nerve. He also saw that the pattern of the eruptions enabled him to map the sensory field of that nerve more clearly than anyone had previously done. It paralleled the embryonic development of the nerve. Thus a botched procedure became an opportunity for another publication.

In the paper he wrote on this case, Harvey wanted to include both a diagram of the distribution in embryo and a diagram of the nerve field in an adult male portrayed in a fetal-like stance. His friend Max Brödel, the Hopkins medical artist, had no model for such a diagram, so Harvey volunteered. Brödel made a pen-and-ink drawing of the 'rear elevation' of a bent-over Cushing, which he labeled 'a good likeness.' It was used as the basis for the stylized sketch and nerve-map in the article. Cushing inserted Brödel's original drawing in his master collection of his published reprints. It languished there unnoticed until I discovered it nearly a century later. The drawing is accompanied by a snapshot of the rear end of a horse.[28]

Cushing's success with his ganglion patients was a cheering contrast to the pathos of so many brain-damaged victims. He was immensely proud of the operation and his almost perfect results. Whenever he had a 'ganglion' scheduled he urged Kate to cross her fingers for him for luck. The luck held. The Spiller-Frazier matter was so frustrating because Cushing thought the operation was nearly perfect as he had developed it, or at least in his hands, and he hoped to attract private patients who could afford to pay decent fees for the relief he gave.

In these early years of marriage and professional independence he hoped to pay his way in surgery, but the money did not roll in. The first fee he collected for a ganglionectomy came from his seventeenth patient, all the others having been charity cases. 'I might in time make some money out of medicine,' he told his father. Two years later Kate commented, 'Why are all ganglions impecunious I wonder? Anyhow all ours are.'[29]

Part of the answer to Kate's question was that by the time most of the sufferers got to Cushing, they had exhausted their resources. One of the first who had not was Gerald A. Birks, whose family owned one of Canada's major jewelry stores. Birks developed a classic case of trigeminal neuralgia in 1900 at age twenty-eight. His local doctor, the best in Montreal, gave him huge doses of the painkiller phenacetin but warned against relying on opiates. Birks vainly sought relief from unnamed doctors in Philadelphia. 'Birks, you're a fool,' he was told, 'you have but two choices – opiates or suicide.' Birks went to London, where the famous neurologist David Ferrier, determined to find something that would work, prescribed more drugs, electrotherapy, and the services of a hypnotist. Ferrier had heard of the ganglion operation but considered it, Birks remembered, 'as a last desperate resort – a sort of polite way of committing suicide.'

About the time of Cushing's trigeminal presentation in Montreal, Birks's doctor took him to Johns Hopkins to consult with Osler and Cushing. Osler, ever surgeon-friendly, suggested an immediate ganglionectomy, but Cushing hesitated. This would be his youngest case, and he preferred to try attacking the trigeminal nerve directly. He was still nervous about the more total procedure, Birks thought. When Birks's trouble returned six months later, Cushing decided to go ahead. 'I did Mr Birks this a.m. – major operation – always gives one cold feet,' he told Kate. 'Can't tell yet how he will do.'

When it was clear that Birks was doing just fine, Cushing wondered how much he should charge this very rich man. Some American surgeons, including Kelly and Halsted at Hopkins, charged all the traffic would bear for life-saving operations, notoriously billing their rich patients as much as $10,000 (the equivalent of perhaps $300,000 a century later). 'Mr Birks is doing well. If I was the Professer,' wrote Cushing,

'I would charge him $10,000 – otherwise $250 which is enough for the cat family.' Birks, who knew Cushing had saved him from a living death, could not believe his surgeon's reticence about the fee: 'The financial side seemed to be his greatest worry – not for his, but for his patient's interest. When I at last got him to name a figure, which seemed to me a small price to pay for what he had done for me, I had to assure him over and over again that it would not inconvenience me, before he would accept my cheque. I remember saying to him that as a business man I was going to return the compliment by prescribing for him. I pointed out that he would be just as good a surgeon if he were a better business man.'[30] Birks was later decorated for his service in the First World War and became the head of his family business and a major philanthropist. He outlived Cushing by more than a decade.

~

The only reference to their sex life in Harvey and Kate's many intimate letters comes in December 1902, when Kate was visiting in Cleveland. Harvey writes that her absence causes him to work harder: 'Going to bed is no longer an event so I am apt to dally here at this heaped up desk always thinking it's a good thing to do just a little more.'[31]

In fact, Kate had just become pregnant. She gave birth to their first child, a boy, on August 4, 1903. He was officially named William Harvey – after William Osler, Harvey Cushing, and the immortal William Harvey. His godfather Osler, an obsessive nicknamer and Rabelaisian, called the baby Pius, after the pope who was chosen on the day of his birth; also Gargantua or Gargy. Grace Osler wrote to Kate that she and William were 'dancing and singing for joy' at the happy news. (She also told her young friend, 'Take the advice of a strong woman and stay *flat* on your back as long as you can. You will never regret it and rarely have such a good excuse. Men – *husbands & doctors* – are always in such a hurry to get one up and it does make a difference later – And don't forget about the bandage if you want no stomach'.) Grace stood in for her out-of-town husband at the baby's christening. Harvey's father was too late with the suggestion that the baptismal water might come from the bottle that grandmother Cushing had brought back from the River Jordan in the 1860s. The Oslers, too, had baptized their firstborn with Jordan water (it is still on sale to Christian pilgrims in the twenty-first century), though Grace remembered that she had boiled most of the water away, leaving mainly wet sand.[32]

The generations came and went. A few months before William Cushing's birth, Harvey's brother Alleyne, the closest to him in age, was found dead with a bullet in his head and the revolver by his side in Douglas, Arizona. He had drifted around without doing much in life, and no one in the family had seen him for ten years.[33] His mother's letter to Harvey telling him of the sad news was also one of the last he received from her, for in the summer of 1903 she began to experience serious problems with headaches, balance, eyesight, and appetite. Having been tirelessly vigorous all her life, she would not cut back. 'Great thing if she would only retire from business, after the manner of HKC,' Harvey's father wrote him, 'but she will, I have no doubt, go down with her flag at the main.'

The Cushing doctors were not sure of the cause of Bessie's problems, which she judged would be her final illness. Ned thought she valued her husband's loving attention so much that she had stopped trying to get better. But he also suspected a brain tumor and, disregarding his father's view that he would rather not know if something positively bad was wrong, discussed that possibility with Harvey.[34] There is no record of Harvey's views or advice or of any operation on Bessie. She went downhill very rapidly, dying on October 21, 1903, at the age of seventy-five.

Bessie's body was laid out in her nightdress in her bed at home. Harvey told Kate of the scene in Cleveland:

> Just a big wreath of autumn leaves outside the door and nothing black – just like mother. But oh! So still and cold. I hardly realized it till I saw her. No one was there but father. I was glad because I behaved pretty badly. No one knows but you and he and mother how near the surface lie my emotions. Father is

always there – perfectly calm and under control. I hope nothing will snap when he goes back alone. I don't think he has slept any and looks thin and worn. I have been with him most of the afternoon. He talks a good deal about mothers last days and how keen she was and playful with him – I suppose just as they were fifty years ago.

After all the visitors had gone, Kirke came in and covered his wife's cold hands, and he talked to Harvey late into the night about how busy the hands had been all the years of their marriage and how she had held things together during his sicknesses. 'Well she must have been made of iron ...' Harvey told Kate. 'I'm glad she saw and held our little boy before she died. I hope that she passed on to him some of her absolute unselfishness and rare qualities of other sorts which his father missed.'[35] Betsey Maria was buried in the Cushing family vault beside Alleyne. There is no record of an autopsy. A biographer might imagine a relationship between Bessie's suspected brain tumor and her son's relentless pursuit of tumors for the rest of his life, but there is not a hint of supporting evidence. Harvey's course was probably set before his mother's last illness.

Relatives remarked on the especially close relationship between Harvey and his father – he was the only one in the family who would go up and put his arm around the old man's shoulder. The retired father and the brilliant son shared common interests and worldviews, as well as a temperament marked by reticence masking deep affection. Harvey described parting from his father in Cleveland a few months before his marriage: 'We went up to the station and tramped up and down alone and I tried to be cheerful but don't remember saying much except "Be good to Kate for me" – and we both blew our red Cushing noses and talked about other things, Baltimore oysters I believe.'[36]

Father and son shared a passion for old books and medical history. Harvey thought he could remember pricking up his ears at talk about rare books when he was just a child. Now that his father had more time to dabble in his literary interests, and Harvey had the money to build a library, exchanges of books, bookplates, and book lore became a staple of their correspondence. Kirke gave Harvey valuable old medical volumes, and he fed Kate's interest in eighteenth-century English literature. Harvey tried to get his father to write medical history, including their own family's, and was delighted when Kirke became an expert on aspects of the iconography of Benjamin Franklin.

The more time Harvey spent in Baltimore, the more the father-son relationship became triangular, with William Osler as the hypotenuse. Osler was a kindred spirit to Dr Kirke Cushing and a surrogate father to Harvey. Osler shared and personified all of the Cushings' reverence for the medical calling. In his writing and friendships he championed the role of old-fashioned general practitioners such as Drs Erastus and Kirke Cushing (and Ned Cushing, too, whose image in pictures is uncannily like Osler's). From his lofty perch at the top of American medicine in Baltimore, Osler did more than anyone else to advance the career of the new-fashioned surgical specialist, Dr Harvey Cushing. He had not 'pushed' Cushing into neurosurgery, but he had pulled Cushing along at practically every stage.[37] Cushing's respect and admiration for William Osler were matched only by the feelings he came to have for Grace Osler. Kate, too, fell under the spell of their neighbors, who took her under their wing whenever Harvey was away and also when he was not.

Osler, who was accumulating a great personal medical library, would invite Cushing and the other latchkeyers to inspect the latest leatherbound first editions that had arrived from Europe – the works of Harvey, Linacre, Locke, Sydenham, practically every famous name in English-speaking medicine, and many others – or to consider the offerings in the latest catalogs from the great British and continental book dealers. Osler assumed that Cushing would take a special interest in the greatest of all anatomists, Andreas Vesalius, and urged him to write about and collect Vesaliana. Saturated with book talk and medical history from his year in Europe, Cushing needed little prompting. Following the trail of Vesalius became a lifelong hobby, pursued with characteristic ferocity.[38]

Osler, Welch, Kelly, and other Hopkins men displayed their books and their literary-medical-historical erudition at meetings of the Johns

Hopkins Historical Club. Cushing fitted it perfectly. There was a memorable gathering at Osler's house in 1901 when the doctors' collections yielded up five copies of the Editio Princeps of Vesalius's *De humani corporis fabrica*. There was Cushing's own presentation to the club of his spare-time investigation of the life of Samuel Garth, physician and much-beloved poet of the Kit-Kat Club during the reign of Queen Anne. It was an essay written with considerable scholarship and authority and in an agreeable literary style. Perhaps as befitting a Yale graduate, Cushing's was a more serviceable style than Osler's. With far less formal education than Cushing, and perhaps a more deferential personality, Osler tended to overquote authorities in his widely read essays. No one else among the second-generation Hopkins men – Thayer, Finney, Barker, McCrae, Jacobs, W.G. MacCallum, and others, whose collective output of textbooks, memoirs, biographies, and even verse would eventually become prodigious – came near to being Cushing's equal as a writer.

To express his gratitude to Osler, both professional and personal, Cushing organized a dinner in his honor in May 1903 at the Maryland Club. He supervised every detail, including the design of the special menu. The Hopkins house staff presented their chief with a set of the just-completed sixty-three-volume British *Dictionary of National Biography*. Cushing told his father that the young staff were also considering finding a way to honor Halsted, perhaps through a *Festschrift* that would publicize his contributions to surgery: 'He has not done much of anything for us but he has done still less for himself in certain ways and there are lots of things of great surgical value which ... we can claim for him.'[39] Nothing came of this project.

Kate appreciated the Oslers' help when Harvey was out of town, though she much preferred to have him back. 'Dr Osler came over after dinner – They are so attentive while you are away – Aren't they just dears? ... My little boy is well, but I want my *boy* so much. I *must* get used to your being away, but I think about you every minute ... I have that usual cut in half feeling that always comes when I'm away from you.'[40] Harvey was away on the frightening day of the great Baltimore fire of February 7, 1904, which for several hours seemed to be about to destroy all the residences on Franklin Street. The Oslers gathered in Kate and the baby and prepared to evacuate their homes. Just as they were ready to leave, the wind shifted and the danger passed.

Osler himself became a thorn in Kate's side a few months later when he persuaded Harvey to join him on a transatlantic junket to Britain. The trip was to follow the usual round of June medical meetings in Atlantic City and other eastern centers. Kate took the baby to Cleveland, where he came down with some kind of fever. Between trips, Harvey told Kate he was wracked with remorse at their separation and also with his travel plans. He carried on with his surgery, including the Birks operation, and his writing, found time to check the household accounts and criticize Kate for leaving unpaid bills, and forgot their second wedding anniversary. He had told her that if she really needed him in Cleveland she had only to telegraph and he would rush up. She, of course, would not admit to that much dependency.[41]

He finally made it to Cleveland for a few days in July to say goodbye. The parting was not easy – hard things were said between the young wife, who probably did not want him to go, and the willful husband. From the *Campania*, where he shared a cabin with Osler and Tom McCrae, Harvey tried to make it up: 'Oh peaches – its been such a mistake and made us both feel so bad and so often. After what was said it seemed on the whole better to go – perhaps easier for you that I should go though I have no heart for it – at all – only a great lump in my throat and wet eyes. I hope no one will see me ... Please care for your boy – I don't quite see how you can – so much as before. I miss you awfully. How interesting every thing would seem if only you were here.'

He resolved to put his marital misery behind him and make the best of things: 'Now that there's no withdrawing I'm going to try and get as rested and as well as possible on this trip and be more patient and less querulous with everyone and everything when I get back. I think my girl too will feel lots better next fall if she gets out and takes some physical exercise every day.'[42] The crossing became memorable for the good fellowship the traveling doctors enjoyed as they met over drinks and tobacco two or three times a day to hold facetious sessions of their 'North Atlantic Medical Society.' Harvey started another detailed travel diary, in which there is no mention of concern about the situation at home. There was sightseeing in Dublin, then a day talking about the brain with Sherrington in Liverpool, then 'a great sensation to be in London again.'

Cushing was surprised to have a ringside seat at one of the decade's major North Atlantic medical stories, the British wooing of America's greatest physician. Before leaving for England, where he was to get an honorary degree from Oxford during a British Medical Association meeting, Osler had been sounded out as a candidate for the regius professorship of medicine at Oxford. Only Grace knew of the possibility until Osler told Cushing about it on their first day in London. Harvey immediately wrote to Kate: 'Dont you dare tell but Dr O has been offered the Regius Prof at Oxford. May take it. Says it will be a great place for Mrs O to become a fat dowager and himself to. A synecure – no work big salary – nothing to do but give one lecture a year and drink port the rest of the time – perhaps write the history of Medicine.'[43]

Cushing sightsaw indefatigably in Oxford, which he found beautiful, traditional, and sleepily scholastic, and also in Cambridge, which by contrast was 'awake, modern, scientific.' He took in the BMA meeting and dismissed English medical men as 'a bit tiresome, except the neurologists.' The American surgeon clearly did not have the temperament to be an Oxford regius. Did Osler, the Anglo-Canadian? Harvey was in the audience at Oxford's Sheldonian Theatre for the awarding of honorary degrees, and he witnessed the tremendous applause that Osler received for an address that seemed to bridge tradition and modernity, British gentility and American energy: 'Dr O stirred them all up by ... talking of the necessity not only of tradition and ideals but force to carry out ideals.'[44]

Cushing and McCrae could not figure out whether Osler would take the British offer. He teased them by showing part of a telegram from Grace advising him not to procrastinate. On the second day of the

homebound passage, Cushing recorded in his diary that while alone in
the cabin he straightened some loose papers of Osler's and noticed a
sheet referring to his chief's acceptance of the Oxford job. The news
was overwhelmingly depressing to Cushing. When it became public –
Osler wrote to all of his friends from shipboard – the Hopkins community was thrown into despair at being virtually deserted by their professional, moral, and spiritual leader.

The Cushings were losing their patrons, neighbors, friends, and William Harvey Cushing's godparents. Grace Osler had urged her husband
to take the chair (her full telegram read, 'Do Not procrastinate: Accept at Once') because of her fear that his health was being imperilled
by overwork. She shared her feelings with Kate, one medical wife to
another: 'These have been very trying weeks – Such a serious matter
settled and now I am in possession of an Oxford Professor. My heart is
heavy & light in turn ... I am trying only to look on the bright side and
think of the many advantages of comparative ease for Dr Osler and a
charming chance for Revere. Please forgive us – and remember how
easy it is to cross the sea.'

Having seen her husband go all the way to England and back for a
single conference, spending about a month away, Kate already knew
how easy it was to cross the sea. Maybe the trip had been good for
Harvey – at least he thought so:

> I feel so well now and vigorous and 'different – in the head' from the way I
> have been feeling all the spring. I knew I ought to go but now that I am
> having a good time it seems so selfish. I didn't expect to enjoy it but if I had
> puttered about at home doing and thinking much the same old things I
> would have been just dull and stupid all the time trying to work for con-
> science sake without accomplishing or having any heart in anything, and we
> would both have been out of sorts in consequence. After this we can take the
> kitten and go anywhere cant we? Please understand peaches girl.[45]

Whatever Kate understood about her husband's rationalizations, after spending time together in Cleveland that August they again sepa-

rated as he went back to Baltimore and worked through the heat of September. Their letters have apparently not all survived and their language is sometimes ambiguous, but the friction seems to have been reasonably serious. One day Mrs Goodwillie asked Harvey when Kate would be coming back. He said he didn't know, 'to which she gently added "I suppose you don't care."' Early in October, after again chewing Kate out for having run up unpaid bills, Harvey turned to their situation: 'Oh! Peaches – you are so far away and I am so cross with a bad cold and with wondering whether you wouldn't really rather stay in Cleveland. Five weeks today since I came back here. I'm afraid I'm not very understanding. If you will come back next Monday and share my humble home "all will be forgiven" and if you want me to I will go out Saturday night D[eo] V[olente] and come back with you. I love you and want to see the kitten.' Soon after this letter Kate returned.[46]

∽

The Cushings were fascinated onlookers as the Oslers went through their final, extremely hectic winter in Baltimore, a time of portrait painting, textbook revision, after-dinner speeches, house cleaning, seeing old patients and old friends, and trying not to see reporters. Avoiding the press became practically impossible for Osler in the aftermath of his injudicious farewell speech at Johns Hopkins in which, carried away with the idea that aging professors should know when to move on, he facetiously advocated euthanizing sexagenarians.

Harvey's good neighborliness included playing the villainous Guy Fawkes, caught skulking in the cellar in a gunpowder plot to blow up Revere Osler's home at 1 West Franklin. He also tried to raise money to save the house, slated for demolition, hoping to preserve it as a library. Neither plot nor philanthropic plan succeeded. Nor did Cushing have any effective role in the choice of Osler's successor at Johns Hopkins. He was drawn to a quixotic scheme to have William Welch named Physician-in-Chief and Professor of Medicine as a kind of modern Hippocrates. The idea gained no support, least of all from Welch.

Cushing was delighted when it was finally decided to call his old friend Lewellys Barker back from Chicago to take Osler's place.

Harvey uncharacteristically passed up the grand farewell dinner in New York at which the American medical profession said good-bye to Osler. He had been traveling a lot and was short of money, he claimed. Nor did the Cushings host any other farewell function for the Oslers. Kate may have considered it not yet her place to be a medical hostess in Baltimore, and she probably still did not like the city. But Grace Osler very much liked her, and from the ship she thanked Kate warmly for having been so 'angelic' to them all winter: 'I shall always be grateful to you ... You knew without my saying what pleasure you brought into our neighborhood and I have so often expressed what a source of thankfulness that you have been always ready & willing to fall into our cosey life. Fancy what you might have been!'

Kate wanted a house of their own in Baltimore. After the Oslers left, Harvey began looking while she again went to Cleveland to avoid the heat. He could not find anything suitable in the summer of 1905, was still not making much money from his surgery, and wrote to her about the possibility of settling back home. 'Will make more money when we go to Cleveland, Peaches, and have lots and lots of patients and stop writing papers about things we only half believe and other people don't believe at all.'[47]

After a vacation together in Canada, they took a summer house in the Maryland countryside, and for several months Harvey commuted to Hopkins while Kate helped the servants with the housework and cooking and read Walter Scott novels. It turned into an idyllic time for both of them, summed up by Kate in a long letter to her father-in-law:

> I have enjoyed the three months here almost more than anything else I ever did – and the baby is bouncing and actually red cheeked. And Harvey full of energy. He has been very busy, starting his clinic, and took two flying trips in the last week, one to the Perkins in Virginia, and one to Ridgefield, Conn where he was called to see Ray Tod Balkley's child. They are here now, and he is going to operate next week ...

He has had three or four ganglions this fall and every thing seems to have gone well – Those things seem to come in waves, just now a wave of good luck. He has an assistant this year, just graduated from the Medical School, a great big tall chap named Gilman, and a great friend of ours. He does all sorts of things, from meeting the Balkleys at the station, and escorting them to their hotel, to overseeing the finishing of the dog house.

We are packing up to go to town ... No 3 is all cleaned, a new carpet in the nursery, and telephones in almost every room![48]

In January 1906, as Harvey's career continued to careen ahead, Kate gave birth to their second child, Mary Benedict.

～

Cushing had earned the right to an assistant by his outstanding contribution to the teaching of medical students at Johns Hopkins, and by creating the 'dog house' – the Hunterian Laboratory – as an innovative center for both teaching and research.

Surgical instruction at Hopkins had been haphazard and inept, partly because of Halsted's negligence and partly because no one knew how to handle surgical teaching in medical school. As Cushing had experienced in Boston, would-be surgeons learned best through apprenticeship. Med school starter courses on cadavers were not at all satisfactory. Students working on dead bodies had no incentive to take asepsis and patient management seriously or to learn to control bleeding or handle tissues gently. When Cushing returned from Europe, he took over a Hopkins cadaver course that J.M.T. Finney had been giving, and he immediately decided to replace dead humans with live animals. He remembered how the students had watched his abortive research with Halsted on dogs and how he personally had benefited from doing animal surgery in Europe. Better to learn the basics of surgery by being surgeons to the living.

Cushing divided students into teams of five: a 'family physican,' a surgeon, his two assistants, and an anesthetist. The family doctor was to do a history and diagnose a problem with a dog and call in the surgical team to operate. They would be gowned, gloved, and masked, use proper anesthetics and full aseptic procedure, keep their ether charts, do post-op follow-ups, and write final reports. Before surgery, the students prepared dressings and sterilized their instruments. During surgery, they developed 'the proper feeling of responsibility for the general welfare of the anesthetized patient.' After surgery, they cleaned up, having learned 'carefully and with tears' the work that nurses and orderlies did. If there was a fatality, they did an autopsy.

Cushing's role as instructor was mainly to give advice on handling the scalpel, coping with hemostasis, and performing ligation, suturing, and other procedures. One student remembered that Cushing watched him at work and commented, 'I could do better surgery with dirty hands than you are doing with gloved hands.' The quaking beginner expected a chewing-out. Instead, Cushing quietly gave him a lesson in antisepsis: 'You put your finger against the brain. The glove may have been sterile when it came out of the basin of bichloride, but during the time you have been wearing it, it is possible that organisms have landed on the finger. I would rather trust the tip of an unsterilized Halsted clamp than I would a rubber glove which is being smeared all around in a wound. Try to be as sterile as possible in all ways, but always assume, in handling tissues, that you are "dirty."' A student who complained to Cushing about the problem of getting the ether cone over a dog's big menacing muzzle was told that he was like a golfer blaming his golf balls.[49]

His aim was not so much to make surgeons as to familiarize would-be doctors with the basic principles of this area of medicine. His brilliantly innovative course was an instant success, unique in that and most other eras. Year after year, practically everyone in the medical class tried to sign up for Cushing's elective in surgery, which was remembered by those who took it as 'something wonderful.' This was remarkable in a school whose teachers, other than Osler, did not do much for their students. In 1903 the third-year class delegated a special committee to thank Cushing for his 'originality in methods of teaching, the close personal attention and the clearness of presentation' of his course. Each spring, Harvey offered a postgraduate course in operative surgery along the same lines.[50]

Cushing occasionally practiced and researched surgical procedures on dogs, sometimes demonstrating for his students. His friend Councilman pointed out that he was really doing exercises in comparative surgery. By 1905 he was lobbying hard for a new building, even offering to do the fundraising himself. When the Hopkins trustees, flush with extra money from donations after the Baltimore fire, agreed to build a joint animal house and pathology lab, Harvey took Welch's advice and named it the Hunterian Laboratory of Experimental Medicine, after the great British investigators and collectors.

Cushing encouraged some of the better medical students to do serious research at the Hunterian, and had several series of their papers published in the *Johns Hopkins Hospital Bulletin*. From the beginning of his animal work he was sensitive to the antivivisection movement, which was apt to flare at any time in any state or city, and he went to great lengths to show that his animals were treated humanely. He invited Baltimoreans to refer seriously sick animals to the experts at the Hunterian, developed something of a consulting veterinary practice, and even gave a course in animal surgery to veterinarians. One of Baltimore's most militant antivivisectionists was won over, he claimed, when they removed a disfiguring tumor from her pet poodle.[51]

Cushing arranged to have his assistant, Philip Gilman, take over most of his teaching responsibilities (and receive most of the $500 Hopkins now paid for the course), and began using the Hunterian solely as a research laboratory. Its success became a model, both in teaching and in the use of animals. 'Many expressions of interest have come from outside sources,' Harvey told his father. 'We seem to have mapped out or started out a new claim and others want to follow suit.' In 1908 he agreed to serve on a high-powered Council in Defense of Medical Research being established by the American Medical Association to fend off antivivisectionist pressure. He was not happy with the council's use of 'defense' in its title, for he felt they had nothing to be defensive about.[52]

~

Others had begun studying Johns Hopkins's 'claims' in medicine, re-search, medical teaching, and surgery. By about 1905 distinguished visitors to America were making Baltimore the high point of their in-vestigations of New World medicine. They came to see Osler, Halsted, John J. Abel's pharmacology lab, Franklin Mall's work in embryology, and, in increasing numbers, Harvey Cushing's surgery. 'Every one has a foreigner now-a-days,' Harvey wrote during a particularly heavy influx in 1904. Four years later he told his father, 'Such a lot of foreigners ... The "centre of gravity" seems to be shifting this way though it will be long before it gets on this side of the Atlantic. I rather think surgery attracts more over than other things.' One of his most welcome visitors in 1907 was Albert Kocher, son of the master surgeon in Berne. Cushing invited him to observe one of his ganglionectomies. Theodor Kocher closed the circle, as it were, in thanking Cushing for the hospitality to his son: 'He has now ... a much fresher idea of the earnestness, con-science and ability with which scientific work is done on the other side of the ocean, although I was fully aware already ... that the United States are the place where we have to go and learn more than we are able to show to the many men coming over to see us. Our turn now to admire others!'[53]

The admiration for Cushing by other American physicians and sur-geons led to a stream of invitations to leave Johns Hopkins. W.W. Keen, tried to lure him to be his successor at Philadelphia's Jefferson College. He could write his own ticket back to Cleveland – one of the family's rich friends said he would build Cushing six dog houses in Cleveland, but not one in Baltimore. In 1906-7 the president of Yale urged Cushing to come home to New Haven to help build Yale's struggling medical school, which was still handicapped by the lack of a good teaching hospital with good clinical material. Cornell's medical school, in New York City, which had an abundance of patient material but a nonchalant approach to everything except making money, also tried to lure him.

He took only the Yale offer particularly seriously, mostly out of college loyalty. This prompted his Boston friends to remind him that Harvard, in the midst of planning a great expansion, was still very much a possibility. He toyed with going to Yale as a prelude to a move to Harvard, but Welch advised strongly against the idea. Hopkins, anxious to keep him, gave him the right to admit his own patients to its wards and to appoint his own resident. With the hospital, the Hunterian, and his assistants, and with more patients coming to him, Cushing decided he could accomplish more in Baltimore than anywhere else. Apropos of one of the offers, Kate told his father in 1906, 'We are so happy here and Harvey is doing the kind of work he likes, and that nobody else can do, and every one is nice to us, and it is hard to go out into the cold world.'[54]

So the Cushings seemed almost settled in Baltimore. The Oslers stayed with them on their return visits, and in December 1906 Kate hosted a glittering tea for William and Grace, entertaining hundreds of guests at 3 West Franklin in rooms fragrant with American Beauty roses. A party of forty stayed for dinner.[55] The next spring the Cushings bought their first home, a rambling New England–style frame house at 107 East Chase Street. From Cleveland, Harvey's proud father asked him to arrange to have his portrait done in oils by 'the best artist that Baltimore, Philadelphia, or Washington holds forth, and will pay cash on demand.'[56] They eventually chose Edmund C. Tarbell, paid him the very large fee of $2,500, and were rewarded with the fine formal study reproduced on the dust jacket of this book.

The serene formal face of Cushing success masked continuing tension between Harvey and Kate. Snippets of their troubles exude from old letters like whiffs of disagreeable odors. At the end of May 1907, for example, Kate left for Cleveland with the children so abruptly that she forgot her golf clubs and the keys to her luggage. Harvey wrote her unhappily but coldly:

It's very dreary here without you and so empty of kittens. It doesn't seem as though I could bear it another day: but something has been wrong for so long that I think it is much better for you to be away. If we are going to be happy together we must learn to be more patient with one another. Its awful to think that we both hesitate about living alone without a third party – that we are glaring and reticent unless someone else is about – that its easy to 'play fair' with other people and difficult at home. Its hard to understand inasmuch as I'm sure we love one another.

He wrote to her about the medical meetings in Atlantic City, Albert Kocher's visit, his ganglion work, and William the butler – and then had to apologize for having forgotten their fifth anniversary.[57] Her letters to him from these weeks, if she wrote any, have not been found. He worked on in Baltimore, putting in fifteen-hour days on his head surgery manuscript, telling her that he was lonely and depressed and that he loved her and her real home was with him. They finally reunited at a rented cottage at Little Boars Head, New Hampshire, on the Atlantic coast north of Boston, where they conceived another child, Betsey, who was born in May 1908.

～

In the spring of 1908 Cushing had to decide what to do for a thirty-two-year-old teacher-farmer he had operated on three times in 1906 for a suspected tumor. The patient took anesthetic badly and bled a lot. Cushing had had to withdraw on the first operation, removed a blood clot and a small cyst the second time, and could not find any tumor the third time, despite employing a process of cortical stimulation, adapted from Sherrington, to try to locate growths below the surfaces of the brain. When the patient's convulsive symptoms returned, he begged Cushing to try again. Against his better judgment, Cushing agreed: 'It seemed unfair to deny the poor fellow the more extensive exploration which he so earnestly solicited.'

The patient again took anesthetic badly, and bleeding forced Cushing to stop this fourth operation. He could not close up, but simply put gauze and a dressing over the hole exposing the brain. For the fifth attempt, knowing that the brain tissue is insensitive, he resolved not to use anesthetic. He removed the dressing, used cortical stimulation to decide where to cut into the brain, and found a small cyst, a degenerated tumor, about a centimeter below the surface. He was able to dissect it out, found another cyst right below it, got it out too, filled the wound with saline solution, and closed it. During the whole three-hour operation the patient was fully conscious, unimpaired, alert to what was happening and able to share his thoughts and sensations with his surgeon. Even Cushing thought it was 'a startling thing' to see the post-central convolution, the area of the brain generally believed to be particularly concerned with sensory perception, painlessly incised and tumors removed from its depth: 'It was truly remarkable in this patient to find that the extensive manipulations which were essential to the removal of the tumor could be carried out while the patient was perfectly conscious, was chatting and was taking a lively interest in the progress of the operation.'[58]

Cushing had only had about ten successful tumor removals by the time of this demonstration of the amazing possibilities of brain surgery. One reason for such meager results was the comparative scarcity of brain tumor cases, even at Johns Hopkins. Before Cushing began to publish his multiple reports detailing what knowing colleagues – the Keens, Oslers, and others – realized was an astonishing medical saga, many patients with brain tumors had been undiagnosed, misdiagnosed, or written off as hopeless. Now a surgeon at America's best hospital offered real hope to some of these sufferers.

He was also starting to publish a new series of articles on how ophthalmological examination could easily disclose the 'choked disc,' which he could now prove was pressure on the retinal nerve, a sure symptom of a tumor problem. With Cushing proclaiming, 'The diagnosis is written on the patient's retina,' more ophthalmologists were able to diagnose tumors. They were also more likely to refer the patients to the surgical genius in Baltimore.[59] In 1909 some sixty-four brain tumor cases came to Johns Hopkins, more than in the preceding twenty years combined.[60] Even more came in 1910, the year of the Leonard Wood operation.

Cushing kept track of all of his patients and their records, and had begun to develop a statistical profile of his operative results. The statistics would always be difficult to interpret because of changes in the condition of his patients and in his surgical boldness. Sometimes the figures are hard to fathom. Revisiting the 'special field' of neurosurgery in 1910, five years after his first 'apologia,' Cushing reported these results on his tumor patients:

> In our last one hundred cases, over a period of eighteen months, there were eight operative fatalities in the first fifty and only three in the second fifty; there were only ten extirpations or six cyst evacuations with practical cures in the first fifty, and there have been twenty in the last fifty. In the entire one hundred, therefore, there have been thirty apparent (to all intents and purposes) cures, thirteen operative deaths and sixty-seven measures which have been definitely palliative. There has been a complete absence of the old-time post-operative complications. A meningitis or fungus cerebri is almost inexcusable today.[61]

While it makes sense in this summary that Cushing did 110 procedures on his 100 patients, he seems to misstate his operative deaths and offers no definition of cure.

He continued to broaden his work, exploring the physiology of the cerebrospinal fluid, the phenomenon of pressure on the optical nerve, and the nature of the tumors he was removing. With helpers and with the Hunterian Laboratory as his fiefdom, he was expanding into both neurosurgical research and the education of bright young men who would become America's first deliberately trained neurosurgeons. He also became less sloppy in presenting statistics.

Where was the progress taking them? Most obviously, they were moving deeper into the brain. Through the rear of the box Cushing was beginning to attack tumors of the cerebellum, having developed a special 'cross-bow' incision and entry, as well as a special 'outrigger' for placing patients face-down during surgery. Exactly how they would approach the bottom of the box was still unclear, but Cushing and his students were preparing to confront one of the most little known but intriguing of all organs, the hypophysis cerebri or pituitary gland. In 1905 Cushing had thought it barely imaginable that someone would succeed in operating on the pituitary. Five years later he was ready to try.

The main reasons for Cushing's success in laying the foundation for neurosurgery were homely and unspectacular. 'The men who are making aerial flight a thing of the near future are not the "spellbinders," thrilling as their individual flights may be, but the men who, like Langley and the Wrights, are working at principles,' he wrote. To an audience at the University of Liverpool, the American explained the innovations that made a new field of radical surgical intervention possible: 'Earlier diagnoses and more prompt interference, a wider experience in overcoming the technical difficulties of these cases, coupled with the courage to work slowly and painstakingly, these things will lead to increasingly better results in this responsible work, the success of which depends so greatly upon detail, patience, and the expenditure of time.'[62]

For the rest of his career, Cushing would struggle to keep finding the time to expand on his remarkable achievement as the founding father of neurosurgery. He would be less successful at finding time for his responsibilities as a husband and father.

SEVEN

The Bottom of the Box:
Interrogating the Pituitary

~

The assistants and students who worked for Cushing were always pleased when the Chief invited them to his home. 'Mrs. Chief' was a warm, gracious hostess and served a perfect tea. Remarkably, Cushing himself often failed to appear, having been tied up at the hospital or in the lab. A young Bostonian, John Homans, who had been sent to train with the man Harvard considered to be America's most promising surgeon, recalled, 'I had never seen anyone work like Cushing before, and found it difficult to believe that he could enjoy life on this basis ... His pace never varied, unless it became accelerated.'[1] Kate longed for the old days when she could look forward to having her husband home for tea and conversation.

Harvey turned forty on April 8, 1909, the age by which William Osler thought that a man's best work had been done. From then on, one coasted. Cushing could have been more than content with his achievement as the founder of a new surgical specialty. Writing to his father three days after his fortieth birthday, he did boast a bit: patients were now coming to him, mostly with brain tumors, from all over the United States and Canada.

In the same letter Harvey told his father about new work he and his assistants were doing on the pituitary body, a ductless gland deep in the brain whose secretions play a fundamental role in human development:

'It seems to be an important gland and one which is surgically acessible.' He had just had his first clinical case, a man whose pituitary he had operated on for acromegaly: 'It is quite extraordinary how he has improved – quite a brilliant affair all around ... I think it is the first case in this country.'

Two months later, in Atlantic City, he delivered the Oration on Surgery at the sixtieth annual meeting of the American Medical Association. It was a report on his pituitary work – 'The Hypophysis Cerebri: Clinical Aspects of Hyperpituitarism and of hypopituitarism' – and was one of his most brilliant intellectual performances. George Crile judged it the best presentation the AMA had ever heard. Here was a surgeon giving a paper that integrated experimental and clinical data to present a new paradigm of the physiology and pathology of one of the body's most mysterious organs.

In the next few months Cushing, an American surgeon, came to be recognized as one of the world's authorities on everything to do with the pituitary – and, of course, began to attract many more patients with suspected pituitary problems. Even as he continued to refine and elaborate his methods of attacking tumors through the top and sides of the 'closed box' of the cranium, he was also working on surgical procedures to get at the pituitary through the bottom of the skull – entering through the face and across the sphenoidal bone. 'I think of little else than the pituitary body nowadays' he told his father in 1909. By 1912 he had enough data, including forty-eight clinical cases, to form the basis of a remarkable 322–page monograph, *The Pituitary Body and Its Disorders.*[2]

With his mastery of the pituitary, he automatically became a pioneer in the exploding field of knowledge about the body's glandular, or internal, secretions. Cushing became a founding father of endocrinology, one of the most exciting areas of medical science in the first half of the twentieth century. He tried hard to push his pituitary work into even more exotic new territory. In 1912 he did what may well have been the world's first pituitary transplant.

Of course it did not work. Many of Cushing's ideas about the pituitary did not quite work. The concepts for which he is known today did not emerge until late in his career (described in chapter 13). Founding neurosurgery by being progressively conservative and endlessly patient was one kind of challenge; theorizing and surgically tinkering in the dark about an organ of stunning complexity proved far more difficult, even for the brilliant, driven workaholic Cushing had become.

~

In earlier years he had not paid much attention to the pituitary gland. A little nut of an organ, weighing about half a gram, it sits at the very bottom of the brain in a small saddle of bony tissue, the sella turcica. For many centuries anatomists had thought the gland, formally known as the hypophysis cerebri, was somehow responsible for the excretion of brain wastes through the nasal cavities. *Pituitarius* is Latin for 'phlegm.' The gland was of no interest to surgeons because it could not be reached in living subjects. They only encountered it at autopsy.

This had been the case, for example, with one of Harvey's earliest neurosurgical failures, a noticeably sexually underdeveloped woman with failing vision who died in 1902 after his third unsuccessful operation. She was found to have a tumor at the base of the brain that had enveloped both the pituitary and the nearby chiasm of the optic nerves. Three years later he had better luck with another woman, who was suffering from headaches, vision problems, and menstrual cessation; a bilateral decompression (opening the cranium on both sides) apparently allowed the brain and tumor to lift away from some of the affected nerves, relieving the patient's symptoms.

Suspecting another pituitary problem in this case, Cushing began to study the literature on conditions associated with pituitary lesions. For about twenty years, investigators had been aware of peculiar disorders involving abnormal pituitaries. Some patients suffered from forms of excessive bodily growth, including acromegaly. Some women failed to develop sexually or ceased menstruating. One of Cushing's friends from his *wanderjahr*, Alfred Fröhlich, had published a famous case of a pituitary tumor apparently causing a boy to become sluggish, fat, and sexually immature – what came to be called Fröhlich's syndrome. In 1906 Harvey read a paper to the American Neurological Association setting his two cases in the context of this literature. It seemed to him that the combination of sexual infantilism and optic atrophy could now be interpreted as evidence of a tumor affecting the pituitary. The paper was a modest contribution – 'feeling in the dark,' Cushing noted a few years later.[3]

Researchers moved surprisingly quickly to penetrate the barriers that blocked understanding of the pituitary. They realized, for example, that x-rays, normally no help in locating brain lesions, could provide circumstantial evidence of pituitary problems by showing deformities in the sella turcica caused by pressure from tumorous or swollen glands. Working with animals and experimenting with various routes to the organ, a number of European surgeons, including Horsley in England, were able to reach the pituitary and begin attacking tumors. Cushing, having forecast this development in his 1904 survey of neurological surgery, also intended to go there.

But the organ was so mysterious, so little studied, that it was not clear what a surgeon should do after he got to it. How should an enlarged or damaged pituitary be handled? Take it out like a diseased appendix or a stone-filled gallbladder or cancerous ovaries? Excise it like a goiterous thyroid? There are many organs and appendages that the body can do without. But is the pituitary one of them?

The body's ductless glands include the pituitary, the thyroid and parathyroids, the thymus, adrenals, ovaries, and testes. Their secretions began to interest researchers in the 1880s and 1890s. Internal secretions from the ductless glands (in 1902 the term 'hormone' was coined to describe them) were in some cases essential to sustaining life. An animal that lost its thyroid or adrenals (or its pancreas, a gland that seemed to have both internal and external secretions) always died. For someone contemplating surgical work on the pituitary, it was vitally important to know what would happen if the whole organ was excised. The early reports were fragmentary and contradictory, not least be-

cause of the technical problem of getting the surgery right. If a hypophysectomized animal lived, perhaps the surgeon had failed to get out
the whole organ. If it died, perhaps the surgery had caused infection or
hemorrhage or had nicked some other vital area.

In late 1907 or early 1908 Cushing assigned to one of his surgical
students, Lewis Reford, the problem of determining whether the pituitary is essential to life. Cushing himself took an unusual personal interest in Reford's project. They found that the best work was being done
in Romania by the physiologist Nicolas Paulesco, who had developed
what seemed to be an ideal surgical approach to the pituitary of dogs.
Perhaps coincidently, it involved the same bilateral decompressive
methods that Cushing had used on his 1905 patient. Using and refining
Paulesco's technique, also applying the extreme antisepsis and care that
Cushing required for surgery on dogs and humans alike, Reford, soon
joined by Samuel J. Crowe and John Homans, removed pituitaries from
dozens of dogs. They mastered the operation and could do it in less
than an hour; their speed and their unlimited supply of dogs – they
eventually depituitarized more than a hundred – generated more experimental results than anyone else had the luxury of studying.[4]

Most of the dogs died, apparently confirming Paulesco's findings and
the view that pituitary secretions are essential to maintaining life. Cushing
was thus positioned to put down the famously impetuous Chicago surgeon, John B. Murphy, who enthusiastically predicted to the American
Medical Association in 1908 that within the next year there would be
twenty-five pituitarectomies. If so, Harvey commented, there would
be twenty-five deaths in twenty-five cases.[5]

More important, Cushing began asking other questions about the
gland. The pituitary has two lobes, anterior and posterior. Are both
lobes or only one essential to life? His experiments seemed to show that
dogs could live without the posterior lobe but not without the anterior.
What exactly happened to animals and humans when their pituitary
glands went awry but continued to function? The literature was puzzling: it associated both the conditions of acromegaly and adipose sexual
infantilism with pituitary damage caused by tumors. A foggy debate

was underway about whether tumors affecting the pituitary had the effect of inhibiting or stimulating whatever the pituitary secreted.

'The whole thing burst on me one day at the laboratory,' Cushing noted a few months later. Others corroborated that there had been a sudden flash of insight. Cushing was examining an experimental dog that had been depituitarized but was clinging to life – perhaps, they thought, because a little bit of the gland was still present. The dog had become fat, lazy, and asexual. 'Here is Fröhlich's asexual adiposity!' Cushing exclaimed. Since the animal had almost no pituitary, its lack of maturation and energy must be due to deficient pituitary secretion. Conversely, excessive growth, notably the acromegalic condition, must be due to an excessive secretion. So tumors could cause two completely different functional disorders of the gland.

In this respect, the pituitary seemed to be almost exactly like the thyroid gland, for whose disorders the terms 'hypothyroidism' and 'hyperthyroidism' had been coined. Very familiar with the thyroid work Halsted and others had done at Hopkins, Cushing coined the terms 'hypopituitarism' and 'hyperpituitarism,' arguing from his dog studies and the model of the thyroid that each condition created a distinctive symptom complex.

This was the new pituitary paradigm that Cushing outlined in his major paper to the American Surgical Association in June 1909. The pituitary somehow controlled growth. Oversecretion would cause fast growth; oversecretion in infancy would lead to gigantism; after puberty, it would lead to the extension and thickening of bone and tissues called acromegaly. Undersecretion in infancy would prevent the onset of puberty; after puberty, it would lead to asexual regression and adiposity.[6]

Within this simple framework, Cushing realized, there were many mysteries. It was not clear exactly what the pituitary secreted and from which lobe. How did rates of secretion vary under normal and abnormal conditions? Did the pituitary's secretions affect the body directly, or did they do so indirectly through their action on some of the other ductless glands? Or both ways? If the pituitary really did behave like the thyroid gland, would it be possible to compensate for deficient secretion, as doctors did with hypothyroidism, by feeding patients extracts of the gland? Thyroid gland therapy had sensationally cured cases of cretinism and myxedema. With cases of hypersecretion, on the other hand, as in goiterous thyroids, perhaps surgical treatment would stop the excess.

Cushing applied his ideas to patients faster than he could publish papers. In March 1909 he examined a thirty-eight-year-old farmer, John Hemens, referred to him by his Minnesota surgical friend Charles Mayo. Hemens suffered from headaches, intolerance to light, dizziness, and tingling in his extremities. For several years his lips and tongue had been thickening, and his jaw, hands, and feet had been growing, the classic stigmata of acromegaly; x-rays showed that the sella, the pituitary saddle, was enlarged.

Cushing decided to try to give Hemens relief by excising part of his swollen pituitary. The patient's tongue was so thick that Cushing did a preliminary tracheotomy to facilitate anesthetization. The operative route they used to reach the dog pituitary would not work safely with humans, so Cushing chose a 'transphenoidal' route that had been pioneered by a European surgeon two years earlier. He entered at the bottom of the forehead, cut through nasal bone and cartilege, folded the nose back as a kind of frontonasal flap, and passed through the nasal sinuses to reach the sphenoid bone at the bottom of the cranium. Using an electric headlight to illuminate a dark field, he located the area of the sphenoid that was the floor of the sella, came up through it, split the dural sheaf of the enlarged pituitary, and removed about one-third of the anterior lobe.

Cushing was able to close without incident. He was surprised by how little bleeding there was and how easy it had been to reach the pituitary. We might be surprised at his being able to sew the nose back in place without totally disfiguring the patient. Hemens was walking three days after the operation, his headaches apparently gone and tissues beginning to shrink. 'The chap walked in to the clinic on his sixth day after operation when our Surgical Club was here,' Harvey exulted to his father, 'as much to my astonishment as theirs.' Hemens was discharged and got on with life, minus only his sense of smell. Cushing described his case triumphantly to his fellow American surgeons in June 1909, and made it the basis of his presentation to the Sixteenth International Medical Congress in Budapest later that summer.[7]

∽

Cushing liked to refer to the pituitary as a 'stowaway gland,' which had now been brought to light and was being interrogated. For three years he spent much of his time, both in the clinic and the Hunterian Laboratory, giving the gland the third degree. He asked every anatomical and physiological question he could think of about the pituitary. How is it vascularized? How do the lobes relate to each other? Do its secretions empty into the bloodstream? Into the cerebrospinal fluid? What is the relation of hypo- to hypersecretion and to the secreting lobes? How do the secretions affect the blood pressure, carbohydrate metabolism, the functioning of the other ductless glands?

As more patients came to him with what were apparently pituitary disorders, the clinical-pathological interrogation became more urgent. Could hypopituitarism be eased by feeding the patient pituitary extracts? If so, extracts of the whole gland? Or of the anterior lobe? Or the posterior? Was pituitary dysfunction always caused by tumors, cysts, or abscesses? Were these most likely to be lesions to the gland itself, lesions in the neighborhood of the gland, or distant lesions somehow compressing the pituitary? Could pituitaries go haywire of their own accord, becoming functionally erratic? What exactly were the signs and symptoms underlying the diagnosis of pituitary disorder? Of hypopituitarism? Of hyperpituitarism?

What were the best surgical approaches to pituitary problems? Was there a better route to the organ? Should the route vary according to the suspected location of the lesion? Were there more radical therapies? Could x-radiation on its own shrink tumors? If Halsted, Kocher, and others could experiment with grafts or transplants of thyroid and parathyroid tissue, why not try grafting with pituitary matter? Try everything first on dogs.

The stowaway gland, whose first answers had seemed relatively straightforward to Cushing, turned out to be maddeningly elusive, deceptive, complex. For his time, Harvey was a master interrogator of the pituitary and a brilliant interpreter of the data it seemed to provide. But the story he thought he had obtained (which he published in numerous articles) proved less than satisfactory. To change the imagery: Cushing and other pituitary and endocrine researchers in the early years of the century were like traders or missionaries who had discovered a dark, lush new continent which they were trying to explore, map, develop, and improve, all at once, on foot and with limited understanding and tools. Or they were like concertgoers who had never heard anyone play more than one instrument at a time, let alone the music of a symphony orchestra. Cushing's very early pituitary research fell prey, as he gradually realized, to misconceptions, simplifications, wishful thinking, and dead ends.

His genius was to have grasped the concept of the pituitary as the gland whose secretions control growth. In 1912 he wrote about 'the hormone of growth.'[8] In fact, it would take many more years before human growth hormone was isolated as a pituitary secretion, by which time it was also understood that the pituitary secretes a whole choir of hormones. Many of these are under the control of what in 1912 was still a completely neglected glandlike portion of the brain, the hypothalamus. Lacking techniques to isolate or purify any of these hormones, lacking knowledge of the hugely complex relationship of pituitary secretions with those of the other glands – indeed, knowing next to nothing about the body's endocrine system – Cushing and his students offered hypotheses and speculations most of which were quickly consigned to the dustbin of hormonal history.

They tried feeding pituitary extracts to their dogs and their patients. They used a range of extracts – whole gland, anterior lobe, posterior lobe – sometimes making the substance from pituitaries purchased at the slaughterhouse, sometimes relying on products that drug companies were beginning to offer, or those made by the meat-packing giant, Armour and Company, in trying to market its byproducts. By today's standards, these extracts were unstandardized sludges of hormones and ground-up tissue and other contaminants, and were inert or inconsistent. They were not at all comparable to the much simpler thyroid extracts, which could work remarkably well. The pituitary proved to be no more analogous to the thyroid gland than an orchestra is to a musical duo.

When Cushing's team thought they were seeing beneficial effects from feeding extracts or grafting bits of gland, they were actually being led astray by wishful thinking, placebo effects, inadequate controls, unrelated transitory phenomena, and other factors. Publishing very quickly, Cushing tended to jump to conclusions based on favorable interpretations of very short-term results. His 1909 surgery on John Hemens for acromegaly, for example, turned out not to be such a clear success. By 1912 most of Hemens's problems had returned. 'It cannot be said that the experience is anything more than suggestive of what may possibly be accomplished in early and aggravated cases of acromegaly,' Cushing wrote carefully.[9]

His belief that implants of bits of gland in some of the hypophysectomized dogs had been beneficial led Cushing to his most radical surgical experiment, the attempt to transplant a pituitary. He found that William Buckner, a forty-eight-year-old Cincinnati real estate developer, had had his pituitary almost completely destroyed by a cyst. Cushing cleaned out the area surgically and prescribed large doses of pituitary extract. When the somnolent, nearly comatose patient continued to deteriorate, Cushing (apparently at Buckner's wife's urging) in February 1912 implanted the gland from a newly deceased baby in the subcortex of Buckner's temporal lobe. 'From all clinical indications it would seem that the implanted fragment remains viable and has assumed a sufficient measure of functional activity,' Cushing wrote a few weeks later as he rushed his book to completion, having the sense to add, however, that 'the whole [transplantation] question is very unsettled.'[10]

He never revisited this question. It won him ridiculous notoriety when reporters learned of the operation and wrote it up in the New York newspapers, grafting their own suppositions onto the bare bones of the story. 'Broker's Frayed Brain Replaced with a Baby's,' claimed the *Herald*:

> In view of about a score of professors and students Dr. Cushing performed his greatest operation. After administering the anesthetic he removed the back of Mr. Buckner's skull and with great care took out the entire brain, which was placed on a piece of linen beside the head and could be seen to pulsate with each heart beat of the patient. The diseased portion was then very carefully severed from the minor brain, and while Dr. Cushing was severing the diseased section another surgeon was transplanting the infant's brain. The major brain was left untouched. After the transplantation the entire brain was restored to its proper place and the section of the skull which had been cut out was replaced.

Johns Hopkins issued an indignant denial that any such procedure had ever taken place. What really happened was that the unfortunate Buckner enjoyed a period of apparent mental impovement, managed to get home for a few days, and then relapsed. Cushing did a second transplant, to no effect. Buckner died, a lethargic, twitching wreck, a few weeks later.[11]

Cushing's real and substantial surgical achievement in the early pituitary years was to develop an improved transphenoidal route to the pituitary area. After two entrances through the nasal area and several frustrating attempts to enter laterally through subtemporal openings, Cushing in 1910 adopted a sublabial approach, which had first been used by Albert E. Halstead of Chicago. The patient's upper lip was drawn back, an incision made in the soft tissue between the upper lip and the gums, and the surgeon inserted his way between the mucous membrane of the nasal cavity on the one hand and the cartilaginous septum on the other. Using a speculum and headlight, he could reach the sphenoid bone, find the sellar floor, come up through it, and then respond to the situation he found.

'The mere technical triumph of exposing the contents of the sella turcica by one or another method is far from the most important consideration,' Cushing warned. 'The crux of the situation lies in the manner of dealing with the pathologically modified gland when it has been brought into view ... The lesions, themselves, and their neighbourhood manifestations, are so variable that there can be no one standard operation applicable to all cases.' The surgeon might remove an infrasellar tumor, evacuate a cyst, be content with the considerable palliative benefits of sellar decompression, or, if absolutely necessary, partially extirpate a pituitary tumor or swelling – though many such tumors were simply not operable. Bleeding was easily controlled 'with the exercise of sufficient patience,' withdrawal was straightforward, drainage unneccesary, and the incision closable with two or three sutures. The patient – face and nose intact and unscarred – could be back at work in a matter of days.

Cushing's specialized anesthetist, Griffith Davis, developed an ingenious tube that made tracheotomies on acromegalic patients unneccessary. Max Brödel made memorable drawings of Cushing doing his transphenoidal approach to the pituitary in 1912. Harvey occasionally had problems with the operation (the surgeon could get lost trying to locate the pituitary fossa region of the sphenoid bone, or the mucous membrane could tear and meningitis develop), but four deaths among his first twenty-seven patients was, at 13.7 percent, a comparatively low mortality rate. He may not have been able to get all the answers he wanted, but now he was interrogating the gland, as it were, face-to-face.[12]

~

To publish detailed case histories of forty-eight patients with literally one-in-a-million disorders of an organ many clinicians had never heard about, as Cushing did in his 1912 book *The Pituitary Body*, was a major triumph. Many of these patients had been misdiagnosed, often by gynecologists or pediatricians, and some had been surgically mutilated or otherwise mistreated. Women complaining of amenorrhea and adiposity with headaches, for example, were apt to have their sex organs removed after exploratory surgery. 'With an open abdomen,' Cushing commented tartly, 'some surgeons cannot resist the impulse to guillotine some organ on the chance that it may be the culprit.'[13]

Harvey organized his cases according to the patients' signs and symptoms: signs of tumor, such as headaches and visual problems, almost always accompanied the growth disturbances caused by abnormal secretions. He concluded his book with a discussion of incidence, symptomology, and treatment. He was still optimistic about glandular therapy and was characteristically cautious about surgical treatment.

He made significant mistakes. Pictures and descriptions of some of his cases suggest a tendency to overclaim for his organ, that he may have been too eager to label a fat boy or a big man a pituitary problem. There were so few glandular symptoms in one case, for example, and so little visual improvement after a sellar decompression that it is no surprise to find, in Cushing's papers, follow-up correspondence indicating that his patient's real problem was tertiary syphilis.[14] Still, the exceptions underline the achievement in drawing attention to the pituitary as a potent mischief maker. In his monograph, Cushing for the first time presented clinicians with a guide to the disorders they could now associate with the pituitary, making it a seminal work in the literature of endocrinology.

When he was at a loss about a patient's symptoms, Cushing erred on the side of doing no harm. He did nothing, for example, in the case of John Turner, a thirty-eight-year-old, 275-pound giant, estimated to be about 8 feet tall, who was losing the use of his legs. By the time Cushing saw Turner, he had realized that his theoretical distinction between hypo- and hyperpituitarism did not hold up well in the real world. It appeared that a patient could be hyper- at one time in his life, hypo- at another, and perhaps both at the same time. Many giants and acromegalics had been hyper- but now seemed hypo-, having stopped growing and begun to run to fat and weakness. There was no point in trying to excise their swollen pituitaries, which might do them more harm; perhaps they needed pituitary extracts to stimulate their growth. In practice, Cushing realized that he had to simplify his classification and accept that many patients suffered from what could only be labeled 'dispituitarism,' a disordered pituitary.

For the rest of his career Cushing was fascinated by the problems of the pituitary and by the gross growth disorders that created giants, dwarfs, circus fat ladies, and other 'freaks.' He hoped to keep his most extreme acromegalic, John Turner, under observation at Johns Hopkins until death. When complaints from the nurses, the superintendent, and Turner himself led to the poor man's release to his home in Washington, DC, Cushing's fallback position was to be sure he was in on the autopsy. It was conducted, he wrote in his book, 'under most inauspicious circumstances.' Sam Crowe, Cushing's house man, elaborated:

> Word came from Washington one night that John had died. His body had been taken by relatives and was in an undertaking establishment awaiting burial the next day. Also that the family would permit no post-mortem. Dr. Cushing was frantic. After much telephoning, the undertaker, for the good of science and a consideration, agreed to permit, on his own responsibility, the removal of John's brain and pituitary gland ... I was routed out of bed and armed with a supply of instruments and a large sum of money, arrived at the mortician's about 3 o'clock in the morning. This was necessary because at that hour there was less likelihood of the family's appearing and interfering with the proceedings. It was impossible to remove John from his coffin and I was warned to leave no signs that would indicate an autopsy had been made. It was finally accomplished in a manner fairly satisfactory to all parties.

Crowe thought it would be unseemly for this story to be published in Cushing's official biography but told his first biographer, John Fulton, that it showed how Cushing 'would stop at nothing to gain his ends. He was so eager for accurate knowledge that he was entirely ruthless as to how he got them.' Cushing had an easier time persuading the curator of the Hunterian Museum in London to dismantle the skull of the institution's famous 'Irish giant' so that the sella could be studied. It proved to have been grossly enlarged, and there was other evidence of a pituitary tumor.[15]

The Pituitary Body and Its Disorders was a dated book within two or three years of its publication (its author began changing his views on the functions of the lobes, for example, and conceded that the gland technically was not essential to maintain life), and it became something of an embarrassment for Cushing when he found physicians still citing it twenty years later. It had become the clinical guide to the pituitary, not least because of its 321 illustrations. Harvey's old interest in 'kodaking' had by now become a passion for keeping visual images as well as written and x-ray records of his patients. All his articles contained numerous illustrations – pictures, x-rays, perimetry studies – often published at his own expense. The most remarkable picture in *The Pituitary Body* was of the naked John Turner towering over the 5 ft. 8 in. S.J. Crowe. Crowe said that for years he was recognized medically in America and Europe as 'the man with the giant in Dr Cushing's book.' Ironically, as a writer in the *Journal of the American Medical Association* pointed out a quarter-century later, the picture gave fairly clear visual evidence that Cushing erred in stating in his text that Turner had been 8 ft. 3 in. tall. Studies of Turner's bones corroborated that he was probably no more than 7 ft. 1 in.[16]

Reviewers welcomed Cushing's monograph as an American triumph, a model of scientific exposition, and a presentation of cases that read almost like a novel. 'Your book has the great advantage of being an all round one in anatomy, physiology, pathology and surgical treatment, just like its author,' a European friend wrote. An even friendlier writer in the *Maryland Medical Journal* decided that Harvey had written 'an unique and masterful piece of work' that would place him among the medical immortals. Some critics wondered if Cushing was a little too speculative, a little too enthusiastic. A shrewd writer in the *Cleveland Medical Journal* asked pointedly exactly what had been achieved when the notions of hypo- and hyperpituitarism had to be collapsed back into the noncommittal concept of 'dispituitarism.'[17]

Still, there was a strong sense that Cushing had become the master guide to an intriguing new field of inquiry. As the author himself put it, 'We are, of course, only at the threshold of understanding these matters.' He was very pleased at the reaction to his monograph, writing to a friend, 'I'm quite set up, and think I must be a literary character in disguise. But I'll never try it again.'[18] In fact, there was no doubt that Cushing would have much more to report on the subject of the pituitary and its disorders. He had led the way in interrogating the stowaway, mapping the continent, recording the music.

∾

Cushing had now developed the three fields of surgery that occupied him for the rest of his operating career: ganglionectomies for trigeminal neuralgia, intracranial procedures to attack brain tumors, and special approaches to the pituitary region.

During the attack on the pituitary he had continued with his other operations. His series of ganglion removals mounted without a setback, and the tumor work generated the triumph on Leonard Wood. Throughout the rest of his career he made many contributions to the enormous preoperative problem of diagnosis and to postoperative issues of tumor analysis and classification. From time to time he made important innovations in surgical technique. Hundreds of lives were saved or prolonged or made less miserable in his operating rooms and during the First World War in his operating tents. If none of these things had happened, he would still have been celebrated for the work he did in his years of maximum creativity, 1900–12. He had become the acknowledged leader on one of the ultimate frontiers of surgery, known and respected around the world.

He was now the master, the 'Chief,' held in fear and awe by his underlings, but also the model for students wanting to learn his esoteric trade. How did the great Cushing do it? What were his 'tricks'? What was the secret of his success?

Anyone could learn quite a bit about Cushing from his publications and his presentations at meetings. He was constantly describing his methods. He was now perhaps more often a senior craftsman than a brilliant innovator – though there was always room for such improvements as his development of silver clips in brain surgery and his use of bits of living tissue and blood clots to inhibit bleeding. Again and again he emphasized how delicate the work had to be:

> The slow separation of brain from tumor, working now here, now there, leaving small, flattened pads of hot, wrung-out cotton to control oozing for the time being from a given area, until it can be again attacked ... slow, blunt dissection with the right hand, while an assistant keeps the field clean by the careful use of wet cotton pledgets ... The tearing out of a growth by the insertion of the fingers means a fragmental removal, extravasation and oedema from unnecessary damage, and blind points of hemorrhage.

He put even more emphasis, if such were possible, on the need for careful attention to detail. To the American Surgical Association in June 1911 he argued at length that the stirring, slap-dash, and spectacular in surgery was giving way to the quiet, patient, and undramatic performance. There was nothing wrong with being slow and fussy, because fussiness was the concern for detail that made everything possible: 'The successful consummation of any critical operation often depends upon seeming trifles ... the scrupulous observance of surgical minutiae that makes possible the safe conduct of major intracranial performances – performances which a few years ago were attended in most cases by a veritable dance Macaber.' (He still did not pay enough attention to spelling minutiae.)[19]

His co-workers at Hopkins remembered Cushing as an almost impossibly exacting and demanding taskmaster to whom, with one notable exception, they were almost fanatically loyal. He took pains to surround himself with good people on whom he could rely. They ranged from his special anesthetist, 'Griff' Davis, to his first operating-room nurse, Helen Adams, to Jimmy, the wizened little Welshman who looked after the dogs in the Hunterian Laboratory. Once, when Jimmy was urged to cut some Cushing-imposed red tape, he replied, 'Orders is orders, and if Dr. Cushing says that the building should be burned down, in well nigh half an hour there would be little of the building left.'[20]

The essence of a good operating-room nurse was (and is) the ability to know what to do without being told. Helen Adams prided herself on knowing which instrument or dressing Cushing would need next, 'and handing it without his asking – making the operating – quiet. He *greatly* appreciated it.' Nurses and trainees who did not measure up during operations were treated with withering scorn and sarcasm, and sometimes fled in tears. After the tension in the room had eased, Cushing usually went out and apologized. While some nurses refused to work for Cushing, the tough ones such as Adams chalked up his moods to the stress of the long, difficult operations. This is a very old story in surgery. Cushing's tendency to sarcasm, the Hopkins people thought, was probably picked up from Halsted.[21] Osler was no longer around to remind him to keep it in check. Less articulate surgeons were known to release operating-room tension with profanity and by throwing instruments.

Cushing generally picked his assistants from the bright medical students who took his dog surgery course. The chosen one would first serve a year as a surgical fellow in the Hunterian Laboratory and then work on the wards as the chief's resident or house man. Lewis Reford, Samuel J. Crowe, Emil Goetsch, Walter Dandy, and Conrad Jacobson all took this route. All of them, along with John Homans of Boston, became involved in his pituitary research and shared authorship with Cushing in many of the publications. According to Jacobson, 'Cushing's man' (as he was known throughout the hospital) was expected above all to have 'geist' – spirit, verve, energy – almost as much as Cushing himself: 'Every little detail regarding the patient ... and pertaining to new and exacting operations was a personal affair with Dr. Cushing. He was an extremely hard taskmaster and drove his man incessantly, almost to the point of exhaustion.' The assistant was responsible for doing multiple examinations of patients, writing up the histories, helping at each day's very long operations, making dressings, supervising Cushing's patients' special diets, and being on duty at night. 'His assistant led a strenuous life,' Sam Crowe remembered, 'but Doctor Cushing's days were far more strenuous.'[22]

Nurse Adams recalled how Cushing dealt with his men:

> The fact that the interne during the day had assisted in two or three operations of three hours each, made not the slightest difference. He [Cushing] often called up about midnight and again later in the night, asking in minute detail about what had been done. If conditions were not satisfactory, he'd ask the interne *why* he had not relieved the pressure by numerous punctures, and if they had been done, he'd ask the blood-pressure or symptoms noted. Woe to the interne or nurse who couldn't answer *which* arm or leg the patient had moved, or in which *direction* the eyes were turned!
>
> Words like the following were never spared, – 'Dr. – just *why* did you take up this line of work, if you are not sufficiently interested to watch the symptoms more closely.' Sometimes the interne would be called at intervals for punctures or symptoms for two or three nights, catching sleep at intervals, and in the morning be required to assist at Operations as usual. Dr. Cushing in times of stress, never saved himself or spared his assistants, by word or deed.

One of his assistants, William Sharpe, remembered a horrible contretemps with Cushing over postoperative care. When Sharpe attempted to hold a nurse partly responsible for the problem, Cushing snapped at him, 'Don't blame it on the nurse. You're yellow!' They nearly came to blows, but patched it up the next day.[23]

He liked to work on holidays when there was no competition for the operating room. Roy McClure, subbing for one of Cushing's men in 1908, remembered spending an alleged holiday holding retractors from morning to late afternoon as Cushing did three ganglionectomies. Other assistants spent their days off wrestling with articles in foreign languages – Cushing expected them to read science in any language – or checking footnotes in their draft articles for fear that he would get to the library and check them first.[24]

There was sometimes no sound for hours on end in Cushing's operating room. 'If assistants moved unnecessarily or if a head turned aside,'

Jacobson remembered, 'Cushing would mutter "Keep your eyes on the wound; keep your eyes on the ball."' Another assistant recalled having been startled when blood suddenly squirted into his eye. 'Dr. Cushing remarked without looking up, "That was a bad reflex." "Well," I said, "Dr. Cushing what *should* I do when blood squirts in my eye?" Without looking up he retorted, "Shut your eye."'[25]

A Cushing performance was artistic, and he knew it. He told his men that surgery was hand work, just as precious carving was hand work. Almost ritualistically, he insisted on shaving the patient's head himself, draping the patient's head himself, and doing his own closing. He was especially pleased if there were no blood stains on the drapes when the operation ended. The younger men noticed his conservatism in resisting mechanical innovations, such as electric drills for trephining. When he finally did convert it was a minor sensation. His students of course joked about how any bad luck they had with a case was blamed on their bad surgery while things that went wrong with Cushing's cases were acts of God.[26] In fact, no one was harder on himself when he lost a patient than Cushing was. Gods dislike making judgment errors.

To the staff of the hospital, Cushing was the crotchety perfectionist who was making their lives miserable with all the brain cases he attracted and his almost eccentric attitudes about their care. Probably from his early interest in intestinal asepsis, he had pronounced ideas about patient food intake and evacuation. The hospital staff were expected to make sure his patients' bowels moved regularly, and Cushing always checked the defecation charts. A bad chart led to a severe reprimand: 'He would say, and I think with conviction, that any house officer responsible for such a record on the defecation chart was careless, irresponsible, and would never make a good doctor.' He was acting on an apparently well-founded belief that straining at stool – say, to relieve constipation – could have serious and even fatal consequences for patients with certain brain conditions.[27]

Cushing insisted that his patients be served an egg (preferably softboiled), bacon, toast, and marmalade every day for breakfast. The marmalade was to be faintly bitter. They were to have a purée of spinach at

lunch and prunes stewed in senna tea at supper. Samuel Crowe remembered how after a hard day's work Cushing flew into a range when he
learned that Crowe had forgotten to order the spinach for a certain
patient: 'I reacted with an equal rage, said I had done the best I could
to help him and to carry out his orders, and that I would pack my bags
at once and leave the Johns Hopkins Hospital and Baltimore forever.
Immediately Doctor Cushing clapped me on the back and said in the
most fatherly way: "Sam, forget it. Do you think I would waste my time
talking to you if I didn't think you were worth it?"'[28]

The medical students heard stories of his sharp temper and driving
manner, but for those who did not work under him Cushing seemed
simply to be one of the great men – perhaps the very greatest now that
Osler was gone – at America's very greatest medical school and hospital. His brilliance was already legendary. Many who met him outside
the hospital grind found him charming, considerate, and extraordinarily wide-ranging. A few wondered how to reconcile their experience of
an erudite gentleman with their friends' dislike of an overbearing dicta-
tor. Nurse Adams and others argued that all of Dr Cushing's demands
were made in the interests of his patients. Another nurse told McClure
how Cushing would be cross and peevish in the operating room, 'but at
the end of the long day, he would turn to them with a smile, saying that
they must be very tired, and this smile would more than make up for all
their trials and tribulations.'[29]

And there were those kind invitations to tea at Dr and Mrs Cushing's
home, sometimes even on Sunday afternoons. On the weekends Dr
Cushing usually made it home for tea, though sharply at four o'clock
he would excuse himself and go to his study to work. He still liked to
play sports and occasionally challenged his assistants to a set or two of
tennis. He played with the same determination to win that he displayed
in the operating room.

A Baltimore surgeon, Bertram Bernheim, who had worked in the
Hunterian Laboratory and knew him well, summarized Cushing in these
years as 'a tough hombre,' the kind of man you could work with, admire, and respect, but not one you would like:

Not many men down here liked him – not, that is, in the way they liked Dr. Finney. He rode roughshod over them and was ruthless. Yet he had his moments and could be as charming and delightful as anyone else. Only there weren't many such moments – chiefly, I suspected, because he was so tense and so occupied in mind with so many different things at one and the same time. I could never understand how he stood it all – physically. Yet tired, jumpy, bitterly critical, frightfully busy, if you caught him just right he'd give you hours of his time and spare no pains to orient and instruct you.

Tough hombre. Yeah, but one of America's immortals.[30]

It was Kate, of course, who saw and lived with all sides of Harvey, Kate who, as Grace Osler put it, had the 'privilege' of having married him. While he worked, she was expected to raise the children and manage the household, supply a shoulder for him to lean on when he was professionally despondent, and be hostess to visiting dignitaries, students, and surgical colleagues. In the long summers, when Baltimore heat was unbearable, Kate had to do all of this – except the socializing – at a distance, usually from Little Boars Head on the New Hampshire shore, while Harvey worked in Baltimore and attended medical meetings.

Here is Kate with the three small children at 'LBH' in June 1909. The baby, Betsey, comes down with something like whooping cough. How much help is her doctor husband? 'Your letter about the w-coughing just came' Harvey writes, 'I have only a second to answer before going to Wilmington to see poor Dr. Green who has a broken back from an automobile accident. So there are worse things than whoops, dear Peaches, though they are bad enough. Cheer up. I am sure everything will pass out all right. If Betsey has it we all have had it probably and it's been a pretty mild dose thank Heaven.'

Kate had to manage the household accounts. Harvey knew he could be a scold – the hemorrhoids that afflicted him in the spring of 1909 could not have soothed his disposition – but he could not seem to stop himself from nagging her about money and bills:

> Peaches you know how I hate this sort of thing. I don't see how you could have mistaken your bank acc't to this extent. If there is one thing in this world to be punctillious about its the *prompt!* payment of debts. It troubles me more or less all the time to feel that you let your bills lie about unpaid ... Whenever you are behind you can come to me and get funds as you know but this pushing off of settlements until the last minute when there is no wherewithal to meet them is paralyzing and destroys your and my credit with the bank and trades people ... Its poor economy as well as a bad principle. It's one of the things I want firmly grounded in the childrens minds as they grow up.

Possibly to have more time with her husband, Kate left the children with the Goodwillies and accompanied him on a six-week European junket in the late summer of 1909. Typically, he found he could not make it to Little Boars Head before their sailing date. But he did have his hemorrhoids removed – his barnacles scraped, as he put it – and had recovered his equanimity after one of the most strenuous years of his life. Aboard the *Lusitania* he bounced back nicely, Kate reported to her mother, adding that for her part she always felt like a caged lion on these voyages.[31]

In England they went sightseeing together, visited the Oslers, and dined on pigeon pie at the Cheshire Cheese. It almost worked for Kate: 'Harvey is enjoying it all so much and I am too – only I can't quite lose that sense of uneasiness – I thought I was going to – I simply *ache* for the children.' On the Continent he was a tireless traveler and surprised her by never getting cross or flustered. While he haunted bookshops 'and did his Doctor business,' Kate cultivated an interest in Dutch interiors and art, and polished her skill at smiling politely and being pleasant. Harvey took her to his old haunts in Berne, where they visited the Kochers and Kroneckers before moving on to Budapest and the Sixteenth International Medical Congress, where he gave his paper on his first surgical treatment of acromegaly. 'My! Harvey is a big man over here!' Kate exclaimed to her mother.[32]

Harvey considered the congress a great success, and Kate found the whole week 'a mad whirl of gayety.' They moved on to Italy for more rubbernecking, shopping, book buying, and good eating. 'We are full of Savonarola, Andreas, Botticelli, spagetti, Medicis, fromage cum fungi, figs, which are ripe and good – true of all the fruit – Strozzis Palazzo, costale con spinache, and Filippo Lippi,' Harvey wrote to his father from the Grand Hotel in Florence. 'Still, not so confused as the inebriate who asked a London "bobby" – "Scuse me, is this Bond Street or Wednesday."'[33]

When they landed back in America, Harvey went to Baltimore and Kate went to the children at Little Boars Head. Betsey had got over her coughing and, according to her mother, was 'more beautiful than the day.' Although Harvey had not seen his youngest child for about four months, he took Kate's word for it. A year earlier, Kate had commented hopefully to her father-in-law that Harvey took more interest in Betsey than in either of the other two children.[34] On this trip she became pregnant with their fourth child, Henry, born in May 1910.

The American medical world's interest in Cushing came to a head early in 1910 in an intense competition to lure him away from Hopkins. As Americans liked to say in those days, big men were on the verge of doing big things, in medicine as in many other areas of life. Harvey Cushing, America's most brilliant surgeon, would be one of the biggest catches of all for an ambitious medical school.

Everyone with a big vision of the future of medicine in the United States based it on the model of Johns Hopkins, the finest product of which was Harvey Cushing himself. At Hopkins, whose initial growing pains had long since receded, a great medical school was based in a great hospital, supported by a great university. All were dedicated to excellence, and the frontier of excellence was the creation of new knowl-

edge through research, both pure and applied. Hopkins's lavish endowment helped create an environment rich in personnel, rich in laboratories, rich in time for study and research, and rich and comfortable in
the spirit of inquiry. The medical and philanthropic leaders of the United
States and Canada – vast, wealthy countries – wanted to build more
institutions just like Hopkins. In his well-publicized 1910 report to the
Carnegie Foundation on the state of North American medical education, educator Abraham Flexner weighed every school against the
Hopkins model. He challenged every faculty and every community to
rise to Hopkins-like standards or give up and close down.

Even before he published his report, Flexner, a Midwesterner, was in
cahoots with the Midwesterner who ran most of the Carnegie philan-
thropies, Henry S. Pritchett, to promote the building of a great medical
school in the great city at the heart of the continent, St Louis, Missouri.
The powers behind Washington University, especially the dynamic St
Louis merchant Robert Brookings, were eager to transform their sec-
ond-rate medical faculty into the Johns Hopkins of the Southwest. The
way to do it was to use Brookings's enthusiasm and money to build a
new hospital and to recruit the best physicians and surgeons they could
possibly find. In January 1910 Cushing was summoned by telegram to a
meeting at the Carnegie Foundation in New York. Brookings, Flexner,
Pritchett, and David Edsall – an outstanding professor of therapeutics
who was being plucked from Philadelphia to be dean and impresario of
the Washington faculty – presented him with their vision and offered
him the chair of surgery. He could virtually write his own ticket. Would
he move west?

'Very alluring but rather sudden. Kate rather limp about it,' Harvey
wrote to his father. Still, the irrepressible and undoubtedly committed
Brookings was almost impossible to resist, and the time had probably
come in Harvey's career to move on. He was formally subordinate to
Halsted at Hopkins and was having trouble with the hospital about the
large numbers of beds he required for all his patients.[35] Two weeks after
this meeting, he had the great surgical triumph of the Leonard Wood
operation.

Sadly, immediately after that event he was called to Cleveland where his father lay gravely ill; he died on February 12, of strokes and heart failure, at the age of eighty-two. On the last day of his life Dr Kirke told his family, 'I do not know what will happen, but it is all right for I have already said all that I wished to say about everything.' In his will he left his substantial properties to his children, who several years earlier had created the H.K. Cushing Research Laboratory at Western Reserve University in his honor. Osler wrote Harvey that his father had had a fine life, with nothing to regret, and 'a son after his own heart ... It is a great thing to come of such good stock.' He urged Cushing to look over the St Louis ground very carefully before making up his mind.[36]

Harvard Medical School, which already considered itself a great institution, had its own Hopkins-like planning well underway. The principal innovation was to be a new university-affiliated hospital, endowed by the estate of the millionaire merchant Peter Bent Brigham. The assumption that Harvey Cushing would eventually get an offer from Harvard had been current for years. Word of the St Louis possibility, and perhaps of Cushing's achievement with Leonard Wood, now galvanized the Bostonians. At the end of March, President A. Lawrence Lowell of Harvard told Cushing that an offer was being drafted. When it came it was for the head of surgery at the new Brigham Hospital, with the understanding that Cushing would also succeed Maurice Richardson as the Moseley Professor of Surgery at Harvard.

Cushing weighed his options 'in great turmoil' through the spring of 1910. He was having to choose, both socially and medically, between the wide-open opportunities of the West and the conservative culture of the East. He could have anything he wanted in St Louis, where they were, in effect, starting anew. 'Come to us and be as free as the Prairie air,' Brookings wrote. 'Organize your department to suit yourself and have the whole western & southwestern country back of you.'

In Boston he would either have to fit into an established system, rich in tradition and slow to change, or he would have to find a way of changing it. 'The Boston folk are queer cattle,' brother Ned wrote, 'and I can imagine many an annoying and disturbing factor in organizing a surgical department there.' Despite his Harvard medical degree, Harvey would be an outsider in a town where birth still mattered a lot, medically as well as socially (his friend Allie Porter, for example, was an eighth-generation physician), where clinical research was still neglected, and where hospital and other institutional rivalries had deep roots. The Harvard Medical School was not Johns Hopkins: it had less money, less 'geist,' many more conflicts about curriculum and priorities, and was having to compromise its formal, Hopkins-like admission standards in order to attract students.[37]

Many of Cushing's friends, both inside and outside Boston, counted on him as the newcomer who would shake up the staid Harvard ways. J. Collins Warren, a Boston medical brahmin hoping to undermine tradition, told Harvey he would be their 'surgical Messiah' in building up 'a great and ideal medical university.' A former classmate, Joe Pratt, told him he would be 'the Joshua to lead us into the Promised Land.' W.T. Councilman, a crusty outsider in Boston, had for years championed the former student to whom he had given perfect marks. Young stars at Harvard, such as psychologist Robert Yerkes and the physiologist Walter B. Cannon, hoped he would come and support their interest in change. He was warned, though, to spell out all his requirements before agreeing to come, because afterwards it would be difficult.[38]

While Ned Cushing was noncommittal in his advice to Harvey, the Oslers, both William and the very Bostonian Grace, emphatically urged him to choose Harvard. The crunch came at the end of April: Harvey was at the train station to go to meetings in Boston when Brookings and the chancellor of Washington University intercepted him to display blueprints of their proposed hospital. He got to Boston, was pushed to exhaustion operating on patients there (a rare breaking of his 'home turf only' rule), and was followed home on the train by other Bostonians pleading the case for coming to Harvard. Then he was met in Baltimore by Midwesterners pleading for St Louis. Some of his Hopkins colleagues, notably William Welch and the psychiatrist Adolf Meyer, tried to persuade him to stay in Baltimore – but Johns Hopkins did not try nearly as hard to keep him as Cushing thought he might reasonably expect.[39]

He procrastinated for a few more weeks but in mid-May finally decided: 'I wish to announce my engagement to Miss Peter Bent Brigham.' Looking back on the situation a few years later, he noted that David Edsall's decision to jump ship from St Louis that spring and stay in Philadelphia had been a factor. So had his father's death, which greatly upset him. Ultimately, while he had Midwestern roots, most of the United States that he was familiar with was on the eastern seaboard. 'St. Louis seemed very far away,' he noted. Most of his friends thought he had made the right decision. Only Brookings grumbled that he had chosen Harvard's 'prestige and marble buildings' over the open-minded and enthusiastic institutions in St Louis. Cushing had turned his back on the idea of moving farther west, as his New England ancestors had done. He would settle in Boston.[40]

Boston and Harvard did not prove to be exactly the Cushings' cup of tea, but Harvey had probably made the right choice. Washington University's medical faculty in St. Louis went through a period of intense conflict and turmoil, failing to fulfill its promoters' aspirations for many years. It is hard to imagine Cushing lasting for more than a year or two there. David Edsall of Philadelphia had the misfortune to change his mind again, took a chair of preventive medicine at Washington in 1911, and within a year became so disillusioned that he too landed in Boston. Ironically, the role Edsall ultimately played at Harvard would add to Cushing's frustrations.

∾

The Cushings did not move to Boston until the Peter Bent Brigham Hospital was much further advanced in construction, more than two years later, in September 1912. Kate Cushing is the nearly invisible principal in the story of Harvey's indecision. Except for her early doubts about St Louis, the sources are silent on her views.

Mild biographical mystery envelops both Harvey and Kate in the

summer and autumn of 1910. With two possible and important exceptions (undated letters that appear to have been misplaced in 1911 files),
there are no communications between husband and wife in that period, in fact hardly any letters at all signed by either of them. Kate
seems to have gone to Little Boars Head, though, and Harvey's operating records show that he was sometimes in Baltimore. He may also
have gone to Europe.

It seems to have been a time of serious strain in their marriage. In
one of the undated letters, written from Little Boars Head, Kate offers a
few pleasantries and then says, 'Now, I'm going to complain a little.'
She complains a lot, revealing all the cracks in their marriage, all her
frustrations. Here is the price that the Cushing family was paying for
Harvey's career:

> I hate such long separations. I remember your saying once before we were
> married that it was a good thing for married people to have plenty of vaca-
> tions away from each other. I think so too – many and short. It seemed to me
> that we were completely out of touch. You weren't a bit interested in any of
> my concerns, aside from the children's affairs. And I may have seemed indif-
> ferent to your affairs. I don't see how it is possible to avoid such a condition
> when there are long separations and when you said something about your
> going to Boston and my staying in Baltimore, my heart sank into my boots.
> Peaches, don't you know that we have got to do it together? Is it necessary
> that we should be apart in order to make the move to Boston? In both going
> to a strange place to live, unless we make our interests one, unless we talk to
> each other, and take a little pain with each other, it's going to be perfectly
> ghastly.
>
> And I'm sort of scared. I'm not going to have Mary [Goodwillie], I'm not
> going to get intimate with any one right away, and if you aren't interested in
> me, I have no one. You were not interested in me one bit – when you were
> here – there wasn't a thing you cared to talk about with me – You like to talk
> to Mrs. Goodwillie & Mary – so do I – we fled to them whenever we could
> – If we haven't even the little affairs of daily life to draw us together, as we
> wouldn't have during any long separation we would simply drift further and

further apart – you absorbed in your work. I – in my work and possibly somebody else who happened to be interested in me a little. I don't mean any nonsense you know that, but it's too easy to get into the habit of turning to some one person for a little human interest.

I thought about it all last night, and then decided to tell you, because last spring you told me to tell you things. Why I couldn't any more have told you when you were here! An absolute pall descended over me I couldn't speak. You never spoke but to criticize. You couldn't have realized it. I have *wrastled* with Billy and Betsey all summer. I have put my whole mind and all my energy in looking after the children mentally morally and physically – not one word of commendation did you give me – nothing but little critical remarks and you thought me very touchy and ill tempered I think, when I was trying to bear them ... I couldn't talk to you Harvey – you weren't interested.

There are so many wretched marriages – people tugging apart, instead of trying to pull together. It seems as though I couldn't bear it to have ours go that way. I have tried so hard – fought so many battles with my own evil moods and jealousies sometimes won sometimes not, but this sort of gradually drifting apart – each one self sufficient without the other – I can't do this alone – we've got to do it together.

I'm scared about the winter I don't want to go home very much. Everything is dust and ashes to me unless I have your interest your sympathy and help. I don't lean heavily on you. I don't lean heavily enough – and this separation business isn't safe. Those long silent dinners – when no one is there – not the silence of understanding, but the silence of constraint. And that after being away until seven o'clock – from nine in the morning. No more nice afternoon teas that I looked forward to all day, with you coming in and sitting on your stool – You don't realize how little you were at home all last winter and spring. I didn't realize how Willy and I missed your coming. I can't stand it Peaches this winter if it's like that. I try to fill up my life as other people do, with women friends and with the children – but its awfully dry bones when you grow more and more absorbed and silent – more uninterested and indifferent. Why I'd be a different woman if you ever gave me a word of commendation for anything – a sympathetic pat on the back. One thing I'm going to do, and that is to do some outside work. Some charity organization work or something of that sort. Please don't think I'm criticizing and blaming you – but I truly don't want you to slip away from me – and I don't want to slip away from you – Your own girl.[41]

A letter of Harvey's, which apparently refers to this letter, is very gloomy:

An awful day – hot and muggy – a bad ganglion case – several foreign visitors on my chest – patients throwing fits at unfortunate moments – people who want to be put to work – a shortage of dogs for the Hunterian – patients who need attention – a cold in the head – and not the least your depressing letter ... My desk is piled high with things undone. I think I'll give it up and crawl off somewhere to die. 'In his 42nd year a young man of great promise &c' Only you would know that he gave up because he had bitten off more than he could chew – alone.[42]

To compound the mystery, Cushing's comings and goings in July, August, and September 1910 are murky. He was operating at the hospital from time to time but otherwise disappears from the record. His official biographer John Fulton presumed, on the basis of a few paragraphs which Cushing wrote years later, that he went abroad that summer on the Society of Clinical Surgery's excursion to the United Kingdom. In fact, he was not on that trip. His name is not on the lists of attendees in the Crile Papers, nor is it mentioned in their travel diaries, and a letter of Osler's indicates that he was not present when Osler entertained the group at Oxford. We have no letters from Harvey to Kate or anyone else that summer, and no travel diary.[43]

It was one of the most stressful times of Cushing's life. He mentions in one of his memoirs how upset he was after his father's death. He had been working at an astonishing and constantly accelerating pace for years. Friends worried about whether his health could stand up. At times, he did too: 'I wish something would force me into a few months vacation and rest,' he wrote around 1909.[44] Most of his life he had been prone to short periods of depression, a pattern that recurred in his later years. Now he was at mid-life and had made a major, extremely diffi-

cult decision to relocate from Baltimore to Boston. His wife was showing signs of deep unhappiness in their marriage.

There is no explicit evidence that Cushing faltered in his routines –
but the absence of his usual high volume of mail, and the nearly total
absence of letters to Kate, is suggestive. The Cushings may have gone
through a major reconsideration of the terms of their marriage. Harvey
may have gone off by himself somewhere in the United States or Europe. There is an outside possibility that he had some form of break-
down that summer of 1910, perhaps a period of depression, perhaps
just a long period of rest and seclusion before pulling himself back together. He would have deliberately covered up any signs of cracks in
his public façade. As a surgeon, as a brain surgeon, and as a Cushing,
he would have been determined not to show weakness or failure. (About
this time, according to the memoirs of the psychiatrist and psychoana-
lyst Ernest Jones, Cushing consulted him in Toronto, but only about his
anxieties before operating; Jones may have misremembered or Cushing
may have been fishing for help.)[45]

There is no evidence that anything changed in Harvey and Kate's
relationship as a result of the airing of grievances or whatever passing
depression he may have suffered. Perhaps they understood one another and the terms of their marriage a little more clearly. In June
1911 Kate was again left at Little Boars Head while Harvey went on a
journey by train across the continent to medical meetings on the West
Coast – his first trip to California. He wrote her his usual observant
and sometimes affectionate notes, describing the wonderful natural
beauty of the landscape and his distaste for high society and the need
to dress for dinner.[46]

There had been yet another blow a few months earlier that year.
'Neddie is dying in a near room in a most beautiful and ecstatic euthanasia,' Harvey wrote on March 22, 1911. His forty-eight-year-old brother
had inoperable bowel cancer. All Harvey could do was compile a written record of Ned's last days, his 'very Cushing' calm approach to death
('euthanasia' was used to describe a good death), and his hope that
Ned's physician's 'touch' would pass on to his son, Pat.

Pray God he has for it must go on somewhere – too rare to be lost in any family that has it. Some Cushing doctor of the next generation may know what I mean – the thing that puts a patient almost immediately under your control and in your confidence with a trust that fails not. I can see that [George] Crile doesn't have it – fine as he is and fond as Ned is of him – Pat at 13 quieted him in a moment, George and the others – all falling over themselves in devotion – made him jumpy. This is something quite apart from the spirit of research which is in our modern type.

Until Pat was trained in medicine, Harvey would be the last of the Cushing doctors. He thought Ned, a brilliant and totally dedicated professional, a general practitioner who had become one of the most popular and respected, civic-spirited, doctors in Cleveland, was the best physician he had ever known.[47]

Anticipating that Harvey would be in despair after Ned's loss, Amory Codman wrote him, 'You have gone so far now that you are responsible to mankind and have got to go on and work whether your best friends are here to help or not.' Over in England, Osler worried that Cushing habitually carried too much sail: 'He gets an extraordinary amount of work out of himself and others, and it would be a thousand pities if he broke down.' Harvey's close friend Jim Mumford advised him to temper his ambition and learn to relax: 'Don't, don't forget how to play.'[48]

～

Cushing played vigorous games of tennis for exercise, while otherwise drowning his sorrows in more work – especially his pituitary studies – and in preparing for the move from Baltimore to Boston. One of the many issues he had to deal with was personnel. Which of his eager young assistants would he invite to follow him from Baltimore to Boston?

If he had been going to St Louis, perhaps the most natural fit would have been Walter Dandy. Dandy, who would eventually become Cushing's bitter rival and the second-most important figure in American neurosurgery, hailed from the railway town of Sedalia, Missouri, and in his youth was as unformed and ambitious as the West itself. His parents, John and Rachel Dandy, were immigrants from England who had come to America in the 1880s. Rachel was a dressmaker, John a railwayman. Neither had much in the way of formal education. The Dandys owned a modest home in a blue-collar neighborhood, worshiped as Plymouth Brethren, believed in America as a land of opportunity for people with the grit to challenge the rich and powerful in the race of life (John was always inclined to vote the Socialist ticket), and invested unlimited emotional capital in the prospect that their only child Walter, 'the best and brightest boy on earth,' would become famous and rich.[49]

Walter himself completely internalized, both genetically and culturally, his parents' ambition for him. 'I am what you made me and evolved me,' he told them in 1914. As a little boy he wanted to win every game he played and cried if he lost. He always wanted to get top grades at school – his father once reminded him of how angry he had been when he felt he had been graded unjustly: 'You was defiant and said with rage in your little face I can beat her.' It was something of a refrain in the Dandy home whenever Walter announced, 'The first place is mine' or 'Mama I have got it.'[50] After graduating from Sedalia High School as class valedictorian, he enrolled in a program at the University of Missouri that would have led to a medical degree, then soon aspired to learn at better schools. A finalist in one of the earliest Rhodes Scholarship competitions, he took the advice of William Osler and others and applied to Johns Hopkins, where he was admitted into the second-year medical class in the autumn of 1907.

Dandy seized opportunities to do summer research and at the end of third year asked to work with Cushing. His parents urged him on. 'That Dr Cushing is certainly a great man,' his mother wrote. 'While reading about him and his wonderful operations I felt myself wishing wouldn't I like to hear of my boy doing these wonderful operations. I believe some one someday will say just such grand things about you as you have said about Dr Cushing ... I believe he would be glad to help a young man like you.'[51] In 1910, after disappointing himself by graduating only seventeenth in a class of eighty-five, Dandy landed the plum of being Cushing's research assistant in the Hunterian laboratory – with the prospect of becoming his resident in the hospital the following year.

As Walter began doing dog work in the Hunterian, concentrating on the pituitary studies, everything seemed to go well. He reported to his parents that Dr Cushing 'treats me fine, is very enthusiastic and gives me absolute authority and complete charge. He is so busy operating he doesn't get around much now when in town.' The proud parents assumed that Walter would move to Boston when Cushing did or else would take his place at Hopkins: 'Either is pretty good.'[52]

As Cushing began making typical demands on his time, Dandy responded enthusiastically. 'Dr Cushing came over last night at 6 p.m. just as I was going to supper and said come on Dandy and help us do an autopsy on a baby who died of hydrocephalus. When we got there he said go get your supper. I came back and worked till 10 o'clock, then got up at 7 a.m. and worked until 6 p.m. with about 1/2 hour off for dinner. He seemed very enthusiastic about the work.' Dandy was invited to the Cushing home for a Sunday supper. Cushing said he wanted to beat him at a game of tennis soon. 'I told him I didn't think he could do it.'[53]

Dandy intended to make a mark from the beginning. Early on, he complained to Cushing that one of his predecessors was taking credit for his work. That was quickly smoothed over. Only a few weeks later, in December 1910, he was able to boast to his parents that he had 'stumped' Cushing himself on a procedure the chief thought was impossible:

He was around when I was operating on a dog. Asked me what I was trying to do. I told him to produce a tumor in the aqueduct of Sylvius, one place never before reached, and have the animal live. He says why you can't do that. The animal is sure to die. I said I think I can. About an hour later I called him, showed him how I did it. He was tickled and got extremely enthusiastic. Said it was wonderful and called in a couple of doctors to see it. I asked him if he had ever done it. He said my no, no one ever had nerve to try such a thing and beamed all over. He sure was tickled. I told him we would develop a method of examining the interior of the brain by means of a light and this catherization of the aqueduct of Sylvius. He smiled a little and hesitated to say anything.

He is preparing a Harvey Lecture in New York, the biggest in this country. Quite an honor for him. He is great. [54]

This event had momentous consequences. Under Cushing's direction, Dandy's work on pituitary secretion had segued into an interest in the circulation of the cerebrospinal fluid – the clear, colorless, watery liquid that bathes the brain. Neurologists still had little idea how it moved through the brain, from production to reabsorption or drainage back into the bloodstream. It was obviously important to begin to understand this circulation, not least because blockages of the fluid's flow cause its excessive accumulation, the usually fatal condition known as hydrocephalus, or 'water on the brain,' and other deformities, such as spina bifida.

Cushing thought that knowledge of the cerebrospinal circulation was about as primitive as the understanding of blood flow had been before William Harvey's work. He had been puzzling about it ever since his days in Berne. At Hopkins, Lewis Reford had begun to work on aspects of the problem with Franklin P. Mall as early as 1904. There were huge experimental obstacles, though, such as the problem of finding ways of manipulating the channels through which the fluid moved. In a technical masterstroke, this is what young Dandy had achieved with his 'tumor' (actually, a cotton pledget), which he was able to insert to block the midbrain canal that connects the third and fourth ventricles.[55] That Dandy in his exuberance also thought he could get a light into the canal, illuminating the interior of the brain, no doubt caused Cushing's slight smile – though in a strange way, as we shall see, it became one of the most prophetic comments in the history of neurosurgery. For now, it hardly mattered that the kid from the Missouri semi-pro league was boasting about great things to come. The fact was that he had made a home run in his first turn at bat in the research league.

Walter's mother cautioned him to be wary about the frustration he would inevitably feel working with such a hard master as Cushing: 'Don't let anything come between you and Cushing that would spoil your future. His wonderful operations must be very trying on his quick irritable temper so you must overlook his temper. It is the great strain of his work that makes him so irritable. Probably you would be the same if in his position ... Why I am saying these things is I was afraid you might let your temper get the best of you and quit.'[56]

Dandy held his temper, though there were several difficult incidents during his year at the Hunterian. Years later, Dandy remembered how he had delighted Cushing by telling him that their experiments stimulating certain nerves had produced glycosuria. Only after Cushing had heralded the accomplishment did Dandy think to add that experiments with severed nerves, as a control, seemed to do the same thing – whereupon Cushing wounded him with a sarcastic comment of the 'Nobody but you, Dandy ...' variety. Other residents remembered Dandy and Cushing clashing over similarly minor matters, largely because their personalities were so alike.[57] They also disagreed on the significance of Dandy's artificial 'tumor'. Walter thought the experimental hydrocephalus he had produced was identical to the main form of the disease in humans, but Cushing, who had a different theory of hydrocephalus, doubted it. He may also have criticized some of Dandy's ideas about where to take the research. But the friction was not enough to deter Cushing from advancing Dandy to be his chief clinical assistant during the 1911–12 year. A comment to Kate that 'Dandy still smacks his lips and eats with his knife' suggests that Cushing was more concerned about his resident's social rather than surgical skills.[58]

'Glad you have such good work and do so well as first asst. that Dr Cushing does not cuss you,' Walter's father wrote in the autumn of 1911. 'That is getting pretty near the top,' his mother added. 'I am looking forward to the time when Dr W.E. Dandy will be the biggest man in the U.S.A.'[59]

Dandy was an enthusiastic baseball player who would take any risk in an effort to win. In the spring of 1912 he leapt for a fly ball and smashed his valedictory watch and nearly smashed himself against an outfield wall. That same season in the operating room at Johns Hopkins he was exactly like a rookie ballplayer waiting for his chance to show his stuff and take away someone's starting job. He measured himself against Cushing and assumed that if he did well, Cushing would be chagrined. So did his parents, his fanatical supporters. Rachel Dandy to Walter, 1912: 'Never satisfied with all these years of hearing of your great success. Still wanted to hear *more, more, more*. Never satisfied, I guess till we hear of you being No. 1 in the USA. Not Cushing's equal but his superior.' John Dandy to Walter, 1912: 'He may have taught you but it won't be long till you surpass him and, instead of you chasing him for the chance to get to work for him, he will be watching the world give you the chief honor. You will be coming before the crowned heads and International Congress of Sciences as a leader of science and art.'[60]

Dandy began to get his chance in the spring of 1912. In remarkable letters to his parents, he gushed and boasted and worried about his successes and how Cushing might react to them. The first case was an English sailor, suffering from severe epileptic seizures after a fall. According to Dandy, Cushing said the case was untreatable and recommended institutionalization:

I told him I took an interest in the boy and wished he would try and see what he could do. He said well you can try it if you want to. I did and so far the boy is perfectly well, has not had another convulsion. If he should get well it would be a wonderful thing, something which is almost unknown.

It is only 3 days now and while I feel good, am almost afraid to believe it, and hoping. I told Cushing he was doing well and he tried to throw cold water on me but I refuse to yield until shown. I don't think he has ever cured an epileptic. Everyone is astonished at the result so far. But it is too soon to crow. It was a very delicate operation in the most difficult part of the brain, where the largest vessels are present and the very smallest touch improperly placed or slip of the knife would have meant fatal bleeding. But slowly the thing cleared up without any bad effects. It took about 2 hours to free the adhesions which were clinging to the brain and which had to be very carefully separated. Had many an anxious moment, expecting at any time to stir up a haemorrhage which might be fatal. Of course it would look pretty bad for a beginner to have had any serious trouble, and fortunately it pulled out well.

If the result is good, he may be more careful about letting me have any more cases, as it reflects a little on him. He did not expect when he gave me the case, to have me take any such chances as I did, but since he was not there, I went ahead on my own responsibility. I certainly hope the boy gets well. Something which is scarcely known to happen. And which I have never seen happen.

The sailor apparently recovered. 'Dr C. had better look well to his laurals or robes or they will be placed on the young surgical king,' John Dandy exulted. Walter soon had another triumph, of sorts, and was so competitive that he could not resist being pleased when Cushing's cases went comparatively badly:

This has been a great week for me and a hard one for Dr Cushing. My Epileptic boy has not had any more attacks and is going away tomorrow ...

Dr Cushing gave me another big case, one of the hardest and biggest brain operations. It turned out to be the most wonderful case we have seen this year ...

The thing that pleases me most was the fact that there were three cases almost alike in the hospital at the same time. Dr Cushing operated on two and gave me the third to do myself ... He didn't find anything in his 2 cases and I found this most remarkable condition in mine. But the best of it was both his cases did so badly that he had to go in and operate a second time on account of a blood clot formation but mine did splendidly and is still doing so. As you see the big men do not always do the best work. If I had done what he did it would have been sufficient excuse to have never given me anything more to do. But I was very fortunate. He may not give me so much now because they are talking some about the difference which does not look so good to him.[61]

The string of triumphs continued. Dandy would be in awe of Cushing on one day, then try to match him the next – like ballplayers in a hitting contest:

> Well this has been the most wonderful day and the most wonderful week I have yet put in. Today Dr Cushing removed a tumor as large as a big orange from a man's head and he is still living and going to get well. It's one of the most successful cases on record. It left a tremendous hole in his brain ... It was a very spectacular thing to see Dr Cushing pull this big tumor out of the man's brain and still live with half his skull gone in addition ...
>
> I have done 3 big operations myself ... One of them was a very severe operation about as difficult as it is possible to get ... It is the case Dr Cushing started to do two different times and something happened each time, so I think he thought it might be hoodooed. But I sailed into it without fear. It took 3½ hours. I began to realize the responsibility on an operators shoulders by the time it was over. I guess I looked pretty well worn and one of our private patients said she was glad her husband was not a doctor as I looked like I had gone through a lot of responsibility. It is quite a strain, a good deal like the strain on an engineer with his cargo of human freight behind him. Dr Cushing has certainly been good to me and I think I have justified his confidence if he had any.[62]

Dandy continued his research on cerebrospinal fluid and hydrocephalus. He began to inject colored liquid into the brain's cavities to study the fluid's movement. He hoped to prove that Cushing's views about its circulation and blockages were wrong.[63] While this work was proceeding fitfully, Dandy wondered where his immediate future lay. Would Cushing invite him to Boston? Would it be better to stay at Johns Hopkins? Should he get some training either there or somewhere else in general surgery (for he had leapfrogged directly into working on the brain)? There were opportunities in St Louis and Detroit – should he move west? Cushing was characteristically noncommittal about the future, and in June 1912 he went to Europe for six weeks without giving Dandy any hint about what would happen that autumn.

Cushing's absence from the game was the rookie's ultimate opportunity, and by his account – these are some of the most fascinating letters in the history of surgery – he took absolutely maximum advantage of it. Walter Dandy to his parents, July 14, 1912:

> I have had a bully week as far as operations are concerned. Have done 3 or 4 this week. One a hypophysis. Cushing's hardest and most delicate operation and so far this man is doing nicely, though too soon to crow. Imagine Cushing looking at me in resentment and disdain when he finds I have done a hypophysis operation and got away with it. Never had a bit of trouble and did it almost as quickly as he does it. This is the operation where you go back through the nose to the middle of the head. The least deviation from the normal course will lead you to the wrong place and may mean death. The hypophysis is about the size of the tip of your little finger and drilling back to the center of the head to find it is no easy task. The men looked at me in amazement when I posted the operation. Why that was something no one but almighty Cushing would think of doing. They came around to see it. It was as pretty as anything he ever did. I think there is a world record in a man of 26 doing the operation.
>
> I slipped another over him last week. A man with a big brain tumor came in to see him a year ago and he wanted to operate then but the man refused and now came back to have him do it, but he was in Europe. He wanted to wait. I persuaded him not to wait. He said he didn't know anything about me and he did Dr Cushing ... His wife and six children came up next day and begged me guarantee he would not die and would come out alright ... I knew he [Cushing] could not do it any better than I could (in my own conceit) though I was not anxious for the responsibility. The delay was bad for him so I did it. I ran into a great big tumor, great big blood vessels etc. The least little moving or false move meant death almost certainly. It was the hardest operation I have yet had. The tumor was of a kind which could not be removed. But it relieved him of all his symptoms and saved his eyesight as well as Cushing could have done himself ...
>
> Well I am about to slip another over on him next week ... an operation on the backbone. This is another of Cushing's exclusive operations. I think I

will do it in a couple of days rather than wait until he comes back. Gee won't he be sore to think a young sprout is stealling his thunder. I won't tell him much about them when he comes back. I am not at all boastful ...

Dr Geotsch was very much surprised when I was going to do the operation. I showed it to him when I was through. He said, well it isn't so exclusive after all as he would have us believe. He did not have the nerve to do any of these things. Cushing had him bulldoged. I feel as though I can do most any operation that Cushing does now ...

Did I tell you about Dr Cushing leaving a piece of cotton in a womans neck at operation. The wound broke down and has been discharging ever since, about 2 months ago. He went to Europe and left her to incur expense and discomfort here until he came back. He remitted her operation fee of $500 but I think they are going to sue him for damages.

Walter Dandy to his parents, July 21, 1912:

Dr Cushing comes back tomorrow, my harvest is over, I am again a servant rather than master but I am young and cannot expect so much. I slipped some over on him this week. I did the broken back man and made a bully job of him ... I did the operation as nicely as ever he did one and almost as quickly. It took two hours. The men stood around amazed at my nerve and talk a great deal about it, giving me numerous compliments ...

The superintendent of the hospital called up soon after to see how the patient got along, also first thing the next morning. Evidently thinking I was treading on dangerous ground but he never said anything to me. Cushing could not have done better ...

If ever I lacked confidence and nerve, I think I have settled that forever. I have done practically everything Cushing does and so far have not had a death or bad result even to the smallest degree; whereas if I had had, I should not feel so very bad because Cushing has made some big ones himself ... Well it is nice to talk a lot about yourself isn't it.

Cushing was apparently not as jealous of Dandy's achievements (such as they were; there is no corroboration or follow-up of his claims) as the twenty-six year old had assumed. The evidence from Cushing's papers is that he was much too busy in the summer of 1912 to pay attention to Dandy. He was putting the finishing touches on his pituitary monograph, packing up for the move to Boston, and learning to drive. Kate and the children were at Little Boars Head.

On the evening of August 26, Cushing did make some time for Dandy and apparently told the young man that he would not be coming to Boston with him. 'He would never do,' Harvey told Kate. 'I've got enough green ones as it is.' This may have been the occasion when Cushing suggested, according to Dandy, that 'I had no imagination, that I was not in the proper environment in the east. I should go west where the requirements were not so high.' There may also have been an incident in the lab about this time when Cushing began packing up Dandy's research notes to take them with him to Boston. Dandy objected that they were his, and Cushing flared up but then dropped the matter with a comment that they probably did not amount to anything anyway.[64]

Dandy and Cushing ended their last day as colleagues with a set of tennis. There were no tie-breakers in those days. The forty-three-year-old surgeon and his twenty-six-year-old assistant played evenly, game after game. Neither could get more than one game up and win the set. After twenty games, the score stood 10–10 and they declared their match a draw.[65]

EIGHT

Adieu the Simple Life

The Cushings were taking their lives and Harvey's career to a new level by moving to Boston. He would have major new professional responsibilities at an important new hospital and at one of America's greatest medical schools. Boston was an intellectual and cultural center in ways that Baltimore would never be. Harvey and Kate would have a place near the upper rung of one of the more exclusive social ladders in America. His surgical prominence would attract patients to his clinic from across the continent. The Cushings would live in a much grander house and own a grand automobile.

'The simple life slips away, alas,' Harvey wrote to Kate in the summer of 1912, dazed with fatigue after staying up all night with a dying senator and then finalizing the deal to buy a $40,000 house in the exclusive suburb of Brookline. The Cushing purchase made news in Boston. Sending Kate a clipping about it, Harvey returned to the theme: 'Adieu the simple life. They will all be saying that we used to be pretty good until we allowed ourselves to slide into a high gear.' Maybe they would get away with it, he joked, if she wore quieter hats and he grew some whiskers to hide behind.[1]

He had no intention of hiding professionally or from the kind of medical socializing he enjoyed. Leap forward exactly one year, to August 1913: Harvey and Kate are in London, the capital of the world's greatest empire, for another professional Olympics, the Seventeenth International Medical Congress. Seven thousand physicians attend from around the world. Royalty and cabinet ministers are among the dozens of speakers at the opening ceremonies. There are banquets, receptions, fêtes, garden parties (the Canadian high commissioner hosts five thousand at his), and conversaziones galore. All the London hospitals entertain. Churches put on special services. There are excursions to Oxford and Cambridge and on the Thames. Osler, now Sir William Osler, baronet, and in the fullness of his stature as Regius Professor of Medicine at Oxford, plays godfather to the congress. He takes a whole floor at Brown's Hotel, and he and Lady Osler entertain guests for ten straight days. 'Every body you ever heard of is in London,' Kate Cushing writes to her mother.[2]

Harvey Cushing is everywhere, usually in the formal dress he normally despises. Fresh from having received an honorary degree from his alma mater, Yale University, he is admitted to honourary fellowship in the Royal College of Surgeons of England. At the professional sessions he gives one presentation on the organs of the internal secretion, another on pituitary diseases, a third on brain tumors. These are small potatoes compared with the major oration he has been invited to give at a plenary session in the Albert Hall, one of only three such congress events. He speaks on 'Realignments in Greater Medicine: Their Effect upon Surgery and the Influence of Surgery upon Them.' It is a sweeping overview of the rise of modern medicine, the flowering of surgery, the growth of specialism, the role of science, experimentation, laboratories, and much more. The brash forty-four-year-old American – astonishingly young to be an elder medical statesman – condemns the 'discouraging blight' put on British medical research by antivivisection legislation, discreetly but pointedly chides his hosts for their slowness in responding to innovation, and names only one institution as a model of surgical excellence – the Mayo Clinic in Rochester, Minnesota.

Cushing's critical comments on British medical education spark controversy in the *Times*. In Osler's view, and that of many of his friends, Harvey is the outstanding figure at the congress. 'This has certainly been the week of our lives!' Kate gushes. 'They all seem to think he's the biggest thing at the Congress!'³ (Kate is furious at being barred by her gender from attending Harvey's induction into the Royal College of Surgeons. She may secretly support the cause of the suffragettes who demonstrate at the congress in favor of votes for British women. Woman's suffrage is also an issue at home in the United States; Harvey is solidly against it). After the congress, Harvey and Kate have a week's holiday with the Oslers in Scotland and then sail home on the *Lusitania*. After they land, Kate goes to Little Boars Head to be with the children, while Harvey stays in Boston to work.

～

Like many high achievers who become celebrities, Cushing blew hot and cold about his prominence, his mood depending on how frazzled he was by his workload. He cherished what for him was the simple life – day after day in the operating room and laboratory, and at his desk. He hated interruptions in his routine, and when overcome by them he became irritable to the point of irresponsibility. From the time it was announced in 1910 that Cushing would leave Baltimore for Boston, planning his professional transplantation was an added strain.

He had so much to wind up at Hopkins, so much to begin in Boston. It was not just a matter of moving his research work – as well as some of his researchers, his practice, and several assistants – but also of handling the duties falling on the chief surgeon of a major new hospital. To start with, the Peter Bent Brigham Hospital had literally to be redesigned.

In many medical and philanthropic minds, including Harvey Cushing's, the aim was to recreate the Johns Hopkins experience in Boston. When Peter Bent Brigham, a classic self-made merchant (who had peddled oysters from a wheelbarrow and amassed millions in real estate) died in 1877, he directed that his estate be allowed to accumulate for twenty-five years and then be used to establish a hospital for the poor folk of Suffolk County, Massachusetts. Thus, 1902 was the magical year when the spending of his benefaction could begin.

Peter Bent Brigham had not seen himself as Boston's answer to Johns Hopkins – his bequest was a smaller sum for a relatively old-fashioned institution – but others were alert to the possibilities. Harvard's Medical School needed to expand, and in the eyes of some of Boston's medical leaders it desperately needed its own teaching hospital. Its working agreements with the independent Massachusetts General Hospital and Boston City Hospital did not always work smoothly, for these institutions were conservative, decentralized, and dominated by tradition. All their appointments went to local men, for example. This meant that Harvard could not recruit outsiders, for it could not guarantee them a hospital berth.

Beginning in the late 1890s, complex discussions at Harvard and with the Brigham trustees finally resulted in a grand plan to relocate the Harvard Medical School on a twenty-six-acre tract of land in the town of Roxbury, southwest of downtown Boston. The Brigham hospital would be built on the same site in the closest possible cooperation with Harvard. Other medical institutions would be welcomed into the family, and a great center of health care would take shape.

Harvard's medical reformers, most notably the surgeon J. Collins Warren, rode a crest of enthusiasm for state-of-the-art medical research, commitment to excellence, and interest in advanced training, the same spirit that had driven Hopkins's success. The new hospital and the medical school would collaborate to advance all these good things. They would be a magnet for first-rate talent, wherever it could be found, and a model of medical education, including a full-fledged residency system. Both medical school and hospital would be richly funded – Harvard went outside the city to enlist financial support from J.P. Morgan and the Rockefellers – and both would have first-rate research facilities. Boston's crust of tradition, parochial contentment, medical inbreeding, and what president A. Lawrence Lowell had called 'promotion by senility' would be broken. Harvard would at least keep pace – in the eyes of many, would maintain its lead – in the American race for medical excellence in the fullest sense of the word.[4]

Winning the competition to employ America's leading surgeon was only one sign of the Brigham-Harvard dynamism. An earlier and equally important appointment was that of Henry A. Christian, a Virginian and Johns Hopkins graduate, to be Physician-in-Chief of the Brigham Hospital. Christian, five years younger than Cushing, was moving laterally, getting back to practice after serving a difficult few years as 'boy dean' of the factious and rather troubled Harvard Medical School. Christian and Cushing knew and liked each other and expected to work well together in giving the new hospital both the structure and the spirit they had soaked up in Baltimore. The éminence grise who had lobbied influentially for both appointments was the former Johns Hopkins pathologist who had been wooed to Boston many years earlier, William T. Councilman. 'Counce' became chief pathologist of the Brigham.

The very bricks and mortar of the Brigham would resemble Johns Hopkins, it seemed. The trustees had hired Hopkins's architect, John Shaw Billings, who designed a structure for them in the same pavilion style as the Baltimore complex. That style had already been out of date when Hopkins was stuck with it in 1889; thus one reason for the delay in actually building the Peter Bent Brigham Hospital was the need to go back to the drawing board and plan a more up-to-date structure. (Another reason for the delay involved lawsuits by Brigham heirs trying to block the marriage to Harvard). Cushing had the opportunity literally to design his new workplace.

Hopkins had been short of money in its early years. So Cushing and Christian both favored skimping on construction in order to conserve endowment money to support the Brigham's operating costs. The two doctors cooperated in cutting out frills and signed on to the 'grandly simple style' of the redesigned Peter Bent Brigham complex: coldly functional red-brick buildings hiding behind an imposing columned façade. From the outside the Brigham looked more like a temple of finance than a hospital, but its homage to classicism complemented the grandiose marble quadrangle that was the new Harvard Medical School. They were – and still are – temples of medicine, temples of health, temples of education, and temples of American wealth, philanthropy, and ambition. 'He found our Medical School brick and left it marble,' the faculty said of President Charles Eliot when it made him an honorary MD.[5]

In the Brigham case, the ambition had become much grander than simply serving the poor of Suffolk County. One of Cushing's very first demands – others also raised the issue – was to expand the mandate of the hospital beyond being a charitable institution. If hospitals were becoming temples of medical salvation, especially through surgery, then everyone had an interest in being able to pass through their gates. The well-to-do could afford to pay for their hospital services, though of course would expect to be well served in special quarters. Most good physicians and surgeons needed hospital accommodation for the patients in their large private practices. Doctors who served in hospitals solely for the indigent had to become split medical personalities, spending private time at private hospitals where they could service private patients and make their living.

Johns Hopkins had always reserved some beds for its staff's paying patients, though almost never enough. Many Hopkinsites, including Cushing, had occasionally had to serve patients in other Baltimore hospitals. In Boston, Cushing and Christian intended to do all their practice at the Brigham and therefore insisted that the Brigham have space available for patients to come from all over America and the world. All modern teaching hospitals, including the new Barnes Hospital in St Louis and the Toronto General Hospital up in Canada, were going in this direction. The Peter Bent Brigham would have private beds available to anyone who could pay for them, especially the patients of its chiefs of staff.[6]

Christian and Cushing would appoint the rest of the staff, their decisions to be rubber-stamped by the hospital board. Organizationally, the Brigham was to be hierarchical, with layers of assistants and residents – like Johns Hopkins and in contrast to Harvard's other, much more decentralized, hospital affiliates. While some Bostonians muttered about the 'Johns Hopkinsization' of Harvard, the university and the Brigham trustees were committed to managerial as well as medical excellence.

They also endorsed their medical leaders' enthusiasm for first-rate laboratory and animal research facilities, and adequate support staff. About
the only issue on which the chiefs did not get their way was a request
that all Brigham patients consent on admission to being autopsied if
they died in hospital. Medical desiderata took second place to sensible
public relations.

The major sticking-point about the move, a serious one, was the
slow pace of construction during a hectic economic boom. Cushing
had known in the spring of 1910 that he would not leave Baltimore for
a year or two, but by the end of 1911 he was volubly upset at the
continuing uncertainty about exactly when and how he would move.
He wrote increasingly sharp letters on the matter to the chairman of
the Brigham's board, Alexander Cochrane. The best the board could
do was promise Cushing a salary from October 1, 1912, and offer to
subsidize foreign travel and research for him and some of his staff from
that date until the buildings were ready.

Complaining that he could not afford to have his team and his practice disrupted for what might be a period of many months, Cushing
began to make veiled threats about staying in Baltimore until after the
Brigham had actually opened, or perhaps not moving at all. He offended Cochrane, who complained to Christian, who knew Cushing
well enough to stand up to him. Christian told the work-obsessed surgeon that it would be foolish to stay in Baltimore and let others shape
the environment where he would be operating for the rest of his active
life:

> You cannot simply walk in and pick up the reins of the team; you have got to
> know your horses before you can drive them successfully, and the time be-
> tween your arrival in Boston and the settling of your family on the one hand,
> and the opening of the Hospital on the other, will be a splendid time for you
> to do just this thing ... Perfectly frankly, I do not think it will hurt your
> machine and your research work if it does rest for a time. It will probably do
> you more good than otherwise to get out of it, and bump up against these
> various problems good and hard ... You are looking at the proposition too

much from the point of view of your research and your team, whose importance I do not deny, but I do think it will do you all good to shake loose for
a while and do something else.[7]

Cushing responded to the dressing-down, as prima donnas and bul-
lies sometimes do, by immediately giving way. He was agreeable to a
fault, rubber-stamping hospital plans and giving almost no thought to
the optimal design of his work areas, a strange lacuna for a surgical
perfectionist. On the other hand, he got credit for something like a
diplomatic coup in taking Christian's advice to appoint John Homans
and David Cheever, blue-blooded Bostonians, as his two general surgeons. They smoothed the way for the prickly outsider, Harvey Cushing,
and the several neurosurgical assistants he would be bringing with him
from Baltimore.[8]

Cushing evidently sought Christian's assurance on another matter,
the delicate issue of race. At Johns Hopkins, like many other hospitals
at the time and for many more years, there were separate white and
'colored' wards. The medical and nursing staff were white. In proudly
abolitionist Boston there would not be many black patients or students, but there would be no overt discrimination or segregation. We
have only Christian's reply to what must have been an expression of
concern from Harvey:

> Do not get worried about the color question. The trouble with you Yanks is
> that you get more rabid than we Rebs are, because you do not understand the
> darky well enough in his internal mechanism. When I was doing the ward
> teaching at the MGH I not infrequently had some negro students for exer-
> cises of one kind or another ... As the Northerners would not have the darkies
> around, they had to be turned over to me, and I always managed to run them
> without much trouble. Within certain limitations this can be done, and I
> anticipate no trouble on that score at the Brigham Hospital. As you probably
> know, I do not like the black man any better than most Southern people, but
> I think I can get along with most of them without much difficulty, and I do
> not think you will have any trouble at all in the matter.[9]

Amazingly, Cushing's worst mistake in planning the Boston move involved the terms of his own appointment. The Brigham Board of Trustees appointed him Surgeon-in-Chief to the hospital. Harvard's corporation appointed him Professor of Surgery. In the early negotiations he expected to receive Harvard's one endowed surgical chair, the Moseley professorship, which was held by one of his mentors, Maurice Richardson. Richardson's formal retirement date was not yet at hand, however, and rather than create bad feelings by trying to force the issue, Cushing contented himself with a generic chair until Richardson's departure. When Richardson died suddenly in the summer of 1912, Cushing became Moseley Professor of Surgery at Harvard.

He thought that his chair was the senior one in surgery at Harvard and carried with it headship of the department, just as Halsted, Surgeon-in-chief of Johns Hopkins Hospital, was also head of surgery at the medical school. When Harvey asked President Lowell for confirmation of this, a carefully phrased reply by a senior member of the medical school assured him that he would not be subordinate to anyone and would take 'the leading part' in developing surgical teaching. Cushing did not ask for further clarification, possibly because William Welch may have suggested it would be rude to press further, or because he thought things were clear enough.[10] He was much more of a hospital surgeon than a university teacher anyway. He had never done much formal teaching in the Hopkins medical school and told Christian that he planned to do even less at Harvard: 'I hope to shunt just as much of the teaching as I possibly can on to other men, for too much of it is not compatable with the continuance with problem work.'[11] He would later bitterly regret having been too polite or too sloppy to get everything clear with Harvard.

The happiest part of the Cushing relocation was probably the decision to buy a beautiful high-ceilinged colonial home on a large wooded lot at 305 Walnut Street in Brookline. Half-hidden by trees, the rambling frame house, yellow with white trim, had a library, two parlors, a music room, dining room, two bathrooms, six-second-floor bedrooms, servants' quarters on the third floor, and a stable that could accommodate both humans and horses. The Cushings had their own tennis court, fruit trees, and vegetable and flower gardens. There were private schools and colleges and tennis clubs nearby, and the hospital was only about a twenty-minute walk away. The neighborhood was changing, but expert opinion held that the people buying and building small houses farther down the street were 'a very good class of Irish' and that eventually the property might be made even more valuable 'for cutting-up purposes.' The house was on the market for $40,000. Cushing offered $35,000 and got it at $37,500. Today it would be a multimillion-dollar property on what is still a lovely residential street, but it has long since been 'cut-up.'[12]

He bought his first automobile, a Cadillac, in Baltimore the summer before moving to Boston. Surgeon's fingers and equanimity were not much use to him behind the wheel, driving lessons notwithstanding: 'I enjoy it, but feel as though I had an elephant on my hands. Some day it will step on me and squnch me.'[13] He obtained a licence to drive but had the car shipped to Boston to save time. He did his last operation at Hopkins on a Friday morning early in September 1912 and caught the train north that afternoon. Kate and the children came down from Little Boars Head to meet him at their new home.

∽

Trains, steamships, automobiles. The mobility of Cushing's generation of physicians and surgeons, well before the age of practical air travel, helps explain their achievement. Medicine was being transformed, by mobility, from local melodrama (the country doctor, the city medical school, the county medical society, the region's special disease) to high national and international theater. While Cushing was not quite adventurous enough to relocate to St Louis – and while he never forgot his roots in Cleveland, New Haven, Boston, and Baltimore – as a surgeon he was a citizen of the whole United States, with aspirations to influence the world.

He sought, worked with, and taught talented colleagues wherever they could be found. The surgeons had a passion to see one another at work, to share the tricks of the trade, learn by observation, drive themselves to excellence. Those finishing-school trips to Europe had been the highlight of many American medical lives – often they were once-in-a-lifetime travels – but for Cushing they were only the beginning. Even though he stopped operating in other venues, he traveled constantly. When he was not working hard at home, he was away from home.

He was not yet hobnobbing with other neurosurgeons, because there were none to hobnob with. Charles Elsberg, who kept to himself, began doing mostly spinal cord work at the Neurological Institute in New York in 1909. Ernest Sachs, a young New Yorker of Jewish descent (as was Elsberg), studied medicine at Hopkins, worked with Victor Horsley in London (just before Horsley effectively abandoned surgery for left-wing political crusading), and was hired at Washington University in St Louis to do neurosurgery there in 1911. Sachs happened to become America's first designated professor of neurosurgery. Philadelphia's Charles Frazier operated often on the brain but only under a neurologists' direction; he spent most of his time on other procedures and as an administrator. Cushing was vastly senior to Elsberg and Sachs and had little regard for Frazier. He saw himself as a surgeon who happened to have become a neurosurgeon, and he never lost interest in issues of general surgery.

His favorite peripatetic American group was the Society of Clinical Surgery, which he had helped found in 1903 and hosted at its first meeting. The point of the organization was to learn by traveling and by watching one another at work, rather than listening to papers. The society had instant success among the brightest young surgeons – and with certain canny veterans, such as William Osler, who flattered it by founding the copycat Interurban Clinical Club of physicians to visit one another's clinics. In its early, years the surgeons went on trips to New York, Buffalo, Cleveland, Boston, then west to Chicago, and considerably farther west to the unlikely destination of Rochester, Minnesota.

The point of the Rochester excursion, which Harvey found time for
in 1905, was to see the remarkable 'clinic in a cornfield' that William
Worrall Mayo and his surgeon sons, Will and Charlie, had created in
association with a local hospital in a little crossroads city. Building on
their father's general medical-surgical practice, the Mayo boys brilliantly
rode the opportunities of this first golden age of surgery. They were
both skilled and enthusiastic general surgeons; they had a happy knack
of finding and getting along with talented associates; they had a passion
for surgical excellence and the Westerners' determination to learn what
the East did well and then improve on it. Like Cushing, the Mayos took
the time and had the money to travel constantly in search of new procedures, better methods, and new approaches.[14]

Harvey may have come to know the Mayo brothers, a few years his
senior, on some of their early visits to Johns Hopkins. They were fascinated by Halsted's technique – such an improvement on the rough-
and-ready work of the Chicago-based fathers of Midwestern surgery:
Christian Fenger, Nicholas Senn, and the controversial showman J.B.
Murphy. When Harvey compared notes with Will Mayo and W.S.
Ochsner outside the medical congress meeting in Paris back in 1900,
he found kindred spirits. The Mayo brothers became charter pillars of
the Society of Clinical Surgery. 'He's a good one,' Harvey wrote privately of Will Mayo in 1904. When he saw the Mayos working in their
surgical fields on the 1905 trip, he was even more impressed. The Chicago surgeons he had seen were not very thorough and seemed to be
biting off more than they could chew. But the Mayos, he told his father,
'have built up a wonderful operative clinic and are well protected by
an able staff of internists, specialists etc and are little likely to make
mistakes. Both of the Mayos are charming fellows and lead a simple life
in a simple community. They do as good and as much surgery in their
own particular lines as any other two men in the world. It has become
... quite a Mecca for medical men.'[15]

Trains brought sick people and doctors from all over America to the
Mayo clinic, then still affiliated with a local Catholic hospital, where
the Mayo boys and their helpers in 1905 did some four thousand op-

erations. High volume improved their results – they did appendectomies, hernias, gall bladders, goiters, and all the other standard procedures, though nothing yet on the brain. Their reputation had become
national and was becoming international, and they were enjoying the
distinction of becoming surgeons to other surgeons. Surgery already
had its star system, much like professional sports.

In these years the Mayos concentrated on clinical work, leaving research to the more academically inclined. One of these was Cleveland's
George Crile, another founding member of the Society of Clinical Surgery. Crile, a product of rural Ohio and a third-rate medical school,
had pulled himself up by his bootstraps performing what he called 'al-
ley cat surgery' at half a dozen Cleveland hospitals while doing animal
research in his spare time – research that had jibed so nicely with
Harvey's early interests.

By the early twentieth century, Crile had risen to the top of the
Cleveland profession at that city's Lakeside Hospital while carrying out
ever more elaborate investigations at Western Reserve University. Crile
became the most important American to experiment with blood transfusion, a procedure still very primitive in the absence of both technology and blood typing. Recognizing few limits to the power of research
or his own energy, Crile explored the problem of restoring vital functions after they seemed to have stopped. When a patient appeared to
have died on the operating table or from drowning or electrocution,
could medicine bring him back to life? Could he be resurrected? It was
not Frankenstein surgery – not yet – but Crile did aspire to understand
the meaning of life and death.[16]

Cushing had heard about other exciting experiments that were being conducted by a young Frenchman at the University of Chicago. As
the surgeons' society passed through Chicago on its way back east in
1905, Cushing rounded up everyone who had a few more hours to wait
for trains, and they trooped over to a lab where Alexis Carrel, a recent
immigrant from France via Canada, hoped to show them the amazing
things he could do with the blood vessels of dogs. Crile killed Carrel's
first dog by overanesthetizing it, but the young surgeon's demonstra-

tion of his technique for suturing blood vessels – vascular anastomosis – dazzled the visitors. Carrel could reconnect severed veins and arteries, could graft blood vessels within the body, and was en route to trying to transplant whole organs and reattach body parts.

Cushing and Crile were both fascinated by Carrel. Here was another virtuoso surgeon doing the previously impossible. They spread the word about his work, and they encouraged Carrel to think about moving east. Cushing brought him to Baltimore to give a talk. Nothing came of a scheme to make him head of the Hunterian Laboratory or of Cleveland prospects; but Cushing's Hopkins friend Simon Flexner had become research director of the ambitious Rockefeller Institute in New York, and William Welch was its chairman, and in 1906 Carrel moved east to the Rockefeller Institute's splendid laboratories. He spent the rest of his career there, working on tissue culturing and transplantation and spare parts problems, and pondering the nature of life.[17]

In preaching the dawn of an era of tissue and organ interchangeability, Alexis Carrel came closer to Dr Frankenstein than anyone outside central Europe. His early work inspired Cushing to have a student experiment with vein grafts to try to drain hydrocephalus, also to experiment with putting a new hind leg onto one of his dogs, and to try his pituitary transplant. Crile began suturing the veins of blood donors to the arteries of recipients to facilitate blood transfusions. The Frenchman had an odd personality, though, being prone to wild and sometimes crude enthusiasms divorced from scientific common sense. Some of Cushing's friends quickly dismissed him as just being very good at sewing.[18]

When European surgeons visited America, their train tickets always included stops in Baltimore, Cleveland, and Rochester, Minnesota. New York had good surgeons too, but medicine there was notoriously commercial. Philadelphia had always been a great medical center, featuring such pioneers of American surgery as W.W. Keen, who carried on agelessly, but there were conflicting opinions about the city's superstar, Charles Frazier, who tended to dissipate his energies in deaning at the University of Pennsylvania. Boston was reputed to be living on its past standing.

Harvey's closest surgical friend in the town, classmate James Mumford, was the permanent secretary of the Society of Clinical Surgery but was more interested in teaching and writing than operating. Mumford's free spirit and his several volumes of light essays on the surgical life greatly appealed to Harvey, perhaps fueling his own literary interests. The Bostonians had worked so hard to get Cushing because his reputation would put their town back on the surgical map. 'Some one ought to take our faculty and our students by the hair,' Mumford wrote to Cushing in 1912, 'and tell them something about the great seething life which is waiting for medical care & direction in every town and hamlet of the country. There never were such chances in any country and in all history.'[19] Sadly, within three years Mumford died of tuberculosis.

Having first gone abroad as students, the Americans now returned to Europe as confident equals – perhaps in some minds, as surgical conquerors. In 1910 members of the Society of Clinical Surgery (George Crile, president) visited the United Kingdom – the trip Harvey was not on – and in the summer of 1912 (Charlie Mayo, president) they toured the leading medical centers of Germany and Austria. Harvey was an enthusiastic member of the motorcade that year, the summer when Walter Dandy filled in for him in Baltimore.

As arranged by Thomas Cook & Son, ten motor cars of camera-sporting American surgeons and their families – though not Kate Cushing – visited clinics in Hamburg, Berlin, Leipzig, Jena, Vienna, Munich, Tübingen, Stuttgart, Heidelberg, Würzburg, and Frankfurt. Harvey missed several sessions when he made a quick trip to Lausanne to see the sick father of an American friend, and he also detoured to Berne for the celebration of Theodor Kocher's fortieth year as professor of surgery. The Swiss held a grand jubilee party, not least because a few years earlier Kocher had become the first surgeon to win a Nobel Prize for discoveries in physiology or medicine. Harvey endured two nights on a German sleeping car to have the day in Berne, rejoined the 'Cookers,' and filled pages of his travel diary with notes of their visits and snapshots from his Kodak. As he commented to Kate, there came a time on these trips when food and sleep didn't matter.[20]

In Europe in 1912, Cushing was impressed by some clinics, appalled by others, and most enjoyed talking with Viennese neurologists as an equal. 'I was terribly pleased that they all seemed to know so much about our hypophyseal work,' he told Kate. The wealth and organizational efficiency of German clinics and hospitals still impressed the Americans; the Europeans' treatment of their patients still did not. When old Emile Roux operated on Cushing's American friend in Lausanne, for example, he did use half a pair of rubber gloves – a glove on his left hand – but completely soiled it as he rooted around in the patient's rectum and other cavities.[21]

The British Isles seemed to be more surgically conservative than Germany. On their 1910 trip the Americans saw several British surgeons using archaic antiseptic and anesthetization procedures from Lister's day. The most impressive English surgeon, Berkeley Moynihan, admitted to having 'picked up quite a few American tricks.' (During his first American trip Moynihan had stayed with the Criles; following English practice, he routinely left his shoes outside his door every night for polishing. Having no servants, George and Grace Crile shone Moynihan's shoes themselves.)[22]

Nor was it only the Americans who looked askance at Old World medical practices. In 1911 Harvey asked a young Australian who was going to London after visiting Johns Hopkins to write to him about his impressions of surgery in the imperial capital. The verdict was anything but flattering. The British were ten to fifteen years behind Australia in their surgical practices, L.W. Jeffries wrote:

> That operations should be carried on with the use of marine sponges, rinsed out by nurses wearing no gowns or caps; that assistants should wear no caps, & operators not always change their gowns between operations, and a hundred other glaring faults would have seemed incredible had I not witnessed it. – I saw one man passing catheters on a row of men standing up. On the table was a jug full of instruments; he took one, passed it, wiped it on a towel held in his hand & dropped it back into the jug: and so on down the line using the same instruments & the same towel all the time.

Australians in London were annoying the British by their enthusiasm for American surgery.

Back in the United States, the Society of Clinical Surgery had been so successful that Franklin Martin, a Chicago gynecologist who in 1905 founded the important journal *Surgery, Gynecology and Obstetrics*, decided to invite all American surgeons to observe the best of the profession. In 1910 he organized the first Clinical Congress of Surgeons of North America, an event whose tremendous success (200 were expected, 1,300 came) is judged by historian Ira Rutkow to have 'crowned the process of professionalization for surgery in the United States. From that time on, surgery, as a specialized branch of therapeutics within the whole of American medicine, could never be denied.'[23] In 1912 it was announced that Alexis Carrel had won a Nobel Prize, surgery's second, for the innovations he had made while working in America. The next year saw Cushing's triumph at the International Medical Congress in London. On that occasion Will Mayo, George Crile, and Chicago's John B. Murphy were also made honorary fellows of the Royal College of Surgeons of England.

Franklin Martin built on his successes in 1913 by founding the American College of Surgeons as a body that would, like the British royal colleges, raise the moral, educational, and professional standards of the profession. At first Cushing and his friends, whose standards needed no raising and who were comfortable in their closed societies, tended to look down on Martin as a crude *arriviste*. But as it became clear that he was doing great things for their profession, almost everyone finally was persuaded to support his projects.

These developments underlay the rising American confidence and New World impatience with the slowness of the Old World that provoked Cushing's critical comments on British medical research, education, and surgery in his 1913 London address. The Americans had more than caught up to Europe; the British, especially, were in danger of falling behind. As Cushing and his colleagues planned to take advantage of their opportunity to start afresh yet again with their new hospital in Boston, the institution they studied most carefully was neither in

Europe nor along the eastern seaboard. To find out how 'easy' surgery
could be, to find the 'esprit de corps' that they should emulate in Boston, David Cheever spent six days in 1912 at the Mayo clinic. One
traveled west to find excellence.[24]

~

The Cushings moved to Boston in September 1912 and had nothing to
do. The Peter Bent Brigham Hospital was nowhere near opening. Their
house was in the midst of renovation. Fortunately, Harvard's surgical
research laboratory was available. Harvey also did some operating in
private hospitals, including the one that Amory Codman had founded
after leaving the Massachusetts General Hospital in protest against its
rigid seniority system. Cushing's motoring career ended abruptly, however, in what his first official biographer describes as 'an unhappy motor
accident (in which he was not at fault) that resulted in the death of an
elderly female pedestrian.' There is no reference of any kind to this
incident in his surviving papers or in Boston's leading newspaper. Harvey
apparently never drove again. His gardener, Gustave Schneekloth,
became the family's chauffeur.[25]

In January 1913 the first makeshift ward was at last opened in the
Peter Bent Brigham Hospital. The first surgical patient, a woman with
varicose veins, was admitted on January 27.[26] Informal opening ceremonies of sorts were held at the end of April, but only to take advantage of one of Sir William Osler's American visits. Osler gave his protégés
a gentle medical pep talk, including the sage advice that working
through their 'preliminary worries and troubles' would do them good in
the long run. For many more months the surgical superstar of Boston
and Harvard made do with a temporary operating room and control of
fifteen beds at what amounted to a hospital construction site. 'Cushings
hospital is not yet open,' Walter Dandy wrote to his parents from Baltimore in February 1913. 'I would have wasted all this time and a year
more if I had gone with him so everything seems like the best so far
doesn't it.'[27]

The Brigham finally formally opened on Founder's Day, November 12, 1914. Its 220 beds were soon filled. Some of the early worries and troubles involved friction between the hospital and the university, and there was much dissatisfaction with surgical working conditions. 'What a God Damn ugly building! What a God Damn ugly building!' the irreverent W.T. Councilman said to one of Cushing's residents. 'I cannot see how Dr Cushing could allow such a building.' Jim Mumford thought the emphasis on steel, cement, and linoleum in the Brigham's interior nicely reflected Cushing's personality.[28]

During construction of the hospital, Cushing's research and production of articles proceeded almost without interruption. The puzzle of the pituitary continued to fascinate, as he toyed with leftover pieces from the Baltimore work. (To the chagrin of the Hopkins administrators, he had taken many of his patient files with him, as though they were his personal property.) He also added new pituitary projects in Boston, where Harvard had given him a special laboratory to study metabolic issues relating to the ductless glands. Knowing the power of pituitary secretions – 'Aint nuthin' the hypophys cant do,' he joked to Kate[29] – he was vulnerable to the temptation to find evidence of their action everywhere. And he was determined to proclaim a unified theory of the gland's function, maybe even a unified theory of the mind.

Surely, for example, if pituitary secretions had such a powerful physical effect, certainly influencing behavior, they must also influence one's mental state. The search for physical determinants of human emotion had become a hot topic in Cushing's research circles, and in many others. George Crile, for example, was fascinated by the nervous system and by evolution and was beginning to build elaborate models of the bases of emotional and intellectual behavior. One of Cushing's most brilliant and closest colleagues at Harvard, the physiologist Walter Cannon, was deeply engaged in the problem of chemical mediation of nerve impulses and eventually became particularly famous for his work on the production of epinephrine (adrenalin) in emergency situations – what became known as the 'fight or flight' response. Cushing supplied Cannon with surgical techniques for suturing nerves.

If the adrenals could be so related to the emotions, why not the pituitary? Cushing seemed to see it as the great mediating gland. Its secretions seemed to be directed by the sympathetic nervous system, and, he now sometimes speculated, the secretion from its posterior lobe into the cerebrospinal fluid perhaps acted as a control over mental states – a kind of primitive hormone of the brain. He hoped he could show, for example, that the mental lassitude of patients suffering from hypopituitarism (including hydrocephalic patients whose cerebrospinal circulation was blocked) centered on a failure of that secretion.[30]

Chasing these psychobiological theories led him a long way from his surgical comfort zone – into studies, for example, of the extreme lethargy of hibernation, which he thought might be caused by the pituitary effectively shutting down. A New England scientist shared with Cushing his collection of woodchuck brains and pituitaries, which were examined at Harvard's surgical lab in the hope of proving the hypothesis. Thus, one day in 1914 the world's leading brain surgeon takes time to do an autopsy on a woodchuck as part of studies that will lead to the publication of a major paper trying to establish hibernation as a pituitary-controlled phenomenon. In it he almost, but not quite, claimed sleep for the pituitary too.[31]

From woodchucks to Freud. In April 1913 Cushing returned to Baltimore for the opening of Johns Hopkins's new psychiatric clinic – he had become good friends with its young professor of psychiatry, Adolf Meyer – and gave one of the most ambitious overviews of his career on 'Psychic disturbances Associated with Disorders of the Ductless Glands.' Researchers of his ilk had seldom found common ground with experts in mental illness, he admitted. Perhaps Hopkins's Phipps Clinic would now be the meeting place. It was certainly wrong, as colleagues like Crile were realizing, to view patients as 'solely visceral organisms.' A Massachusetts asylum superintendent had read his pituitary book and thought it described some of his patients, particularly the dull, lethargic ones. Harvey thought he could detect serious mood alterations in his pituitary patients, especially those suffering from hypopituitarism (hyperpituitarism seemed to sharpen emotion and intellect – or so he speculated on the basis of some of his observations of acromegalics, plus his reading of Rabelais). Cannon's work, along with everyday observations of mood changes during, say, puberty and pregnancy, underlined the power of the ductless glands and their hormones to affect behavior. With evidence now linking pituitary secretions to sexual development, perhaps the physical basis of the strange behavior described by the Freudians was becoming clear:

> With this conception we may find some physiological or pathological basis for what is regarded by many as a psychotherapeutic phantasy; for the various neuroses and asthenias may arise primarily as the result of some disturbance of internal secretion which paves the way for the dreams, symbolisms, neurograms and other acrostichal manifestations dissected by the psychoanalyst.
>
> If therefore we are to swallow the Freudian doctrines whole – a difficult morsel for many – and are to interpret hysteria and the psychoneuroses solely as the resultant of early mental conflicts and compromises between the libido and its repressions it will be easily seen that any secretory deviation which on the one hand excites or on the other diminishes, sexual activities must be an important element in modifying the terms affecting the ultimate compromise.[32]

Cushing knew he was stretching a long way, probably too far. He told Simon Flexner that in the hibernation paper he was masking uncertainty with 'readabalness' and probably should submit it to the journal of ephemera, *Popular Science*. In the psychic disturbances paper, published in the *American Journal of Insanity*, he warned that the 'rush to the opened door' of internal secretions might lead to clinicians pushing quack remedies, as in the bad old days when Brown-Séquard proclaimed discovery of the elixir of life. He had little luck experimenting with pituitary extracts on patients, was buffaloed when other investigators and his own students challenged his concept of pituitary secretion into the cerebrospinal fluid, and tilted at no more Freudian windmills.

A view spread by some of his associates that Cushing had a tendency to cling doggedly to unprovable hypotheses is not quite accurate. In the real world of diagnosis, when examining patients who had been sent to him because of his pituitary reputation, he relied heavily on quantifiable evidence, especially damage to the optic chiasm.[33] His ophthalmologist associate, Clifford Walker, followed Cushing to the Brigham, where for several years they continued their long series of important studies of impairment of the visual fields in pituitary disorders.

His first new research fellow at the Brigham, Lewis Weed, was put to work on a major study of the cerebrospinal fluid, which Cushing sometimes characterized as the brain's bathwater. He hoped to find where it came from – the source of the tap – and where it drained. In elaborate dog experiments Weed built on techniques that Walter Dandy had worked out under Cushing's supervision at Hopkins. Weed confirmed the fairly well-established view that the fluid originated with the choroid plexus in the third and fourth ventricles of the brain, and he supplied powerful evidence, forcing Cushing to modify his own theories, that it was absorbed through protrusions of the arachnoid lining into the dura.

It happened that Walter Dandy was pursuing his interest in the same problem in Baltimore. Dandy burned with determination to prove that the man who had slighted, abandoned, and scoffed at him and his work was all wrong on cerebrospinal fluid and hydrocephalus questions. 'I am anxious to get even with Cushing as much as possible,' Dandy told his parents.[34]

Their disagreement was this: Cushing thought most cases of hydrocephalus in infants were caused by misfunction of the absorption mechanism out of the subarachnoid space. Dandy, on the other hand, thought obstructions in the brain's canals, such as he had been able to create experimentally, were probably the most common cause. By injecting fluid into the ventricles of hydrocephalic infants and tracking its migration to the urine, Dandy proved his point to his own satisfaction. He was able to differentiate between 'obstructive' and 'communicating' types of internal hydrocephalus *and* to devise a practical diagnostic test. Dandy's seniors at Hopkins realized that the young resident had made a truly important discovery. The various causes of hydrocephalus had to be understood before intervention could be tried.

Dandy had begun this work under Cushing's supervision, and he knew that the master disagreed with some of his theories and perhaps with his eagerness to rush to conclusions. In an apparently positive letter from Boston, Cushing advised Dandy to rework his material and consider publishing under his own name. Dandy hesitated, was advised by Hopkins friends to go ahead, and finally decided to be independent and challenge Cushing. 'I think I will write Dr Cushing and tell him I am going to publish my work on hydrocephalus and let him get as sore as he wants to,' Walter told his parents in June 1913. 'I don't expect any favors from him anyhow. I think I am already a better and stronger man from his antagonism than I would be under his tutelage and at his feet.' Men grew strong through struggle, Walter had earlier remarked to his parents when they advised him to be more temperate. Now they urged him on, hoping their David would humiliate the Goliath and be awarded the Nobel Prize.[35]

Dandy tested his presentation at the Johns Hopkins Medical Society, where he received a warm response. According to him, John Howland, the professor of pediatrics, observed that it was the best piece of work ever to come out of America. Dandy gave his paper to the world, Harvey Cushing in attendance, at a meeting in Philadelphia on December 29, 1913. Here is Walter's account of the occasion, written late that night:

Well I went, saw and conquered, I think at Philadelphia. I bored it into Cushing hard and he was sore as a pup ... I met him before the meeting and greeted him with a smile feeling very self assured but I could get no return. He glided by grazing my hands and never said boo ...

At the meeting I was the first paper. I don't believe anyone ever made a more rattling speech. I was sore to the bone and eyed him during my entire speech. And what did he do, never looked up at me. He followed me, made a most lamentably weak speech I have ever heard. I expected to meet antagonism, but none there was. He said he 'could not agree with Dr Dandy's theories' but beyond that it was a very weak thing. When talking he could not once look at me. He knew he was guilty. It was the most puerile demonstration of a big man's actions I have ever seen.

Well several men went up to see a scrap but none turned up. They said it was the best speech they had ever heard and Cushing was shown up like a baby. Well nothing could please me more nor will do so now than Cushings enmity and antagonism. It has made me fight and he will know that I cannot be subdued as easily as he thought once. Once when he told me I had no imagination, that I was not in the proper environment in the east I should go west where the requirements were not so high ...

One fellow asked me why I looked at Cushing all the time. I said I was sore. He said if that was what was wrong, someone ought to beat me before every meeting I talked at, for it was almost perfect.

Dandy's presentation received major newspaper coverage, with talk of the possibility of a cure for those poor swollen-headed babies. Within days, Dandy began hearing from desperate parents. He was cock of the walk at Johns Hopkins, with everyone praising his work. Cushing's correspondence, on the other hand, contains no account of the occasion and no reference to Dandy's paper. A diary shows that Harvey left the Philadelphia meetings early with a case of bronchitis. In January he wrote Dandy a very friendly letter complimenting him on a just-published study of the nerve supply to the pituitary.[36]

Cushing did not think that Dandy and the issues he raised were central to his own investigations. Through the grapevine Dandy heard that Cushing had told Lewis Weed, who was writing up his work for publication, to pay no attention to Dandy's Philadelphia presentation. In fact, there is a passing citation to the first published summary of Dandy's paper in the series of seven 'Studies on the Cerebro-Spinal Fluid and Its Pathway' that Cushing, Weed, and Paul Wegefarth sent to the *Journal of Medical Research* in the summer of 1914. They were careful to credit Dandy with his innovation in producing experimental hydrocephalus and several times mentioned that they disagreed with his views on absorption of the cerebrospinal fluid. They said nothing about his conclusions about blockage and hydrocephalus or his diagnostic test. Cushing may have been skeptical about Dandy's research base, which consisted only of seven dog experiments and seven human cases. Or he may have been the distracted parent, ignoring the insights of the clamoring adolescent.[37]

Walter Dandy got on with his work in the spring of 1914, hoping that his 'victory over Cushing' would support his ambition to take over neurosurgery at Johns Hopkins. He worried that in hydrocephalus he had to face competition from two of Cushing's old rivals, Spiller and Frazier in Philadelphia. He was reassured after seeing Frazier work: 'A bum operator ... even I could do better than what I saw him do.'[38] If he had time, he told his parents, he would visit the Mayos and learn a little from them. 'It was the best thing that ever happened to me when I broke with Cushing ... But there is a long battle ahead yet, in fact it is only beginning.' Still, Dandy thought his antagonist was probably over the hill: 'I think Cushing has passed his highest mark and is now only marking time and making money or reaping the harvest.'[39]

~

Whether or not Cushing had passed his highest mark by the time he turned forty-five in 1914, there is no doubt that he was a fixture in Boston and was an American medical celebrity – indeed, a global one. The flow of patients with serious brain ailments followed him north; neurosurgery instantly became the one specialized field in which the Peter Bent Brigham Hospital was renowned. Otherwise, as Harvey said in his Founder's Day address, his hope for the Brigham was that it would be a 'centripetal' rather than a 'centrifugal' kind of place, in which everyone would work in harmony across disciplinary barriers, areas of specialty would shift with changing personnel, the staff would give all their time to work at this one institution, and energy would not be frittered away in extramural professional pursuits.[40]

Of course there would be a certain amount of extramural socializing in a city renowned for its residents' intellectual and cultural accomplishments. A neighbor and fellow Ohioan, the distinguished American historian James Ford Rhodes, befriended Harvey – who had told him of his interest in the history of medicine – and became his guide to the delicacies of club life in Boston. He urged Harvey to accept all invitations at first, then winnow his commitments to a minimum: 'I hear on all sides that you are the greatest brain surgeon in the world. I know well what I should do were I that and only 45 years old. I should make everything subservient to my operating work. I should do as little administrative work as possible. I should leave the history of medicine to others. Administrators and historians are plenty. A truly great operative surgeon is rare. And think of it to have the brain for your province!'

Harvey joined Boston's two most exclusive dining clubs, the Saturday Club and The Club. Twice a month he shared food and talk with about half of the best minds of Boston (there were no women present), and in the case of the Saturday Club, which was endowed, did not even have to pay a bill. For a time he also attended the Royce Club, presided over by philosopher Josiah Royce, which featured a monthly evening of abstract discussion. Kate called it the Brainstorm Club. 'I was wholly outclassed,' Harvey admitted.[41] He had no other interest in the still flourishing world of men's clubs, and even less in the hectic social lives led by many high achievers in the socially sensitive city.

Lewis Weed remembered a quiet meal with the Cushings at 305 Walnut Street being interrupted one night when Harvey had to rush out to a dinner that he had forgotten about. Within a year of their arrival in Boston, according to Kate, Harvey went on strike against any more dinner invitations; people who understood this invited his wife to luncheons instead. When he could not escape socializing, he could be delightfully voluble. At one dinner party he was full of funny stories about how he should have excised the speech center of one of his suffragist patients. He did not realize that the merriment level was particularly high because one of the other guests was a noted suffragist.[42]

Kate gave the impression of being as perfectly suited to running the household at 305 Walnut as Harvey was to doing brain surgery. 'He could always come back from the terrific strain of work at the hospital to a peaceful home and a serene wife who had intelligent understanding, a grand sense of humor, and who supplied the creature comforts which only a good house-keeper can provide,' a neighbor and close female friend remembered. 'She not only forestalled all his needs, but was in every way the perfect companion for him, for not only having a fine character she also carried herself beautifully and had a beauty of face and expression.'

Kate's private letters indicate that her beauty of face and expression was often a mask for insecurity, fatigue, and disdain. While the house-keeping was being made easier by such labor-saving devices as electric vacuum cleaners, Kate found the social obligations so strenuous that she in fact supported Harvey's withdrawal from dinner parties: 'I'm SORRY. I simply cannot get rest here. When I come in from a luncheon drained of every idea and thought I *cannot* go to my room and rest for an hour, in order to be a little fresh to dine out!' The worst occasions were when Harvey required her to socialize with visiting foreign doctors or, even worse, put them up. While the American medicos were no doubt honored by a visit from one of Europe's surgical societies in the spring of 1914, to Kate Cushing it meant the ordeal of having some of these 'terrible Germans' as house guests.

Almost as bad were the required events outside their home, including a lunch put on by the notoriously social-climbing Mixter family: 'The Mixter lunch was a mess ... it was a perfectly good meal, but nothing attractive pleasant or dignified about it. So many people huddled into a small house – the tea at the Medical School was not much better. They had imported some attractive young ladies for the occasion ... who spoke various languages, and then they were not introduced to any who spoke their particular language ... Of course I think every one realizes now that they really all wanted to see Harvey – at least he was the chief attraction – he was very tactful.'[43]

~

Harvey's bread-and-butter work, day in and day out, was the hunt for brain tumors, abscesses, or cysts, punctuated by the occasional ganglionectomy. With his tumor operations numbering in the several hundreds, with probably more pituitary experience than anyone in the world, he began occasionally to stand back and reflect on the results and their statistical significance. This seems a logical next step for an intelligent surgeon, but Cushing may also have been influenced by Amory Codman, now a leading Boston orthopedic surgeon (though he destroyed his career in a spectacular 1915 attack on the Harvard/MGH surgical establishment). Codman was a pioneering and quixotic crusader for measuring outcomes in medicine, or what he called the End Results Idea. In those days and for many years later, it did not naturally occur to hospitals or surgeons to do follow-up studies of discharged patients.[44]

At the 1914 American Medical Association meeting, Harvey delivered a long, somewhat gloomy commentary on a paper by a brain surgeon from Breslau – perhaps one of Kate's terrible Germans – summarizing the work that had been done there. Cushing pointed out that most statistics on intracranial operations were virtually meaningless. They lumped together disparate procedures, ignored quality-of-life issues, and sometimes fudged the cause of death or the meaning of recovery. On a truly strict construction, he pointed out, probably no more than 5 percent of tumor patients were actually 'cured.'

The mortality rates from brain surgery that the Europeans were reporting – from a low of 38 percent in Vienna to well over 50 percent by Horsley and his associates at the National Hospital in Queen Square – were 'staggering,' said Cushing, especially when compared with his own Boston rate of about 8 percent in some 140 cases. He was not sure that the series were statistically comparable ('I can hardly imagine an optimism sufficient to carry a surgeon into a class of work in which one out of every two or three patients dies obviously from one's intervention'), but he thought there was little doubt that on virtually any basis his methods were being vindicated: 'The effects of concentration of work show themselves in our results, which depend so greatly on such details as perfection of anesthesia, scrupulous technique, ample expenditure of time, painstaking closure of wounds without drainage, and a multitude of other elements, which so many operators impatiently regard as trivialities.'[45]

As he reaped the harvest of his work, Harvey had the opportunity, mentioned by Dandy, to get rich. He could charge his private patients many thousands of dollars for his astonishing surgical feats. Halsted and Kelly at Hopkins had soaked rich families huge sums for procedures that were almost hackwork by comparison. Will and Charlie Mayo had become rich and lived in grand mansions in Rochester. Many other surgeons did very well in their profession, being handsomely paid whether or not they saved the patient's life.

Harvey had no sooner reached this pinnacle – immense reputation, tremendous earning power – when he and many of his academic colleagues found themselves caught in the whirlwind of a movement to cap their incomes. It did not come from patients or insurers. Rather, it was led by the philanthropic bureaucrats who administered John D. Rockefeller's millions, notably Simon Flexner, his educator brother Abraham, and their mentor and hero, William Welch of Johns Hopkins.

The Flexners had bought into an idea that had originated in a mix of envy and principle among the scientists at Hopkins. Living on fixed salaries, and with few opportunities for extra income, they (especially Franklin P. Mall, a dark figure in the history of American academic medicine) concluded that the private medical practices of the leading members of the clinical staff of the hospital and medical school, especially the surgeons, were too tempting and should be controlled. Clinicians should not be part-time employees, free to moonlight on their own and at other institutions (some surgeons ran their own private hospitals), but should be full-timers – full-timers like the scientists, like employees of law firms and the executives of most businesses. If seeing patients was integral to doctors' work at a medical school or hospital, then compensation for it should be part of their salaries. Any extra fees charged to the Hopkins clients in the private-patients wards should be payable to the institution.

Abraham Flexner became an instant powerbroker in American medical education as a result of his 1910 Carnegie Foundation report, *Medical Education in the United States and Canada.* When the Rockefeller philanthropists asked his advice on the next step towards greater excellence at Johns Hopkins, he suggested offering grants to convert the leading clinical positions to full-time. Once Hopkins had adopted this model, surely all other good medical schools would follow.

The problem was that many of the leading clinicians at Hopkins, including Osler's successor Lewellys Barker and the dynamic gynecological surgeon Howard Kelly, had no interest in giving up private practice to go on full salary. They would lose not only significant income – the proposed salary levels would not nearly compensate for lost patient fees – but also personal autonomy. A fierce and bitter debate raged almost out of control at Johns Hopkins, even drawing in Osler himself, who from semi-retirement in Oxford scathingly denounced the full-time idea as a denigration of the professional values he had always championed.

Having left Hopkins just before the storm broke and having arranged that he would be able to service his private patients on their own ward at the Peter Bent Brigham, Cushing was comfortably sidelined through the first stages of the furor, which he followed with interest and a certain amount of self-satisfaction. He and Christian had finessed the issue, it seemed, by agreeing to limit their private practice to the Brigham itself: they would do no moonlighting outside the hospital but would give their full-time to the Brigham, where patients who could afford to pay would come to them and pay their professional fees. This practice, which came to be called 'geographical full-time,' seemed an ideal compromise between two extremes.

It did not satisfy Flexner and the Rockefellers. Cushing suddenly was sucked into the debate when Harvard decided in the spring of 1913 to apply for a major Rockefeller grant to improve its clinical teaching. The grant was approved on condition that the school, working with its hospitals, convert its chief physicians and surgeons to full-time salaries. The fat was in the fire: Would Harvey Cushing, Surgeon-in-Chief at the Peter Bent Brigham and Moseley Professor of Surgery at Harvard, agree to work on a full-time salary from Harvard and the Brigham of about $15,000 a year – a 50 percent increase on his current wage but far below his normal earning capacity?[46]

For almost a year there was intense discussion, argument, and negotiation at the highest levels of the university, the medical school, and the hospital. An air of intrigue, petty academic politics, and deep personal antagonisms hung over much of the debate. Dean Edward H. Bradford of the medical school, a conservative Bostonian, appears to have had little use for Cushing, and vice versa. Cushing, who knew the Rockefeller group very well, told a Boston businessman that the whole problem stemmed from the fact that Abraham Flexner was a socialist who wanted everyone to be content with $5,000 a year.[47] Abraham Flexner was in many ways an inflexible clone of his brother Simon, whose desire to promote their alma mater, Johns Hopkins, and the projects of William Welch was almost boundless.

Too much was at stake, though, and there were too many possibililties for compromise for anyone to sit too rigidly on his high horse. Cushing often professed agreement with the principle of full-time – saying that no one should neglect his teaching and research to go whoring after money – and his own record at Hopkins was probably the cleanest of any surgeon. On the other hand, he did not see why he should put control of his professional future and income in the hands of a board of hospital trustees and a board of university governors. The two boards had only a gentleman's agreement to cooperate, were not cooperating smoothly, and in neither case promised to safeguard the independence of their professional staff. What would stop a hospital board from exploiting its salaried staff to maximize the institution's income? Surely the geographical 'whole-time' practicing that Cushing and Christian had agreed to at the Brigham was a reasonable compromise with the doctrinaire 'full-time' system.

Harvey's notes, made at the time and afterwards, stressed the prob-

lem of the Brigham-Harvard relationship, along with his 'apprehen-
sions that we would be likely to be enslaved by this arrangement even
though we might live comfortably enough on the offered salaries and
would be free from responsibility.' He politely told President Lowell
that if full-time on the Hopkins model was going to be implemented at
Harvard, he would resign rather than stand in its way – which, of course,
meant that he was standing in its way. Lowell understood perfectly that
he could not afford to go ahead and lose Cushing, and probably Christian too, so in the spring of 1914 decided to let the matter rest.[48]

So much money was at stake that it did not rest for long. By early
1915 the full-time question was being forced at Johns Hopkins, where
it sparked Lewellys Barker's resignation and caused many years of dis-
ruption and difficulty. With other universities apparently starting to fall
into line, many of the faculty at the financially stressed Harvard Medical School came to believe that only Harvey Cushing was standing in
the way of their getting the money they desperately needed to preserve
their leadership.[49] In March 1915 Lowell reversed himself and suggested
that Cushing go ahead and resign as Surgeon-in-Chief at the Brigham
but maintain an appointment there as a visiting surgeon as well as his
Moseley professorship. At some point in their discussions, Lowell had
also informed Cushing, to the latter's surprise and annoyance, that he
was not head of Harvard's surgery department – Harvard surgery had
no head – but was only one of the several professors of surgery, each
with a hospital appointment.

Cushing's canny move in the delicate game was to convey the
president's desire to the chairman of the board of the Brigham, Alexander
Cochrane, indicating that he was perfectly flexible except that he would
not accept full-time as it had been implemented at Hopkins. The members of the board thought about the matter for a month, gathered advice from other physicians, decided that the current 'whole-time' relationship with their staff was working perfectly well, and concluded that
it would cause too much friction if they had to replace their chief surgeon. The hospital told the president of the university that it would not
make any change in its staffing arrangements or its system of compen-

sation.[50] The president had no choice but to tell Flexner and the General Education Board that Harvard was turning down the Rockefeller grant because it would not meet their conditions.

The first time I studied this conflict, in my biography of William Osler, I concluded that Harvard's rejection of Rockefeller money was an example of a university taking a firm stand on a money issue – such a rarity that I created an index entry, 'Harvard ... courageous, principled.' This was naive and wrong. In fact, the episode demonstrated Harvey Cushing's stubbornness and his prestige in his new surgical milieu. He defeated Lowell and his colleagues in the medical school by having won the support of the independent board of the Peter Bent Brigham Hospital. Faced with that situation, money-hungry and troubled Harvard turned tail.

One of many underlying ironies in the affair was the fact that Cushing was among the least likely of American surgeons to shirk his responsibilities for the sake of money. Being independently wealthy, he did not need to make much money from his surgery, nor did he want to professionally. He had many other interests in life than simply operating to earn fees. During the final stages of the rather sordid drama of Rockefeller bullying, Harvard obsequiousness, and Brigham obstinacy, Cushing was not even operating in America, and certainly not operating for fees from anyone. He had gone to France to help save the lives of soldiers wounded in the great European war.

NINE

Adieu America: Cushing Goes to War

~

Cushing took a rare holiday in early August 1914, a few days salmon fishing in Canada with a group that included one of his house men, Elliott Cutler. While they were gone a war broke out in Europe: Germany and Austria-Hungary against Russia, France, and the British Empire. Harvey later joked about how the world fell apart when he went on vacation.[1]

It did not fall apart for Americans that summer of 1914 because their country, unlike the British Dominion of Canada, simply stayed out of the affair. The United States was officially neutral. The few Americans who paid attention to events in far-off countries had strong opinions about whether or not German militarism or British imperialism or a volatile mix of Great Power rivalries had caused the conflict; but hardly anyone believed that it was vitally important for the United States to get involved.

As he went on with his work in Boston, Cushing, like many educated Americans, tried not to be influenced by the propaganda from either side. He had strong personal and scientific ties with both sides. British friends wrote to him of their determination to fight to the last man. On the other hand, his old friend from Hopkins, Max Brödel, urged him not to believe the mistruths spread by the 'All-lies.'[2] Very quickly, though, stories about the brutal methods the Germans were using to subdue resistance in the formerly neutral country of Belgium began to influence opinion among many Anglo-Americans, especially New Englanders.

German destruction of the Belgian university town of Louvain, including the burning of its beautiful library, was a special outrage. Harvey had visited that library in 1912 to see its editions of the works of Vesalius, and he had planned to return to Belgium that autumn for celebrations of Vesalius's four hundredth birthday. Now those books had been reduced to ashes, and Cushing found himself supporting international efforts to help Belgian refugees. Many of the Louvain faculty and their families had fled to England and were being helped at Oxford by the Oslers and other friends, with financial support from America.

'Try as we may to be neutral as a nation, we can not be neutral as individuals,' Harvey wrote apropos of Belgian relief in November 1914, 'and the most extraordinary wave of sympathy and indignation has swept over the entire country here.' He urged Henry Head, the distinguished British neurologist and editor of *Brain*, to take comfort in knowing that 'ninety-nine out of a hundred people over here are very much on your side and one hundred percent of the Cushing family.'[3] He was speaking for Kate too. Both Cushings regularly corresponded with the Oslers, who had thrown themselves into war work. Sir William had wondered informally if he might get Harvey to come over.

~

Americans in Paris, who numbered in the thousands, naturally sympathized with the French as they faced another invasion by Germans. The American colony in Paris had done its bit more than forty years earlier, helping serve the sick and wounded when the city was besieged during the Franco-Prussian War. In September 1914, with the Kaiser's armies again approaching the suburbs of the city, Americans literally mobilized, a number of them driving their automobiles out to the battlefields on the Marne to try and help bring back the wounded. They may have done little more than add to the confusion, but as the fighting stabilized, a beautiful myth grew up of how the people of Paris, its taxi drivers, its rich Americans, and others had saved the city and the country. *Vive la France!*

The current and previous American ambassadors to France, Myron T. Herrick and Robert Bacon, organized their countrymen to graft a special hospital for wounded soldiers onto the existing Paris facility for sick Americans. The government donated a new high school building, the Lycée Pasteur, in the suburb of Neuilly-sur-Seine. A few patients were handled in August, and in the autumn plans evolved to create a serious military hospital, an *Ambulance américaine*, with a capacity of 450 beds. As the front stabilized and the armies dug their trenches all the way from the English Channel to the Swiss border, the charitable Americans looked homeward for financial and medical support.

The touring president of Paris's American Chamber of Commerce asked George Crile in Cleveland if he would be interested in serving in their new hospital. Crile said he would have to take his staff with him. It occurred to him that others would be interested in serving – perhaps leading American medical schools and their hospitals could send surgical teams on, say, a three-month rotation. Crile and other volunteers from Lakeside Hospital–Western Reserve University would lead the way. Crile hoped that Pennsylvania, Chicago, Harvard, and Hopkins would also organize units. He had his own group ready to leave by the end of December and wrote to Cushing wondering if Harvard would be interested in going next.[4]

Harvey replied immediately that he thought Harvard's surgery department would have no problem organizing a team. He would be happy to lead it, as long as an outstanding personal matter (full-time was at a boil) did not interfere. Harvard University officially had no objection to the endeavor, as long as it did not have to pay the estimated $10,000 cost. The Brigham trustees were also cautiously agreeable. Either on his own or through connections, Cushing found a well-to-do manufacturer of cartridge belts, William Lindsey, who offered to fund the mission to a total of $20,000. As soon as Crile reached Paris, he began peppering

the Bostonians with advice about Neuilly and how they should organize themselves.[5]

The more Harvey learned about the Paris affair that winter, the more
skeptical he became. No longer neutral about the war, he was still not
sure that there was a real need for his services: 'We of course all know
that the French and English physicians are perfectly well prepared and
able to take care of the wounded and it has seemed to me a little pre-
sumptuous of the Americans to establish a hospital to supplement their
work.' He heard sentiment to the effect that the Parisian Americans
were creating 'a sort of hôpital de luxe,' in which the French profession
actually took little interest but where volunteer Americans could do
feel-good work. Crile, who stayed at the *Ambulance américaine* for six
weeks, admitted to Cushing that the workload might be light unless a
big battle developed and that most neurological cases would probably
be treated elsewhere. Harvey should think of himself as a sort of soldier
of fortune, with no professional expectations. Just being able to see
Paris and tour the front, Crile told Cushing, had been one of the most
profound and depressing experiences of his life.[6]

There was no trouble recruiting volunteers at Harvard and the
Brigham, and there was much local lionizing of doctors and nurses going off to help heal the wounded of all nations. Cushing, however, told
many of his friends, apparently sincerely, that he did not want to inter-
rupt all his work and projects – 'Glory be darned!' He thought it his
duty, though, to head a Harvard unit: 'It would have been rather humiliating for us to have Crile go over in charge of the Western Reserve
Unit and to send some junior man here in charge of ours.'

Kate was lukewarm too. She was pregnant again. Harvey would face
many dangers, not least the threat that Atlantic steamers might be
torpedoed by German submarines. Crile told Cushing that the danger
was exaggerated:

The Cunard office told me – as they told everybody – when I bought my
ticket, that the Germans would sink the *Lusitania* at sight if they could ... But
when I was told of the limitations of their submarines and the very slight
chance of their doing anything at this time, I had no hesitancy and believe

my staff will not, and will plan to come home the same way April first. I think
traveling on the sea is very safe and never has been so interesting. The passenger list was bereft of Jews and traveling folk, and was filled with a serious
minded and very interesting collection of people.[7]

The Harvard unit, thirteen surgeons and four nurses, booked first-class
passage on an old English steamer, the *Canopic*, which sailed from Boston on March 22, 1915, for Gibraltar.

However unenthusiastic he was, Harvey naturally would keep a detailed diary of the experience. He began it with a few lines from a
Mother Goose rhyme:

> Mother may I go to war
> Yes you may my son
> Wear your woollen comforter
> But don't fire off your gun.

∾

'She seemed very low in the water – the *Canopic* – when we found her
hidden behind the new Commonwealth Pier.' He took an interest in
everything – everything he saw and heard, everything he did, all the
people he met – and he wrote it all down, eventually compiling a massive, quarter-million-word war diary, one of medical history's major Great
War journals. In 1936 a condensed and slightly expurgated edition of
the diaries was published to good critical response. On this first crossing, Harvey comments on the weather, the seasickness, the very English tea breaks (even the ship's engines stopped at teatime), the group's
musicales – Virginia reels, 'darkie songs,' national anthems, 'The Son of
God Goes Forth to War' – a visit down to steerage to treat a sick child,
and the Americans' attempts to learn French. The passage was stormy,
everyone caught colds, he did wear his woolen comforter, and there
was no submarine threat.[8]

After landing, the Harvard group journeyed to the war by the backdoor, sightseeing and 'kodaking' through Spain. In Madrid, Harvey got to see the Prado, where he was most impressed by the work of Antonio Moro. As the Americans approached Paris by train, they began to see encampments for convalescent wounded, and girls at stations selling tricolor buttons '*pour less blessés.*' An English Red Cross nurse on leave warned them of dreadful sights to come, 'men shot in the head and crazed and screaming, awful infections ... atrocities.' The blue-and-grey-garbed French reservists they saw in the station at Bordeaux reminded Harvey of pictures of American Civil War veterans, except that they looked small and forlorn – 'not much *élan* here.'[9]

The first patient they examined at the *Ambulance américaine* – or the American Ambulance, as they called it – on April 1 was a paraplegic, a Frenchman who had been shot in the back by a French bullet. No wonder *élan* was low.

> It is difficult to say just what are one's most vivid impressions: the amazing patience of the seriously wounded, some of them hanging on for months; the dreadful deformities (not so much in the way of amputations, but broken jaws and twisted, scarred faces); the tedious healing of the infected wounds, with discharging sinuses, tubes, irrigations and repeated dressings – so much so that grating and painful fractures are simply abandoned to wait for wounds to heal, which they don't seem to do; the risks under apparently favorable circumstances of attempting clean operations.[10]

The hospital had every variety of wounded and sick, from paraplegics and the hopelessly mutilated to influenza sufferers and malingerers. Most were French soldiers, with a few 'Turcos' (Algerians in the French army) and a smattering of British 'Tommies.' Earlier, the Ambulance had admitted a few Germans in a pretense of neutralism, but now there were none.

The Harvard unit immediately went to work, taking charge of some 160 beds. A few new cases arrived each day, and Harvey spent much time classifying them and studying how injured soldiers were triaged, ticketed, and transported back from the front. Every wounded man had a story; Harvey wished he could understand French better. On his forty-sixth birthday, he wrote for the *Boston Medical and Surgical Journal* a description of the American Ambulance, which he thought was undoubtedly the best of the several hundred auxiliary hospitals in Paris. 'All the talk about de luxe and society is gossip,' he told Kate. He concluded his article with an appreciation of American volunteers in action:

> To follow a poor wounded devil in his dirty uniform, brought in in a Ford ambulance by an upstanding young ambulance driver – a college graduate likely enough – from some distributing point, to see him recorded by the indefatigable Mr. Kollman, then stripped and given a bath, well lathered in a tub by one James Jackson, formerly engaged in some mercantile pursuit, ... then taken to his bed, where he quickly falls into an exhausted sleep, by orderlies who may be young architects or artists or sons of aristocratic families, shaved and clipped by a barber who accepts no fee, cared for in countless ways subsequently by attractive, skilled and effective attendants, men and women of all walks, but serving with whole-souled devotion – it all is a most creditable thing for American enthusiasm and prompt action to have put through.[11]

Harvey's young friend Elliott Cutler, serving with the unit as a house officer, gave him a box of cigarettes for his birthday.

The Americans were told that they still had no idea of what the real war was like. So Harvey's colleague Richard P. Strong wangled a pass to visit the front, also getting the day's password and a car and driver. Strong and Cushing spent a long Sunday speeding through the French countryside. The Germans had conquered huge sections of Belgium and France and had been stopped only a few score miles from Paris before digging in for what would prove to be years of bloody stalemate. The American doctors saw villages devastated during the great battle on the Marne ('all the descriptions and photographs I have seen of pillaged villages fail to give any conception of what it all meant'), climbed around abandoned trenches ('strange warfare, fit only for weasles, moles, or rats'), and watched the big guns pounding German lines. Everywhere they passed out cigarettes to Allied soldiers. A doctor told them that all the wounded men begged to go to the American Ambulance where, they had heard, they would be pampered.[12]

Cushing's more systematic medical touring was expedited by his friend Alexis Carrel, who had volunteered and was well placed in French medical circles. Harvey was able to inspect a crude front-line French *ambulance* (field hospital), with adjacent burying ground, rustic altar, and a stake for the executions of malingerers. Behind the lines at Compiègne he saw a 1,200–bed military hospital where specialists were working on soldiers with punctured eyes and ruptured eardrums. The ancient royal palace at Compiègne had also been turned into a hospital, its famous Salle des Fêtes now lined with beds full of African troops sick with typhoid, malaria, and other fevers: 'Of the makeshifts for water and baths and toilets for the sick, the less said the better. Louis Quinze didn't put in much plumbing,'

Volunteer and freelance hospitals had sprung up everywhere in the French cities and countryside in the early days of the war. Cushing visited chateaux whose owners had converted them to *ambulances*, hiring whatever medical help they could get and scrounging around in their motor cars to collect wounded. French inspectors were gradually sorting out the useful from the marginal facilities. 'Society dotes on the excitement of war and loves to provide – however badly – for the wounded,' Cushing remarked, 'particularly if they are presentable and can be wheeled in to afternoon tea.' He dined in splendor one night at the converted chateau of a Mrs DePew and listened to her complaints about how hard it was to hire a good surgeon, while cannonading could be heard in the distance. He thought the French were more intimidated by this fierce American woman than they were by the Boche.

Alexis Carrel, Nobel laureate, was in charge of a special *hôpital complémentaire* in a once-fashionable hotel on the edge of the Forêt de Compiègne. Rockefeller Institute money and a large staff, including Swiss nurses supplied by Theoder Kocher and racing-car drivers serving as chauffeurs, supported Carrel's elaborate studies of wound treatment. Cushing saw some of the work that Carrel and Henry Dakin were doing irrigating wounds with bactericidal fluids, a procedure that soon became one of the more significant and controversial innovations in wartime medicine. Madame Carrel presided over this 'research hospital *de luxe*' as its iron-willed housekeeper.[13]

Cushing spent late April 1915 doing serious surgery at Neuilly. He operated frequently, usually but not always on head cases. These were all too common as a result of trench warfare. Facial surgery and especially dental reconstruction, not high priorities in the British and French armies, were among the specialties at Neuilly. While Cushing was there, an unusual number of shattered skulls and jaws started appearing at the hospital. One of its ambulance drivers, a certain Washington Lopp, had been a peacetime tango instructor and social organizer to the political wives of Paris, and he had, as Cushing put it, 'many ears to whisper into.' Hearing that the Harvard unit wanted head cases, Lopp whispered, and the wounded came.[14]

The American maestro dazzled observers with his technique. Instead of searching for tumors, the main job was to extract fragments of bone, clothing, dirt, and shells from head wounds. X-rays helped locate shell fragments, but it was often hard to get them out. French surgeons at the American Ambulance had been famously experimenting with a magnet to suck shell fragments from wounds, and Harvey became the first to use the magnet successfully on heads. The most memorable occasion was a day when he had attracted a large crowd of onlookers as he and Cutler tried to find a metal fragment deep in a soldier's brain. They used a six–inch nail to make contact with the missile, then magnetized the nail, withdrew it, and hoped that the particle would come out too. Three elaborate efforts failed. Visitors were giving up and leaving, and Cushing was grumbling audibly ('as when one begins to scold his golf ball') when on a final try, the nail emerged with a little rough steel fragment on its tip. 'Surely the most interesting foreign body experience I have ever had,' Harvey wrote in his diary that night. 'I told Cutler the other day never to show any signs of elation when you remove a foreign body for it's a particular characteristic of certain kinds of surgeons to make much of spectacular opportunities of this kind – but here I *had* to grin and show my satisfaction.' The French marveled at the 'invisible scars' left by Cushing's handiwork.[15]

He pasted in his diary clippings about the ordnance used in the fighting, especially the shells and cartridges he confronted at his end of things, and he mused about the process: 'There are two parties in warfare with the soldiers between. One party busies itself with the elaboration and manufacture of destructive agents which have the greatest possible man killing or man wounding powers – the other party receives them thus wounded and with scalpel and forceps and gauze & plaster tries to repair them.'[16]

The main problem he saw with repairing head wounds was that battlefield first aid – attempts at cleaning and sterilizing by inexperienced personnel – often led to secondary infection. In a major article after his Neuilly experience, Cushing argued that it was often better to refrain from trying to treat head wounds at the front and concentrate on moving the victims to centers that had the expertise to treat them well. Describing his experience with the magnet in that article, Harvey offered one of his most striking images: 'The brain of course is not a pie, even though it may in the past have been treated as such by the little Jack Horners of surgery.'[17]

The Paris days were even more surreal than Cushing's normal life as a brain surgeon. He would go directly from the Ambulance to formal dinner parties with members of the American establishment in France: Ambassador Herrick, who had known his brother Ned; the former ambassador, Bacon, who had become a senior Red Cross worker; a college roommate of his brother Harry, who turned out to be Colonel Edward House, an intimate adviser of President Wilson. American army officers and bright young men from the embassy talked trench warfare and French and German strategy – the gossip was that the Germans were concentrating their forces near Ypres in Flanders – while female dinner companions bent his ear about the politics and finances of the hospital and how the men were taking it over. 'Women make no concessions,' he noted, 'and when their dander is up they cannot be reasoned with –

at least some women – and more women than men.' His own woman at home worried too much about him being in danger, and he had constantly to reassure her: 'As I wrote you we are further from any of the *horrors* of war here than you are at home – of course not from the pity of it ... Please get out of your mind that this is dangerous and heroic business.'[18]

Suddenly on April 24 the American Ambulance was told to send all its motor cars to La Chapelle station to receive wounded. It was a rare midday distribution, for the government did not like to be seen moving casualties through Paris streets. As the disembarked soldiers appeared in the station, first came the *petits blessés* who could still walk, then men in wheelchairs, and then the *grands blessés* on stretchers:

> The impressive thing about it is that it is all so quiet. People talk in low voices; there is no hurry, no shouting, no gesticulating, no giving of directions ... And the line of wounded – tired, grimy, muddy, stolid, uncomplaining, bloody. It would make you weep ... Those with legs to walk on had heads or bodies or arms in bandages or slings, in the hurried applying of which, day before yesterday, uniforms and sleeves had been ruthlessly slit open. Not a murmur, not a grunt – limping, shuffling hobbling – in all kinds of bedraggled uniforms ... home troops and African Zouaves, and occasionally a Marine ...
>
> The wounded all have their tags dangling from a button somewhere ... and in addition each has been chalked somewhere on his coat with a big B (*blessé*), or an M (*malade*) so that they can be sorted readily.

Many were coughing. People whispered that these men had come from Ypres and that the Germans had used some kind of asphyxiating gas on them. Harvey could hardly believe it and thought he had misunderstood – the men probably just had the usual bronchitis. They did not. These *blessés* told horrifying stories of the cloud of suffocating 'smoke' that had rolled down from the German trenches at Ypres, smelling like ether or sulphur, killing hundreds of African Zouaves. 'There's devil's work going on around Ypres,' Cushing noted.[19]

Within a day the Ambulance had every bed filled and was turning away patients – much to Harvey's dismay, for he thought many of the convalescents could be put on straw mattresses on the floor. Newspapers carried accounts of the German offensive near Ypres. It had begun with the release of chlorine gas, the first use of poison gas in modern warfare. The only good news was that a Canadian division had managed to hold on and counterattack – the Germans had already nicknamed the kilted Scots Canadians the 'ladies from hell.' Harvey knew that a Canadian friend from Johns Hopkins, John McCrae, Tom's brother, was somewhere in France with his unit, and he penciled a note in his diary hoping that Jack wasn't in this affair.[20]

Harvey talked about returning to France later in the year for more service. Sir William Osler and several prominent Americans were promoting the idea that American medical units could staff one or more of the thousand–bed base hospital units that the British forces were erecting on the French coast. Cushing leapt at a suggestion that he investigate the British situation, and planned to leave Paris early in May. He went on a last sightseeing outing with the junior staff of the Harvard unit, taking one of the popular Sunday rail excursions to the Marne battlefields. The killing ground was being picked over by souvenir hunters and young boys gathering shells, cartridges, canteens, caps, and buckles to sell on the streets of Paris. There were shallow graves everywhere, mass burial sites and individual markers: 'It was particularly sad to see the clusters around the last year's haystacks where men must have sought shelter from the hail of missiles in their advance across open fields.'[21]

∼

The British military did not bother with mysterious passwords for those who journeyed through the territory they held, but neither did they tolerate sightseers snapping 'kodaks,' and you also had to learn your way through their alphabet jungle of RAMCs, GHQs, DGMSs, and so on. Harvey had a quick three-day tour of the whole British medical system. It started at the front, where battlefield stretcher-bears took wounded soldiers to a regimental aid post; then on to a field ambulance or dressing station; then by motor or train behind the lines to a casualty clearing station; finally, unless they had died or been returned to the fighting, to one of the temporary base hospitals on the Channel coast. The luckiest and those most badly maimed were shipped home to a general hospital or convalescent unit, or to be discharged. Others, having been patched up, were sent back into action.

Harvey was astounded by the sheer number of casualties the British were handling. The standard base hospital had 1,040 beds, and most were filling up with serious cases from Ypres. 'Our leisurely job at Neuilly ... seems child's play.' At No. 13 General Hospital in the converted casino in Boulogne, he marveled at all the head and spine wounds and the opportunity they were giving two of his British neurological friends, Gordon Holmes and Percy Sargent, to contribute to medical knowledge.[22]

The Royal Army Medical Corps made extensive use of medical volunteers and consultants from private practice, among whom Harvey was right at home. He talked wounds, antiseptics, and infections, for example, with the famous immunologist Sir Almroth Wright of St Mary's Hospital, who was known for his development of vaccines and preventive sera but is now best remembered for being caricatured by Bernard Shaw in *The Doctor's Dilemma*.

He talked late into the night with his British friends – shop talk about head wounds and spinal paralysis; war talk about the Germans and their ruthlessness; doctor talk about malingerers and the large number of wounded left hands they were seeing, and about the small number of bayonet wounds, indicating that few prisoners were taken (actually, it indicated that there was little use of the bayonet). Gas talk, too. The Germans seemed to be using a kind of cheap commercial chlorine; the British were rushing primitive respirators to the front, and they were resisting their soldiers' demands for retaliation. The general mood was gloomy and was made worse for Cushing when he saw some of the gassed soldiers coughing their lungs out, then studied their ruined lungs at autopsy. The horrors of gas attacks were not being exaggerated.

On May 5 Cushing was taken to a rural hilltop to get a glimpse of the Ypres battlefield: 'It would have been interesting enough as a simple, lovely, pastoral view across the Belgian countryside; but here we were watching a distant struggle for a city – one of the most desperate as yet in the greatest of world wars.' They could see the remains of the city and a hill southeast of town that the Germans had attacked that day under cover of gas. Big guns, said to be Canadian, were firing near them. Harvey learned only later that Jack McCrae, a doctor serving as a combatant with the Canadian artillery, was somewhere out there, having been in the thick of the action every day since the battle known as Second Ypres had begun. Only a few hours earlier, during a lull in the fighting, McCrae, dabbling in light verse as many literary doctors did in those years, had scribbled some lines in memory of a comrade fallen in that Flanders field. The verses, published a few months later, became the most famous poem of the war. At the field ambulance near his vantage point, Cushing was shown men too sick to be evacuated, men in sheds about to die and join the others buried in Flanders fields. It was enough to shake even very strong men: 'We do not care to examine them in any detail – it's too harrowing.'

Harvey had arranged to sail home from England on May 8, 1915, on an American ship, though he considered switching his booking to one of Cunard's flagships, the *Lusitania*, scheduled to leave a few days later. 'Whatever the liner may be I don't think you need have the least anxiety,' he wrote Kate, 'no more than in ordinary times.' His first visit in wartime Britain was to the Oslers in Oxford. Although Grace Osler was an American – indeed was a great-granddaughter of Paul Revere – and their only son, Revere, was about to become of military age, they had never considered withdrawing to America. In their mid-sixties and often depressed by the war, William and Grace had thrown themselves into volunteer service of every kind. When Harvey arrived, the dinner talk was deliberately about rare books and manuscripts and Revere's growing bibliophilia: 'W.O. finally turns in, only to be aroused by news that Poynton's son has been killed – news which he must transmit to the family. And then Lady O. and her sister and I sit up long, talking the sort of gossip of the war to which W.O. never will listen, for he says he hears all he can bear during the day.'[23]

Harvey went to London on May 7 to meet with the Director General of the Medical Services to discuss American participation in British hospital work. In an otherwise amicable discussion, Cushing apparently mentioned the wonderful research opportunities he had noticed and was told bluntly that this was a serious war, not an occasion for scientific research. Harvey often found British attitudes puzzling. If the war was so serious, why was London so normal? Why did no one go to work before 9:30 or 10:00 AM? Why, apart from the uniforms in recruiting posters and shop displays, was there so little khaki to be seen in the streets compared with Paris?

He was shopping in a London arcade when a bobby suddenly poked his head in the door and yelled, 'They've got the *Lusitania.*' The sandwich-board men in Trafalgar Square confirmed the news of the great liner's torpedoing. Huge crowds gathered in front of the Cunard Line's office. 'Wot'll they do next?' Harvey's taxi driver exclaimed. 'When will England wake up?' said Cushing. 'This may arouse them – and us!' The *Lusitania* carried 1,959 passengers and crew, of whom 1,195 were killed; 124 of the dead were Americans, including a daughter of William Lindsey, who had financed the Harvard unit's service in Paris.[24]

Cushing left for America the next day on the *St Paul*. The Liverpool docks were a scene of stunned, sometimes hysterical, confusion. Harvey was gloomy and pessimistic: 'Liverpool is a dirty ugly place with loads of people and men on the streets and a mighty small sprinkling of khaki. And the place where we embarked was disgracefully dirty and unswept and the porters looked like cut throats ... And these are the fellows who must beat the Germans.'

The *St Paul* raced away from England, many of its American passengers wearing life jackets and bellicosely damning the Germans for their murder of innocent civilians. (In fact, the *Lusitania* had also been carrying British troops and munitions, and Germany had published warnings in American newspapers before it sailed.) On their first morning out, most passengers were at church service and Harvey was writing in his cabin when a friend told him to come up to the forward deck:

> This I did, but rather wish I had not. We were going through the *Lusitania* wreckage – had been, indeed, for the past hour. Steamer chairs, oars, boxes, overturned boats – and bodies. As I came out we passed quite near a collapsible boat which was bottom side up, with the body of a woman and a child floating alongside ...
>
> All told, I believe some fifteen bodies were counted, and this was only in our immediate lane; the wreckage must have been strewn for some twenty miles or more – we at least were passing through it for considerably over an hour. Once we veered off to get a nearer view of the only boat which was seen to be right side up; but the officers, all of whom were on the bridge scrutinizing everything with their glasses, appeared satisfied and we went back on our course.
>
> That was about all. No, there was something else: a single little trawler a long way off on our port quarter, evidently patrolling for corpses – at a guinea each – on this sunny Sabbath morning.[25]

Despite his country's outrage at the sinking of the *Lusitania*, Woodrow Wilson managed to keep the United States out of the war, at least for the time being. This was the occasion on which he proclaimed, 'There is such a thing as a man being too proud to fight.'

Harvey was back in Boston. The rest of the Harvard unit served out its three months in Paris and came home, replaced at the American Ambulance by a team from the University of Pennsylvania, then one from Wisconsin. Johns Hopkins, located in a city with a large German population and with many of its leading researchers German trained, never sent a unit to Paris.

The idea of American university support for the British army's medical work through what were sometimes called Osler units was taken up in Boston – Harvey did all he could to encourage it – and in the summer of 1915 a second Harvard Surgical Unit sailed to France, where it took over an old British base hospital, No. 22, on the coast at Camiers. A Johns Hopkins group was supposed to relieve it a few months later but reneged on that commitment as well, the trustees not wishing to risk, Cushing was told, 'the alienation of the German friends of the University.'[26]

Harvey told George Crile that his trip to the war, about which he had been so dubious, had been an experience not to be missed. He would have stayed much longer had it not been for Kate's pregnancy. He looked forward to going back in another Osler unit rotation, though on balance he thought the American Ambulance was a better venue. The British had not been well prepared for the Harvard group that had joined their service, and at first it had had little to do.[27]

Cushing threw himself back into his work in Boston, noting a month after getting home how quickly the Ambulance episode had faded from his mind. Harvey and Kate's fifth and last child, Barbara, or 'Babs' or 'Baby,' was born in mid-July 1915. Harvey's days centered on the operating room at the Brigham and the constant and growing parade of patients with desperate neurological problems. Most had suspected brain tumors, but there were always the trigeminal neuralgia cases who were hoping to benefit from Cushing's almost routine operation. In September, 1915, for example, Cushing did a ganglionectomy on the mother of his former prize patient, Gerald Birks. 'She has done splendidly, as the last two hundred or so of these cases have done,' Harvey told Osler. Birks was now fighting in France, his face permanently anesthetized from the surgery done eleven years earlier: 'If he gets hit in the face he won't know it.'[28]

The ruction at Harvard and the Brigham caused by the full-time debate had ended, but new friction developed at the hospital as Cushing became increasingly irritable with its administration and its indifference to the need for more resources. Brigham beds and staff were equally divided between the medical and surgical services, but pressure on the surgical side, especially neurological, was steadily increasing. 'Even if we disregard the physical strain of surgical operations, a disproportionate burden of work is thrown on the surgical staff, and this will have to be remedied,' Cushing wrote in his annual report for 1915. 'Particularly is this true of the members of the staff in charge of the patients with neurological disorders, which represent possibly 15 or 20 per cent of our admissions, for there are no conditions which demand a more time-consuming preliminary study, more nerve-racking and exhausting operations and more detailed after-treatment.'

He expanded his capacity to study his patients by hiring support staff, often paying them out of his own pocket. He needed a good personal secretary to supplement the surgical stenographers the hospital supplied, and in 1915 he struck gold by hiring Julia Shepley, a young woman of impeccable Boston breeding whose family inhabited the same social circles as the Cushings. Cushing wrote to a friend that Julia was 'tip top' and he only worried that she would tire of long hours, low wages, and having to get along with him. 'I fear I am a good deal of a martinet and some day when I'm weary and peevish she may think she's had enough.'[29] Cushing hired other support women to do photographic and art work and to organize the large amount of histological and pathological data being generated from the tumors he extracted. He did not know it at the time, but he again struck it rich professionally with the bright and eager secretary he hired in 1915 to handle his technical writing, Louise Eisenhardt from New Jersey.

Harvey's expansion of his personal staff involved him in exasperating disputes with the hospital administration over large matters and small. He fought for his staff's right to have access to the nurses' lunch room, his researcher's right to live in the hospital, and his own right not to have the stenographers fired without his consent. Administrators and trustees at the Peter Bent Brigham found that they had a very irascible head of surgery. Cushing could get upset about unimaginably petty details, such as whether the hospital's stationery matched its envelopes. He was aware of his irritability, which he would occasionally regret. 'It is, I know very foolish of me to become annoyed at people and things,' he wrote George Crile in the summer of 1916. 'I should remember the jingle,'

The cow is in the hammock
The cat is in the lake
The dog is in the bedstead
What difference does it make?

The Brigham's administration was cut from old-fashioned, watch-the-pennies-distrust-the-staff cloth at a time when the hospital had to decide whether to expand or stagnate. Both Cushing and Henry Christian thought that the 'natural' development of the comparatively small hospital would be to grow – to add more residents, nurses, and research workers, expand the physical plant, raise salaries, and also put Cushing's personal helpers on the payroll. Early in 1917 the two chiefs drew up a detailed memorandum to the trustees, expressing their vision and urging action. These hard-driving, ambitious doctors, who had earned tremendous influence and power as national leaders in their profession, were frustrated at not being able to chart the course of the institution where they did their everyday work. Instead of running the place, they and their staff were being treated like outsiders who had to be overseen.[30]

They were not appreciably happier with the situation at the Harvard Medical School, for it also seemed disorganized, unbusinesslike, and adrift under the weak leadership of Dean Bradford, no friend of Cushing's. The biographers of Harvey's colleague Walter Cannon conclude that in these years Harvard's Medical School was 'in a state of perpetual administrative crisis.' Nor would Cushing ever get over his frustration at learning he was not head of surgery at the school. Could western-born men like Cushing and Cannon ever be more than 'outlanders' in contented, inbred Boston?[31]

Cushing's unhappiness with the Brigham and Harvard, and perhaps Kate's unease about social life in Boston, sometimes translated into thoughts of another move. In February 1916 he concluded a business letter to Crile with a wistful postscript: 'Don't you want to get Mr. Hanna to endow a department of neurological surgery and bring me home again? I sometimes think I have had enough of running a large machine, for I find it makes one very unproductive.' A year later he gave some thought to an invitation to take the chair of surgery at New York's Columbia University, writing to a Baltimore friend: 'My present job is interesting enough and there is plenty to do, but it has its very serious drawbacks, and just now the Trustees who are a very remote group of people seem to have reached the end of their tether and appear to be satisfied with standing pat instead of going ahead.' On reflection, he feared leaping from a frying pan into a fire, and noted in his diary that his hooks were in too deep to leave the Brigham, 'though it is far from all one could wish.'[32]

Cushing had now operated on more patients with verified or suspected brain tumors than any other North American surgeon, probably any surgeon in history. By February 1917 his series comprised 337 patients from his Baltimore years and 447 in Boston. In 468 of these instances he had been able to verify the presence of a brain tumor, either at operation or, unfortunately, at autopsy.[33] Cushing's case records were a mine of information, particularly rich because of the care with which they had been compiled and preserved. He possessed detailed histories, detailed operative reports, follow-up studies, extensive photographic records, and, whenever he had been able to locate a tumor during an operation or after death, tissue specimens. It was a unique collection of data about neurosurgical patients and their diseases, which he now began to organize and reorganize, study, sift, and refine. What could his experiences and his records reveal about his surgery? What could the data reveal about brain tumors themselves?

Before neurosurgeons had begun to have occasional successes in locating tumors, the growths could only be studied at autopsy. Traditional methods of removing the brain in postmortem examinations, however, included first stripping away the meninges, or linings, which often destroyed tumors and certainly distorted pathologists' understanding of them. By about 1910 Cushing was accumulating better postmortem data by having the whole brain 'fixed' for study through intracarotid injection; much more importantly, he was generating specimens of fresh tumor tissue from his operating room on at least a weekly basis.[34]

The triumphs of surgery in these years were creating many new opportunities for histological and pathological study of organs and tissues. To Cushing it seemed self-evident that a neurosurgeon should garner all possible knowledge about the nature of his enemy. Where and how did tumors grow? Which were benign, which would recur, which would metastasize? How could tumors best be classified? And, of course, how could they be diagnosed and found?

Cushing had always worked closely with histologists and pathologists at Hopkins, but had been possessive of his records and specimens and had taken most of them to Harvard. In his early Boston years, he was especially close to his old friend and mentor W.A. Councilman, who as chief pathologist at the Brigham supplied Cushing with elaborate analyses of the specimens sent for examination. By about 1916 Cushing had decided to undertake a major study of meningeal tumors – those springing from the linings of the brain, as opposed to the gliomas arising from the nervous tissue itself. Soon he became sidetracked by a peculiar kind of tumor over which there had been much histological dispute at the Brigham; it seemed to be both meningeal and gliomatous, yet generated a unique set of signs and symptoms which made it potentially relatively easy to diagnose and locate. These were tumors of the nervus acusticus, the acoustic nerve, which originates deep in the hind brain in what is called the cerebellopontine angle, where the cerebellum meets the pons at the upper end of the spinal cord.

As with his pituitary work, Cushing's ability to get to and attack tumors in this hard-to-reach suboccipital area led to his becoming the original expert. In 1916 he began work on what would become his second book, a monograph on the tumors of the nervus acusticus and the territory of the cerebellopontine angle. When it went to press in 1917, he was able to report on a series of twenty-nine verified cases, the largest number anyone had ever studied.

It was a story of very limited success. Everyone who went after tumors in this region of the brain had reported horrifying mortality rates, 70 percent and upwards. Victor Horsley, Cushing claimed, had lost five of the six acoustic tumor patients he had operated on in 1903. Cushing's own early suboccipital work, which he began in 1905–6, was very tentative; he had to learn such basics as how to secure the head and shoulders and how to anesthetize a patient lying face down. 'The situation, as now recalled,' he wrote in 1917, 'brings up a picture of the patient's head insecurely held by an assistant, the anesthetic awkwardly administered to a subject having respiratory embarrassment, and an inexperienced operator attempting to expose the cerebellum in a wobbly and bloody field.'[35]

His basic approach to cerebellar problems, a bilateral exposure from a 'cross-bow' entry in the middle of the back of the head, was first used solely to give decompressive relief. When he started exploring and first 'stumbled upon' acoustic tumors, he found them so deeply involved with nerves and blood vessels that he thought they could not be totally enucleated, or removed. Then he was emboldened by good results from partial enucleation, scooping out bits of tumor with a long-handled blunt spoon. Thinking that excessive caution had probably led to unnecessary death, he went after whole tumors, only to conclude that this also caused death. 'The cerebellopontine angle, like the fence corner of the Gettysburg battlefield, might well be called the "bloody angle,"' this most literary of surgeons suddenly comments more than two hundred pages into a technical monograph.[36]

Cushing doggedly recorded lessons from each failure. His judgment about how to attack acoustic tumors improved with experience, and his mortality rate fell from 40 percent in his first ten cases in Baltimore to only one of his most recent ten patients in Boston.[37] Most important – and the justification for his monograph – was that he had learned how to correlate verified acoustic tumors with patient histories to the point where he understood the unique symptomology of this kind of growth and thus could set out the criteria for a differential diagnosis.

X-rays were still not very helpful, and there was no other way of looking into the head. Everything depended on reasoning based on a

patient's history of signs and symptoms. If a patient had suffered deaf-
ness in one ear, accompanied by tinnitus (ringing or wave sounds) and
vertigo, followed by facial numbness, certain visual defects, occipital
pain, distorted gait, and other problems, the probability of an acoustic
tumor was very high. And Cushing could go in and get at it, and at
least help the patient buy more time.

Nothing was easy, despite the improved incidence of patient survival. The operations were long, the tumors impossible to remove in
toto, and even the most cocksure diagnoses and prognoses could be
confounded. Cushing's 1917 monograph, *Tumors of the Nervus Acusticus
and the Syndrome of the Cerebellopontine Angle*, dedicated to Councilman, was only slightly less ambitious than his pituitary book and was
more lucid in its presentation and reasoning. But after 280 pages of
brilliant, careful analysis, Cushing still ended with uncertainty: 'One
cannot gauge the benefit of operations from figures nor can one chart
or tabulate such factors as relief from pain and preservation of vision,
and so long as this equation must be taken into consideration, statistics
regarding the results of brain tumor operations in general are deceptive
and can be made to prove almost anything the author desires, no matter how honest he may be.'[38]

He had a very honest reservation on one key point. 'I doubt very
much, unless some more perfected method is devised, whether one of
these lesions can with safety be totally enucleated.' He was almost certainly too involved with other matters – the war again – to notice in
one of the Hopkins journals that Walter Dandy in 1916 had exhibited
a patient from whose brain, he said, he had been able to totally enucle-
ate one of those lesions.[39]

⌁

The European war continued to generate great battles, incredible numbers of casualties, and no victories. Especially after the sinking of the
Lusitania, the Cushings' circle was as morally committed to the Allied
cause as Bostonians had been to abolishing slavery in the days of John

Brown and Harper's Ferry. So long as Wilson's policy of official neutrality resonated with public opinion, however, those who wanted America to fight had to be content with urging that Americans become better prepared to fight. Republican politicians and such military leaders as Cushing's former patient General Leonard Wood led the 'preparedness' campaign, which gathered steam through 1915 and 1916. It involved citizen participation in quasi-military training, lobbying for more spending on the armed forces, advocating all aid to the Allies short of war, and supporting pro-British, anti-German propaganda in the United States.

The Boston-Harvard medical community had its second surgical unit serving in France, and Harvey also continued to be in close touch with the affairs of the American Ambulance in Neuilly. He served on several committees to mobilize support for American war charities in Paris. As well, he was an adviser to and promoter of the work of the New England Surgical Dressings Committee, a volunteer women's group formed early in 1915 to supply the Harvard unit and the American Ambulance with the elaborate muslin and gauze dressings used liberally in wound treatment. Kate Cushing and her friends were deeply involved. Housed in the Brigham's outpatients building from the autumn of 1915, the committee shipped millions of 'Boston tins' – sealed biscuit cans containing sterile dressings – over the next few years.[40] At work, at home, and in their clubs, the engaged Americans circulated news of the activities of volunteer ambulance drivers and aviators, of Canadian friends such as Jack McCrae and the other McGill doctors, and, of course, of the Oslers at Oxford with all their connections and hospitality. Harvey had also volunteered for membership in the newly created Army Medical Reserve Corps.

Cushing's war work became more official in September 1915 when he received a request from the United States Army's Surgeon General, W.C. Gorgas, to become involved formally in medical preparedness. Gorgas was worrying about the need for a vastly expanded medical service if the country went to war. George Crile inspired him to consider creating volunteer hospital units such as the ones Crile and Cushing had taken to Paris. He asked the two surgeons to begin reforming their units, each with a capacity to staff a 500–bed base hospital, as a model. The volunteer medics were to be enrolled in the Medical Reserve Corps, ready to be called to duty in time of war. Perhaps for political reasons, the European war was not mentioned in the early letters. It was suggested only that the hospital units might serve in Texas if problems with Mexico worsened.

Cushing responded enthusiastically. But the enterprise immediately bogged down in paper power struggles involving Harvard's President Lowell, who wanted to control and shape any Harvard unit, the Brigham trustees, who wanted credit for any contribution coming mainly from their hospital, and the American Red Cross, which was determined to maintain its prewar monopoly of medical relief work. By the spring of 1916, not one but three hospital units existed on paper in Boston, one for each of the major city hospitals, all officially under Red Cross auspices and all short of volunteers, equipment, or training. Cushing's Brigham unit included the medical school and was formally called the Harvard University Base Hospital Unit, or Base Hospital No. 5. Cushing, its director, had found army bureaucrats almost impossibly difficult to work with. George Crile had moved slightly more quickly in putting together his Cleveland team; in October 1916 his Western Reserve University unit held a two-day trial mobilization, complete with army tents, during surgical meetings in Philadelphia.[41]

The whole preparedness cause was seriously set back that autumn when Woodrow Wilson was reelected on a platform reaffirming American neutrality. The next winter was passed with many meetings and much correspondence about the base hospitals and hardly any progress, Harvey wrote in his history of Base Hospital No. 5. He endorsed Walter Hines Page's later comment that these were the years when Americans held their heads low.[42]

Shortly after Wilson reached a new low by calling on the belligerents to negotiate 'peace without victory,' Germany threw caution and American sensitivities to the winds by announcing that on February 1, 1917, it would resume unrestricted submarine warfare, which had been suspended after the *Lusitania* outrage. American neutrality seemed impossible to maintain. The country now appeared to be squarely on the road to war.

Washington began preparing for serious mobilization, mostly by appointing committees. Harvey served on a Surgeon General's Committee on the state of surgical instruments. It found chests of old instruments in Washington, some of them dating from the Civil War. In the meantime, recruiting for the hospital units was going from bad to worse as volunteers began to have second thoughts about making a real commitment. Cushing decided in mid-March that about the only way to publicize the cause was to stage a dramatic appearance by the Boston units. What better place to do it, for both convenience and publicity, than right in the heart of the city, on the parade ground of Boston Common? Put up tents and a few portable huts, supply actual medical care to city accident cases, work out defects in the organization and equipment, garner useful publicity, recruit more support workers, and it would be on its way to becoming a serious outfit. It would surely be just a formality to get official permission for such a display of practical patriotism. War was probably only a matter of days or weeks away; many other organizations and patriotic societies in the city were becoming more active.

Harvey threw himself into the mobilization scheme with his usual energy, drawing up plans, meeting with officials, raising money, recruiting, ordering tents and outbuildings, and attending flag-waving patriotic meetings, all while maintaining his surgical schedule and enduring painful side effects from having set an example by volunteering for antityphoid inoculation.[43] On April 6 the United States declared war on Germany, in Wilson's words, to make the world 'safe for democracy.' Despite the preparedness movement, the country had remained woefully unprepared and was at war only on paper. Everyone knew that it would take many months to recruit and train American armies for service in France, so there was plenty of time for useful experiments like Cushing's little sideshow. Washington and the Red Cross were supportive. Harvey expected to have the medical units officially up and running by May 15.

Obstacles grew like the weeds on Boston Common. The Red Cross hesitated to use new equipment that would then have to be disinfected and sterilized. Medical volunteers for the hospital units did not want to disrupt their work lives. Student volunteers had second thoughts about disrupting their studies. Lay volunteers wondered about wages. 'I am ashamed to send the lists with so many scratched names,' Harvey wrote in his reactivated war diary. 'While *theoretically* many in this community are bubbling with patriotism, *practically* many of them spend their time scolding the government because they think it isn't doing what they want.' In a fit of temper, he told a reneging second-year medical student that he was 'yellow' and had 'cold feet.'[44] He later titled this chapter of his diary 'The Battle of Boston Common.'

The city's normally exuberant Irish American mayor, James Michael Curley, had coolish feet about having a military hospital on the common. Curley bent in the patriotic breeze, but leaked the project to the newspapers, leaked his concern that the encampment might become permanent, and suggested there were better locations. Then it turned out that Cushing's gung-ho enthusiasm was not shared by the directors of the other two Boston base hospital units, who were so hesitant during a meeting with the mayor that Cushing announced he would go it alone. 'It will be a big job,' he told his diary. 'Many will be glad to see it fail.' Even good friends and colleagues could not understand all this 'hysteria' about preparedness in a country that, war or no war, was obviously never going to be invaded.

Hearing that Leonard Wood was paying an incognito visit to Boston, Cushing decided to use the army's ranking officer to force the mayor's hand. Wood was agreeable. Cushing organized a meeting of Wood and other VIPs with prominent Boston friends in the mayor's office. The needful pressure was applied, and pledges were made to donate $20,000 to cover the cost of the mobilization. Curley appeared to buckle, even matching Cushing's own pledge of $1,000. Elliott Cutler's father served as the unit's treasurer.

Cushing had not reckoned on Boston public opinion. Lovers of Boston Common got it into their heads that the creation of a 'temporary'

military hospital on their green would soon lead to the permanent desecration of their great park. Editorialists viewed it with alarm. Little old
ladies from Beacon Hill mobilized, pledging to shed blood if necessary
to stop a sacrilege about as serious as vivisecting animals. Cushing was
deluged with complaints, angry visitors, and critical comment at his
clubs: 'An experience out of a novel ... Very funny – if it had not been
so serious.' The army reneged on its promise to supply canvas, for the
whole United States was now desperately short of tents. President Lowell
let Cushing know that the Harvard Corporation had no opinion about
the hospital mobilization; in other words, it would not support him.
Injunctions were threatened.

Kate Cushing passionately believed in the righteousness and moral-
ity of the Allied cause. She was at least as caught up in the wave of
patriotism as her husband. The Cushing children were already doing
war work, being paid ten cents an hour to dig up the front lawn of their
Brookline property to plant potatoes. Trying to explain the mobilization to some of her friends, Kate received, in Harvey's words, 'a most
uncomfortable not to say discourteous reception at a luncheon among
the [Beacon] Hill tribe where she learned from idle brained women's
gossip where lies the opposition ... KC and I about ready to give up and
live somewhere else.'

They saw how different their values were from ordinary Bostonians'
when they attended a parade of Harvard's student regiment along Beacon Street. It was escorting newly arrived French officers who had been
sent to train the citizen soldiers: 'A fine sight, but the bystanders showed
little enthusiasm. KC threw a bouquet of Mayflowers into one of the
motors and the French officer caught it and saluted smilingly. The only
flowers thrown! People interested of course but no cheering or waving
and practically no one saluted the flags. Cold roast Boston.'*

Was Boston – which stood thirty-third among the states in fulfilling
recruiting quotas – all patriotic talk without real action? Were the

---

*The reference is to Bostonians' habit of serving cold roast beef to their families, and guests,
on Mondays, the cook's day off.

Cushings more true to real New England values than this generation of Bostonians? 'Brought up in a Western city,' Harvey told his diary, 'my traditions of the Boston parade ground are sounder than theirs.' His memories, familial and historical, stretched back to the beginning of the Civil War. 'This mobilization business is nearly breaking my back,' he wrote Leonard Wood on April 27.[45]

On Saturday morning, April 28, Cushing had a late start in the operating room, but a transfrontal pituitary operation went unusually well as he found and treated a congenital suprasellar cyst. Afterwards he joined an unusually large gathering of Boston's male elite at a Saturday Club luncheon. The former Harvard president, Charles Eliot, made a point of asking Harvey to sit beside him, and over the oyster course began lobbying him on behalf of the friends of Boston Common. Cushing defended his project calmly at first – surely Harvard's volunteer soldiers were going to need competent medical assistance – but then he responded to complacency and obscurantist conservatism with mounting anger:

> I saw no food after the oysters – only blood. Told them individually what I thought of them and of their regard for an historically dead instead of a living Boston Common ... Slammed out at poor Jim Curtis – at Sturgis Bigelow who wanted to bet that there would be a stone annex of the city Hospital on the Common before the summer was over – refused to talk to poor Mr. Higginson and Dr. Walcott (in joke) as they had not stood by me at the Corporation Meeting ... Sturgis Bigelow somewhat flushed bustled up and would defend the Common against this sacrilege and I shook my finger at him and said I hardly expected this from a doctor but that he was absolutely typical of the Bostonians, who would put a plot of grass no matter how holy above their country's needs.

The militant surgeon-soldier was well on his way to burning friendships and bridges in his adopted city when he was interrupted to take a telephone call. His secretary read him a telegram just received from Surgeon General Gorgas. How soon could Cushing mobilize his unit?

Not for service on the grass of Boston Common but somewhere near Flanders fields. The American doctors and nurses were needed in Europe. 'Will get ready immediately for earliest possible sailing,' Cushing replied. In his forty-ninth year, Cushing was going to the war again, now as a medical officer in the United States Army.[46]

~

It is not well known that the first American army units sent to Europe in the First World War were base hospitals composed of doctors and nurses and their support staff. Many months passed before the fighting men of the American Expeditionary Force, enlisted or conscripted, were equipped, semi-trained, and ready to sail – indeed, it became a bitter joke in Europe that the Yanks were coming, coming, coming. In these very early days, however, an official British mission to Washington to discuss war needs requested medical help because unrestricted submarine action in the English Channel meant that hospital ships were no longer safe, and it was decided to add more hospital beds in France. Washington agreed to mobilize whatever base hospital units it could – Crile's, Cushing's, and four others seemed more or less ready to go – and rush them across the Atlantic.[47]

The patriotic medics raced to comply, to bring order and uniformity out of their organizational chaos, and to go down in history as the first Americans officially to serve in the war zone. The contest really was between the two surgeons who had first served in Paris and had founded the first two base hospitals. George Crile had had one trial mobilization of Base Hospital No. 4; Cushing, in losing the battle of Boston Common, had given Washington the impression that Base Hospital No. 5 was morally ready to go. In practically every other way, both units were unprepared. The volunteer doctors and nurses had virtually no support personnel, only a mish-mash of medical supplies on hand and on order, no uniforms, and in most cases no military experience. Everyone seemed to proceed on the shaky assumption that anyone who could treat patients at home could immediately do the same at war. This was more or less what Harvey and his friends had done behind the lines in Paris.

Washington must have liked the value of the gesture of rushing American healers to the war but did not want to alert German submarines by playing up the units' departure. Cushing, who rushed to Washington for consultations, persuaded the authorities that it was necessary to get publicity in order to recruit staff. He received a personal shock, probably a considerable embarrassment, to find out that after two years service as 'director' of his unit, it would have to be under the formal command of a regular army officer, Major R.U. Patterson. Cushing was to be immediately activated and commissioned a major, with indeterminate responsibilities looking after surgery. In effect, he carried on as director of the Boston end of the operation.[48]

Cushing and the tireless Elliott Cutler – a young enthusiast trying to be like his chief in every way – decided to commit Base Hospital No. 5 to be ready to sail within a week. Now that an early trip to France was a certainty, volunteers lined up at the Harvard Medical School to sign on as orderlies, waiters, cooks, carpenters, electricians, and other artisans. They were given their medical exams and typhoid inoculations and began drilling, still wearing civilian clothes as there were uniforms only for the officers. Boston's Committee of Public Safety and other volunteer groups gave money, transportation, telephones, secretarial help, and flags. The army, issuing a flurry of contradictory orders, finally decided that the base hospitals would not take any basic supplies, neither tents nor bandages, but would have these provided in France.

A few of the academics, researchers, and physicians who had casually agreed to serve for the duration of any war now had trouble getting released from their jobs. When Harvard's President Lowell, whose continued coolness to the scheme infuriated the Cushings, objected to the loss of several of his valued professors, the professors simply threatened to resign. When the star of the physiology department, Walter Cannon, first came home wearing a uniform, one of his children exclaimed, 'Mamma, look, here comes Father dressed up like a Boy Scout!'[49]

Harvey, also in uniform, was on the job every day till midnight: 'Very little food, very little sleep, and incessant cigarettes. A bad combination, but somehow it went along.'[50] Former opponents in the Battle of Boston Common now embraced the noble volunteers and wished them every success.

The Reverend Endicott Peabody, legendary headmaster of the very exclusive Groton School, asked Cushing to take his son Malcolm as hospital chaplain. Cushing decided to have a special church service to mark the unit's departure. On Sunday, May 6, 1917, the 25 doctors, 65 nurses, 3 secretaries (including Julia Shepley), and 150 enlisted men of the U.S. Army Medical Corps Base Hospital No. 5 marched across Boston Common in cold rain to St Paul's Episcopal Cathedral. Many dignitaries, including the governor of Massachusetts and Mayor Curley, were on hand. Police held back overflow crowds.

The processional hymn, played by the Harvard band, was 'The Son of God Goes Forth to War':

> The Son of God goes forth to war,
> A kingly crown to gain:
> His blood-red banner streams afar:
> Who follows in His train?

Both Endicott and Malcolm Peabody addressed the congregation, talking of the bleeding in France and this unit's mission of mercy. Bishop Lawrence of Boston presided over the dedication of the colors. The 'banner' of course, was star-spangled, a special American flag, in a journalist's words 'as bright and handsome as silk and skill could ever make it.' It was the first Boston flag to be sent to a battlefield in Europe. Women wept during the singing of 'The Star-Spangled Banner' and 'The Battle Hymn of the Republic.' With their children, Harvey and Kate Cushing sat tearless, vindicated. 'It was the proudest moment of my life,' Kate told her mother. 'En famille we ... marched out of the church with our heads in the air! ... I've never in my life felt less like weeping.' Harvey's 'only moment of distress,' he told his diary, 'came when Henry reached over and put a little warm hand in mine, while "America" was being sung just before we filed out.'

The medical warriors marched with their flag back across the common. Veteran onlookers were reminded of parades half a century earlier at the beginning of the Civil War. After his midday meal Harvey went back to the Brigham to finish up his work.[51]

∾

Early the next morning, Boston's South Station was bedecked in Union Jacks and French tricolors as Base Hospital No. 5 embarked on a train for an unknown destination. Now there were no tears, Cornelia Cannon reported, 'except those shed copiously by Dr. Cushing's chauffeur [Gus Schneekloth], who was inconsolable.' After a few days of basic training at a military base, Base Hospital No. 5 sailed from New York aboard a munitions ship, the SS *Saxonia*, on May 11. By four days they had lost the race with George Crile's hospital to be the first unit to sail. Crile's group, Harvey noted sourly, had been bundled aboard, 'undrilled and without uniforms or flags.' Both of the surgeon-patriots, of course, were in effect going to the war for the second time.[52]

TEN

An American Surgeon at Passchendaele

❧

Hazebrouck, France, 3:10 AM, June 7, 1917. Harvey Cushing, billeted with a French family, is jolted awake by the largest manmade explosion there has ever been. British engineers have detonated more than a million pounds of high explosive in tunnels under the German lines at Messines Ridge, near Ypres. The noise is heard one hundred and fifty miles away in London.

The German advance positions are utterly destroyed, and the British Second Army easily captures the remains of Messines Ridge. Even so, there are casualties, though fewer than expected. Harvey is one of a number of surgeons sent up from base hospitals to handle the wounded at casualty clearing stations a few miles behind the lines. Late that day he settles in to work at a New Zealand unit. Wrapped in a rubber apron and wearing his boots, Major Cushing does his first head case, a soldier named Dark. 'And it was. No X-rays, a poor light and a bullet in the knee which I didn't get, and another likewise in his side which had reached his lower spine ... All this incidental to his cranial wound which we repaired and closed.'

Next morning, the New Zealanders have assembled more head cases for Cushing's attention than he can possibly handle. 'The unusual experience for me of operating alone on heads with a strange anesthetist using chloroform ... Much too great loss of blood, poor if any X-rays, practically no neurological study. Luckily most of the cases went well with flaps and closure. Most of them really favorable.' The results one might expect when the famous neurosurgeon operates on the battle-field.[1]

Observers soon realize that Cushing's exquisite precision and care create an odd problem: he is too slow. Given the volume of wounded, his operations are too long, in a way too good. Harvey Cushing doing brain surgery at a casualty clearing station is like a master chef working at McDonald's. Sir Anthony Bowlby, the chief British surgical consultant on the Western Front, finds the situation embarrassing and asks George Crile, who happens also to be in the area, how to handle the Cushing problem. Crile advises that it's worthwhile to have one such perfect technician on hand as a model. Let Cushing do his thing, and organize other groups around him to handle the overflow.[2]

Every few days during this and many later battles and during all the quiet times on the Western Front, Cushing writes or dictates long diary entries. Being interested in practically everything, he accumulates volume after volume. He has an artist's eye for scenes, a writer's interest in imagery, and a historian's passion to record events. He has a Zelig-like knack of being around when history is being made.

~

As their ship zigzagged across the Atlantic in May 1917, the 243 men and women of U.S. Army Base Hospital No. 5 slept fully clothed and with orders to wear life preservers at all times. Nearing Britain, they passed through the wreckage of a ship torpedoed only hours earlier. Most of the earnest Americans decided on the voyage that in lieu of drinking alcohol during their tour of duty they would sing drinking songs. Many took an official temperance pledge circulated by their commanding officer. They passed the time reading, drilling, playing cards, drilling, and being inspected. 'Mother never meant that I should be a soldier,' Walter Cannon exclaimed at the end of a long day. When they took revolver practice, Harvey noted, they all succeeded in hitting their target, the ocean.[3]

The *Saxonia* docked in Falmouth in fog. The enlisted men went to Blackpool for further training, while the doctors and nurses took a cold night train to London, arriving tired and disheveled. The group was more impressed with its own importance, Harvey wrote, than were the British, who had not been officially notified that any of these Americans were coming. George Crile's Base Hospital No. 4, which had arrived one day earlier, received a somewhat perfunctory formal welcome from the king and queen; Base Hospital No. 5 was worth greetings only from a royal nephew. Cushing did stumble upon King George V and Queen Mary when he wandered into a reception at the Officers' Club – the guests of honor were Canadians, combatants from the beginning of the war, whose great victory at Vimy Ridge a month earlier was being celebrated. Cushing always felt comfortable in Canadian company: 'The only ones really jubilantly cordial to us,' he noted in these early days. 'Stop us in the streets. Talk their own language. The English say – "Oh when did you land?" But they are glad too in their way.'[4]

The Oslers and Sherringtons and other Oxonian medical families also welcomed the Harvard folk. Oxford on a weekend in May 1917 was spectacularly beautiful, even if the punts on the Isis held mostly convalescents. Those in the know realized that most of the smart young student cadets about to leave for France would not return. Two of Osler's nephews had already been killed. William and Grace's only son, Revere, an artillery officer, had survived six months of battle and had just been home for his first leave. His parents were oppressed by the fear that they would never see him again.

Base Hospital No. 5 was assigned to take over the operation of one of the Royal Army Medical Corps's hospitals in France. Harvey, who seems to have expected special treatment for his unit, was 'very much disturbed' to learn that its site was a run-down British tent hospital, No. 11 General, part of the vast encampment on the French coast near Camiers. The Americans crossed a cold, foggy English Channel on May 30, 1917, standing in their life jackets all the way, listening to their

invisible destroyer escorts groaning and shrieking at one another with
their sirens. They were taken fifteen miles down the coast to their new
home, given a frugal supper in a cold mess hall, and fell into bed. A
convoy of incoming casualties arrived in the middle of the night. The
departing team of British doctors looked after these wounded, not happily, while the newcomers slept.

～

They had the poorest site of all the hospitals and troop encampments
on the Camiers-Etaples plain, south of Boulogne. It was a dense, dirty,
down-at-heel tent city on low ground completely surrounded by other
units. An exhausted, demoralized British medical unit, which had treated
some eight thousand casualties from the spring offensive, was being
withdrawn. Except for some surgical instruments, the Americans had
no equipment of their own, not even a vehicle. Their thin U.S. Army
uniforms did not keep out the biting Picardy cold. There were no bathing facilities, and four men were assigned to tents meant for one. They
did not fly their silk star-spangled banner. Their American identity was
submerged as they became workers at just another British base hospital
– though they were peculiar and puritanical by British standards, having gone officially 'dry.' A week after the unit's arrival, its harried quar-
termaster, in broken health, gave up and shot himself.[5]

   Genuinely puzzled at their treatment by the British but not wanting
to seem complainers, the Americans settled in to make the best of a
very bad situation. They wrote and telegraphed home to arrange shipment of some of the supplies, including motor cars and prefabricated
wooden huts, which had been assembled for their aborted mobilization. 'Possibly it is not a bad thing for us to have been piled into this
poor place, for it will give us a chance at least to show how industry can
make even such a hospital as this is better than it has been,' Harvey
wrote home. 'The Britisher does not begin work until ten, and we gave
the men we are to succeed a shock last night by posting an order that
the entire staff is to be called at 7.15.'[6]

After only a week at Camiers, Cushing was summoned to duty at the casualty clearing stations in the Ypres salient, and he had his initiation into battlefield surgery during the attack on Messines Ridge. A First World War casually clearing station was a recognizable ancestor of the American Mobile Army Surgical Hospitals, or MASH, units. In his diary Cushing often marveled at the stoicism of the wounded soldiers, the disfigured and the dying, who always said they were 'doing very well, sir' or 'not so bad, sir.' On June 12 he observed the emergency amputation of the hand of a British general, who lay on the table wearing the ribbon of the Victoria Cross he had won at the Battle of the Somme. When he came out of the anesthetic, General Congreve protested at being relieved from duty for such a trifle as losing his hand. Later in the war, Congreve also lost his son – who also won the Victoria Cross.

When Cushing was not operating, he went on orientation tours of other neighboring facilities with Sir Anthony Bowlby and other medical officers. The British army was building up for another offensive – encouraging news because of all the stories circulating about the French, whose soldiers had lost the will to fight and had mutinied: 'France indeed in an impossible state – fizzling out.' Cushing happened to meet Field Marshal Sir Douglas Haig, Britain's commanding officer in France, who expressed great satisfaction at the Messines victory. 'He's a stunning creature,' Harvey told Kate.[7]

Cushing saw survivors of Messines and other engagements who were so 'shell-shocked' that they fell into uncontrollable convulsing at the sound of artillery. He also saw what the Canadians had gone through on Vimy Ridge:

> Words fail to give any conception of the desolation. No convulsion of Nature could have done what man and man's machines have done ...
>
> It was an upheaval of sandbags, accoutrements, broken rifles not worth salvaging, entrenching tools, cartridge clips and machine-gun ribbons, food tins, water bottles, helmets, trench mortars, unexploded shells of every size, hand grenades, to which we give a wide berth, a human tibia exhumed from

somewhere, bits of clothing – and often smells, though two months have given ample time for burials ... It recalled the view two years ago out over Ypres – too vast to comprehend. Impossible to contract anything on such a scale down to one's own experiences; it is far easier to magnify small things in the imagination and thus get some conception of what had been going on.

He scrambled into a dry shell crater:

Among the canteens and food tins and fragments of tools and weapons was a broken stretcher, and alongside of it a British helmet with a through-and-through rifle shot – also stains on the band within to show what happened to the poor chap who now lies buried and unknown in the bottom of the crater in which he had fallen ... At one place we came upon some rough graves marked C.D. 24, probably the 24th Canadians, but burials for the most part must have been shallow – often in holes already made.

∾

Sent back to Camiers during the lull, Cushing continued to operate, though in a less urgent atmosphere. The unit was very busy, since a staff planned for 500 beds found itself with as many as 1,800 patients under canvas. Their site was rat-infested and appallingly drained, and their tents leaked. Harvey spent an evening dining at the nearby No. 1 Canadian Hospital, where he marveled at its superb location in pine woods, its beautiful wards, splendid operating rooms, perfect lighting, dressing rooms and bathrooms, hot running water, and tennis courts. 'One can talk to the Canadians and Australians as to one's own people.' The Canadians and Australians told him that the British had given the Americans the worst site for a hospital in all of France and warned him to expect indolence and indifference when he suggested reforms or innovations. The only way to get official action was to kick continually.[8]

The Americans tried to bypass official British channels and get private help from Boston. To their chagrin they found that Washington now required them to use only official channels. Their prefabricated huts and motor cars were never shipped, and they had to wait months for reinforcements from home, relying in the meantime on British support workers. But parcels of warm clothing and food did get through, and Cushing had many friends in the American community in Paris. He went there for help.

With his usual flair for timing, he arrived in Paris on the Fourth of July, 1917, just in time to attend celebrations welcoming General 'Black Jack' Pershing and the first battalion of American combat soldiers. *Vive L'Amérique!* American troops paraded through Paris streets to cheers and flowers, and one of Pershing's officers proclaimed, 'Lafayette, nous voici.' Harvey recorded that his countrymen were 'a disappointing looking lot, despite the enthusiasm. Nothing like the Australians or Canadians, but I hope better ones will follow.' The Americans marched in squads, not yet trusting themselves as platoons. It was not clear whether they would be nicknamed 'Sammies' after Uncle Sam or 'Teddies' after Theodore Roosevelt.[9] Strangely, they were soon being called 'doughboys,' an obscure usage dating from before the Civil War. Cushing never used 'Yanks' or 'Yankees' to describe Americans.

He found everyone running round in circles at the U.S. Army's new Paris headquarters and decided 'in about five minutes that it was useless to talk to them further, and far better to stay with the British for the rest of the war and do what we can with our outrageous camp.' Friends in one of the private American ambulance services that were about to be replaced by the military offered Base Hospital No. 5 a sky-blue Ford ambulance, 'the last one in the world,' a godsend. Cushing packed it full of supplies, ranging from linoleum to live rabbits (for research – not, as the French thought, for eating), and set out with a driver back to the coast. Just outside Paris the Ford broke down. Harvey tried to telephone for help and was upset at not being able to get through. A French observer commented, 'Monsieur n'a pas beaucoup de patience ... Monsieur must be Américain, – we thought him Anglais but he is not sufficiently content to be Anglais.'[10]

Being a surgeon and being Harvey Cushing, a kindred spirit to frontiersmen and surgeons named Hawkeye, he was not particularly content with anyone. 'I wish I dared say in a letter what I thought of the waste, the incompetence and the antiquated methods of business of the British Army ... An energetic people would do in 1 year what they do in 2 and with only half the expense & bother,' Harvey said in a letter to Kate – part of the fair amount of grumbling going on through official and unofficial channels. All the hospital's water had to be boiled because of bacterial contamination. So many men broke the unit's quixotic temperance pledge that it was officially called off.[11]

Good weather soothed American spirits well into July. Decent food and warm clothing and the intense interest the doctors took in their work sustained the unit. The only completely insoluble problem appeared to be keeping socks darned. The British RAMC leaders, who were doing their own grumbling about the bother the Americans were causing, made plans to relocate No. 5 in a better setting.[12] There was time for midsummer relaxation – a colleague noted in his diary that Cushing sang in an octet at a YMCA concert, played tennis, and at least once returned 'quite cheerily' but otherwise none the worse after an evening's carousing.[13] On July 21 Harvey was watching the finals of a tennis tournament when he received an order to be ready to leave for the front at 4:00 PM. He had three minutes' notice.

⌇

Field Marshall Haig had massed half a million troops and thousands of guns for another all-out offensive, intended to be one of the decisive battles of history. After a massive bombardment, the British Fifth Army was to smash through the German lines in the Ypres salient and break out into open country. The shattered and demoralized enemy would then retreat and surely sue for peace.

As part of the buildup, the Royal Army Medical Corps prepared some fifteen casualty clearing stations at road and rail junctions just behind the lines; these received cutely medicated designations, such as Mendinghem, Bandagehem, and Dosinghem (both Endinghem and

Kuringhem were vetoed).[14] Cushing headed one of many surgical teams sent up from the base hospitals – he brought with him an assistant, an anesthetist, an orderly, operating gear, and a supply of 'Boston tins' of dressings. He was stationed at No. 46 Casualty Clearing Station at Mendinghem near the village of Proven. It was normally a 200-bed temporary hospital, with a capacity to handle as many as 1,300 patients in a rush. A major part of the job would be triage – deciding which of the wounded to evacuate to base hospitals, which to prepare for immediate surgery (the rough guideline being to operate on anyone who needed relief within twenty-four hours), and which cases to set aside and quietly succor until the moment of death. As far as was practical, soldiers with serious head wounds would be directed to No. 46 CCS for Major Cushing's attention. Other American surgical teams from the base hospitals were also brought up.

Aerial battles and preliminary bombardments had already started when Cushing's team arrived in an ambulance on July 22. They were greeted by officers running for cover from explosions, one of which blew out the windows and electricity in the operating room. 'This is evidently a warm corner we've come into,' Harvey wrote. An ominously busy one too. No. 46 CCS had just taken in a thousand men suffering from the effects of a new German weapon: artillery shells loaded with mustard gas. The foul yellow poison blistered and rotted skin and eyes and lungs, and caused panic among hospital orderlies as it spread from skin to clothing and from clothing to skin. Qualms about retaliation had long since disappeared. The British replied to the first use of mustard gas shells with 70,000 phosgene shells. And the real battle had yet to begin. Harvey noted that the gassed men were under no illusions about how hard 'Fritz' was going to be to beat.[15]

In the final quiet days before zero hour he worked on head cases, operating into the small hours of the morning, trying to get used to a strange and uncomfortable environment. He decided he needed his magnet and managed to commandeer it from his unit over his commanding officer's objections. With all their teams and equipment in place, the medics waited, hanging on every scrap of gossip. Wounded pilots from the Royal Flying Corps confirmed rumors of a tactical German retreat from their advance positions. The aviators – 'mere kids' to Cushing – had inspected the German trenches at a height of about 600 feet. 'They would have hit us with a beer bottle,' a downed flier told his doctor.[16]

'More operations this morning, and our first try with the magnet – unsuccessful,' Cushing wrote on Sunday, July 29. 'The country is simply swarming with men, munitions, and mud, for it rained hard this morning. A bad thing for the advance if it keeps on ... The evening spent in a futile endeavor to resuscitate disconsolate Johnnie Morton's first patient, who had a respiratory failure from a spreading intracerebral hemorrhage.' Monday the thirtieth was overcast: 'Very quiet – practically no guns – nothing in the air. Still waiting for zero day and hour.' Word spread that the battle would begin early the next day. 'Let us hope there will be no more rain, for it adds enormousy to the sepsis.' At 3:50 AM on July 31, in a deluge of rain, the Battle of Passchendaele finally began.

~

He called it a 'summer of strange situations.' From August to the end of October Cushing was almost constantly on duty at No. 46 CCS, doing hundreds of operations as wave after wave of British and Empire soldiers – he lists thirteen separate attacks – threw themselves futilely, suicidally, at the German positions. From the earliest hours, rain and shells and a shallow water table turned the Flanders lowlands into a horrible sea of mud. At the end of the first day of fighting, the pre-op hut at No. 46 was packed with untouched cases 'so caked in wet mud,' Harvey wrote, 'that it's a task even to strip them and find out what they've got.'

> *August 2* Pouring cats and dogs all day – also pouring cold and shivering wounded, covered with mud and blood. Some wounds of the head, when the mud is scraped off, prove to be trifles – others of unsuspected gravity ... One

can't possibly keep up with them; and the unsystematic Britisher drives one mad. The news, too, is very bad. The greatest battle of history is floundering up to its middle in a morass ...

Operating from 8.30 a.m. one day till 2.00 a.m. the next; standing in a pair of rubber boots, and periodically full of tea as a stimulant, is not healthy. It's an awful business, probably the worst possible training in surgery for a young man, and ruinous for the carefully acquired technique of an oldster ... Finished up an hour ago with an extraction of a large piece of shell from a man's badly infected ventricle with the magnet ... A lot of wounded must have drowned in the mud.

August 3 Continuous downpour for the fourth consecutive day ... In the early afternoon a large batch of wounded were unexpectedly brought in – mostly heads – men who have been lying out for four days in craters in the rain, without food. It is amazing what the human animal can endure. Some of them had maggots in their wounds ... Many muddy bystanders from the adjacent hospitals looking on and fairly sitting on the instrument stands ... They think I'm killing Miss Gerrard. She does double work – anesthetist and instruments too – moreover, like me, has no regular schedule of hours.

August 4 Another night helping Johnnie and Blake as long as I could stand up ... Urgent operations on more rotting men.

Strange situations. In the middle of this, the RAMC's Director General of Medical Operations, Sir Arthur Sloggett, appears and insists that Cushing draft a letter to him denying that Cushing or Base Hospital No. 5 have been badly treated by the British in the matter of the location of their hospital. There have been threats to raise the issue in Parliament back in England. Sloggett, who wishes the Americans had never come over, has to cover himself. Cushing writes an appropriate letter and goes back to work. At night, dead tired, he finds that a long and locked ambulance train blocks his path back to his tent: 'There are two alternatives – to feel your way around in a sea of mud or to crawl under. I crawled under to-night and nearly cracked my head.'[17]

He knew that despite the willingness to tolerate his special techniques, he had to handle more cases. It often took three hours or longer
to extract bone and shell fragments from a soldier's brain and then
close the wound, and with a run of patients dying of infection (he was
losing more than half of the men he tried to help), it hardly seemed
possible to take shortcuts. His first reaction was to resent British incompetence:

> I am driven to distraction by the British dilatoriness, the everlasting stopping
> for meals. Someone is eating all day long – orderlies, sisters, noncoms, offic-
> ers. As a result there is only about an hour between any two meals – breakfast,
> lunch, tea, dinner, late supper – when the team as a whole can work together.
> In the other operating room they stop also for broth and biscuits at 11 a.m. As
> most of these men breakfast at nine, this means quite a gastronomic day, and
> most of them eat more meals than they operate on patients. I shall try to drive
> our American team into eight head cases a day or bust.[18]

He almost 'busted' getting through six in a day, then started taking lunch and tea in the operating room, which saved another hour.
He revved himself up with morning coffee, sent by Kate, and went
through a daily pack of cigarettes, Fatimas, also sent by his wife. He
told her that he had never done more work on less sleep, had never
felt better, and was gaining weight. In the operating hut he arranged
to have the next case being prepped for him while he worked so
that he could switch instantly. By mid-August he could do eight
serious cases in a day, averaging two hours each: 'It's amusing to
think that at home I used to regard a single major cranial operation
as a day's work.'[19]

He was conserving medical manpower by using a nurse anesthetist,
a practice the British were reluctant to adopt. Most important, both to
save time and to improve antisepsis, Cushing and his team learned a
new way of handling penetrating wounds of the head. After opening
the scalp, he encircled the whole wounded region of the skull and lifted
out the fractured area and its depressed bone fragments in one piece.

Then, with a catheter, he cleaned the tract the missile had taken, employing Carrel's special disinfecting fluid. It was an important innovation to use the catheter to suck out bone fragments. The magnet would get pieces of steel.

Writing up his record day in his diary, Cushing found time to reflect on the contrast between his seventh case – a big square-headed German prisoner – and his eighth – 'a little eighteen-year old Tommy from East London – scared, peaked, underfed, underdeveloped. He had been in training six months and was in the trenches ... *just ten minutes* when he was hit.'[20] Harvey was now doing most of his cases under local novocaine anesthetic, talking to the soldiers while he tried to clean and stabilize their brains.

Strange situations. Casualty clearing stations and hospitals were sometimes bombed or shelled. At a neighboring CCS the doctors sandbagged their tents and made dugouts for the nursing sisters. One night the women took refuge in ditches dug by Chinese coolies in a nearby cemetery. At Harvey's CCS, the officers all dug 'funk holes' about two feet deep beside their tents and prepared to sleep in them. To Cushing, they looked like little graves. No one was quite sure whether painting red crosses on the roofs of the medical encampments gave better protection or made them easier targets.[21]

Long before the phrase became common, Cushing tried to save the life of an 'unknown' soldier, an unconscious man who had been brought in without any identifying tag. It was a hopeless case. On August 19 they had a crying baby in the operating room and treated the wounds the baby and its mother had received in an air raid. There were cheerful, gossipy dinners at regimental messes, with no one mentioning that at dawn the men would follow a barrage into something worse than the Inferno. There were midnight bitching sessions when the surgeons, having sent their exhausted nurses to bed and cleaned up the hut themselves, wound down over eggs and tea in the mess. 'We've spent another hour discussing the English,' Harvey told his diary, 'who we think are lazy, and without manners.'[22]

The strangest situation? On August 26 Cushing received a letter

from Grace Osler telling him that Revere was coincidentally somewhere in the same neighborhood: 'How awful you would feel if you saw
him with a bad head wound – but what a mercy it would be for him.
The anticipated horror is very wearing.'[23] Harvey began trying to locate Revere for a get-together. He was exhausted and ready to turn in
after a long day on the twenty-ninth when at 10 PM he had a message
from a fellow American surgeon: Sir William Osler's son was seriously
wounded at No. 47 CCS, Dosinghem. Come immediately.

An ambulance took him in heavy rain the few miles to Dosinghem.
Revere had been brought in that evening. His artillery unit had been
wiped out by a casual shell burst. His own wounds, Cushing wrote,
'could not have been much worse, though there was a bare chance –
one traversing through the upper abdomen, another penetrating the
chest just above the heart, two others in the thigh.'

By midnight (this is hard to believe but true), four of the most skilled
surgeons the United States could offer – Cushing, George Crile, and
William Darroch and George Brewer from New York – had assembled
to operate on twenty-one–year-old Revere. Crile gave transfusions,
Cushing tracked his pulse, Brewer and Darroch opened his abdomen
and cleaned and sutured his wounds. They did not expect recovery.
'His condition remained unaltered,' Cushing recorded the next day
(though in a later letter he said he thought there had been a brief rally),
'and about seven this morning the world lost this fine boy, as it does
many others every day':

> We saw him buried in the early morning. A soggy Flanders field beside a
> little oak grove to the rear of the Dosinghem group – an overcast, windy,
> autumnal day – the long rows of wooden crosses – the new ditches half full of
> water being dug by Chinese coolies wearing tin helmets – the boy wrapped
> in an army blanket and covered by a weather-worn Union Jack, carried on
> their shoulders by four slipping stretcher-bearers. A strange scene – the great-
> great-great grandson of Paul Revere under a British flag, and awaiting him a
> group of some six or eight American Army medical officers – saddened with
> thoughts of his father ... Some green branches were thrown in for him to lie

on. The Padre recited the usual service – the bugler gave the 'Last Post' – and we went about our duties.

Cushing had cut a button from Revere's tunic. He had wired the family, breaking the news, and now he gave instructions to have the grave marked. Later he told Kate it was his worst experience since Ned's death.[24]

Back in Camiers, the Harvard unit had been been working flat out since the beginning of the offensive, its beds full, its staff stretched to the limit and beyond. Its commanding officer, Major Patterson, fended off constant calls from Cushing and others for more help at the casualty clearing stations. On September 4, German bombs fell on the tent city of Base Hospital No. 5, killing an officer and three enlisted men and wounding twenty-two. These were the first Americans to die while officially serving their country in the war. Cushing rushed back to base, but there was nothing he could do: 'There were of course a number of critical and urgent operations. MacLeod, the nice young chap who brought over our last reënforcements, lost both legs, and the next day had a double thigh amputation, high up, for fulminating gas-bacillus infection. To Cutler's great credit he promises to recover.' Cushing's desire to be first in the field knew no limits: 'If casualties were to be had,' he told Kate, 'I'm not sorry that we stood the brunt of the first ones.'[25]

Low in spirits and feeling vaguely ill, Cushing managed to get a few days' rest during the early September break in the fighting. He used these to work on his case records, hear how the war was going, nip into Paris, sightsee the ruins of Ypres, and get to know the pilots at a nearby airfield, a group of cocky 'perfect children' whose heroics in aerial combat fascinated him. On the afternoon before the offensive was about to resume, Harvey set out for a long walk with one of his assistants, Gilbert Horrax. He found himself bothered by a strange bout of sharp pain in the calves and felt humiliated in having to turn back. He thought he had some kind of 'duckboard' ailment caused by weeks of walking on narrow planks over Flanders mud. An orthopedist colleague he spoke to about the problem thought it was just a matter of a short Achilles tendon and advised that he wear higher heels. Examining himself, Cushing began to suspect a circulation problem. In fact, it was the beginning of what would eventually be very serious trouble in his legs and feet.[26]

~

He was on duty at No. 46 CCS during September and October as Haig threw his forces against the German positions in attack after attack, big push on big push, bombardment upon bombardment. There were nights in the operating hut when it sounded as if the whole world was exploding, as bombs fell, munition dumps were hit, and the buildings rattled with shock waves from the big guns. A few hours later an eerie quiet would be broken by faint notes from the old piano someone was playing in the mess, then the clatter of footsteps on duckboards, reminding Harvey of notes on a muffled xylophone. Cold wet weather set in. The night before the (eighth) 'big push' of October 4, Cushing dined with men of the Scots Guards. The talk was gloomy – how quickly the crows, the frogs, the maggots could pick a dead body clean. Pipe Major Ross suggested that the next few weeks would show whether Britain could have won the war without American help. Harvey asked Ross for the name of the tune he played for them that dreary evening. It was 'The McIntosh Lament.'[27]

As the eighth, ninth, tenth, eleventh, twelfth, and thirteenth attacks were all thrown back, the mud and pessimism and weather all worsened:

October 8   Everything is wet, sodden, and cold.

October 11, 1 AM   Done to a frazzle after our final case ... Murphy wants to know how I manage to keep warm. I don't.

October 12   Worse than any morning we have seen, if that is possible ...

One wonders how men could long survive even were there no fighting.

October 21   In the afternoon to Dosinghem to see Revere's grave ... It's dreadful to see that place grow – a thousand burials in the past three weeks.

October 26   Salvation Corner on the way to Solferino Farm ... French graves with their red and blue circle on the wooden cross ... desolate beyond words ...

I have just been talking with a young subaltern of the 50th Division, who, shaking and trembling, is pretending to smoke a cigarette in his bed in the officers' ward. His battalion went in last night, following a muddy tape. They got absolutely scattered and lost – had no idea where they were – many wandered directly into the enemy's area ... there was practically nobody left.

It's easy to play the game from the grandstand; but I can't help feeling that this show in view of the downpour ought to have been called off.

October 27   Almost all the wounds are minor ones ... This means either that we were driven back and left our more serious wounded, or else only the walkers survived to get away and out of the mire.

Ironically, the surgical results were getting better. Continuing to operate on the most serious head cases, with Horrax usually assisting him, Cushing's techniques for debriding wounds – encircling the wound, sucking out foreign matter and pulped brain tissue, cleaning the track, then closing – were so effective that his mortality rate for wounds that penetrated the dura fell from 54.5 percent in the first month of the battle to 28.8 percent in the third. On Sundays, while other surgical teams relied on nursing sisters to change patients' dressings, Cushing, Gil Horrax, and Gertrude Gerrard, his nurse anesthetist, did it themselves. To him, the other surgeons were 'partly inexperienced in this kind of work and partly – well lazy.'[28]

Cushing had no illusions about the success of the battle, but he was proud that he was there, practicing surgery in strange, incredible situations while keeping meticulous case records in the midst of the chaos and even illustrating them with before-and-after photographs taken with his contraband Kodak. The Battle of Passchendaele was unspeakably awful, to be sure. In the grand sweep of things, the surgeons had no hope of stemming the hemorrhaging of the British armies – in some ways, the death of the British Empire. But to be there was to be on the edge, just as he so often lived on the edge in the operating room. It was to be like the young pilots who put their lives at risk in every flight and whose feats in their frail little aircraft fascinated the middle-aged brain surgeon.

On Sunday, October 28, he left Horrax to do a couple of stray head cases and spent the afternoon with a friend touring the battle zone, struggling to find words for what so many had found indescribable:

> The salient is a waste unbelievably littered with débris of every kind, dead horses, derelict tanks, fallen and crumpled aeroplanes, cordite cans, shells, mortars, fish-tail bombs, broken and abandoned limbers, barbed wire, old trenches, water-filled craters, strips of old road camouflage, gravestones and tumbled cemeteries, sheet-iron fragments of old Nissan huts, fallen trees, frames of inverted A-shaped trench supports, and I can't remember at the moment more – except the gooey mud.

When the shells actually started exploding near him, Cushing felt an existential, animal thrill: 'The savage in you makes you adore it with its squalor and wastefulness and glorious noise. You feel that, after all, this is what men were intended for rather than to sit in easy chairs with a cigarette and whiskey, the evening paper or the best-seller, and to pretend that such a veneer means civilization and that there is no barbarian behind your starched and studded shirt front.'

He told Kate that his tour of the front had been 'very exciting': 'I'm afraid I like it – the real savage in me.' When he published his diaries nineteen years later, he did not change a word of this startling entry.[29]

On their last afternoon in the salient, Cushing and Horrax again visited Ypres. They spent two hours in the ruins of St Martin's Cathedral and the Cloth Hall, picking up bits of fallen stone and marble and glass, noting fragments of human bone from a disturbed grave and rusted dud shells. Harvey tried to word-paint the 'noble ruin ... with the tottering pinnacles and arches between us and the reddish streaks of light from the broken western sky ... the row of ugly balloons, like partly curled-up black maggots.' A party of New Zealand soldiers who were living in the ruins showed them the big cathedral bell, half-buried in sandbags, a ragged hole in its side. With wax and paper, the American doctors made rubbings of the figures round the top of the bell: Death beckoning to a bride, Death taking an old man by the arm. The old bell had seen many dances of death, Harvey thought, but this was the most horrible.[30]

Cushing left the salient on November 1. To finish the story he later inserted a footnote in his diaries mentioning the final push by fresh Canadian troops early in November that enabled them to seize the ruined village of Passchendaele and control the high ground. There had been no breakthrough.

∾

'I am really over there in spirit with you – It is all so real to me. And this life here, rather unreal, except my work and the children.'[31] Kate Cushing was as existentially captured by the war as Harvey. If she had had any doubts in 1915, she had none by 1917 and had completely supported Harvey's campaign for preparedness. She had decided that Germany was a barbarous threat to all the values of home, family, and country and dear friends like the Oslers – that she treasured. She totally approved of her husband's decision to leave her with the five little children and go to war; this time, he was leaving them for the best of reasons. The tensions and frictions of their marriage dissolved into patriotic enthusiasm.

They wrote every three or four days. Kate poured out her feelings:

I told you once I didn't know how it feels to be patriotic – well that's all changed now ... I have still the strangest feeling of gladness that you are first in the field, and that you are out of this nagging place ... I am so proud of what you have done and of what you are going to do ... I wouldn't have missed that great week [before sailing] for any thing – it was the crowning week of my life, to feel so absolutely at one with you, your ideas and aims ... I have never been quite so happy in spite of the loneliness, because we shall always have it and it is a guarantee for the future. I feel so sure of you and of my self. And now I want to do, even in the smallest things, every thing that you would wish me to ... I'll try to be patient and work hard for you here, and not use a cent more money than I have to, so that when you come back you can have a good rest, and never have to work any more if you don't want to ... I would willingly lay down my life for you.[32]

Kate took a course in home nursing, folded gauze for the Surgical Dressings Committee, tried going from door to door selling Liberty Loan Bonds ('It's a rotten job'), grew vegetables at home and at Little Boars Head, observed days of meatless, wheatless, and porkless dining, and dusted off her canning skills. 'We are going back to those primitive things, knitting, sewing & cooking for our men folks – We shall all be happier for it.' She sent her man parcel after parcel of tobacco, biscuits, chocolate, soap, maple sugar, soap mislabeled as maple sugar, coffee, family pictures, string, hair lotion, thumb tacks, pencil sharpeners, warm pajamas with sewed-in feet, just like the children's, and special red, white, and blue woolen socks. 'Love is certainly in every stitch.' She passed on all the home-front gossip: 'This country looks entirely different since May 11th ... The sons of half the women I know are in camps – Don't let them think over there for a minute that we're not in it up to the hilt – and think what we've accomplished since Apr. 6th in spite of the politicians!'[33]

The wives of the Harvard unit met regularly and read each other excerpts from their men's letters. Kate read and sometimes circulated expurgated versions of Harvey's diaries. She lunched often with Julia Shepley's mother, another source of news. The women of that era proudly used the phrase 'Keep the home fires burning.' Kate told Harvey about all the children's little problems and achievements – Bill's adventures at camp, Betsy's grown-up sense of humor 'which will save her life some day,' Henry's missing front teeth, Mary reading *Pride and Prejudice,* and the radiant beauty of baby Barbara: 'I never saw a child so full of the joy of life. Her sweet little voice chatters from morning until night. She is the most entrancing two year old baby I ever saw.'[34]

'I get tired of the children, and eagerly seek my kind, get enough of them, and go thankfully back to the children! Sewing circle is rather sickening this year – they are still talking about things like suffrage and damning the administration.' She went to patriotic meetings and fundraisers, and now the tears streamed down her face during 'The Marseillaise' and 'The Star-Spangled Banner.' She confessed to loathing, hating, despising the Germans, despite Harvey's having cautioned her against such feelings:

> If I didn't feel that the war was necessary, and that it was necessary for you to sit by your fire in France for an indefinite period, while I sit by my fire here – the children growing up & we all needing and wanting you most frightfully – I should go mad – & I must keep it before me night & day that to win – to gain freedom for all countries, we must all put our backs into it for all we are worth – save our money for Liberty Loans & war taxes & using every bit of energy we possess and all the time we can give, outside of ones necessary household duties, to working in one way or another toward that one end – and not indulge ourselves in high flown thoughts as to the origin of war or the settlement afterwards ... You must keep up my courage once in a while by saying that all this is true – *do my* job ...
>
> I price beef carefully & bend the chickens breast bones, as in early Baltimore days.[35]

Was Harvey keeping warm and dry? Was he getting enough to eat? 'If only you keep well – wear your winter underclothes and take your medicine as Wendy says to Peter Pan.' Kate had bitter contempt for doctors who were not volunteering to serve, including so many of the Johns Hopkins crowd, especially their old friend Lewellys Barker. Having heard that Cushing's wife was a 'madwoman' on the subject of Germany, Barker breezed in one night with the greeting, 'To hell with the Kaiser': 'He did say at dinner that he felt like a slacker, with you and all those men over there – whereupon you might have cut the silence with a knife, and I piped up & said 'Well you know Lewellys, there's yet time.'[36]

Outside of medical circles, Kate was charming and composed. Henry Lee Higginson, one of Boston's grand brahmins, wrote Harvey: 'I never saw a woman who kept her poise or cheerfulness more than she does, and I was struck with the beauty of her hair the other night. Like a thoroughbred, I am sure she hides all her aches, and smiles as a matter of course ... We shall never meet an angel that is more delightful company or more healthy in every way than Mrs. Harvey Cushing.' Of course, Higginson agreed with Kate about the war.[37]

When the slaughter took Revere Osler, Kate could hardly stand the grief and had to stay in her room, weeping and writing to her husband: 'This morning I can't seem to face the world, it's so dark. I miss so and sorrow so for my friends. Can we not give up just one day to grieving for our friends. The children think I have a cold, and don't mind and mother sits like a youthful watch dog down stairs and fends people off ... My heart is simply breaking for them. I can't think or write of anything else.'[38]

✎

The surgeon soldiers were contemptuous of Americans who had found ways to bootleg their wives over to France. They saw a lot of 'concealed wives' at dinners and other social events in Paris, where they went from time to time in the winter of 1917–18 for meetings of a joint Anglo-American committee on war-related research. 'An altogether bad thing in principle this wife business,' Harvey noted, 'and people spend a good deal of time in apologia which indicates that they agree – at least as regards the other man's wife.'[39]

He often told Kate, still his 'Peaches,' how much he missed her and the children. He occasionally wrote to them – especially to Bill, usually about the flyers and their battles – but told Kate it was all he could do to keep up his diary and write to her. Knowing how long six months is for a child, he wondered if they would remember him and said he knew he wouldn't recognize baby Barbara if he saw her on the Ypres road. A few of Betsey's wartime letters to her father survive: 'I am terribly lonesome without you fah ... you must not think that we will forget you, because we won't just as long as we live ... Almost everybody asks me who I've got in the service, and I proudly say father ... I am so lonesome for you.' Kate told him that two-year-old Barbara talked to the picture of him in the upstairs hall: 'Morning Father ... Hello Father.'[40]

Harvey felt vaguely ill and depressed for a month after leaving the Passchendaele battlefield: 'shivery sensations, aches, and a weazened brain.' He thought it was partly a touch of 'grippe', and partly a letdown from the intense life of No. 46 CCS. It was probably more than that. As a doctor and a soldier and a stoic, Cushing tended to ignore illnesses. In February 1918 he admitted to his diary that he was 'bedridden in Boulogne,' suffering from what he considered 'bogus pneumonia.' Kate received letters from people who knew him saying it was the real thing. [41]

Strange bacilli and viruses, and mental pathogens too, were everywhere in France in those years, and few soldiers came out completely untouched or unbroken. When Harvey met up with Jack McCrae, author of 'In Flanders Fields,' he found him transformed by the Ypres experience from a sunny, companionable colleague into a brooding, asthmatic loner. Soon Cushing again visited McCrae, who was on his deathbed in a nearby hospital, suffering from atypical pneumonia and meningitis, 'a bright flame burning out.'[42] Harvey noticed members of McCrae's McGill hospital unit hunting for winter poppies to put on his grave. Another funeral in the diary, January 29, 1918:

We saw him buried this afternoon at the cemetery on the hillside at Wimereux with military honors – a tribute to Canada as well as to him. A large gathering of friends – all who could get there, even from a distance ... We met at No. 14 General – a brilliant sunny afternoon – and walked the mile or so to the cemetery. A company of North Staffords and many R.A.M.C. orderlies and Canadian sisters headed the procession – then 'Bonfire,' led by two grooms and carrying the regulation white ribbon, with his master's boots reversed over the saddle – then the rest of us.

Six sergeants bore the coffin from the gates, and as he was being lowered into his grave there was a distant sound of guns – as though called into voice by the occasion. An admirable prayer by one of the three Padres who officiated. The Staffords ... fix bayonets, and instead of firing over the grave, as in time of peace, stand at salute during the Last Post with its final wailing note which brings a lump to our throats – and so we leave him there, underground but in sunshine.

∿

It was a comfortable winter in Base Hospital No. 5's splendid new quarters. When Cushing rejoined his unit in November, it was being moved to the Channel port of Boulogne, to operate the British No. 13 General Hospital, located in the huge casino. Here the Americans had one of the grandest buildings on the coast, with every convenience – even Sir Almroth Wright's research lab, equipped with Wright himself – and probably the only 'baccarat ward' in France. Harvey stayed with Wright for the first few days, then moved into a rented villa with other officers; the enlisted men bunked beachside in wheeled bathing huts.

There was very little fighting on the Western Front in the winter of 1917–18 and little business at the hospital. Harvey told Kate they felt as far from the war as if they were in Boston. Harvey spent an hour or two on the wards each day but seldom operated; he devoted most of his time to writing a long article about his battlefield surgery. The Americans played baseball and football, held concerts and vaudeville and minstrel shows, saw motion pictures, exchanged visits with other units, often drank too much, and feasted on real turkeys at Thanksgiving and Christmas. Everyone was trying to keep spirits up and not think too much about war prospects. The British and French offensives of 1917 had been bloody failures. Italy had been almost knocked out of the war. Russia had been; the Bolsheviks had seized power and were suing for peace. The Americans were still coming, always coming.

Cushing word-sketched the parade of passing ships in the Channel, the sunsets, the storms. He recorded dinner parties with interesting guests: Almroth Wright 'at his inscrutable best ... simply paralyzing'; the inarticulate Colonel Hamerton loosening his tongue and talking about the varieties of 'niggers' he had experienced in Africa; General Leonard Wood complaining about the disorganized mess of the American war machine. Wood, a very political and almost openly Republican general before the war, was embittered at Wilson's having denied him an active command in France. 'He's got in the habit of kicking I fear thro' his 3 years of preparedness,' Harvey told Kate. 'Very sore at the gov't which is quite natural ... I did all I could to cheer him up.' Harvey could not detect any deterioration in Wood's physical condition almost eight years after surgery, but thought his pessimism was obsessive: 'It's a time when everyone must be an optimist willy nilly. It's one of the unbeatable qualities of these somewhat dull Britishers.'[43]

The war took more old acquaintances, some of them thousands of miles away. Victor Horsley, pioneer of neurosurgery, had died of heat stroke in Mesopotamia. Cushing spent the last night of 1917 listening to a mutual friend tell of Horsley operating on a friend's dromedary and of Horsley operating on his own son for epilepsy. They might have talked about the eccentric surgeon's fatal conviction that an abstainer from alcohol could not be hurt by hot weather. 'What an unbelievable creature Horsley was,' Harvey recalled, 'an absolute believer in himself and no other till the end. Lucky I did not stay and work with him in 1900.' Other old memories came flooding back the day he received two letters from his brothers in Cleveland. Will, the eldest, wrote a cheery, newsy letter, dated December 18, 1917. Harry's letter contained word that Will had died suddenly in his office on December 19.[44]

Cushing saw Leonard Wood twice more in Paris. Once was on a social occasion when Wood invited Harvey to come with him to the French front. Harvey was too busy. Two weeks later he saw Wood professionally. At the front, a mortar explosion had killed four of the French officers with Wood's party, had left fragments in the brain of one of Wood's aides, but had given Wood himself only a flesh wound: 'I found him with his sick-room full of people ... very fit, showing what he could do with his palsied hand ... Expects to go to the front again to finish his observations.' Harvey went driving with Wood in the Bois de Boulogne, where they came upon a carriage with an old French couple, the almost forgotten General Joffre and his wife. Wood, ostracized by the Wilsonians, was trying hard not to go the way of the Joffres.[45]

Cushing spent most of his free time writing about the head surgery he had done at No. 46 CCS. He rushed a summary of his work into print in the *British Medical Journal* in February 1917; a longer analysis was published two months later in the *British Journal of Surgery*. With 126 pages of detailed case studies, drawings, and photographs, it was virtually a book on wartime head surgery – and it did become *the* book when it formed the basis of accounts of that subject in both the American and the British official histories of wartime medical services.[46]

Cushing outlined his techniques and results, hoping his improved mortality rates would serve as 'a score against which others working under similar conditions may successfully compete.' But were these elaborate cranial operations justified under battlefield conditions? he asked. Did they take too much time to be practical in the medical rush? He answered that they were medically justified: the best results could be secured by operating as early as possible; time spent on cerebral wounds was not much greater than on other deep wounds; and physicians had a responsibility to try to save lives. Tribunals could not make snap assessments of the quality of life that soldiers might have after major head surgery, he argued, because all sorts of recoveries were possible. Ultimately, the issue of whether surgeons should give priority to simple or more severe wounds was 'a matter for a military rather than a medical decision.'

Everything about the handling of the wounded had a bearing on survival. The quicker stretcher-bearers were at bringing in the wounded, he pointed out, the more lives might be saved – though a higher proportion of the desperately wounded would consequently die in hospital rather than in shell holes. He did not add that bolder retrieval of wounded might also mean more dead stretcher-bearers. Such issues were canvassed one day at an army medical school session at which he was scheduled to speak. The commanding officer of a field ambulance, one Fletcher, talked about the fine points of clearing a battlefield: how to choose stretcher-bearers, whether prisoners should carry the wounded, how the carrying was done, searching for wounded at night (be sure to warn your side that you're out), the looting issue, and much more. Were duckboards too narrow for stretcher bearing? Fletcher asked. To Cushing's delight,

> a big Canadian sergeant arose and said he would like to show how they carried *their* wounded and could keep to duckboards ... He and four bearers ... came forward – one of them got on a stretcher – the other four swung it up to their shoulders, but instead of its resting on their inner shoulders they put their heads and bodies close together and got the handlebars on the outer shoulders. Fletcher admitted he'd never thought of carrying in this way ... When someone asked about carrying in the trenches, the sergeant said: 'We never uses a trench, sir, we takes over the top.'

When the neurosurgeon followed with his talk on treating head injuries, he could not hold the audience's attention, and he scorned his effort as very feeble.[47]

The Anglo-American medical research committee, whose Paris meetings Cushing liked to attend, also concentrated on mundane problems: scabies, trench fever, delousing, inoculating, disinfecting wounds, antigas procedures, and the new practice of blood transfusion. Colleagues such as Walter Cannon and Richard Strong were doing practical, empirical studies of shock and the role of lice in causing trench fever. George Crile, on the other hand, who continued to be ubiquitous in the Allied medical effort, had gone research mad and proposed a huge project, headed by himself, to study every malady known to warfare and wounds 'and ultra-violet light; electrolysis; radium; intracellular resuscitation ...' 'A great irridescent bubble ... which we had to prick,' commented Cushing. 'George took it like a man. We will now all work in cooperation and try and keep our feet on the ground, and not blow bubbles, but keep our minds fixed on the practical problems concerning the wastage of man power and its prevention.'[48]

Harvey was able to get to England in early March 1918 to take a few days' leave and to submit his long article. The visit was made deeply melancholy by the grief he found in Oxford. William Osler was 'a shadow of his former self,' who did not talk about Revere. Grace, in her agony, could hardly talk about anything else.

Osler took Cushing on his weekly visit to No. 15 Canadian General Hospital on the Astor estate at Cliveden. They inspected the neurological cases and watched Nancy Astor whack one of the wounded Tommies with her riding crop: '"Get up," she said – "you haven't any guts" ... He roars with delight, and the others join in. She is doubtless the best psychotherapeutist in the establishment.' Osler, a different kind of psychotherapeutist, took him on a round of visits to children, 'some of his many darlings who find things in his pockets and cuddle about him while he tells a story before they go to bed.'

Back at the Oslers' house, Osler and Cushing had a late-night talk about rare books and collecting. Osler showed his friend the little notebook in which Revere, following in their footsteps, had listed his book purchases. The last entry in it, on the boy's last leave, was Dobell's *Meditations on the four last things: Death, Judgment, Heaven, Hell*.[49]

Cushing's complaints about Britain and the British gradually softened. As he crossed back to France, for example, he studied two of his countrymen:

> Spick-and-span West Pointers – a colonel and a major – just out of a bandbox – tight-fitting, neatly pressed thin uniforms, paper-soled pointed riding boots – very alert and erect – also very complaining. Such a contrast to the civilian officers of the B.E.F. just returning from leave with all emotions buried behind the *Times* after a 'So long old girl,' and 'Bring back a D.S.O., Charlie,' on the platform. Charlie, like most of the others, in heavy trench boots and

enveloped in a soiled raincoat over a ragged 'British warm' – many of them with wound strips and the spectral Mons-Star ribbon ... indicating long as well as meritorious service.

He was no longer so sure that American cockiness made sense; the West Pointers, he thought, 'have much to learn and they're probably at bottom very brave and capable, though tactless, fellows.'[50]

Nor was it clear with whom he would work for the rest of the war. Both the British and American medical services wanted him to take charge of their neurosurgical effort. He spent several days in March at American medical headquarters in Neufchâteau, east of Paris, where there was something of a Hopkins reunion with old friends such as Hugh Young and W.S. Thayer, now highly placed consultants in U.S. Army medicine. J.M.T. Finney was at the very top of the heap as chief surgical consultant to the army, and he hoped to pry Harvey loose from the British.

Most of his friends had rallied to the flag when America finally abandoned its neutrality. Cushing toured the splendid Johns Hopkins base hospital at Bazoilles; visited American 'evacuation' hospitals, the equivalent of casualty clearing stations, behind lines that American soldiers had taken over in the St Mihiel salient; spent a few minutes in Domrémy-la-Pucelle seeing the cottage where Joan of Arc was said to have been born; and with Finney and others spent an afternoon in Verdun, the site of France's most desperate fighting in 1916–17. Verdun had been an even worse killing field than Passchendaele. The medics toured Verdun's great Vauban citadel and its curiously spared cathedral, examining Roman crypts and murals until incoming shells drove them under cover. They saw American troops moving towards the front and the French coming out. The long lines of Packard trucks along the dusty *voie sacrée* reminded Harvey of prairie schooners. Finney commented that the Americans looked as though they were ready for business. Finney had adopted as their group's watchword that season the title of a popular song: 'It's a great life if you don't weaken.'[51]

~

The Germans attacked in Flanders on the first day of spring, March 21.
Some sixty divisions broke the junction between British and French
lines and poured into open countryside, jeopardizing everything. The
British might be rolled up against the Channel and driven out of France.
Paris was again threatened. A giant German cannon began shelling the
French capital from the astonishing distance of seventy-five miles, firing the first projectiles ever to enter the stratosphere. Weakened to the
verge of panic, the British and French governments created a joint
command under the French Marshal Foch.

Harvey was back with his hospital unit at Boulogne, where at first
there was little to do but sit around and wait for news. Their British
friends were full of self-criticism at being woefully unprepared for an
offensive they knew was coming. But they also told a story of an American soldier being served a mug of beer. 'It's flat, this beer,' he complains. 'Naturally,' says the barmaid, 'It's been waiting for you for three
years.'[52]

The walking wounded trickled in during the first week, then cases
from the casualty clearing stations, and soon the surgeons were working flat out. Harvey had few head cases, though, and was in a kind of
limbo about being transferred to the American Expeditionary Force.
Then he was suddenly needed, both at the casino to help with gas cases
and as a surgeon nearer the front. He had just turned forty-nine and
was worried about the problems with his feet and legs, but when he
slipped on a banana peel on his birthday he was still able to keep his
balance. He and Cutler were ordered up to No. 58 CCS near Lillers
and went to work in the operating hut, where they stood up to the
situation better than he had feared. They were overwhelmed with
wounded, including civilians. Women and children lay on stretchers
alongside the dirt-smeared soldiers. Most of their academic talk about
wound treatment seemed irrelevant. A train full of incoming wounded
was bombed, and when the victims finally reached the hospital many
of them were dead.[53]

Streams of refugees. No hot water. No fire. But in Harvey's billet in a doctor's house in a pleasant village on April 12, the 'blinds open on to a fine sunny morning with the birds gayly chirping in the budding horse-chestnuts.' By the end of the day, No. 58 CCS and all its wounded have been completely evacuated. Its medical teams scatter to other places. A distracted, overwrought general asks Harvey what he wants to do: 'Anything you wish, sir.' He winds up at British No. 7 General Hospital in an old monastery near St Omer, but it too is being evacuated. Everything is a mess. 'With our backs to the wall ... each one of us must fight on to the end,' the panicking General Haig has ordered. From Ypres, Cushing hears that all the ground gained at Messines and Passchendaele has been lost to the Germans in six days.

He finally ends up at No. 4 Canadian CCS near Pernes, where he alternates between working desperately hard and having nothing to do. No one has any idea how the battle is going – Harvey thinks it a good sign when his last head case one day is a German: 'Someone must have made a successful counterattack, else we should scarcely have been receiving enemy wounded.' He feels at home with the young men from the prairies, breezy Winnipeggers, dug in and determined: 'They're the boys – divisions at full strength ... No talk from them of falling back – of the end of the war ... They have had their troubles with the British but say little of it.' From the beginning of the war, Cushing has admired the Canadians, and now he hopes he can stay with them. 'They are all citizen soldiers,' he tells Kate. 'That's why they have been so good from the very start. That's the main reason the British don't like them – the best organized, the most dependable, the best fighting unit on this western front and the Boches leave them severely alone.'[54]

On April 24 Cushing is in the middle of a serious operation when his commanding officer comes in and reads him an order to report to the American Expeditionary Force for 'temporary duty'. That night he leaves for Neufchâteau, where he finds that American disorganization, demoralization, and continued inaction are even more depressing than British incompetence. At least the British keep tidy and clean. In the American army, as in the French, no one seems to bathe: 'The whole army is very lousy ... the soldiers dirty and shabby,' and even the medical officers do not keep a proper latrine.

Cushing has traveled everywhere with a fold-up canvas bathtub; when it finally springs a leak, he manages to replace it. He reflects on how much he has picked up from the British, almost unconsciously, and is not sure that the American approach to being citizen soldiers works: 'Born free and equal there is no one willing to accept the job of proper disposal of his own, far less other people's excreta.' Indiscipline and organizational chaos are everywhere. Harvey records a 'darkie' story about a waiter who, when asked if he is head of the lodge, replies, 'Oh, no ... I'se only de supreme King, dere's seven above me.' He learns that he has been taken away from battlefield surgery and required to travel halfway across France for the sole purpose of giving one lecture to fifty officers in training at a U.S. Army school. 'It's the way we have in the army,' the school's commanding officer tells the angry surgeon.[55]

Cushing decides he wants to stay with the British Expeditionary Force. The BEF is not so sure it wants Cushing. He no sooner gets back to Boulogne than he is recalled to Paris to answer a serious complaint which the British censor has made to the American authorities about Major Cushing's disregard of regulations. He has twice violated the rules governing censorship. The first time, some months earlier, he passed on to Kate some passages from an ordinary soldier's letter that he himself had censored, as part of his officer's duties. Now the censor has found diary notes in a letter to Kate which contain some of the harsh criticisms of the British that have peppered his pages from the beginning of the war. Knowing that his diaries would never pass censorship, Cushing normally sent them home with traveling friends. These pages got into a letter by mistake.

Cushing grovels, writing an abject letter of apology. For a few days he has nothing to do but hang around Paris with his tail between his legs, awaiting his fate, worrying that he may be sent home in disgrace, perhaps even court-martialed. Back at home, his sister Alice has just died. Kate goes to Cleveland to help clean out the Cushing house (Harvey wants just one thing, his father's book of Cushing family genealogy), and then she returns to Boston to care for the children, who are all down with measles. 'I am supremely satisfied with my life, and would not have one thing changed,' writes the wife, who right now is coping better than the husband.[56]

Harvey's troubles soon blow over. There is never any serious thought of court-martialing him; the matter is dropped and forgotten – except in postwar storytelling, where it is blown out of all proportion. On the censorship matter, he has been 'thoughtlessly foolish,' as J.M.T. Finney remarks in his memoirs. But instead of changing his ways, Cushing is simply more careful not to mail his diaries, which also contain very pointed criticism of Finney's competence and that of most of the American military.[57]

Cushing is ordered to return to Boulogne and do a feasibility study of handling neurosurgical cases in both armies. He almost immediately goes over to England to study the situation there – finding little agreement on principles of treatment – and on to Dublin where in a glittering formal ceremony he is made an honorary fellow of Ireland's Royal College of Surgeons. The ceremony is held in the college's bullet-scarred building, which was seized as a holdout by Irish nationalists during the 1916 Easter Rebellion against British rule. In his formal speech Cushing urges the Irish to do their bit in the war.

∽

After a May lull, the German offensive resumed in June. There was now repeated bombing along the coast, with many hospitals hit and much loss of life. Boulogne was frequently attacked. One night Cushing took Crile to see the caves under the city's thirteenth-century citadel, where thousands of people nightly took shelter from air raids: 'To such extremes are the populace driven – underground like moles, into subterranean chambers built for similar purpose six centuries ago – then as now the only safe ultimate refuge ... We agree that we'd rather have our families take the chance of a hit in their own beds.'[58]

Base Hospital No. 5 in the casino came through unscathed. Cushing occasionally operated on special cases and groused about the hundreds of 'sick' American soldiers being foisted on them right off the boat. Most had chronic health problems and should never have been declared fit for service. The good news was that hundreds of thousands of American troops were now pouring into France through Boulogne and other ports, and American units were finally going into battle. In mid-June, just as the British decided to transfer all their head cases to his service in Boulogne, Cushing was transferred to the AEF at Neufchâteau to be its chief neurosurgical consultant.

He was promoted to lieutenant colonel, a small change that reflected a big fight at home between the regular army and the civilian reservists, who had hitherto not been allowed to rise above the rank of major. For the rest of the war he continued to have doubts about the army and its customs and medical officers. 'I gave my seat on the train the other day as there was standing room only to a colonel who graduated from a second rate medical school four years ago and went directly in the regular army medical corps,' he told Kate. 'We got into Paris three hours late – 7 hour trip. Its to laugh.' (In this letter he also had to apologize to Kate for having forgotten their wedding anniversary. 'But why should I remember this particular one when every day is an anniversary for us?' On June 10 Kate had lit a special fire and put flowers in his office, and had written telling him that after sixteen years 'I still think you by far the most agreeable and interesting person I know!')[59]

Formally he had a desk job in the army medical headquarters overlooking the pig market in Neufchâteau. As American troops moved into the front lines, he was almost constantly on the go, organizing surgical teams, delivering supplies, inspecting facilities, and coordinating with the research committee and Red Cross workers in Paris. At the end of June, from a hotel balcony overlooking the Tuileries gardens, he watched Gotha bombers attacking Paris. He wandered the streets wondering if the city was doomed to fall and be destroyed. Could the Americans help save France in the next round of fighting?

Cushing inspected American 'nerve cases' at the former American Ambulance, now a Red Cross hospital, and also visited one of Theodore

Roosevelt's sons, Archie, who was suffering from a puzzling condition apparently caused by botched surgery. He saw a group of Americans, including two Yale students, who had volunteered to get sick for Richard Strong's studies of trench fever. Lice feces and urine had been rubbed on their bodies and injected under their skin, making them very ill but nailing down the etiology of the disease. For a second time Harvey took in the July 4 parade of American troops in Paris – now many thousands of them, some fresh from the Battle of Belleau Wood, marching down the Champs Élysées as the Stars and Stripes flew from the tip of the Eiffel Tower. 'Well, it was a grand and stirring show!' There were rumors that the German delay in relaunching their offensive might be related to an 'epidemic of grippe' that apparently had hit their troops hard.

When the Americans next went into battle, so did Cushing. He operated all day and most nights during the bloody fighting on the Marne in the third week of July, his life becoming nothing but surgery. Eventually he lost track of days and dates:

> We've been operating all night behind the 2nd Division in this newly pitched evacuation hospital which had never seen a battle casualty till forty-eight hours ago and found itself equipped with hospital supplies dating from before the Spanish War – no X-ray, no Dakin's fluid – no nurses, nor desire for any – not a prepared sterile dressing – no sterilizer ... and little compressed bundles of ancient gauze and tabloid finger bandages with which to dress the stinking ruins of these poor lads.

He could hardly believe the appalling mess, utter confusion, and awful chaos of the medical service, a disorder that appears to have reflected the problems the troops themselves faced under the naive generalship that was sacrificing their lives with almost Haig-like abandon: 'Amputations of the thigh – sucking chest wounds – mutilations – German wounded ... Sometime about dawn, while waiting for the next head to be shaved, I lay down on an empty operating table, went promptly to sleep, and fell off.' It was worse than Passchendaele, he told Kate, so bad that for once he couldn't write about it.[60]

Early in August he was behind the Third Division at an unkempt hospital where everyone was still too busy doing emergency repair to bother with special surgery. He persuaded the commanding officer to let him demonstrate what could be done on a soldier who would otherwise be left to die as inoperable. In the middle of the operation, feeling weak, he had to turn it over to Elliott Cutler and go to bed. He soon began to feel feverish and aching. He was driven back to Neufchâteau in an open car in pouring rain and began to suffer what he first dismissed as the 'three days grippe,' then gradually realized it was something worse. It was almost certainly a case of the influenza that was epidemic among the armies and would eventually kill millions around the world. W.S. Thayer told him to stop trying to work and to take a holiday on the Riviera. He got as far as Paris, where he slept feverishly for five days in a hotel room, then went back to work. The good news was that stories were coming in that something was wrong with the Boches, flu or worse. Just possibly, they were about to crack.

As part of the medical buildup for Pershing's St Mihiel offensive, Cushing was able to get a field neurological hospital set up near Benoite Vaux, where he planned to work. Eight of the first ten patients admitted to it were suffering from dilated pupils and hallucinations. Rambling in nearby woods with a field naturalist, Cushing realized they were suffering from belladonna poisoning. Learning that his Hopkins friends, Thayer and Finney, were about to become generals, he thought they too must be delusional. 'La la, How silly will they feel – or will they? They certainly must buck up on their organization, which is too impossible for words. In fact there is none.'

He watched the St Mihiel show from a divisional headquarters and found the American advance exhilarating. Later he inspected the beautifully constructed German defenses and helped interview a captured medical officer. When the German mentioned England's hatred of his country, 'I suddenly got fluent and informed him that so far as I could see there was only one country among the Allies that bid fair to hate Germany and that was the USA and we proposed to have her on her knees for her crimes against us and civilization.'[61] German forces were not yet on their knees at St Mihiel; they walked away before the attack began, a strategic withdrawal, and offered no serious resistance.

Pershing then shifted his armies and their hospitals sixty miles west to throw themselves at the German lines in the Argonne valley. Ever since his 'grippe,' Harvey had suffered from blurring vision. He told no one – a great life if you don't weaken – but realized that he could no longer see well enough to operate. He organized the roadside signage pointing the way to a special neurosurgical hospital at Deuxnouds, where one of his protégés from Boston, Samuel Harvey, led several teams; then he helped triage the wounded and send the head cases to the boys at 'Dough-nuts.'[62]

Sam Harvey and E.B. Towne soon had more work than they could handle – progress in the Argonne offensive came at very heavy cost – and Cushing pitched in to help. On October 1 he was trying to show a new team of surgeons how to do a head case when he had to stop because his eyes were bothering him. A few days later he had to go to bed in Richard Strong's Paris apartment. He was feverish: 'Something has happened to my hind legs and I wobble like a tabetic and can't feel the floor when I unsteadily get up in the morning.'[63]

Walking on legs that seemed asleep to their knees, Cushing somehow managed to get going again. He never complained and stayed at his desk but was fooling no one, especially when he had to use a magnifying glass to read his mail. On October 14 he tried operating again at Deuxnouds, 'but the light was poor and I could not see well enough to do a proper job. All the way home in the car I had spells of diplopia' (double vision). He dragged himself to the office for one rainy depressing day in which most of the talk was of American troops being cut down by influenza and pneumonia on their transatlantic crossing.

Now Cushing's hands were starting to go numb, and he had trouble dressing. Sidney Schwab, a neurologist in charge of a hospital at La Fauche, finally persuaded him to give up and become a 'guest.' For fear of being declared an invalid, Harvey did not want to be officially hospitalized. Schwab's diagnosis was a multiple toxic neuritis, a rare and mysterious syndrome of unknown etiology (Osler said there were about fifty-seven clinical varieties of polyneuritis) but recognized as a sequel to influenza sometimes. It seemed to include a touch of encephalitis, or inflammation of the brain, a condition seen fairly often in those years, which seemed to explain his vision problems. To modern clinicians, Cushing's symptoms are an exact fit with Guillain-Barré syndrome, which was just being delineated in those years and whose exact cause is still unclear. It may have been superimposed on Buerger's disease in his extremities, a condition of vascular inflammation caused at least in part by smoking.[64]

This was the end of his war. Cushing spent the rest of October and much of November in hospital, his feet and hands so numb that he could barely dress himself and totter a few steps. Friends came to poke and prod and learnedly discuss his condition. Julia Shepley, who had worked faithfully at Base Hospital No. 5 and then at Neufchâteau, brought him his mail and took dictation. His main way of testing his reflexes was to swat French flies. He tried to describe his condition: 'The paresthesias are chiefly in soles and palms and I have a vague sense of familiarity with the sensation – as though I had met it some- where in a dream. Like stepping barefoot on a very stiff and prickly doormat – a feeling, too, as though the plantar and palmar fascias had shrunk in the wash and were drawn taught.' In the end he endorsed two old maxims: our sensations transcend our vocabularies, and doctors who observe themselves have a fool for a patient.[65]

He told Kate that he was a typical sick doctor, 'hating to bother people and knowing how little they know anyway and how busy they are – you just want to go off behind a bush ... like a sick puppy dog.' He was very worried that he would be a permanent cripple, unable to resume prac- tice. Schwab, who spent many hours with him, marveled at his courage, insight, and self-understanding. Cushing, he wrote many years later, was 'one of the most delightful and impressive personalities that it has been my fortune to come in contact with during my life time.'[66]

Cushing followed the rest of the war, day after day of Allied ad- vances, with a map, pins, and a ball of yarn. His fingers became so numb that he could not move the pins, nor could he shave: 'Unfortunately missing the last act of the drama ... The news astonishes ... Dynasties are tottering ... more and more amazing every day ... It hardly seems possible ... the American advance ... it is the finger of fate!' When the guns fell silent on November 11, Harvey celebrated with a cup of tea with the hospital matron, the chaplain, and Sidney Schwab.

Late on the eleventh Cushing dictated a long diary entry about the historic occasion – the end of the German empire, twenty million people dead, someone bound to be held responsible. He had occasionally used athletic metaphors to describe the war – seeing the Americans as late-inning pinch hitters for the British and French, for example. Now, straining for effect, he recalled those Saturday spectacles that as an American and a college graduate he knew so well:

> The past few days have been comparable to the last few minutes of a decisive intercollegiate football game at the end of a season. On one side of the field, alive with color and excitement, an exultant crowd, touched by the last rays of a November sun – an unexpected victory within their grasp through an unlooked-for collapse of the visiting team. Across, on the other side of the darkening field, tense, colorless, shivering, and still, sit the defeated, watching their opponents roll up goal after goal as they smash through an ever-weakening line that shortly before seemed impregnable.
>
> Just so, till the whistle, blew ... Surely the Bowmen of Agincourt, the Angel of Mons, and Saint George himself must have appeared yesterday, even as they are said to have appeared in those tragic days of August 1914.
>
> It's a trivial comparison, – a world war and a football game, – but when something is so colossal as to transcend comprehension one must reduce it to the simple terms of familiar things.

∾

A terrible plague of influenza swept through New England and Boston that autumn. Schools were closed, hospitals and doctors and nurses overwhelmed with work. Kate gave the children urotropin as a prophylactic; it made no difference, but they did not catch the virus, nor did she. She soldiered on, wearing farmerette overalls as she did her gardening, spending her private income on Liberty Bonds, spending a day selling Liberty Bonds on a Boston street corner in a booth with a phonograph playing 'Over There' and with Boy and Girl Scouts as barkers. Lewellys Barker, she told Harvey, had continued to be a slacker by staying away from flu patients. As for the Germans, she told Gus the chauffeur that the people driving around with 'To Hell with the Kaiser' signs on their cars were going too far, but she wrote to Harvey that her 'private hate' continued: 'I shall never be able to trust one of them again – or to listen to their accursed language ... Everything about them is loathsome to me.' She remembered his remark, 'There's a good deal of the savage in us.'[67]

She wondered what he would do after the war: 'Will you ever come back to the H. Med School? I doubt it.' She was frantic with worry and fear about his health, forcing him to stop euphemizing and tell her the truth. 'Perhaps we must both be prepared for shocks, when Johnny comes marching home again ...' she mused. 'I should hate to be untouched by the past year – the only wounds I can show take the form of lines & gray hairs.'[68]

When Kate heard the news that an armistice had been negotiated, 'My legs gave out,' she told Harvey, 'and I sat on the floor.' On November 11 she went to St Paul's Cathedral and sang 'The Battle Hymn of the Republic.' That evening, while she and her friends were at the theater, some of their Brookline neighbors gathered in their yard and gave three times three cheers for Dr Cushing. Daughter Mary came out on the porch and thanked them. On November 12 Kate began her letter with the words:

Come home.

We have won the war dearest Harvey, its over. Our supreme moment has come. I think the terms of surrender are soul satisfying ...

To think of those silent guns – the horrible elan ... ended and the enemy beaten out of their boots! America turned the trick – now let me say it once & for all ...

Barbara asks every time she comes in Has Father come home yet? She expects you every moment.

⬥

In France there was a huge backlog of medical work. All the military hospitals were crammed with wounded and with influenza cases. Everyone was weary and wanted to go home. Cushing, who went back to his desk on November 16, wanted to close the war chapter of his life properly, as he would an operation. He hoped that the AEF would set up some kind of institute of neurology to coordinate treatment of the head cases in the various hospitals and ship them to special institutions in the United States. He made plans for an elaborate gathering of surgical data and triaging of the neurological cases at the port hospitals. He and other researchers talked about continuing their meetings to discuss what could be learned from the war.

These plans all collapsed in the rush to get home. 'The regular medical corps has made a worse mess of the home sending of the wounded, if that is possible, than they made of the caring for them during our fighting period,' Harvey wrote Kate on Thanksgiving Day 1918. No one collected statistics, no one made reports, no one was interested in new ideas or any systematic handling of patients. The only goal was to get the sick boys back to their hometowns as fast as possible. Regular army physicians wanted to get rid of the swollen staff of consultants as fast as possible. In mid-December, Cushing was released from his duties and sent back to Base Hospital No. 5 in Boulogne. Before he left Neufchâteau he finished a brief but comprehensive report to the Surgeon General on his work there.[69]

In the last few weeks of December 1918, in Boulogne, he drafted his 118–page history, *The Story of US Army Base Hospital No. 5*, 'by a Member of the Unit,' which was be published by Harvard University Press in 1919. The unit's contribution to the war had been to handle a total of 45,000 sick and wounded. The six American base hospitals that had gone over early and been attached to the British Expeditionary Force had handled a total of 336,600 patients – more cases than the seventy-eight base hospitals with the American Expeditionary Force.

Harvey took final motor trips to Paris and through the French countryside, and to the great battlefields on the Somme, at Vimy Ridge, and at Passchendaele, writing thousands more words in his diaries, and finally becoming redundant. He revisited Revere Osler's grave, 'a sad, muddy and gruesome quest,' and pasted in his diaries a snapshot of Jack McCrae's grave. One of his traveling companions was Almroth Wright's assistant, Alexander Fleming, who later won the Nobel Prize for his work on penicillin. Fleming and Cushing journeyed through 'a country where there is little left but wire and graves.'[70]

Kate and the children were frantically impatient to see him again. Harvey, as he admitted only to her, was extremely worried about his fragile health. He was still very shaky on his feet and afraid that if he tried to do too much, tried to come home too soon, he would wind up on a hospital ship and have to come down the ramp in America in a wheelchair. He thought it best to wait and come home with the Harvard unit. When it was clear that the unit's departure was to be delayed for several more months, he arranged to sail from England in early February.

He spent his last two weeks in Britain mostly in Oxford, at 13 Norham Gardens, where William and Grace Osler were trying to recreate their delightful prewar world of easy hospitality, Sunday dinners in hall, book talk, college talk, history, and tradition: 'Its too lovely here. Sir Wm. in his old form and having regained his weight ... They are certainly wonders – the Os.'[71] With perfect discernment, Osler placed in Cushing's room for bedtime reading a copy of Walt Whitman's *Memoranda during the War*, the poet's experiences as a nurse during the Civil War. Cushing copied out a passage from Whitman, which he used years later to preface the published edition of his war diaries:

> The marrow of the tragedy is concentrated in the hospitals ... Well it is their mothers and sisters cannot see them – cannot conceive and never conceived these things ... Much of a Race depends on what it thinks of death and how it stands personal anguish and sickness.

Harvey left England on February 5, 1919, aboard the *Canopic*, the ship that had brought him over in March 1915. Kate had used her influence with her brother, one of the assistant secretaries of war in Washington, to get him home as early as possible. She met him on the pier at Hoboken, New Jersey, on February 19. They stayed the night in Manhattan and went to the theater.[72]

He was formally discharged from the army on his fiftieth birthday, April 8, a few days before the rest of the Harvard base hospital arrived home. Looking back on the war seventeen years later, he told a correspondent, 'I think all of us who were in the Medical Corps had a little feeling that we were not quite doing our bit.' He said that the greatest contribution had been made by those who served in the front lines. There is no evidence that this sometimes ambitious and self-centered surgeon ever uttered a syllable of complaint about the damage that serving his country and his cause had done to his career or to his health.[73]

ELEVEN

Fathers and Sons

~

'My darling father. I can't wait. I can't wait for that minute when I see your darling face again. It seems as though I had not seen you for a century or longer ... If you come in the night come up in Mary's and my room and take me up in your arms and then I will never let go of you.'[1]

Ten-year-old Betsey wept joyfully when her father, back from the war, stepped off the train in Boston on February 20, 1919. Gus the chauffeur had bedecked the car in flags and brought all the children; he held baby Barbara in his arms. Other friends were on hand. The house at 305 Walnut was filled with flowers. Kate was exhausted. 'How I ever live through these days I don't know,' she wrote in a pocket diary a few days before Harvey's arrival. She had almost been afraid to see her husband again. 'P'raps you won't like me,' she had written to him in France. 'But you can't help loving the children.'[2]

The day after his return he was out seeing people. 'Feel a fearful slump,' Kate wrote on the twenty-second. Soon he was off to New York and Washington promoting his idea of a neurological institute. Then the old social routine resumed in Boston: 'Dinner for Elliott Cutler & Miss Caroline Parker his fiancée, Councilmans, Potters, Dr. Lovatt, A. Homans,' Kate recorded in her diary on May 11. 'Why do we do it?'

He had two responsibilities: getting to know his family again and getting on with his career. He promised Kate and the children that he would spend much time with them that summer at Little Boars Head. As he got busier, his visits dwindled. He promised to take a vacation with the family – Kate had hoped he would take a long rest after the war, perhaps a cruise to the West Indies. When the Cushing holiday came, it lasted four days. 'It was hard to make the children understand,' Kate wrote. 'Something in me was hurt to the core – perhaps it was my heart.'[3]

In December 1919, Sir William Osler, Harvey's surrogate father in medicine, died. A few months later Grace Osler asked Harvey to write Osler's biography. So he took on a third major responsibility and went back to England, to the Osler house in Oxford, in the summer of 1920, less than eighteen months after coming home.

Kate ached in body and soul. Their seventeen-year-old son Bill had had a bad year in school. She took him and Mary with her for a summer stay at the HF Bar Ranch in Buffalo, Wyoming – 'much more my native heath than Boston could ever be.' A letter survives in which she pours out to Harvey her grief about the state of their marriage. She is trying to harden her heart about his treatment of them but doesn't want to have to: '*Don't* let me do it – don't kill the love and tenderness that I have always felt for you – We have a great task before us – we cannot do it if we are estranged and out of sympathy. We must live up to it. We must not fail now. It is a critical time in our lives – either we go triumphantly on to the end, or we miserably fail and drag out a miserable and cheerless life. It is for both of us to decide ... I can't say these things to you. You are always too busy or or too tired.'[4]

∾

Harvey would have preferred not to return to the Brigham and Harvard. The idea of a neurological institute had been on his mind even before the war, and if it had been realized it would have probably taken the Cushings to Washington or New York, for he certainly would have been head of its neurosurgical unit, at the very least. The vision of a unified institute reflected his belief that neurosurgeons needed to know much more about neurology and psychiatric disorders and that psychiatrists needed to root their discipline in knowledge of the brain as a physical organ. Faddism about pituitary and other organic secretions was even worse. Harvey hoped that a national institute of neurology could bring together all serious workers on the brain and become an even better focus for national work than the National Hospital at Queen Square in England or the Salpêtrière in France. In the final months in France the U.S. Army Medical Corps had developed a cadre of leaders and an embryonic organization. Perhaps the Surgeon General could seed its transplantation back to the United States and then Rockefeller or Carnegie money might create an endowment.

Harvey talked up the idea with the military and with the heads of the great foundations, hoping for a ten-million-dollar platform. Early in April 1919 he organized a dinner in New York for individuals whom today we would call stakeholders. There was disappointingly little interest. Other agendas were at play and other organizational initiatives were being promoted by philanthropists and researchers alike. His old friend Simon Flexner, a great power in Rockefeller medical research circles, was particularly and influentially cool to competition from another center. The private New York Neurological Institute already existed, with grand plans of its own. Harvey concluded wistfully, and correctly, that his project was 'a Utopian idea for these fallen times,' and while he still occasionally tried to kindle professional interest in the idea, he gradually gave it up.[5]

He proved ahead of his time by about twenty-five years in having dreamed of the kind of public stimulus to research in the United States that would eventually materialize in the National Institutes of Health. He was prescient, too, about the dangers of psychiatry and other 'disciplines' losing their grounding in mainstream medical science. Just before the war he had been at his most intellectually syncretic and ambitious, speculating about a unified theory of the brain. Harvey's problem was that although he had the prestige to get a hearing for his ideas, he was not politically adroit. He had not helped his standing with the

Flexners and Rockefellers, for example, by opposing them in the full-time fight. As a scion of old Cleveland medicine and old medical values, he was not inclined to kowtow to the nouveaux riches, powerful as they might be, or to anyone else. Defeated, he could always fall back on his personal surgical stronghold in Boston.

Even as Cushing and other veterans returned to peacetime practice, the sense of medicine, like so much else, being in transition, was very strong. Careers were in flux, everyone had been uprooted, younger men were pushing for a place in the sun. The Osler-Halsted-Welch group that had made Johns Hopkins so influential before the war was dying off. Their successor generation, of which no light had shone brighter than Cushing's, was entering its late prime. The next generation was knocking at the door. Given the pace of change in medicine and surgery, everyone was having to refresh his approach to practice every few years. Medical generations move at least as quickly as literary ones, though perhaps with fewer losses.

When Harvey returned to the Brigham after almost two years' absence, he found his establishment 'more or less blown up, as was to be expected.' His chief resident, Conrad Jacobson, had been handling most of the neurosurgery, but not particularly successfully. Jacobson's manic-depressive disposition alienated patients and colleagues.[6] For many reasons it was time for him to move on. Cushing found Jacobson a job at the University of Minnesota and replaced him with Elliott Cutler as chief surgical resident. Harvey insisted to the Brigham trustees that Gil Horrax, a student from Hopkins days who had followed him to Boston and often been at his side in France, should formally be appointed his assistant in neurosurgery. Gertrude Gerrard returned as his anesthetist, and Julia Shepley was indispensable as his private secretary. He badly needed histological help, for Councilman was slipping into retirement and Louise Eisenhardt had left to pursue a medical degree.

The medical schools generated the usual supply of intern fodder, but it was always important to spot exceptional talent. In the summer of 1919 Cushing wrote to the registrar at Hopkins, George Coy, asking for more good men like their most recent import from Baltimore, 'a

very nice gentlemanly fellow named W.G. Penfield, a Rhodes scholar.'
Coy recommended three prospects: a man called, Duffy, who came
near to Penfield's standard, and two others, named Levey and Sachs,
who 'as their names would indicate, are of Semetic [*sic*] origin and
couldn't hide it under a surgical operation.'[7] Cushing had no objection
in principle to working with Jewish students or colleagues as long as the
conditions were right. Penfield spent only a year's internship at the
Brigham, moving on to New York for his residency in surgery – but not
before catching the vision of becoming a neurosurgeon like Cushing.
Nothing developed with the other Hopkins men.

Just how many more brain operations Harvey Cushing would be
able to perform was on his mind as he began trying to pick up the traces
at the Brigham. He was entering late middle age and had experienced
debilitating major illness. He had continuing trouble with his legs and
could not walk very far. He tired easily. He had not operated for eight
months, had not done delicate tumor removals for two years, and could
not be sure of his hands. Elliott Joslin examined him for insurance purposes in 1919 and apparently offered a grim prognosis about impending nephritis or heart disease, suggesting that retirement should be seriously considered.[8] There was a real possibility that his surgical career
had ended.

He first returned to the operating room that April for a case of
trigeminal neuralgia. Jacobson, who had not yet left, stood by to take
over if he faltered. He did not, but he had to apologize for pricking
Jacobson with an unsteady knife. When he tried to remove a large
cerebral tumor from a forty-three–year old Cleveland physician, the
patient died within an hour of closing. With amazing frankness, Cushing
said in his annual report that he ought to have done this return to
tumor surgery in two stages: 'Desperate as these enucleations may sometimes be, far more difficult cases of the same kind have been carried
through with success and the mortality of these procedures should be
very low.' An insider told his first biographer that Cushing was often
close to complete physical collapse when he finished these early postwar operations.[9]

A tired and worried man contemplating passing into history, Cushing in the early postwar years swung between unbecoming pettiness in some matters and surgical statesmanship in others. The pettiness involved letting his concern for his place in surgical history show openly, sometimes crudely. One touchstone was the issue of paternity in the treatment of tic douloureux. Cushing had been privately disgruntled for years about the glory that Spiller and Frazier had garnered in Philadelphia for their 1901 improvement on his 1900 announcement of a new surgical approach to trigeminal neuralgia. The profession, and even Harvey himself, had adopted their proposal not do to a complete ganglionectomy but instead to sever only the sensory root of the nerve, preserving the motor root. The operation was often credited to them and even described as the Spiller-Frazier procedure.

Cushing distinctly remembered that during the discussion of his paper at the Philadelphia conference in 1900 it was Lewellys Barker who had suggested dividing the root. Spiller and Frazier, he thought, had simply acted on that idea (in fact, Spiller had proposed it earlier himself) and had been given undeserved credit for a minor improvement on his own great leap forward. When Harvey learned in the spring of 1919 that the Mayo Clinic was about to tackle trigeminal neuralgia, he told one of his former staffers that he expected they would proceed 'on the lines that I have followed, and they will probably adopt it as their own':

> I have always felt considerably outraged that one or two other people have similarly trespassed, and that the procedure of sensory root avulsion which was first proposed by Dr. Barker of Baltimore at a meeting in Philadelphia, and first carried out in the clinic there, was gobbled up by Spiller and Frazier, and goes by their name. The essential part of the approach and the method, aside from this small point, was adopted purely from my original article. However, this is perhaps all one may expect in this fallen world.[10]

Late in 1919 he returned to Philadelphia to lecture on trigeminal neuralgia, and he raised the credit matter with several correspondents, trying to reconstruct the past and accusing Frazier of having copied several later improvements that he himself had made to the procedure. Harvey announced that he would publish a major paper on his experiences with ganglionectomies, but he never did. 'I found myself confronted by the embarrassing problem of discussing who deserved the primary credit of the sensory root operation,' he mentioned years later, 'and I thought I had better not get tangled up with it.'[11] Knowing better than to pursue these issues too far, Cushing developed in the 1920s a habit of pulling back, tossing off platitudes about credit controversies not being important, even though he had let slip how deeply they gnawed at him.

More collegially and professionally, he sensed the need for better fellowship with America's other neurosurgeons to advance their young specialty. By 1919 about a dozen Americans were operating regularly on the brain. The roster included the veterans, Cushing, Frazier, Sachs, Elsberg, and Howard C. Naffziger – but also newcomers such as Samuel Harvey, who landed at Yale after the war; Gil Horrax and George Heuer; Walter Dandy at Johns Hopkins; and the Mayos' new man, Alfred Adson. Discussing the state of the work with Adson and some of the others in the summer of 1919, Cushing wondered if the time had come 'when we ought to have a neuro-surgical club and get the men together once a year to visit in special clinics.' Early in 1920 he and Sachs organized the Society of Neurological Surgeons. It had only ten charter members and had had to compromise on Cushing's idea of admitting only full-time neurosurgeons. As Sachs explained to him, 'You and I, I think, are the only ones who are doing that exclusively, and though I should like your company, I don't know whether I would be too monotonous for yours!' The society was a far cry from a multimillion dollar neurological institute, but it was a beginning.[12]

Like an aging athlete, Cushing also mulled over his statistical achievements, especially his long series of tumor cases. He categorized and classified them, rehashing the high points and some of the lows. Every time he stepped into the operating room he was going to the plate one more time, as it were, with all the statistical consequences. By May 1,

1923, his series of verified brain tumor cases stood at 868. No one, including Cushing, had any idea how many more surgical home runs he would hit, bases he would steal, runs he would drive in. But it was obviously important to keep track.[13]

~

'The pen is more difficult than the scalpel.' He said he had trouble getting back to writing after the war. He did not like to write or talk about his experiences in France and did nothing with his war diaries. When friends asked him to contribute to a volume of essays to be presented to Sir William Osler on his seventieth birthday, he took a stab at doing a memoir of the old days on West Franklin Street, found it was becoming too personal, and gave up.[14]

In the autumn of 1919 he began hearing from England about Osler's battles with bronchial infection following influenza. Having lived for the psalmist's three score and ten years, Osler died on December 29, 1919, in his Oxford home. 'We are heart broken,' Harvey wrote to a mutual friend. 'But Archie what a beautiful life! Will there ever be another such. Certainly you and I will never know another to compare.' As he leafed through the notes and letters from Osler that he had saved over the years, Cushing took up his pen and wrote a long, loving appreciation of a great physician and a man universally loved for his capacity for friendship. Osler had been Cushing's friend, mentor, role model, idol, and surrogate father. Harvey read his eulogy, 'William Osler, the Man,' at one of his club dinners and published it in a Boston newspaper. It concluded with an Osler quote from Isaiah, which summed up Cushing's own sense of what his friend had meant to him: 'And a man shall be as an hiding place from the wind, and a covert from the tempest; as rivers of water in a dry place, as the shadow of a great rock in a weary land.'[15]

Osler had been a commanding figure in American, Canadian, British, and world medicine. After his death there was a brief debate in England about whether or not he had been the greatest physician in all

history. A major biography of him would certainly be written. Grace
Osler would choose the author.

Grace loved the Cushings more than anyone else in Osler's medical
circles. She felt an especially strong bond with the man who had been
present at Revere's death. And, of course, she was sent a copy of Harvey's
superb obituary essay. She sounded out Kate on whether Harvey might
do the biography. In the meantime, the obvious publisher, Oxford
University Press, made some soundings of its own. David Edsall, now
dean of the Harvard Medical School, recommended Cushing as by far
the best qualified. Harvey himself recommended Fielding Garrison, a
medical historian and biographer, while intimating to Oxford and Edsall
that he had neither the experience nor the time.[16]

'Tanta' Grace's formal invitation to write Osler's biography ('There
is no one here who knows everything – medicine, brain, home, friends,
heart, endurance, in fact all that he was – you know all') arrived in
early March.[17] Harvey swallowed his reservations and instantly agreed.
It was a duty of friendship, it was a duty to medicine, and for a physician with a literary bent, it was a magnificent challenge and opportunity.

Where would he find the time? Harvey must have told Kate and
others that he would make the time. He thought it would probably be
a brief biographical essay, a kind of 'pen sketch': 'I know full well that
the complete story can only be written say fifty years hence.' Literary
friends from his clubs – he consulted Bliss Perry and Mark Howe, who
both had written biographies – advised him that it would take about a
year to do. They warned him that it would be a mistake to try and enter
into any kind of collaboration with a professional writer. He should do
the job on his own.[18] While his qualms did not subside – he had no
experience writing book-length biography, and he did have a time problem – Harvey decided he would do the Osler biography 'or perish in
the attempt.' 'Harvey C. is quite mad with interest,' Grace wrote.[19]

Lady Osler and all of Osler's papers were in England, so he would
have to go over in the summer of 1920. In the meantime, because
Osler had not bothered to keep correspondence, Harvey published a

call for help in major newspapers and medical journals on both sides of the Atlantic, urging everyone with Osler letters and/or recollections to come forward. He wrote to every former associate of Osler's he could locate, to childhood friends and classmates, to publishers, hospitals, and universities asking that files be searched, to booksellers whom Osler had patronized, to Osler's nurse during his final illness, and to some unlikely long shots: 'It would be extremely interesting if the Pope could give a note of his recollection of Osler's visit ... to the Vatican Library and of his own visit to Osler's house and the Bodleian Library.'[20]

The Pope did not oblige, but many others did. To handle the wave of correspondence, Cushing needed more secretarial help. He hired a recent Smith College graduate, Madeline Stanton, in order to free Julia Shepley for the Osler project. Stanton came from a genteel family that had somehow put her through university. She had graduated *cum laude*, but having to support herself she had then taken a commercial course and had found her first job as secretary to the conductor of the Boston Pops Orchestra. Working with a temperamental maestro was perfect training, some thought, for being employed by Harvey Cushing. He paid Stanton's and Shepley's salaries and all his costs of researching and writing the Osler biography (approximately $15,000) out of his own pocket. There was never any kind of contract with Oxford. It would have been unseemly to discuss money in a situation that was mostly about friendship.

He crossed on the *Mauretania* in July, assisting one night at an appendectomy on a seaman. For six weeks Cushing lived at the Osler home, working from 9 AM until midnight, transcribing and organizing documents, jotting down Grace's reminiscences, interviewing British acquaintances. Grace told Kate he worked like a slave. In an age before copying machines, he had three secretaries working on the project. 'To really do the thing well – to Boswellize would take five years,' he told Kate.[21] If he responded to her anguish about the state of their marriage, the letter has not survived. Perhaps he did not find the time. His only break that summer was to collect an honorary degree from Cambridge.

He attacked the Osler biography as he would a neurosurgical case or the subject of a scientific paper, by immersing himself in every detail. He would have to 'saturate,' even 'supersaturate,' himself in Osler. He bombarded friends and family with demands for the slightest scrap of paper or for recollections of the smallest incident and would not take no for an answer: 'I am trying to get inside of WO's skin and I shall want to know these letters and the people he is talking about almost as though they were my own friends.' Grace marveled, 'Was there ever so wonderfully exact & systematic a man?'[22]

When the Canadian Osler family seemed unforthcoming with material on Willie's early life, he began to wonder if they were trying to precensor him, and he developed a case of biographer paranoia. As he explained to a nephew, it was deeply frustrating to have to rely on a family's good will: 'The difference between a biography with all the material and one with as much material as people think the biographer ought to be permitted to see is exactly the same difference that exists between a portrait painted from life and a portrait of the individual painted after his death from an old photograph which in the eyes of the family looks to them like the person concerned.'

Grace Osler's reticence was another obstacle. She had no sooner commissioned him to write the book than she began complaining, teasingly but pointedly, that he had a bad case of 'Biographicitis.' Cushing wanted to see the many letters Grace had written home describing their life in England, but knew she would never agree. He went behind her back, first approaching her sister Sue Chapin for material, then going to the Revere family home near Boston and asking to see letters on the pretext of checking dates. He directed the secretary he took with him to transcribe as many of Grace's letters as she possibly could.[23]

Cushing became a possessive, sometimes peevish biographer. He warned Osler's McGill disciple Maude Abbott, who was collecting Osler reminiscences, to 'keep off the grass' unless she wanted to do the whole job herself. His sharpest exchange was with an Osler cousin, who dared suggest to him: 'As an American I do not think you can even begin to realize the shrinking reticence of an English family ... with regard to their own private personal affairs ... You cannot look on these things with English eyes which open wide with amazement at the blazoning of home life & private affairs in your newspapers.' This was a red flag. 'I am distressed beyond words,' Cushing replied,

> to feel that you have even a thought that I might abuse the confidence which I shall expect the family to place in me as Sir William's biographer ... If you or any other member of the family have the slightest compunctions in the matter, or the slightest anxiety regarding my fitness for this task, we had better have done with it immediately. It, as you know, has been purely a labor of love undertaken at Lady Osler's request, in the midst of a very busy life, and has necessitated giving up a very great many other things which I ought to do ... I do not think, my dear Miss Osler, that you need feel for a moment that your sentiments regarding the privacy of family affairs are any different from those of cultivated people anywhere else in the world; and though an imaginary line may separate Americans from Canadians you may recall that a good many of us have the same ancestry, and it is not well to judge the characteristics of a nation too closely by its newspapers.[24]

He worked on the biography first thing in the morning, went to the hospital and operated, then came home and did more work on the biography late into the night. During holidays he worked all day long on it. By the summer of 1922 a manuscript was beginning to take shape. 'It is a thing of shreds and patches, I fear, in which the scissors and paste pot have played and will continue to play a large part.' He made another quick trip to England and the continent, accompanied by Kate. After giving various lectures and serving as a visiting surgeon (formally a 'Perpetual Student') at St Bartholomew's Hospital, London, Harvey and Kate took Grace Osler to France on a pilgrimage to Revere's grave. The grave was well tended, but the Passchendaele battlefield was still a mess of shell holes, barbed wire, boots, bayonets, and bones. 'Nothing I have ever seen has made such an impression on me,' Kate wrote to her mother. 'We should all see it once.' To Harvey, very little of the real battlefield remained.[25]

∾

Harvey's struggles with his oldest son, William, vied with William Osler for his attention later that summer when everyone else was out of town. Kate had minded the children when they were young, and she would always be much more involved in the girls' lives than their 'Va' (*Vater*). By his lights, Harvey was a proper father to the boys when they began to grow up and think seriously about school and the future. He chose the summer camps they would go to in Maine for toughening up (as he told Kate, 'We're approaching the golf club piazza stage and will have to find some antedote') and the schools they would attend to prepare for Yale.

Bill Cushing was energetic and sports loving, probably intellectually able, but not yet studious or self-disciplined. From France in 1918, Harvey had told Kate that he wished their fifteen-year old could have 'a touch of the war and military discipline much as I hate both of those things.' On his return to Brookline, Harvey fretted that Bill had not been stimulated at the local private school, Milton Academy. Perhaps a switch to Phillips Andover School would be a useful change – not unlike changing one's doctor. There was also the consideration that Milton was basically a Harvard school. 'We are Yale people,' Harvey told one of its teachers, 'and though we do not wish to bring any pressure to bear in the matter feel that we would like to have him go to New Haven. As he is practically the only boy in the school who contemplates such a venture it is perhaps, we feel, a little hard on him that he should not be making friends among those with whom he is likely to be subsequently in college.' The master replied, perhaps with a touch of irony, that Milton understood 'the handicaps under which a boy labors who is preparing for Yale in a distinctly Harvard school.'[26]

Bill played baseball at both Milton and Andover, failed courses at both schools, and also failed the Yale entrance exams. Harvey accepted his 'share of the responsibility for this as perhaps too easy-going a father' and became a stern, disapproving father to Bill: 'The first thing that you must do is to get your lessons absolutely. All other outside activities will have to give way to your lessons ... This means just one thing, my dear boy, that you are to keep up your marks at school or give up the idea of going to College entirely. You are old enough to know that the decision lies entirely with you. There is no excuse whatever for your having such poor marks.'[27]

Bill was on probation at Andover, so Harvey kept him at home in the summer of 1922 to work on his studies while he himself worked on the Osler biography: 'As both you and I find our work somewhat in arrears, we will buckle down the next six weeks and see what we can do ... We can have some tennis in the afternoon.' They also played ball together, took in a game between the Brookline nine and the barnstorming House of David, and set up a wireless radio receiver, with antennae running all over the property. Predictably, there were angry confrontations about Bill's being late for dinner, staying out late, sleeping late, and being pestered by calls from a girl. Harvey claimed to Kate that they really did get along well together except when their temperaments clashed.[28] Their temperaments were probably very similar.

Harvey thought his son had developed an inferiority complex about his studies at Andover. Whatever the cause of his problems, Bill was caught with a crib sheet in an exam that fall and was suspended. His father thought he was 'a perfect ass' and had shot his bolt academically: 'I told Bill that there was just one thing for him to do and that was to get work, and I felt he would feel better if he got his own job.' Bill immediately got a blue-collar job in a General Electric machine shop, became used to rising at 4 AM, stuck it out all year, and reapplied for Yale in the summer of 1923. Despite failing the entrance examinations in English and French, this son of one of Yale's most prominent graduates was duly admitted.[29] He played freshman sports at Yale, maintained average grades, and was lectured by his father about the absolute importance of not going into debt.

When strong-minded fathers try to mold strong-minded sons, intergenerational conflict can be intense. Harvey occasionally realized this: 'I find my children do better if I don't pester them too much.' Second son Henry, 'very much of a home boy,' was allowed to stay at Milton but was encouraged by his parents to spend a toughening summer at a western ranch and meet other Yale-bound men. Otherwise, the boys could choose their courses independently: 'I never even hint to my two boys that I would possibly like to have them or one of them become a doctor to complete the fifth generation.'[30] It never seems to have occurred to Harvey to hint to any of his girls that they might attend any university, let alone join the generations of Cushing doctors.

❧

In October 1920 Cushing addressed one of the largest medical meetings Cleveland had ever seen, on the sweeping topic 'The Special Field of Neurological Surgery after Another Interval.' It was a masterful talk, beautifully framed by an image of medicine as a spreading banyan tree. Some of its branches would develop their own roots if the soil were right. But they must never be mistaken for the trunk, and it must not be forgotten that the whole is one tree. His particular branch-and-root survey heavily emphasized his own contributions – it was really a professional autobiography – until he began dealing with very recent developments. Here the founding father had to acknowledge and appraise the claims of the most prominent member of the coming generation, one of his former students, Walter Dandy.

Dandy had stayed at Hopkins, picked up his missing training in general surgery, moved up through the ranks to become Halsted's resident, and did not join the Hopkins group who went to war. While Cushing was in France in 1917–18, Dandy was working out the basic principles of what became a great neurosurgical breakthrough, the technique known as ventriculography.

The fundamental problem for neurosurgeons had always been their inability to see into the brain from outside. Roentgenography had been of only minor value because x-rays could not differentiate among the tissues and fluids in the brain and could pick up only a very few calcified tumors or occasional bone defects caused by tumors. Dandy's special interest in cerebrospinal fluid led him to hypothesize that it might be possible to inject into the brain's ventricles some circulating medium that would create contrasting shadows on x-ray plates. He experimented with various solutions and finally hit on a substance long recognized by abdominal and thoracic surgeons as facilitating contrast. It was, simply, air. When Dandy replaced cerebrospinal fluid with air in the ventricles of the brain, x-ray photos showed them in fairly clear outline, making it possible to see defects and other abnormalities. His first use of these 'ventriculograms' was to locate obstructions in the ventricles causing hydrocephalus in children. He also located and removed a cerebellar tumor from a twelve-year-old boy.

His classic paper, published in the 1918 *Annals of Surgery*, was forceful, triumphant, and prescient:

> Without a ventriculogram the diagnosis of internal hydrocephalus is frequently guess-work; with the ventriculogram the diagnosis is absolute ... We have not yet applied ventriculography to adults, but expect to do so in all cases in which the diagnosis is obscure ... In adults we should expect the ventriculogram to be at least as sharp or possibly even more so ... Tumors in either cerebral hemisphere may dislocate or compress [or grow into] the ventricle and in this way localize the neoplasm.[31]

A year later Dandy triumphantly expanded on his discovery. Air could circulate in the brain in much the same way as the cerebrospinal fluid, and if injected into the spinal cord it would illuminate the whole subarachnoid space, making it possible to localize even more lesions.[32] Suddenly it seemed possible to do away with the endless, tedious analysis of diagnostic signs and symptoms; the enemy could literally be visualized before the attack began. The concept of ventriculography was obviously a very great triumph. Walter Dandy had his light into the brain.

Practically everything that Dandy published had a triumphant, forceful tone. That was the problem. As he burst into the starting line-up, taking over as the leading neurosurgeon at Hopkins after hitting his towering home run with ventriculography ('You deserve everything they can give you for your splendid work,' Cushing wrote him in a laudatory note; half a dozen universities tried to hire him away),[33] Dandy's confidence and cockiness were practically boundless. He thought he had answers to everything: an operation that would cure epilepsy, an operation that would cure hydrocephalus, a procedure for diagnosing and removing intracranial tumors of the optic nerves.[34] And now, with ventriculography, he had a procedure that should relegate most of Cushing's and other neurosurgeons' diagnostic and exploratory methods – including their palliative decompressions – to the dustbin of history.

The fact that none of his procedures, including ventriculography, had been tried on more than a small handful of cases, sometimes only one or two, did not inhibit his rush to publish. Nor was he inclined to waste his time explaining himself to the defeated establishment. Young, impetuous, impatient, and probably inwardly insecure (also outwardly hampered by severe bouts of sciatica), Dandy did not bother to join the neurosurgeons' club, declining an invitation to become a charter member of the Society of Neurological Surgeons. Cushing and Sachs had hoped he would come to their first meeting, in Boston in November 1920, to discuss ventriculography. Without Dandy, Cushing wrote, it would be like performing the play without Hamlet.[35]

Despite his letter of congratulation, Cushing's response to Dandy's work was conservative, condescending, and paternalistic. In his 1920 overview of neurosurgery he continued to dispute Dandy's views on the role of obstruction in hydrocephalus and suggested that the one tumor Dandy had found by ventriculography might have been located by earlier and more exact perimetry. As for the concept of ventriculography, Cushing was simultaneously complimentary, patronizing, and chastising:

> It is quite certain that in some rare conditions a more exact localizing diagnosis might be made in this way than in any other, and, in the case of tumors situated in silent areas above the tentorium which have led to dilation as well as deformation of one of the ventricles, perhaps only in this way. That

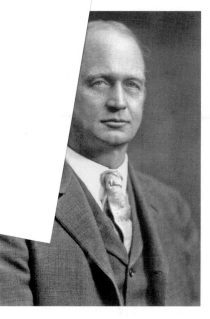

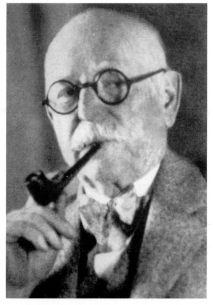

E. Amory Codman,
pioneer of End Results.

William T. Councilman, pathologist.

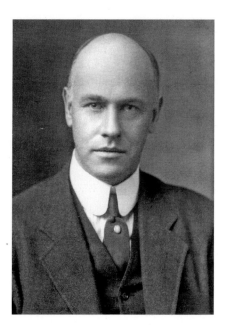

Henry Christian, Cushing's medical colleague in organizing the Brigham.

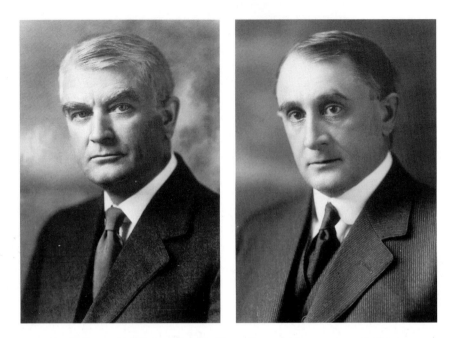

William and Charles Mayo, builders of a great 'clinic in a cornfield.'

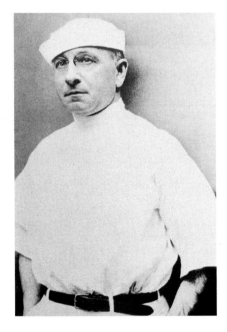

Alexis Carrel: American surgery's first Nobel laureate.

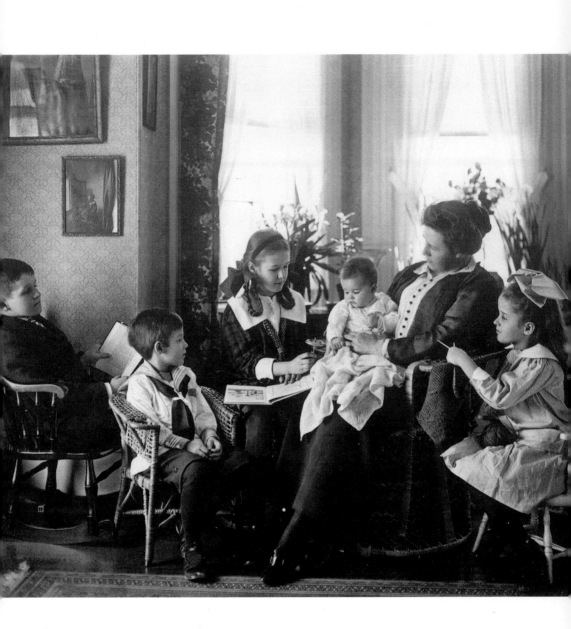

Kate raising the children – Bill, Henry, Mary, Barbara, and Betsey – about 1916.

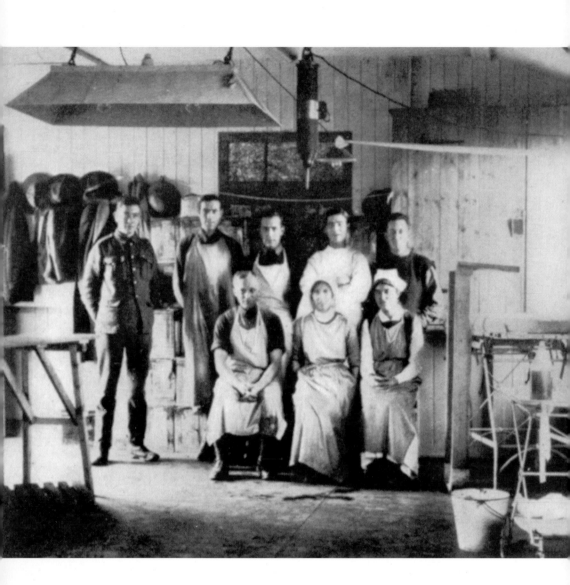

Harvey Cushing and his surgical team, No. 46 Casualty Clearing Station,
after three months at Passchendaele, 1917.

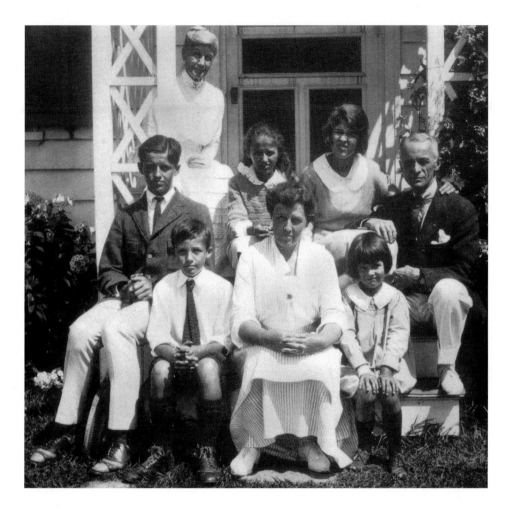

A reunited family, Little Boars Head, 1921. Henry, Kate, and Barbara sit in front of Bill, Betsey, Mary, and Harvey. Caroline Crowell stands.

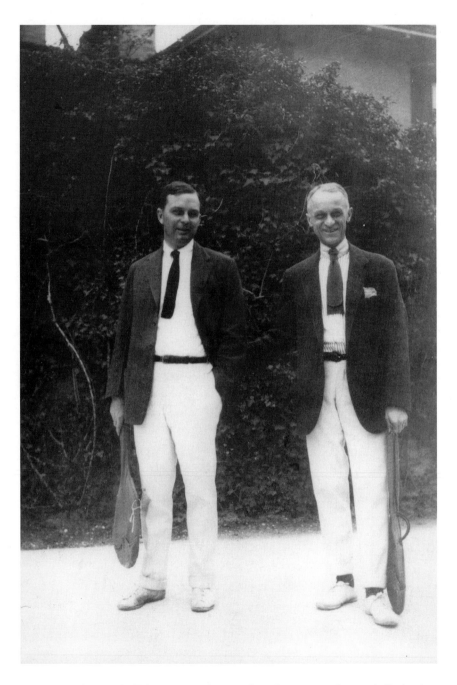

Fierce rivals on and off the court. Walter Dandy and Harvey Cushing, Jekyll Island, Georgia, 1921.

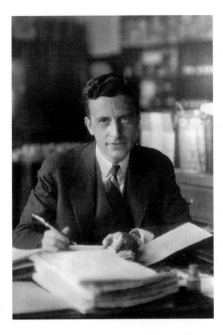

John Fulton, the F. Scott Fitzgerald of
American Medicine.

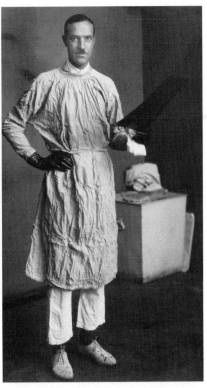

Gil Horrax, faithful assistant.

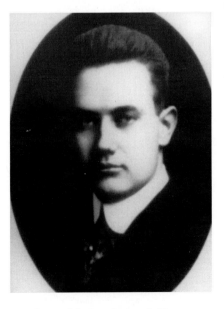

Percival Bailey, Cushing's Tumor
Histologist.

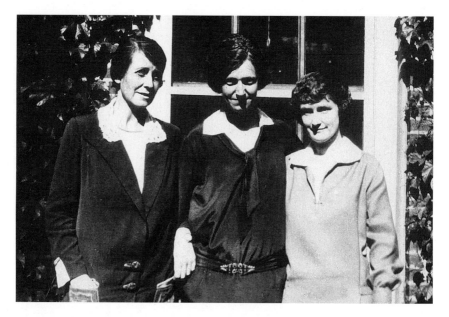

Members of Cushing's 'Harem', ca. 1925. Julia Shepley, Madelaine Stanton, Louise Eisenhardt.

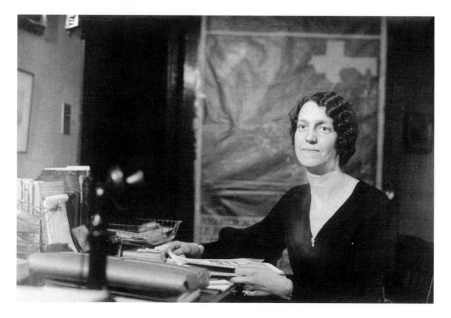

Madeline Stanton at her desk, 1928. The perfect secretary.

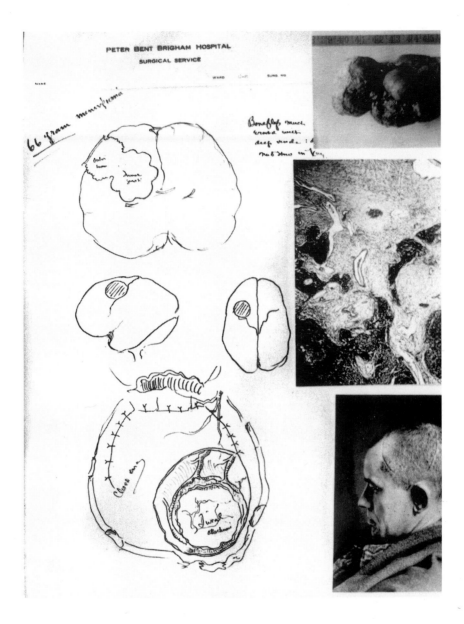

Timothy Donovan, from one of Cushing's composite slides. Cushing operated on him eleven times, removing 1350 grams of tumor.

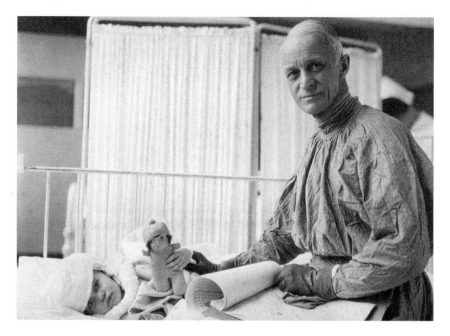

Cushing at the bedside.

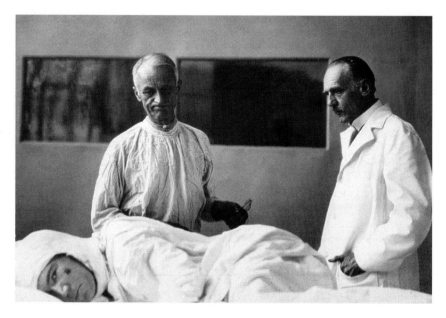

Cushing, Otfrid Foerster, and a worried patient.

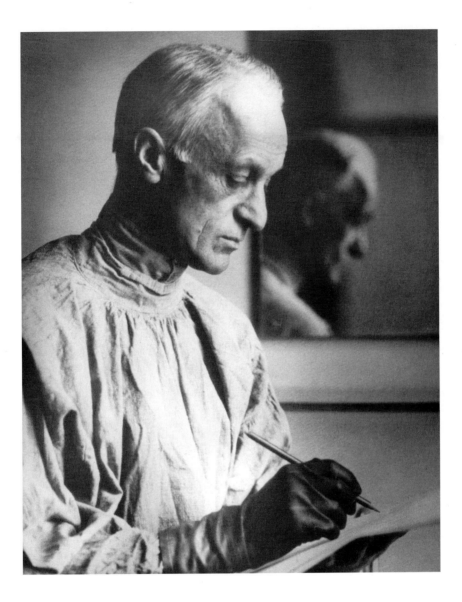

Harvey Cushing, founder of neurosurgery.

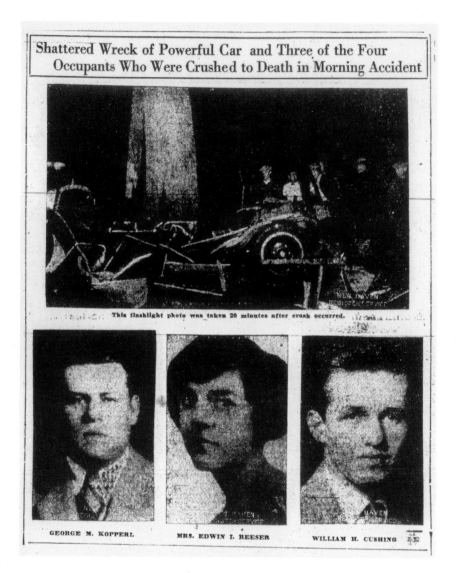

Shattered Wreck of Powerful Car and Three of the Four
Occupants Who Were Crushed to Death in Morning Accident

This flashlight photo was taken 20 minutes after crash occurred.

GEORGE M. KOPPERL   MRS. EDWIN I. REESER   WILLIAM H. CUSHING

William Cushing's death. The New Haven *Evening Register*, June 12, 1926. A Jazz Age
party, alcohol, and a missed curve.

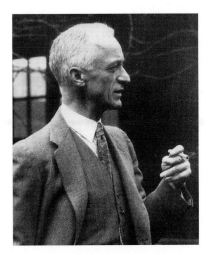

Sixtieth birthday, 1929.

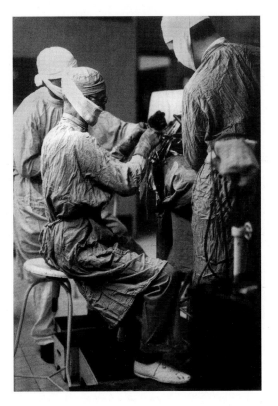

Attacking the 2000th tumor, April 15, 1931. The patient outlived the surgeon.

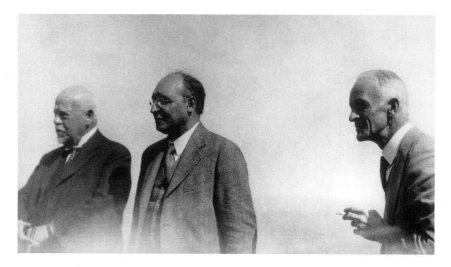

William Welch, Arnold Klebs, Harvey Cushing, Switzerland, 1931.

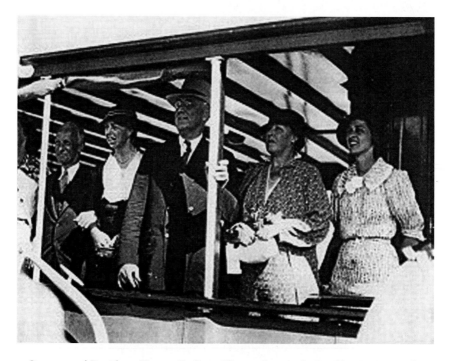

Surgeon and President. Harvey Cushing, Eleanor Roosevelt, Franklin D. Roosevelt, Kate Cushing, and Betsey Cushing Roosevelt, on the *Sequoia*, New Haven, 1934. Like FDR, HC was never photographed with his crutches or wheelchair.

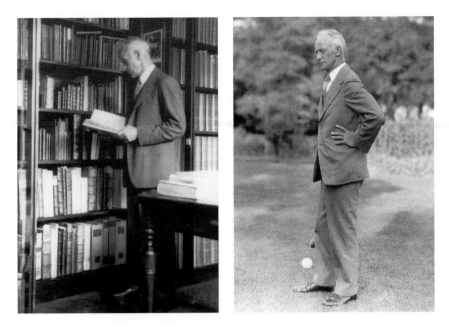

The book collector.　　　　The croquet player.

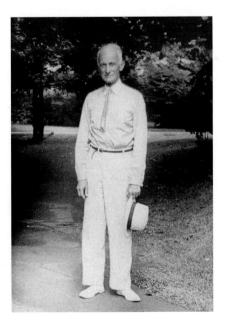

The last picture, 1939.

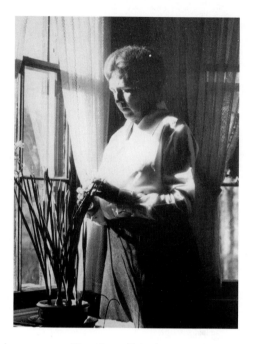

Kate Crowell Cushing.

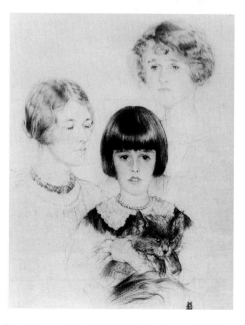

The Cushing sisters. Mary (left), Barbara (center), Betsey (right).

the procedure may be sufficiently developed and safeguarded so that it can be routinely utilized for this purpose is quite within the realms of possibility.

It is still experimental and no doubt it can be left in Dr. Dandy's hands to work out more thoroughly its possibilities as well as its hazards, as he doubtless intends to do ... That there have already been a goodly number of fatalities, doubtless, in the hands of people less expert than the author of the method, is well known. It will soon have a bad repute if so much is expected of it as is given in the author's conclusions, and if the surgeon is encouraged to believe that henceforth he will have less need of exercising his neurologic knowledge in localizing brain tumors.[36]

The ventriculography play without its star was the leading topic of discussion at the historic first meeting of organized American neurosurgeons. 'I am afraid ventriculography did not receive very warm support, and it is too bad that Dandy wasn't here to stand to his guns,' Cushing reported to George Heuer of Johns Hopkins. 'Most everyone who had had any experience at all felt that it was an exceedingly dangerous measure.' Cushing continued to urge Dandy to join the society in the interests of furthering neurosurgery, to which Dandy replied that he was not interested in joining any societies, 'because I feel they are more social than beneficial and I cannot spare the time for them.' He did spare time to be social with Cushing when they chanced to meet on holiday at Jekyll Island, Georgia, in February 1921. They resumed their tennis match. An observer remarked that while Cushing had the form, Dandy won the game.[37]

Form mattered to hard-driving, competitive men, as were virtually all of that generation (and most others) of neurosurgeons. Form was playing by the rules, form was an acknowledgement of the discipline of science, form was professional ethics and basic personal etiquette. One of Cushing's first students, William Sharpe, had fallen into professional disrepute in New York City for publishing popular articles in which he made exaggerated claims for his surgical skills (it is not clear whether he later also overclaimed about other matters in his autobiography, such as the sexual threesome he describes), and he had become non grata.[38] He was deliberately not invited to join the neurosurgical society. Walter Dandy was a brilliant surgeon and was doing spectacularly well at Johns Hopkins, Abraham Flexner wrote in 1919, but he was still 'culturally crude.' Halsted told W.W. Keen that he had tried fruitlessly to teach Dandy how to write scholarly papers and had finally urged him to hire an English teacher. Dandy was also a rough man in the operating room, profane and at times an instrument thrower. He still occasionally dissected out tumors with his fingers, an absolute violation of Cushing's refined technique – much more serious than eating with his knife.[39]

In late 1921 Dandy went way over the top by publishing in the *Journal of the American Medical Association* a sweeping and crude overview of the treatment of brain tumors, mostly their mistreatment by all previous brain surgeons: 'It is useless to deny that surgery has signally failed in its task of curing brain tumors ... Brain surgery has not kept pace ... it is still a crude and bungling effort ... The mention of brain surgery carries a feeling of hopelessness.' Dandy dismissed all diagnostic procedures before ventriculography as mere guesswork. He dismissed virtually all decompression procedures and exploratory craniotomies as harmful; patients would have been better off without them. 'Until the surgeon ceases the bungling indirect operative treatment and strikes for the cause, directly and effectively, the black eye of this field will remain justly merited.' All that the brain surgeon had to do was locate tumors by ventriculography and then go in and remove them, thus curing the patient.[40]

An admiring physician friend wrote Dandy that in this article he had 'Chaplin-like' thrown 'all their Lares & Penates, all their icons and their pet Teddy-bears' at the heads of the whole generation of neurosurgeons: 'To take away their decompression ... & other pet operations and to hold them to rigid pre-operation diagnosis is cruel beyond measure.' Dandy replied that he knew the article was 'rather below one's dignity,' but he had written it, he said, because 'I have been up against the proposition of being banged by all the neurological surgeons to such a degree that I have been forced to paddle my own canoe. It is useless to try to change ... the hide-bound members.'[41]

Cushing and Ernest Sachs were independently outraged, spontaneously writing angry comments that crossed in the mail. Cushing told Sachs that he had read Dandy's article 'with mingled feelings of despair, disappointment, chagrin, and amusement.' Sachs told Cushing that he was 'incensed about it both on account of its form and content' and that he could not understand how Halsted would allow such a publication to come out of Hopkins. 'The less said about it the better,' Cushing concluded. When the editor of the *Boston Medical and Surgical Journal* tried to persuade him to respond to Dandy's radical views, Cushing demurred:

> Dr. Dandy is an old pupil of mine and was for two years my assistant, though I do not believe anyone would know it from reading his article.
>
> I am sorry that he wrote it, for I do not think it will do him good, nor do I think it will do the surgery of brain tumors good, but I think the best way to treat the article is to leave it alone. There may be something on Dandy's side, and time alone will tell. Dandy is young and somewhat radical, and time has a way of curing both of these things – youth and radicalism.

To George Heuer, Dandy's senior at Hopkins, Cushing elaborated:

> There is nothing so bad in the world for any of us as to become insular and to forget that other people are making rapid advances as well as ourselves. It is this which gives individuals a false sense of authoritativeness which can only be corrected by seeing the work of others and having a free exchange of opinions. The Neurosurgical Club was started with this as one of its many objects ...
>
> 'It's a great game as long as you don't weaken,' and the important thing is to keep your head. With all his good qualities, I sometimes think Dandy loses his, which disturbs me not a little for after all I am in a way responsible for his early training.[42]

Ventriculography continued to be the hottest topic when neurosurgeons gathered. They were genuinely perplexed about whether the technique was as good as Dandy claimed. None of his presentations included more than sketchy details of a few cases. Ventriculograms were tricky to read in general, trickier to read the smaller the tumor, and tricky to read because ventricles varied from brain to brain. There were also grave risks. As Dandy acknowledged (but often only in fine print), it was a major, difficult procedure to replace cerebrospinal fluid with air without causing serious and potentially fatal pressure changes in the brain. Some young surgeons, such as Wilder Penfield, visited Dandy, were impressed, and immediately started doing ventriculograms. But in the discussion at the April 1922 meeting of the Society of Neurological Surgeons, 'several of the men reported deaths, and all agreed that the procedure was attended by considerable difficulty ... Most of the men were unable to report as much help from the procedure as had been reported by Dr. Dandy.'[43]

A few weeks later Dandy did appear at the American Neurological Association and gave a slide presentation on ventricular radiography. He also outlined an extremely radical procedure for totally removing gliomas of the cerebral hemispheres and the cerebellum by taking out a zone of healthy brain tissue around them. He was given a very rough ride in the ensuing discussion. Sachs declared that there were few cases in which ventriculography had helped and that the mortality of Dandy's tumor procedure would be very high. Other surgeons chimed in on ventriculography: 'Epoch-making if it can be executed properly' ... 'Extremely hazardous' ... 'Until we have actual statistics we must take the risk blindly.' Cushing was the most explicit:

> I wish that Dr. Dandy would state specifically the number of tumor cases he has investigated in this manner. I believe that he has tended to be overenthusiastic about the procedure and to belittle the risks ... In Dr. Dandy's enthusiasm, he has led many to believe that a shortcut to the localization of brain tumors has been discovered and that all such patients should be subjected to it. I may be unduly conservative, but I have grave doubts of this. If the procedure has been so successful in Dr. Dandy's hands, it is incumbent on him, for the sake of others, to be less general and more specific.

If ventriculography worked for even a small percentage of tumors, Cushing concluded, 'we must eagerly accept the procedure as a very important contribution.'

At the end of the discussion, Dandy had to backpedal and apologize. He had emphasized the dangers in every publication, he claimed: 'In fact the danger is so great that, even with my enthusiasm for and confidence in the method, I have often wondered whether it has not done more harm than good because of indiscriminate use without judgment ... I am sorry that I have not the accurate statistics.' Immediately after the meeting, Cushing wrote him a cloyingly paternal letter saying he hoped they had not been too hard on him: 'It has been an important contribution, but you must be very careful not to over do it, lest you make people expect too much of it, for under these circumstances it is likely to get a black eye.' But Dandy had suffered something close to a public humiliation, which may have been even rougher than the published transcript indicates (there is some evidence that Cushing virtually accused Dandy of doctoring his x-ray images, some of which had been touched up by Brödel before publication). Dandy was incensed and was deeply and permanently offended by what he considered to have been Cushing's personal attack on his integrity.[44]

Then it became Cushing's turn to be furious. In the September 1922 *Johns Hopkins Hospital Bulletin*, Dandy published a very short preliminary report claiming that he had developed a procedure for totally removing tumors of the nervus acusticus. Dandy did not mention Cushing's monograph on these tumors nor that the basic operative approach he described was Cushing's. Nor did he weigh the pros and cons of the procedure or present any information about his cases – even whether he actually had any. He just said he could do it.[45] The article appeared just a few days after W.S. Halsted died. Halsted had been mentor to both Cushing and Dandy. Ironically, the great surgeon died from infection and hemorrhage following gallbladder surgery.

Cushing drafted a pained letter to his professional stepson. Dandy had 'far surpassed' him he admitted but had an obligation to respect the 'amenities' of the profession. His article would be interpreted as 'an unjustifiable bid for cases' unless he expanded it into a proper study of all his acoustic cases and their operative mortality and end results.

Cushing had a habit of drafting angry letters and then regretting them. Instead of sending this letter to Dandy, he sent a franker one to his old friend at Johns Hopkins, W.G. MacCallum:

> Is there anything we can possibly do about Dandy? I have been troubled about him for a good many years, and feel dreadfully that a man with whose training I have had something to do should have such good technique in the operating room but such poor technique as regards the ordinary amenities of the profession.
>
> To my great despair one other man to whom I taught neurosurgical technique, who went to New York, made a bad mess of his professional relationships and has gotten into bad odor.
>
> What has finally led me to express my concern ... is Dandy's last article, if it deserves being called an article, in the recent number of the bulletin. It is not the sort of article or preliminary note that a surgeon with any sense of the amenities of the profession would ever publish. It, moreover, is not the sort of article that the Johns Hopkins Bulletin ought to have accepted. Even if there was something new that he had to describe, not even a man of the John B. Murphy type would have put out a preliminary note saying that he was going to describe a novel operation. Dandy knows full well that his former teacher has written a monograph on these recess tumors and ... further more described in detail the operation which he promises to describe, with a complete series of cases, giving their end results, the ideal, of course, being a total extirpation of the growth when that is possible, which it rarely is without subjecting the patient to unjustifiable risks.
>
> But I care little for this and priority interests me not at all. What does concern me is that an old pupil and a member of the Johns Hopkins surgical staff should have so far lost his sense of propriety as to have published such a preliminary note, and that those responsible for the Johns Hopkins Bulletin should have permitted it to appear. Is there anybody in Baltimore who checks up on Dandy's work? He told us at the American Neurologial Association meeting last year that Dr. Thomas and Dr. Meyer always were

asked to see his patients in case there was an unlocalizable tumor. I asked Meyer about this subsequently, and he told me he thought he had possibly seen two cases with Dandy, whereas Dandy was referring in his address to a series of 300.[46]

Cushing had Johns Hopkins on his mind also because of Halsted's death and the near certainty that he would be invited back as his successor. He had priorities and credit on his mind because on the same day that he first saw Dandy's article he saw an article in another journal by Adson of the Mayo Clinic apparently taking credit for the ganglion operation that Cushing had taught him on a visit a year or so earlier. He complained about this to Will Mayo ('I don't want my young fellows to get into careless habits in this respect, and I am sure you don't want yours') and received an abject apology.[47] Still troubled by these issues, and still trying to come to grips with Halsted's death, he wrote a very angry letter about Dandy's article to the editor of the *Johns Hopkins Bulletin*: 'It is not the sort of article that a member of the surgical staff of the Johns Hopkins Hospital, at least in former days, would have written ... I grieve to say it is by no means his first offense.'

He decided to send this angry letter directly to the offender, adding a handwritten note: 'It is as important for me that you stand in a high plane of professional ethics. I think you are doing yourself a great deal of harm by the tone of some of your publications. You are an independent thinker and worker, and that is not at all a bad thing. But you must not forget your manners, and this last note of yours is in extremely bad taste.'

Dandy snapped back at the man he had once idolized and intended to replace as America's greatest neurosurgeon:

While of course I am not unmindful of your inferences and taunts of dishonesty and your invidious generalizations, at various times, it has seemed far better to ignore them ... They do reflect on you a great deal and in your position you can ill afford it ... There are no statistics or results which I am trying to hide. They will speak for themselves and adequately in due time ...

I feel very sorry for one who is laboring under such an obsession and particularly as it is from one to whom I should now be feeling the deepest debt of gratitude and upon whom I should look with the greatest adoration and consider my friend, guide, and master ... It all seems so unneccessary. It should all be so different.[48]

Dandy probably did not send this letter (the signed original is in his papers, not Cushing's). About a month later, when they had all cooled off, he sent a much more temperate reply to Cushing, regretting the older man's strong feelings and promising to move as quickly as possible to publish his operative work. Cushing then closed the subject with a final paternal intervention:

I wish I could have a heart to heart talk with you re your work in general and the tone of your publications. As long as Halsted was alive and with the feeling that he probably passed judgment on your papers, I felt some natural diffidence re speaking to you about the matter.

You have ability and industry and ought to have a great future ahead of you. Nothing could please me more than this, for your own sake as well as for the fact that you were at one time an assistant of mine.

But one cannot attain the sort of success you ought to attain in medicine if he plays the game too much alone and ignores the work of others.

I thought your brief article was in very bad taste and not the sort of thing a man in your position should have published.[49]

They apparently did have their heart-to-heart talk a few weeks later when Cushing was in Baltimore. Their relationship then settled down into something like a mutually respectful truce. While Dandy would have the eventual satisfaction of seeing Cushing and most of the other neurosurgeons adopt ventriculography (as the technique became perfected, it did enable them to localize many more tumors), their early concerns about its dangers, especially in the hands of neurologists who thought it was as simple as lumbar puncture, were well founded. As Cushing and others pointed out, the mortality rate among patients subjected to early ventriculography was about the same as those operated on for tumor.[50]

Dandy had to admit the validity of these concerns. 'It is a question in my mind, whether I have done more harm than good by the procedure,' he wrote privately in 1921. He eventually also told Cushing that his first claim to have removed an acoustic tumor had been mistaken – it was not a true acoustic tumor.[51] He continued to have a love-hate attitude towards Cushing – emphasis most often on hate – sometimes idolizing him, more often hoping to kill off his father in neurosurgery and take his place. His roundhouse swings at Cushing and most other neurosurgeons and his boycotting their organization and going his own way without collaborators won him no friends and tended to isolate him and Johns Hopkins from the mainstream of his specialty[52] – except that Dandy's brilliance and daring, combined with the reputation of Johns Hopkins, were sometimes sufficient to deflect the course of neurosurgery in the direction he wanted it to go. In the 1920s and 1930s Dandy was seen to represent the 'radical' school of young neurosurgeons who believed in a far more aggressive approach to tumor removal, even at the cost of sacrificing healthy brain tissue.[53]

Cushing, who usually had much more on his mind than the affairs of Walter Dandy, was philosophic about his former pup's intensity. 'I do not think any of us need strive that hard for priority,' he commented to Cutler in 1925 about the acoustic tempest. 'It is largely a matter of background and opportunity, and you and I may be thankful for the parents we chose and for our youthful home surroundings.' He might have added that he could be thankful for having had, as his medical father figure and counselor, William Osler, who had curbed Harvey's own rough edges many years earlier. Cushing had never been nearly as rough-hewn or as nakedly obsessive as Dandy, and the greatest difference between them lay in Cushing's temperamental and surgical caution, contrasted with Dandy's near-reckless impetuosity. Still, there were times when Osler could have said of the young Harvey Cushing exactly what Cushing said of Dandy: 'The poor boy is young – but he's got awful bad manners.'[54] Cushing and Dandy were too much alike for

Osler's biographer to have been an Osler to him. Sometimes Cushing thought about these generational issues: in a biographical obituary of Halsted, written at the height of the conflict with Dandy, Cushing remarked on getting to know Halsted better after leaving his service, 'just as many sons learn to know their fathers not until after they have grown up.'[55]

∾

Cushing was trying to be Osler to the whole profession in the 1920s. Reluctantly but dutifully, he agreed to serve terms as president of the American Neurological Association and of the American College of Surgeons; the key obligation would be the presidential addresses. He also gave major lectures in England and France on his 1922 trip and was Osler's stand-in at the opening of McGill University's new Biological Building in 1923. He was in constant demand as a speaker at Harvard and Yale medical events, in fact, at medical events everywhere in America. He politely declined most but not all invitations.

His most unusual professional involvement was the term he served in 1920–1 as president of the Society for the Study of Internal Secretions, founded in 1917 and flourishing today as the Endocrine Society. He was elected president without his knowledge at a meeting he did not attend of a society dedicated to a discipline that he believed was mostly 'poppycock' and sometimes called 'endocriminology.'[56] He did not see a clinical reason for lumping together treatment of disorders of the very different ductless glands, and he was well aware that much of what passed for glandular therapy was the old scam of peddling replacements for vital fluids. He only agreed to serve because of his ongoing pituitary interest, out of a sense of duty, and to help suppress the quacks.

His 1921 presidential address at the society's Boston meeting began with a beautiful image of the state of the field:

> We find ourselves embarked on the fog-bound and poorly charted sea of endocrinology. It is easy to lose our bearings for we have, most of us, little

knowledge of seafaring and only a vague idea of our destination. Our motives are varied. Some unquestionably follow the lure of discovery; some are
earnest colonizers; some have the spirit of missionaries and would spread the
gospel; some are attracted merely by the prospect of gain and are running full
sail before the trade wind. Traders, adventurers, even pirates are certain to
follow on the heels of exploration. In every profession, even ours, are to be
found those who gather up beads of information of little intrinsic value
which are exchanged for the property of credulous people, as gullible as the
natives of a new-found land. Thus do discoveries become exploited.

The bulk of his talk, an update on the pituitary, was devoted to outlin-
ing how little was known, how little clinical or surgical progress had
been made, the uselessness of giving patients pituitary extract ('The
Lewis Carroll of today would have Alice nibble from a pituitary mush-
room in her left hand and a lutein one in her right and presto! she is any
height desired'), and how wrong it was for a credulous profession to
tolerate 'polypharmaceutical charlatanism':

> This society ... must, so far as possible, through the pages of its journal, keep
> such an exact almanac that those pursuing the subject in the proper spirit
> may be able to avoid unfavorable winds, currents and counter currents. It
> must discountenance the exploitation of the few discoveries which have
> already been made by those who recklessly under full sail plow through a fog
> bank of therapeutics, their horns tooting.[57]

Many in Cushing's audience that day – the society already had more
than fifteen hundred members – knew that the president was attacking
its founder, first secretary, and greatest enthusiast, a California half-
quack named Henry Harrower, who had a major mail-order business
selling every kind of glandular extract. Harvey's post-meeting mail was
thick with congratulatory letters from regular members of the profession, and *cris de coeur* from Henry Harrower.

Cushing was unrepentant and unpersuaded that the internal secretion fad had produced any significant therapeutic breakthroughs since

the 1890s. On January 18, 1922, for example, he told a correspondent that 'the disorders of the thyroid are about the only ones, which, so far as we know, can be very successfully benefitted by glandular administration.' It happened that on the very next day, in a research laboratory at the University of Toronto, a young biochemist named James B. Collip found an effective method of purifying the extract of pancreas gland that Frederick Banting and Charles Best had been experimenting with on diabetic dogs and humans. Within days it was clear that patients were spectacularly benefitted by the administration of what the Toronto group called 'insulin.' Within weeks it was clear that a wonderful medical breakthrough – a much more dramatic advance in endocrinology and therapeutics than, say, ventriculography was in neurology – had taken place. By the summer of 1922, Cushing was writing to the leader of the Toronto team, John J.R. Macleod: 'This insuline business is perfectly stunning ... a great step in advance. It is extraordinary that your predecessors had overlooked it; but then, few people in the world have eyes to see.'[58] Later, he often reflected that he and his own students had failed to see how their interest in metabolism and blood sugar might have led them to insulin. In the meantime, the problem of containing Henry Harrower's enthusiasm for selling to the world tablets of his useless 'Pan-Secretin' passed to the University of Toronto and its lawyers.

Cushing agreed to be president of the American College of Surgeons in 1922–3 only after much persuading and negotiating. Franklin Martin, the tireless founding organizer, put him up for the presidency without consulting him. He tried to withdraw, but friends urged him to take the job to help curb Martin's 'wild stampede' for signing up semiqualified surgeons and creating what W.W. Keen called 'a sort of Frankenstein' society. Harvey's own beef was that in inviting the press to cover surgical clinics, the college had turned its clinical congresses into semi-advertising events. He finally agreed to serve to help make the society a more dignified home for the better class of surgeons. He gave a very Oslerian presidential address on the oneness of medicine and surgery at the plenary Boston meeting in October 1923. At the associated Clinical Congress, he spent much of his talk explaining why they were now banning reporters: 'As a rule, the better the surgeon the more unassuming he is and the more he abhors seeing reference to his work in the lay press ... The College cannot wish to foster the mere spectacularization of surgery.'[59]

Would Harvey Cushing, America's most prominent surgeon, take over America's most prominent chair of surgery and become Halsted's successor at Johns Hopkins – which in a way would also make him Osler's successor? Despite his pro forma suggestion that Hopkins promote its own brightest young man, no one doubted that Cushing would be offered the position. Old Hopkinsites applied much pressure on him to come home to 'family.' He thought long and hard about the prospect, felt very tempted, wondered if support for him was in fact all that widespread in Baltimore, and finally decided against another move:

> My head cautioned me to stay here and my heart drew me back to Baltimore. I have unusual opportunities here and I am far less confident of my ability to stand the strain of a transplantation than I was a dozen years ago ... Though I camouflage the fact before others as well as I can, I am not quite the same fellow I was before my serious illness in France ... Here I can quietly peg along make a few occasional contributions and train some coming young men without my inadequacies being too apparent.[60]

Walter Dandy's name is not mentioned in Cushing's extensive correspondence about returning to Hopkins. W.S. Thayer did warn Harvey that Halsted had not been the best judge of men and had left everything in an organizational mess that would be very time-consuming to straighten out. There was also the thorny issue of the position being a full-time one, with a relatively low salary and no flexibility. Will Mayo, whose advice Cushing solicited, had no doubt about the answer he should give to Baltimore: 'As the first neurologic surgeon of the world you have a duty to perform to all sorts, sizes and conditions of human beings and each should be allowed to pay as much or as little as his circumstances permit ... I get the impression that in clinical things Hopkins is in a sort of an eddy, moving swiftly, but not in the stream.'

Grace Osler, Bostonian to the end, was also firm and telegraphed a play on the telegram she had send to her husband in 1905: 'Do not procrastinate. Refuse.'[61]

A few months later Cushing also refused an umpteenth offer to return to Cleveland, citing his age and infirmities. The Hopkins position went to Dean Lewis from Rush College in Chicago (Walter Dandy did nothing at Hopkins but neurosurgery). Cleveland took Harvey's Boston protégé, Elliott Cutler. George Crile, Cleveland's most prominent surgeon and Harvey's sometimes rival, had removed himself from academic medicine – though never from research – by founding a clinic, the Cleveland Clinic, based on the model of the Mayo Clinic.

∼

To Harvey Cushing, quietly pegging along at the Peter Bent Brigham meant doing about six brain tumor operations a week, occasionally teaching Harvard students, administering the Department of Surgery at the hospital, writing scholarly papers, presidential addresses, and other talks, handling stacks of correspondence, and finishing the Osler manuscript. His total literary output was estimated at five to ten thousand words a day, year after year – astonishing productivity even for a professional writer.[62]

Even his contributions to the hospital's annual published reports, notoriously dreary documents everywhere else on the planet, were lively essays on the state of the institution. One year he would explain the superiorities of the Brigham's geographical full-time system, another year meditate on the dangers of self-satisfaction. He tried to explore the wellsprings of hospital greatness – a balance between tradition and innovation, individuality and community. He indulged his penchant for imagery: Did a hospital have growth stages like a person, its clothes sometimes becoming tight and uncomfortable? Or did it expand like a railroad – adding more trains, then bigger engines, and finally getting serious about improving its roadbed? 'Hospitals from an endocrinological standpoint might be a subject worth elaborating ... Some hospitals start out with unmistakable evidences of gigantism; some later on acquire an acromegalic unwieldiness; and some ... give early signs of progeric senility.'[63]

Every year he worried about his staff not having the time and resources they needed for research. Every year he indicated how the elaborate statistical presentations in most hospital reports, including the Brigham's, were misleading, manipulable, and non-comparable: 'A hospital can make its mortality figures based on the number of operations almost what it will.'[64] In the mid-1920s his reports became more fretful as surgery jostled with medicine for resources at the hospital and as friction with Harvard and the other teaching hospitals increased.

He easily rebuilt his surgical and office team in the early 1920s, drawing on a stream of eager housemen, talented operating-room nurses and anesthetists, and well-bred but needy and usually spinsterish secretaries, medical artists, and photographers. Gilbert Horrax was content to stay on at the Brigham year after year as his principal assistant, even when Cushing urged him to move on to something better. Percival Bailey, a Midwesterner fascinated by neurological histology, took advanced training in Chicago and came to the Brigham to work closely with Cushing on the staining and classification of tumors. Later in the decade, Bailey was replaced by Louise Eisenhardt, who had taken a medical degree at Tufts and graduated at the top of her class.

Cushing welcomed visitors and volunteers, finding financial support and fellowships for some of them and encouraging short-term exchanges at the most senior level. In 1922 the University of Toronto awarded Cushing its Mickle Fellowship for having done the most in medicine in the past ten years 'to advance sound knowledge of a practical kind.' Cushing suggested that the $1,000 prize money be used to support a Toronto graduate during a year's residency with him in Boston to learn neurosurgery. A Scots Canadian doctor's son, Kenneth McKenzie, came to Boston in 1922–3 to learn to become a neurosurgeon. McKenzie was surgically unpolished – 'the sloppiest man I have had for a long time,' Cushing told the hospital superintendent – but he was willing to work and learn, and returned to Toronto to become

Canada's first neurosurgeon, an avowed Cushing disciple for the rest of his life.[65]

Watching Cushing operate was like watching Freud analysing a patient or Osler giving ward rounds or the Pope saying mass. Cushing had created the art. Dandy's views to the contrary notwithstanding, Cushing's overall leadership in neurosurgery was not seriously challenged. He appeared to have stopped innovating technically by the early 1920s but was not so set in his ways that he could not learn new tricks. As the ability to localize tumors increased, he was doing fewer simple decompressions. Many pituitary tumors, he had found, were better approached from above than by his transsphenoidal route, so he did many more transfrontal procedures. In the early postwar years he began to attack some tumors with radiation, a difficult procedure that yielded mixed results wherever it was tried. By 1923, applying lessons from Passchendaele, he was using suction to clear away blood during surgery, a technique that dazzled overseas visitors. One of his assistants, Loyal Davis, experimented with recycling the suctioned (and filtered) blood. So at a time when transfusion was still awkward and uncertain, Cushing's team could replace a patient's lost blood with the same lost blood.[66] When all else failed diagnostically, Cushing also began taking ventriculograms.

The most exciting surgery at the Brigham in the early 1920s, according to Cushing, was not on anyone's brain but on a heart. In what Cushing immediately labeled an 'epical performance,' Elliott Cutler operated on a young girl's heart to attempt to treat mitral stenosis, a valve disorder. This first patient survived the operation – another milestone advance. Back in 1904, Cushing had called the brain the Northwest Passage of surgery. Now he told W.W. Keen, 'There is a new "Northwest" which makes neurosurgery look ancient: namely, the surgery of the heart.'[67] In yet another surgical father-son relationship, Cushing did everything he could to promote Cutler's career, and there was hardly even any friction between them. Perhaps it had something to do with specializing in different organs. Cutler's cardiac work was not ultimately as fruitful as they had hoped it would be – most of his other patients died – but he was ambitious and he knew how to mind his manners.

Cushing's research interests were the pituitary and the characteristics of tumors. Pituitary work was often on hold, as the gland continued stubbornly to resist questioning. The series of tumor cases grew almost daily and, because Cushing's records and samples were so complete, lent themselves to intense analysis. Percival Bailey spent time in Europe mastering advanced staining techniques and then worked with Cushing analysing the clinic's specimens in search of the best way to classify the neoplasms that affected the brain. One of their first conceptual advances was announced by Cushing in his 1922 Cavendish Lecture in London. To bring order out of the 'histological chaos' in categorizing tumors arising from the brain's lining, he proposed to name them 'meningiomas' and went on to outline their characteristics.[68] He also wrote about unusual tumors – primary gliomas of the chiasm and optic nerves, cholesteatoma or 'pearly tumor' – and the strange effects tumors could create, such as the cranial hyperostoses, or growths, that had been so puzzling years earlier with Leonard Wood's meningioma.

The clinic Cushing gave to members of the American Neurological Association when it met in Boston in 1923 was a stunning tour de force. He explained his division of brain tumor cases into verified (a tumor found at operation or autopsy), unverified (a tumor certainly present, but unlocated), and suspected (the suspicion proving incorrect), then divided the tumors into their principal categories – adenomas, meningiomas, neurinomas, and gliomas – and showed examples of patients with each kind. The last patient Cushing showed was a forty-eight-year-old merchant from whom he had removed a gliomatous tumor and cyst: 'The recovery ... is nothing short of a resurrection ... It takes persistence and some courage; but one need never give up hope of doing something to relieve a person with a brain tumor.' Lest they become too optimistic, Cushing concluded by talking about the half-dozen cases that month which his team had not been able to save.[69]

~

He wrote the Osler biography by organizing all the documents in chronological order, choosing the quotations from them that he wished to
use, and then writing bridge passages. Harvey and his secretaries literally scissored and pasted the manuscript into shape in 1922–3. The
manuscript grew at the rate of about a year of Osler's life in a week of
Cushing's. Osler's prose mesmerized him, he had trouble shortening
quotations, and he soon realized that he was assembling an old-fashioned 'life-and-letters' that would require more than one volume.

Cushing found that re-creating Osler's journey from backwoods
Canada in the 1850s to the heights of American medicine at Johns
Hopkins in the 1890s and then to the regius professorship at Oxford
was utterly absorbing. Doing the book taught him more about medicine and life than anything he had ever experienced in his education,
he said.[70] En route with Osler he became fascinated by secondary characters and incidents, refought old battles, and despite his passion for
accuracy, unwittingly retold a few tall tales. After reading one biography that featured too much about the biographer, Cushing decided to
exclude himself from Osler's life. His name would not be mentioned in
the book or the index; when he quoted from his own letters or diaries,
he disguised their authorship.

He knew that as an official biographer he had to be careful to avoid
'treading on what might be tender places' by giving needless offense to
the living. He could not print Osler's view of William Welch as a 'lazy
devil,' nor could he imply that Osler's final illness had been badly
handled by his British physicians. He hoped his account of an angry
dispute about Canadian medical services in the war was sufficiently
tactful: 'The story somehow had to be told and of course those who
know realize who was the nigger in the fence. I sincerely hope his feelings have not been greatly hurt.'[71]

About the only fault he could find in Osler's character was a
Rabelasian streak in some of the gag articles that he wrote under the
pseudonym Egerton Yorrick Davis. Cushing knew that Lady Osler would

never sanction quotations from Davis's published paper on a case of vaginismus (or 'De cohesione in coitu') or his manuscript history of some of the sexual habits of North American natives. But neither did he want to turn Osler into a plaster saint. He managed to insert E.Y. Davis carefully into his pages and played up incidents of conflict that involved Osler, often more dramatically than was warranted. When Grace read the manuscript she only insisted that he remove a letter containing a playful dissertation on bedpans and also Max Brödel's delightful cartoon of Osler as the saint of Johns Hopkins. She was startled to find that Harvey had quoted from her letters home from England and would have preferred that they be left out. But as she told a friend, 'I really could not bother him – he has been an angel for one of his temperament.' There may have been a confrontation that featured Cushing telling her, angelically of course, that if her letters were cut out, they might as well throw the whole manuscript in the stove.[72]

He liked to say later that he had simply started the biography with Osler's birth and finished it seventy years later with his death: 'Nowhere did I undertake to say what I thought were his principal contributions to medicine ... It would have been a faux pas for me to have attempted to give an appraisement of his work which I was incapable of doing or to have asked someone else to undertake to do so for me.'[73] In fact, he began volume 1 with a vivid image of the 'old Canadian trails' used by pioneers such as the Oslers, and he ended volume 2 with the procession of mourners at the Oxford funeral, the living giving up Osler's body to be watched over by the spirits of the medical immortals and the spirits of the young men who had been entertained at the 'Open Arms' (13 Norham Gardens) and then killed in France, 'doubly dead in that they died so young.' The most powerful passages in the biography, which can still move a reader to tears, are the accounts of Revere's death and his parents' grief.

Both the opening and closing images were literary flourishes that reflected more Cushing than Osler. It was Americans, not Canadians, who had moved west along pioneer trails. And Osler, who had thought long and hard about immortality, had never liked to speculate about

spirits watching over the living or the dead. Cushing, of the same generation as Jack McCrae and the men in Flanders fields, liked to sum-
mon spirits for literary and other purposes and may even have vaguely
believed in them. He was more accurate in choosing an introductory
quotation comparing Robert Louis Stevenson's 'childlike mirth' to Osler's
and, at the end, in remarking that Osler had been 'one of the most
greatly beloved physicians of all time.'

By Christmas 1923, Cushing had a manuscript of more than one
million words. 'It is a painful task to use a knife on your own children,' he complained as he struggled to shorten it. His publisher encouraged condensation, one editor telling him that a book, like a
speech, 'should be like a woman's skirt, long enough to cover the
object, and short enough to be interesting.' After taking out about
300,000 words, he gave up and sent the manuscript to England for
critical reading, final corrections, and typesetting. In the summer of
1924 he went to Oxford with Julia Shepley and spent several weeks
making last changes and reading proof. One of his tennis partners
during breaks was a young Rhodes scholar named John Fulton, a
Harvard physiology graduate in love with the Osler mystique. Fulton
had charmed Lady Osler and become the last surrogate son of a medical father he never actually met. Julia Shepley referred to Fulton as
an 'embryo prodigy.'[74]

Cushing barely kept his temper in these final stages. Osler's British
friends were determined that absolutely nothing should be published
that might offend anyone. The Oxford University Press's slow and precise editors and proofreaders were more than Cushing's match at fin-
icky attention to detail. Fortunately, Osler's nephew, Bill Francis, was
in Oxford cataloging Osler's library and outdid everyone in painstaking
pedantry. Hustling Harvey, as Grace nicknamed Cushing, finally went
home, leaving Francis and Miss Shepley to finish the index and fight
final skirmishes about ampersands and 'rat-ridden' versus 'rat-riddled.'
Cushing resisted most attempts to censor his manuscript but did compromise on a few points, such as agreeing to delete Osler's references to
the weak constitution of one of his patients: Edward, Prince of Wales.

Both Julia Shepley's impressions when she met the prince ('a pathetic sight if there ever was one ... I never saw such a scared little rabbit of a person ... such a furtive expression') and the later life of the Duke of Windsor indicate that Osler's judgments had been sound.[75]

~

One of the pleasures and perils of doing biography is the effect that living with a subject comes to have on the biographer. Cushing, of course, had already been profoundly influenced by Osler. Now his secretaries noticed that he was consciously and unconsciously borrowing Osler's turns of phrase. Kate Cushing told Grace Osler that her husband's experience writing Osler's life was good for him 'morally,' which presumably means she thought it made him a better man. One of his few explicit comments about how the book influenced him was in a 1925 letter to a friend at Johns Hopkins: 'Since writing Osler's biography, I have rather come to conclude that personality is the most important thing in the world. It almost always goes with ability, of course, but ability without personality falls like a seed on the desert.' Unfortunately, in the same letter he complained about being surrounded by talented 'Hebrews' with difficult personalities.[76]

As a medical statesman, he ostensibly seemed to be much like Osler in calling for 'a middle ground' in medical education, a balance between laboratory and scientic instruction on one hand and, on the other, the clinic and the art of medicine. In the 1920s it seemed to Cushing that on most issues the pendulum in medical schools and hospitals had swung too far. There was too much emphasis on research and not enough on treating patients, too much medical instruction in science rather than in the real problems of patients, and too much specialization to the detriment of general practice.

When Cushing opened McGill's new Rockefeller-funded research building in 1923, his ruminations on past research triumphs led him in the curious direction of wondering if such splendid facilities were actually needed:

Jenner was a country doctor. Harvey had no laboratory. Vesalius detached from the gallows the body of a criminal and smuggled it to his home to dissect ... Osler made his reputation as a pathologist ... working in quarters a modern pathologist would scorn ...

One sometimes wonders whether the pursuit of knowledge may not possibly be hampered by surroundings too elaborate ... Even to the workers they are not entirely an unmixed blessing, these great modern laboratories. They often bring added responsibilities and administrative burdens which may hamper research ... We have this to contend with in our marble halls at Harvard.[77]

Nor was he impressed with medical schools such as Harvard that had become factorylike in offering standardized teaching in a standardized curriculum – usually two years of preclinical science and then two years of clinical work. In a 1924 talk on the clinical teacher and the medical curriculum, he drew attention to the fact that 90 percent of the students wanted to learn how to practice medicine, not to do research. Perhaps the old ways of teaching them were not so bad after all:

There is much that a present-day medical student might envy in the opportunities offered to a young man of a century ago, apprenticed to such a person, let us say, as Nathan Smith, with the chance to get at the outset an intimate knowledge of people and of people's maladies; to discuss the problems of the sick room with the master while driving him in his gig as he went on his distant house-to-house rounds; to have his collateral reading directed; and subsequently to take a short course somewhere in the so-called fundamentals and get his degree. In our present-day schools, not only is this process rerversed, but the Nathan Smiths, if there are any, scarcely know even the names of their many pupils, whom perforce they meet in a classroom so crowded that the elbow-to-elbow method of teaching and learning is no longer possible.[78]

Cushing called for an earlier emphasis in medical schools on clinical training. He asked what medical education would be like if clinical work came before rather than after science training. In 1923 he tried an Osler-like experiment at Harvard by holding Saturday morning 'observation' clinics for first-year students; the students flocked to attend. Some of his apparently reactionary attacks on medical education in the 1920s actually anticipated by half a century the advent of problem-based medical learning. Why have seven scientists teaching about seven aspects of the pancreas years before a student has ever seen a patient with pancreatic troubles? Harvey wondered in 1924. 'How much simpler to have shown the patient first, to have briefly explained how diabetes came to be recognized and what its complications may be, how step by step the mysteries of carbohydrate metabolism have partly been unraveled and the principles of our present-day treatment established.'[79]

In the 1920s the man who had introduced blood-pressure monitoring into American surgery now complained about excessive reliance on diagnostic tests and machines and inadequate attention to patients. He liked to relate homely anecdotes about baffled hospital specialists x-raying and measuring, counting and ruminating, calling in more specialists, until finally a simple country doctor wanders into the ward and remarks how interesting it is that cases of typhoid fever are still around:

> Careful studies of our patients are not to be superseded by snap diagnoses; yet the incident illustrates ... the over-emphasis laid on the accumulation of often unessential laboratory data, and the underemphasis on what may be learned by a trained observer from a thorough bedside study of the patient ... I do not believe that students can begin to think in terms of the patient too early in their course, nor too early begin to interpret and record what they can see, hear, and touch – perhaps even smell and taste – at the bedside.[80]

Most of the medical trends that Cushing abhorred were famously celebrated by the popular novelist and Yale graduate, Sinclair Lewis, in his 1925 book *Arrowsmith*. Lewis's protagonist, Dr Martin Arrowsmith, turns his back on 'the slimy trail of the dollar' in medical practice (especially surgery) and dedicates his life to research. His models are the idealistic German Jewish scientists at the Rockefeller Institute in New

York. Lewis's medical adviser for the novel, Paul de Kruif, was a close friend of the Flexners and a driven alcoholic. Despite being passingly mentioned in *Arrowsmith* for his brilliant surgical technique, Cushing despised everything about the novel. As a fictional antidote to it, he suggested Sarah Orne Jewett's *A Country Doctor*, published in 1884.[81]

If Osler had been the dominant or sole influence on his thought, Cushing would have held to the middle ground on most medical and social issues. In fact he did not. As a fifty-something descendant of Puritans and generations of traditional family physicians, he was becoming steadily more conservative and disapproving. Though a symbol of medical modernism to the outside world, he was culturally an arch-Victorian. Soon after finishing Osler's life, Cushing wrote a long and partly autobiographical address on his own Ohio and medical roots, which he gave at the opening of a new medical building at Western Reserve University. 'Tradition,' he told his audience, 'is the most powerful binding influence the world knows. It lies deep in most of us, and pride in tradition supplies the glue which holds people and groups of people in cohesion. Pride in family and friends, in Alma Mater and profession, in race and birthplace, in state and nation. The controlling subconsciousness of one's stock and upbringing is something from which time and distance can never wholly wean us.'[82]

Reflecting on the wholesome family and medical traditions that had shaped him in the 1870s and 1880s, Cushing disdained the fads and fashions of the Roaring Twenties. He did not like flappers, bobbed hair, or jazz. He was suspicious of advertising ('anathema to the ethical code of the physician'), business schools, spiritualists, Seventh Day Adventists, antivivisectionists and antivaccinationists, and everything that smacked of frivolity: 'While nations are stewing in their post-bellum troubles, jazz, the "movie," and the *thé dansant* engage the thoughts of the people. The only common ground on which the interests of all appear to meet is the crossword puzzle.'[83]

In the family circle, these attitudes meant that the Cushing children were being raised in the shadow, if not exactly the presence, of a stern, disapproving father. He believed that watching motion pictures was bad for children's eyes, minds, bodies, and morals, and he supported keeping the movies out of Brookline. He believed that women should not smoke in public or drink cocktails – not Kate and certainly not the girls. He continued to smoke heavily himself. There are cigarette burns on pages of his Osler manuscript and the book's galley proofs. He apologized to Kate about being 'testy' with the children and told her that the job she was doing raising them was far more important than his work because it would last longer: 'Don't feel that I fail to realize this.'[84]

∼

The Life of Sir William Osler was published by Oxford University Press in 1925 in two thick volumes. The first 685 pages recounted Osler's life before he left for England in 1905 at the age of fifty-five. A further 686 pages dealt with his fifteen years in England. Cushing dedicated the book to medical students, 'in the hope that something of Osler's spirit may be conveyed to those of a generation that has not known him.' He wrote in his introduction that the volumes were 'merely the outlines for the final portrait, to be painted out when the colours, lights, and shadows come in time to be added.' This seems like an astonishing comment, but Cushing had learned that shorter biographies are often harder to write than longer ones, and they take longer.

Knowing his book's weaknesses, he was apprehensive that reviewers would compare it to such recent well-received works as Lytton Strachey's *Eminent Victorians*. 'I am a humble surgeon and not a Strachey,' he wrote, more than a little disingenuously, to a friend who was reviewing the book:

> Someone who is sufficiently clever with his pen can, and I hope will, write a short biography which will carry the message of his life on for future generations of medical students. But unless someone had made the careful study first, I do not see how it would have been possible.
>
> And even so, I have tried to make it so WO's spirit would show out even in these somewhat detailed chronological chapters. The very fact that for

seventy-five years there were no waves of melancholy and depression is in itself significant. I do not know how you like this Arrowsmith kind of doctor book as influenced by de Kruif, but I should like to propose Osler's life as an antidote to those folks who may think the characters in Arrowsmith are anything more than caricatures.

He was not surprised that some of the reviewers concentrated on the book's excessive length. One of his Harvard colleagues and fellow medical inkslingers, Hans Zinsser, gently pointed out that the Osler biography was three times as long as the standard biography of Pasteur and twice as long as a recent life of Christ: 'Doctor Cushing is a distinguished brain surgeon, and the habit of picking about among the delicate wirings at the base of the human skull breeds a passion for detail that may have run away with him.'[85] (A few years later it would take Zinsser only 228 pages to survey all of *Rats, Lice, and History.*) Morris Fishbein, editor of the *Journal of the American Medical Association,* said it should have been boiled down to two or three hundred pages, and a British reviewer compared it to one of the old bran tubs that English countryfolk paid a few pence to dip into in the hope of finding hidden treasures.

Many more of the reviews were uncritically positive. Osler's life had been intrinsically interesting and his prose powerful and delightful, especially to those who knew the territory and the players. Cushing's connecting passages were often deft, biographically appropriate, and memorable in their imagery. (Medical discovery, for example, in the 1880, was like popcorn popping; after losing Revere, the Oslers 'fathered and mothered, without end, the young soldier-children of their old American friends.') In 1925 there existed no other biography of a contemporary medical personality comparable to Cushing's *Osler.* Even lay readers such as Baltimore's dean of American letters, H.L. Mencken, judged that as 'a collection of souvenirs of Osler the man,' the book had succeeded: 'The curious enchantment that he worked upon all who had any sort of contact with him is visible on every page.'[86]

Soon Cushing began to get letters from Osler's friends, his own friends, and other readers. They came in every day for months. Their verdict was overwhelmingly favorable. Everyone seemed to like what he had done. They told him that he had brought Osler back to life; that the book was a liberal education in itself; it was one of the great biographies of the century, of all time, as good as and maybe better than Boswell on Johnson. Correspondents said they had lost sleep because they couldn't stop reading. Many had been moved to tears, especially by the death of Revere and by the gathering of the spirits at Osler's funeral. Cushing's *Osler* was at once heartwarming, tragic, and inspirational. With family, friends, medical students, and the general public, Cushing had succeeded beyond everyone's hopes. As a friend put it, he had managed to capture 'the shimmer of Osler's wings.' Grace Osler deeply appreciated both the book and the response to it. Sales exceeded everyone's expectations – some 15,000 copies in four printings in the first year alone.[87]

Feeling vindicated by his public, Cushing tried the insecure author's ploy of urging friends to respond to the critical reviews. He toyed with the idea of writing an anonymous review, in which he would quote the favorable letters he was getting and dwell especially on popular approval of the book's length. Then he thought better of it. 'I have other things to attend to, most of them inside of people's heads.'[88]

❧

Cushing's literary output reached a kind of crescendo in 1925–6, for the Osler biography was followed by a small book with Percival Bailey on the gliomas and by the publication of his Cameron Prize Lectures, *Studies in Intracranial Physiology and Surgery*. The collaboration with Bailey broke important new ground in classifying, by cellular origin and composition, the diverse tumors that arise in the brain's own tissue, and correlating types to prognosis. The basic categories – medulloblastomas, spongioblastomas, and astrocytomas – encompassed most gliomas and seemed to have distinct prognoses. Astrocytomas, for example, could be more slow-growing and more amenable to therapy than the other gliomas. The next step, Cushing and Bailey realized, would be to develop quick techniques for identifying tumors. If surgeons could make on-the-spot identifications of the gliomas they had exposed, they would be far better positioned to make their life-and-death decisions.[89]

Cushing delivered the prestigious Cameron Prize Lectures in Edinburgh in October 1925. They constituted, as John Fulton put it, a kind of scientific autobiography. Harvey outlined the history of the three problems that had principally concerned him: intracranial tumors, the pituitary gland, and the circulation of the cerebrospinal fluid. (In the fullness of his career, Cushing had stopped doing ganglionectomies or worrying about credit for what had once been his surgical theme song.) As an elder statesman he went out of his way to give credit to other workers. He dedicated his Cameron Lectures to his research fellows and residents, listing them by name. His discussion of cerebrospinal circulation was notable for setting his disagreement with young Dandy in context. The overview of the pituitary again stressed the baffling complexities of the organ, how little was still known about its secretions, and how pituitary surgery was still in its 'stone age.' Cushing sometimes commented in these years that he no longer thought he knew enough about the pituitary to write a book about it.[90]

The lectures culminated in 'Intracranial Tumors and the Surgeon,' a masterful exposition of progress in brain tumor surgery since the 1880s. He obliquely alluded to recent controversies. Decompression operations, he noted, had served a useful purpose and saved much suffering in their time, and they had stimulated the profession not to accept the inevitability of death by tumor. Ventriculography enlarged the utility of the x-ray, 'but with all said and done, no instrumental aid to diagnosis can equal in importance a detailed and exact hstory of the symptoms in the chronological order of their appearance.' The next step forward would be to develop better, faster knowledge of the brain's lesions, especially at the cellular level. In the meantime, it was important for surgeons to keep score of their tumor experiences, to study each other's scores, to attempt to establish a 'par' for any given procedure, and to aim at lower mortality rates and 'more livable survival periods.' 'A neuro-surgeon's responsibilities would be insufferable if he did not feel that his knowledge of an intricate subject was constantly growing – that his game was improving.'[91]

Cushing seemed to be on top of every facet of his game. Only his physical stamina had fallen off – he could not walk long distances, and he often remarked on the fatiguing nature of long operations. As a surgeon, as a researcher, as a writer, his prestige had never been higher. His former student Lewis Weed, now dean of the Johns Hopkins Medical School, nicely expressed admiration for a medical renaissance man: 'When I read one of your papers or addresses, I think that you should do nothing else but write; when I see you operate I think that you should do nothing else but operate; and when I see you experiment I think that you should do nothing else but experiment.'[92]

In April 1926, about the time of publication of his new books, Cushing learned that he had been awarded the Pulitzer Prize in biography. The criterion (since changed) was 'for the best American biography teaching patriotic and unselfish services to the people, illustrated by an eminent example.' Ironically, yet also as a sign of the impact of the rise of American medicine, the Pulitzer Prize for fiction that year was awarded to Sinclair Lewis for *Arrowsmith*. The terms of that award – for depicting 'the wholesome atmosphere of American life and the highest standard of American life and the highest standard of American manners and manhood' – caused Lewis to turn it down. He said the prize was for obedience to good values rather than for literary merit.

Cushing was amused by the contretemps and delighted to accept his Pulitzer. He had no quarrel whatever with the criteria. William Osler and the examples of his brother, father, grandfather, and great-grandfather had caused him to dedicate his life to service through medicine. On June 5, 1926, he delivered the graduation address to medical students at Jefferson College, Philadelphia, and talked more openly than ever before about his faith in the physician's calling. Cushing was delighted that Jefferson students still took the Hippocratic Oath and still believed in the ties of 'brotherhood' and the guildlike solidarity of the profession.

He restated his view that there was too much emphasis in medicine on laboratory and academic research, too much of Sinclair Lewis's cynicism, and too little concentration on 'the doctor-and-patient relationship.' It was all very well to stress public health and preventative medicine, a current fad at Harvard, 'but say what one will, the time inevitably comes to each and every one, now in the best of health, when he must needs cry out for some experienced and sensible doctor who can alleviate if not cure his particular ailments ... and the kind of sagacity and resourcefulness he will expect and need is less laboratory-born than bred of long and sympathetic familiarity with the anxieties and complaints of ailing, damaged, and worn-out human beings.' He urged the medical students to consecrate themselves to their profession and to the 'practical religion of the physician,' which was 'not the promising of bliss in the future but the giving of health and happiness on earth.' He concluded the address, which he had entitled 'Consecratio Medici,' with a quotation from Stephen Paget's *Confessio Medici:* 'If a doctor's life may not be a divine vocation, then no life is a vocation, and nothing is divine.'[93]

～

Bill Cushing thought more about girls and baseball and hockey at Yale in the mid-1920s than he did about any vocation. Harvey had no special problem with that. Like his father before him, he would bide his time, pay the bills, and wait for the boy to round into form, probably decide to go into medicine. Second son Henry would soon enter Yale. Eldest daughter Mary had finished Westover School in Middlebury, Connecticut, and worked in a bookstore, thought about art school, and had a busy social life. Betsey was still at Westover, fretted about not getting higher marks, and was thrilled when she received letters from her father and when he won the Pulitzer Prize. Barbara was still at home.

Bill Cushing, who had inherited his parents' capacity to be charming, had a good social time and a good athletic time at Yale and still scraped by with average marks. Father and son seemed to understand each other better. Harvey still occasionally lectured Bill on the need to be careful with money, spouting such old-fashioned maxims as 'Better to go in rags than to be in debt.' Bill was desperately contrite about having wasted money, time, and opportunities on women and partying during his first year – which had ended badly with his involvement in some kind of car accident: 'There are a lot of temptations in New Haven. I not always resisted them.'[94]

Nothing worse than failed romances and failing to make the starting line-up of the Yale baseball team befell Bill during his second and third years. When he had decided to continue with varsity ice hockey in his junior year, his father had advised him, 'If you are going in for it I certainly would go in for it hard. Half-way measures never got anybody anywhere.' College sports were a serious business for Cushing fathers and sons. Writing to Bill in February 1926, Harvey repeated the line that also crept into his writing about brain surgery: 'Life all round is a kind of sporting event and the best any of us can do is to try continually to improve our game.'[95]

Inside and outside the operating room, failure and misery, life and death, are one slip, one missed curve away. At the end of the Yale term in the spring of 1926, twenty-two-year-old Bill Cushing and a twenty-one-year-old freshman friend from New York City, George Matthews Kopperl, decide to celebrate. On Friday, June 11, Kopperl, who is not licensed to drive in Connecticut – nor is Cushing – persuades a roomate to lend them a car (an open Willis-St. Claire roadster with a rumble seat) and also a driver's license. They latch onto a couple of dark-haired New Haven beauties, Bernadette Kiernan and Ethel Miller Reeser. Reeser, who is married, tells her husband she is going to visit an aunt, and the four young people drive to the Woodlawn roadhouse near Madison, Connecticut, and dance and drink the night away. Ethel Reeser phones her husband to say she will be spending the night with her aunt.

About 2 AM on Saturday, June 12, residents of Guilford, just outside New Haven, hear a terrible crash by the Boston Post Road. They find the wreckage of the roadster wrapped around a big elm tree and, in a pathetic heap, the bodies of its four occupants. Three are dead of fractured skulls. All of the bodies reek of alcohol. Ethel Reeser lives just long enough to tell rescuers her maiden name.

Driving at high speed on a clear night, at the height of the jazz age, the Yale men had missed the curve.

In Boston, Harvey Cushing received the news later that morning as he was preparing to operate for tumor on a young woman named Murphy. He phoned Kate in New York, went into the operating room and carried out the operation, which was a success. Afterwards, he told his team about the family tragedy and then left for Connecticut to claim his son's body.[96]

TWELVE

Johnson and Boswells: Chief and Harem

Everyone who worked with Cushing knew how he would respond to his son's death. 'Dr. Cushing will hide it all behind a mask,' Elliott Cutler told Madeline Stanton. 'No one will ever see it. Therefore all the worse.'

The mask he put on was almost impenetrable and permanent. The Cushings repressed their grief much more thoroughly than the Oslers had after Revere's death. The hundreds of letters and telegrams of condolence Harvey and Kate received have all but disappeared from their files. Cushing's papers are completely silent about the immediate aftermath of the accident. Harvey never mentioned Bill again to his colleagues.[1]

One letter from Kate to Harvey, written a year later, survives in her papers. In it she talks of how they had steeled themselves during the war and how they did it again when Bill died, 'allowing ourselves no time to grieve, no time to adjust ourselves. The smallest acts of daily life, meeting the butcher the grocer & school master ... months we went about our business raw – with quivering nerves. Thanksgiving Day – Christmas Day – only the night – in which to give way to a natural human grief, and then afraid to – lest they should see the traces in the morning.' Harvey apparently tried to console his wife with the thought, which he may or may not have believed, that Bill was waiting for them to join him. Kate appears to have tried to contact her son's spirit, apparently by occasionally attending seances. People noticed the deep lines of sorrow in Harvey's cheeks.[2]

Cushing could have chosen to slip into semi-retirement after the blow of Bill's death. He was in his late fifties, his legs continued to bother him, and he had become a conservative surgeon whose best work, some thought, had been done years previously. His wife thought it was time to set their house in order, and his four remaining children needed him. His publications in 1925–6 would have stood as the summing up of a magnificent lifetime of achievement.

He did not slow down. Despite having been nearly broken by the awful tragedy, Cushing returned to his game and played it as hard as he could. He threw himself back into his work and in 1926 and 1927 got a second, perhaps even third, wind. He dazzled, intrigued, and sometimes infuriated the self-proclaimed Boswells who undertook to immortalize him in the closing, peak years of his singular career.

~

Cushing had been a surgical innovator without being particularly inventive. Most of the drills and saws and rongeurs and clamps and retractors and hooks and needles and sutures that he used fastidiously and with beautiful outcomes had been initially developed by others. His major technical innovation was probably the use of little silver clips in the war against bleeding. (After a decade or so, his student Ken McKenzie invented a better clip, which Cushing then adopted.) Sets of 'Cushing's Brain Instruments' sold by the Boston firm of Codman & Shurtleff during and after the war were unauthorized knockoffs which he repudiated.[3] His conservatism about such innovations as the use of power drills had been noted well before the war, and he had been volubly cautious about ventriculography. He was fairly early in the field in trying radiation therapy for certain tumors, but by the mid-1920s he had decided that the results, extremely difficult to judge, were only occasionally encouraging. 'I sometimes feel that the consequent loss of hair and bedraggled appearance make this therapeutic measure scarcely worth the inconvenience to the patient and time to the roentgenologist,' he wrote of radiation for glioblastomas. Blind radiation of unverified tumors struck him as a return to a medical dark age.[4]

A number of gynecologists, genitourinary surgeons, and nose-and-throat men had experimented for many years with a variety of electrified instruments to cut and cauterize. Back in 1884, electrocautery had been used in London in the famous Godlee-Bennett tumor removal. Cushing's former associate at Hopkins, Howard Kelly, always an enthusiastic innovator, had taken up the technology and encouraged Harvey to look into it. The brain surgeon briefly tried using an electrified needle to make incisions but decided it was impractical. Also at Johns Hopkins, Walter Dandy was hoping that someone – Kelly or research engineers at General Electric – might make a better cautery that would help him penetrate deeper into the brain.

In the summer or early autumn of 1926, Cushing saw a new electrosurgical device being used against cancers at another Boston hospital. It had been developed by a young Harvard physicist, W.T. Bovie, and combined the cutting and coagulating functions in a small wire loop, which the surgeon manipulated through a pistol–like grip. Bovie's machine also had a strong, reliable current. Cushing saw its possibilities for his work, borrowed 'the Bovie,' and began to experiment.

He first tried the loop on extracranial tumors and with Bovie's help worked his way through some serious technical problems, including the shocks that the current occasionally gave to both operator and assistants. At the first trial in Cushing's operating room, on October 1, 1926, a standby blood donor fainted. A group of French observers coughed incessantly. Hugh Cairns, newly arrived from England, became so rattled that he had to be replaced by Horrax. On later occasions, Cushing tried using a wooden operating table and wooden instruments. One day the current somehow ignited ether vapor, creating a flash of blue flame. One patient was burned by a misplaced electrode, others suffered epileptiform seizures when Cushing first touched the surface of their brains.[5]

As the glitches were resolved, Cushing realized that he had an instrument of tremendous, perhaps revolutionary, potential. He could
cut through tissue more easily than ever before, and in many cases he
could control bleeding far more effectively than with his clips and clamps.
By the spring of 1927 his enthusiasm began to bubble out in correspondence:

> With the aid of Bovie I have been having a most hectic two months taking
> out brain tumors with his electro-surgical apparatus – most astounding and
> revolutionary, the whole business ... It is amazing that either the patient,
> Bovie or the operating staff survive ... Since this machine that he runs for me
> might electrocute anybody any minute, I am trying to make hay while the
> sun shines, viz., that Bovie is around ... Heretofore, these methods have been
> merely used by a lot of specialists who have been fiddling with malignant
> disease whereas its possibilities for general surgery are unfathomed. I have
> been having a perfectly amazing time with Bovie, who has an electro-surgi-
> cal apparatus powerful enough to electrocute a mastodon and pretty nearly
> as big. As a result of this, I have been tackling brain tumors that I never before
> thought I could possibly attack ... I have been sending out for a lot of aban-
> doned cases and having them come in to be redone. I wish I were as young
> and vigorous as you. Then I would feel that I really might accomplish some-
> thing some day for tumors which would make what has already been done
> look like thirty cents.[6]

The Bovie electro scalpel, as it came to be called, was particularly
important in allowing Cushing to attack large, slow-growing tumors
that originate in the meninges of the brain and penetrate deeply into its
tissues. These meningiomas were often so heavily vascularized or so
hard to reach that Cushing had had to be content with buying time by
partial removal or palliation. Back in 1910, the Leonard Wood case
had been a rare example of a simple and apparently complete excision.
More often with such tumors, Cushing had to go in repeatedly to scrape
out new growth. Sometimes he had to give up in defeat. Now it ap-

peared he could triumph: 'I am succeeding in doing things inside the head that I never thought it would be possible to do.'[7]

He also thought he might soon be able to treat victims of pituitary disease in ways no one had ever thought possible. His trail-breaking work before the war, publicized in his famous monograph, had attracted a steady stream of patients with problems apparently stemming from pituitary disorders. But after the failure of his early experiments with pituitary extracts, he had been able to offer only partially effective surgical assaults on tumors affecting the pituitary. His interest in the gland itself had waned.

It came back as a result of new successes by Herbert M. Evans (a former student who had moved to California and later became a leader in endocrinology) and Philip E. Smith, among others, in producing extracts of the anterior pituitary lobe that enabled them to control the growth of laboratory rats. Evans had produced giantism in rats; Smith had shown that extracts could restore growth to rats that had an impaired gland. Other recent advances, including the discovery of insulin and the isolation of parathyroid hormone, were making endocrinology a respectable field of study. By 1926 a new rush to the pituitary was beginning in many centers, and Cushing rejoined the hunt.

One of his research fellows, Leo Davidoff, made an exhaustive study of acromegaly while another, Tracy Putnam, began work with one of Evans's former students on new pituitary extracts. 'We proceeded to elbow our way into the problem of experimental overgrowth,' Cushing wrote a few years later. By September 1926, Putnam was able to display what Cushing called 'some most wonderful giant rats.' Perhaps the team was on the verge of finding a more effective extract than Evans's or Smith's, one that would enable patients with stunted growth to develop normally. Enormous clinical possibilities were at stake, Cushing told David Edsall, Harvard's dean of medicine.[8] In the meantime, Davidoff and Cushing enriched their understanding of acromegaly, now seeing it as a polyglandular disorder caused by an acidophilic adenoma (tumor) of the pituitary.

Cushing's old enthusiasm for 'this amazing structure which conducts the endocrine orchestra' had been rekindled, now with concentration on the anterior lobe. He thought that surgical approaches to pituitary adenomas, which were constantly becoming more effective, might nip acromegaly in the bud, as it were. Effective treatment was highly desirable for a disease which, Harvey wrote, had been conceived by 'Nature in her ugliest mood.' In May 1927 he wrote a rare letter to *Time* magazine, criticizing its frivolous and cruel derision of an acromegalic who was being exhibited as the 'World's Ugliest Woman' in the Ringling Brothers' circus.[9]

That same month he delivered a gripping presidential address to the American Surgical Association on the unpromising subject, 'Experiences with Orbito-Ethmoidal Osteomata Having Intracranial Complications.' The talk was a narrative history of four cases he had handled of strange growths on the ethmoidal bone, replete with references to the shifting boundaries of the Balkan states and his own cowardice in once 'showing a surgical white feather.' He described how he had worked through failure, and had experienced a surgical epiphany ('the cyst was punctured; there was a puff of air, and its walls immediately collapsed leaving an excavation of astonishing size ... I then surmised for the first time ...'), and of how he now had a perfect understanding of these osteomata and their treatment. His old friend Jim Mitchell thought it was one of the best meetings he had ever attended. The talk still conveys the thrill of surgical discovery.[10]

Lecturing in the British Isles in June 1927, he held a large London audience spellbound with a masterly discourse on acromegaly. Then in Glasgow he gave the first Macewen Memorial Lecture, on how electro-surgery 'holds out untold possibilities for the future of neurosurgery.' As a kind of bonus, he gave what correspondents judged the best talk at the Lister Centenary in Edinburgh, a comparison of Lister and Lincoln as emancipators who freed men from the shackles of sepsis and slavery. On this trip he added three more honorary degrees and four honorary memberships to his list of awards.

～

Cushing cut his British trip short so that he could have a medical rendez-vous with his most famous patient, General Leonard Wood. In 1920 Wood, a fierce critic of Woodrow Wilson's conduct of the war, had seemed about to catch the brass ring of American politics as a front-runner for the Republican presidential nomination. Opponents raised questions about Wood's health, hinting that he was a physical and per-haps mental cripple from the surgery Cushing had done on his head in 1910. Harvey had been outraged by the suggestion. He served on Wood's nomination committee and wrote several open letters about the general's good health. It had been a perfectly benign tumor, and the operation had left Wood with just a bit of stiffness in the left foot. Otherwise, Cushing wrote, 'he is the most vigorous and sound human being, mentally and physically, that I ever saw. The procedure did not bother him any more than if he had a broken leg with consequent lameness.' More than ten years after surgery there was no reason to expect recurrence of the tumor. Cushing pointedly suggested that Wood was in better condition to handle the strains of office than Woodrow Wilson, now paralyzed by a stroke, had been in 1916.[11]

Wood lost the 1920 nomination when the Republican convention became deadlocked, and the concept of conniving 'men in smoke-filled rooms' was added to politics as the candidacy went to the obscure Ohioan, Warren Harding. Harding easily won the presidency, and he appointed Wood to another tour of duty as governor of the Philip-pines. Through his early sixties Wood carried on with his usual vigor, ignoring all signs of weakness. He suppressed mounting evidence of physical problems including epileptiform seizures. Whenever he sensed an attack coming on, he locked himself in his bathroom; servants once had to break down the door. Wood was operated on for hernias, banged himself up badly in an automobile accident, and was gradually becom-ing paralyzed on his left side.

Cushing heard that Wood's army doctors were wondering if his brain tumor had recurred. He suggested that Wood see him again. He now realized that in 1910 he ought not to have replaced Wood's bone flap, for the bone itself had probably been invaded by tumor cells; the extirpation therefore had not been complete and the tumor had probably reformed. But there was no need to worry. 'We would have no trouble in taking it out,' the surgeon told the general, 'for I have learned much these past fifteen years about these lesions.' And didn't Leonard Wood have more lives than a cat anyway?

Vomiting, almost paralyzed, and starting to lose vision, Wood still tried to deny he had a problem when Cushing examined him in early August 1927.[12] Cushing told him there was only one choice. 'All right,' Wood replied, 'You're the boss. Can't you do it this afternoon?' Cushing could not, but within two days he was able to get his team together, assemble blood donors, and start work at nine o'clock on a Saturday morning. Hugh Cairns, by now well broken in, assisted, and one of Wood's doctors, Alexander Lambert, observed.

'We had a stupendous task ahead of us, far worse than I had anticipated,' Cushing wrote in Wood's file afterwards. The sixty-six-year-old soldier had become seriously obese, and they had trouble positioning him comfortably. Cushing now did most of these operations using only novocaine as a local anesthetic. As Cushing drilled through the skull, realizing immediately that a massive meningeal tumor had recurred, Wood was awake, talkative, cheery, but fidgety. Fragments of bone engulfed by tumor made it difficult for Cushing to use the electric scalpel to cut tissue and cauterize bleeding points. 'Spurting arterial vessels were everywhere encountered.'

Cushing used his sucker to extract fragments of tumor from its enveloping sac, had better luck than he had feared, and after about four hours was ready for the next stage. He could either proceed directly to remove the tumor's shell or he could stop, close up temporarily, and finish in a second operation after everyone had rested and begun to recuperate. 'I unquestionably should have desisted at this stage for the patient was getting a little restless, constantly changing his head and I do not think that I fully took in the fact that he perhaps had had enough,' Cushing wrote in his operative note.

In fact, Wood was urging Cushing to get on with it, as much for Mrs Wood's sake as his own. Lambert remarked that there were plenty of donors on hand to replace blood. Wood's blood pressure and pulse seemed steady enough, so Cushing ordered a transfusion and kept going, past the point of no return.

After another hour and another transfusion he was just tilting the big emptied tumor sac out of Wood's head, cutting it away from its stem, when he nicked a vein. He had trouble controlling the sudden spurt:

> The bleeding point was with difficulty held, first by pressure with the finger and then by a pack, somewhat insecurely, for in view of the great cavity there was nothing to retain it. There was still no rise in pulse rate and as the bleeding seemed to be checked the wound was loosely closed over the pack.
>
> Fortunately he was not removed from the table for in the course of the next hour the pulse for the first time began to rise and the pressure to fall off so seriously a clot was suspected. So at 5.30 p.m. an emergency reopening of the wound was made and after removing a large clot together with the packing, by the lucky placement of a clip the vessel was this time caught leaving a smooth, clean dry cavity. He was again transfused and picked up promptly. No further bleeding having been set up by this last transfusion, the wound was closed securely (6.20 p.m.) and it was felt that we were safely through.[13]

After almost ten hours, the exhausted team dispersed.

For two hours Wood seemed to be in fairly good condition. Then his pulse started racing, he began breathing quickly and irregularly, and the doctors began to realize that they had lost. Cairns and John Fulton took turns at Wood's bedside, giving cardiac stimulants but mostly feeling helpless. Cushing gave up at 11 PM and went home. Leonard Wood died about 1 AM. 'I liked him almost as well as any man I have ever met,' Cairns wrote his wife later that day. 'And I am sure I've never seen a braver man – a perfectly indomitable man without the faintest trace of fear, and his wife another of the same sort ... No one ever thought he would die because it has been so well known that it was impossible to kill him.'[14]

When Cairns and Fulton did the autopsy that day they found that Wood had been killed by blood seeping into the lower ventricles of his brain. In the end, Cushing had not been able to control the hemorrhage. 'I do not think that I realized that there might again have been a refilling of the wound because I felt that it was quite dry.' He wondered if he should have gone in again one last time that night. 'All told,' he concluded in his operative note, 'it looks like a very bad record of attempting to do too much at a single session but the circumstances were such that we were led on from one stage to another until it was too late to do anything but see the matter through.' A few weeks later he wrote that both his surgical reflexes and his judgment were still rusty after the England trip. If Wood had come to him a few months earlier, he might have been saved. 'He was a great man. I've never lost a patient after operation that so upset me. It was *so* near to success ... If I had used better judgment he would certainly have been saved and no one the wiser. He could easily enough have had another 15 years as good as the last.'[15]

~

He was being watched. Every move Cushing made was studied. It was always so in the operating room: assistants and observers looked on intently for professional reasons, while patients took in what they could through their haze of anesthetic, fear, and hope. But he was also under scrutiny everywhere he went and in everything he did because of his celebrity. Everyone knew he was a towering figure in surgery and medicine, virtually a living legend. You made notes on his surgical technique. You wrote home about him, as Hugh Cairns did the day after the Leonard Wood operation. You jotted down observations about him in your diary. You mentally filed away Cushing anecdotes for retelling at medical gatherings, in your memoirs, or to his biographers.

John Fulton appointed himself to be Cushing's first biographer. He began keeping a diary three weeks after Leonard Wood's death. It was, at first, mostly about Cushing: 'He continues to talk about bad surgical judgment and remarked to Cairns the other day that the only thing he had accomplished since coming back from Europe was to kill an important person. Except for his son's death ... I have never seen him so deeply affected by a disappointment.'[16]

Eventually the people who knew Cushing generated bushels of diaries, letters, notes, observations, and reminiscences. Most of the young men he trained as neurosurgeons wrote or told stories about their experiences with him. Many of his other medical friends and Harvard colleagues recorded Cushing stories, which they passed on to Fulton and others. Some patients wrote to and about him. Tellingly, his family produced least in the way of memoirs, and only a relatively small amount of their correspondence from the years when he was at the height of his fame survives. That lacuna is more than made up for by the gaze of his inner circle: the smart and literate women who called themselves his harem; and the man, Fulton, who saw himself as Cushing's Boswell.

Cushing's harem consisted of his secretaries, Julia Shepley and Madeline Stanton, his histologist, Louise Eisenhardt, and several other female typists, stenographers, medical artists, and photographers who worked directly for him. It did not include nurses, who were independent professionals hired by the hospital. The harem first emerges in a 1924 letter that Julia Shepley, working in Oxford on the Osler biography, wrote to Madeline Stanton back in Boston: 'Regards to the harem & Gilbert the Filbert, & store up the dope conscientiously.'[17] The women in the office, mostly single, mostly New Englanders, spent very long hours working together in Cushing's service. They often got together socially, they wrote to each other on holidays, and they exchanged inside 'dope' about the Chief and the goings-on at the Brigham. There were no overt sexual connotations in their joking about being a harem, though often a sense that they were giving the best part of their lives to serving a very demanding man.

'Gilbert the Filbert' was Gil Horrax, Cushing's permanent chief assistant and, in the eyes of some, a kind of eunuch to the harem (actu-ally, he had married one of Cushing's operating-room nurses) because he stayed year after year, doing whatever Cushing told him to do, ap-parently showing no ambition to get a neurosurgical life of his own. This set him apart from the long series of other Cushing residents and trainees: Conrad Jacobson, Loyal Davis, Ken McKenzie, Percival Bailey, Norman Dott, Leo Davidoff, John Scarff, Eric Oldberg, Bronson Ray, Richard Meagher, Richard Light, and about a dozen others who worked furiously under Cushing for a year or two and moved on into practice or academic medicine.

Hugh Cairns, who came to the Brigham in 1926, was one of the most eager and popular of the novices. Cairns was an Australian war veteran who had won a Rhodes scholarship, married the daughter of the Master of Balliol College, Oxford, and first met Cushing at the Oslers' house. He came to Boston on a Rockefeller Foundation travel-ling fellowship to learn Cushing's techniques so that he could introduce them to English surgery. 'Cairns here for a year as Neurol. Asst. Going to be a great success,' Madeline Stanton jotted in her diary. '*Runs* around everywhere so as to waste no time.' Cairns wrote long letters to his wife at home about his experiences in America in 1926–7. 'Harvey Cushing is a most wonderful man,' he said in his first letter. 'He works us all very hard but himself the hardest.'[18]

John Fulton was a charming, brilliant, and upwardly mobile doctor's son from St Paul, Minnesota, about the same age as F. Scott Fitzgerald (their families had lived in houses on the same street, but apparently did not know one another). He did a BSc at Harvard and also went to Oxford as a Rhodes scholar, studying physiology under C.S. Sherrington. A very quick learner, an enthusiast for the history of medicine, and an Osler worshipper, Fulton made himself so much at home at 13 Norham Gardens that Lady Osler welcomed him as a posthumous 'latch-keyer,' and he became a sort of St Paul to the Osler cult. Fulton and Cairns became friends at Oxford – Fulton had a way of being everyone's friend. He got to know and idolize Cushing during work on the Osler biogra-phy. Julia Shepley described Fulton at Oxford in 1925 as 'so eager and such a deferential hero-worshipper.' Cushing was completely captivated by the young disciple.[19]

Cushing urged Fulton to return to Harvard after taking his Oxford D Phil. He helped get him admitted directly to third-year medicine, writing to the school's admission officer: 'I think he is the sort of man for whom all bars possible should be let down.' Fulton finished an MD in 1927 and, to gain clinical experience, volunteered to work in surgery at the Brigham. He made himself so useful that Cushing gave him an appointment as a special assistant. The Fulton-Cushing relationship became very close because of their Osler connection and their Oslerian interest in medical history and book collecting (thanks to his marriage to a rich Bostonian, Fulton had the wherewithal to build a major library); above all, there was Fulton's burning ambition and his drive to become a neuro-physiologist. Cushing considered him one of the most talented, hard-working, and promising young men he had ever met. Fulton treated Cushing with the adulation that James Boswell had given to Samuel Johnson, and he soon decided to become Cushing's Boswell, much as Cushing had been Osler's. Fulton started to keep a diary, mainly to preserve the great man's doings and sayings for posterity, but also because he was infatuated with words and with becoming a man of medical letters.[20]

Fulton struck up a friendship with Madeline Stanton, who became Cushing's principal secretary in 1925 when Julia Shepley left to open an antique shop on Cape Cod. To the outside world, Miss Stanton was the unremarkable woman at the desk of Cushing's outer office, another plain-looking, plain-dressing, thin-faced, and slightly exophthalmic secretary of indeterminate age (she was born in 1898, a year before Fulton) and rather forbidding formality. In fact, behind the starchy New England veneer was a painfully shy and self-conscious young woman with a superior mind, a superior education, considerable literary ability, a dry sense of humor, and an immense, almost desperate yearning for companionship.[21]

'Mad' Stanton, as her friends in the harem called her (she could also be 'Maudlin' and 'Magdalene'), longed to find a man, longed for a better life than working all day for a pittance and commuting home to care for her invalid mother. She fantasized about romances with the young doctors – first having a crush on Cairns, then on Fulton (both married men) – even as her inhibitions and insecurities held her back. The best that a properly bred New England maiden dared hope for was a little welcome male friendship that might spark harmless fantasies.

She thought that Fulton and the other doctors courted her friendship because she was Cushing's girl Friday, who knew everything about the Chief's schedule, his views and expectations, his life. This was true. In this heyday of the private secretary stenographer, Madeline Stanton spent more non-sleeping time with Harvey Cushing than anyone else did, including Kate Cushing. She perhaps took more interest in him – certainly in his professional life – than his wife now did. Although she privately cursed his quirks and crotchetiness, Miss Stanton idolized the Chief and needed little persuasion from Fulton to begin to see herself as also a bit of a Boswell, or at least a Pepys. Under Fulton's influence, she too began keeping a diary. When Fulton went back to Oxford in 1928 for more work with Sherrington, he emboldened her to write long and frequent letters, mostly about office gossip and the activities of 'Doctor Johnson.' Fulton encouraged Stanton to safeguard every scrap of Cushing's papers, and they both kept all their diaries and letters.

Cushing paid no attention to the foolishness of his staff and probably never knew that the women called themselves his harem. He never had the slightest sexual interest in any of them or apparently in any woman other than Kate. He knew little of the Stanton-Fulton relationship, but like Johnson with Boswell could not help but be aware of Fulton's adoration, which was sometimes cloying and naive. Cushing had a strong sense of his own historic role in neurosurgery; he knew that he was a mentor to a generation of young neurosurgeons; probably, someone would eventually write his biography, as he had written Osler's. If they were all watching him at work, if they were sometimes taking down his table talk or telling stories about him, that was all part of the game.

It was being played constantly, never with higher stakes than in the operating room, where the team fought almost daily with life and death. The cast kept changing, but Cushing's performances went on week after week, year after year, sometimes with good endings, sometimes with a General Leonard Wood or a little child dead in the hospital. The one point of agreement in everyone's diaries, memoirs, and letters is that every time Cushing lost a patient he was morose and depressed. The sources contain only one reference to Cushing mentioning Bill's death – a 1928 diary entry by Madeline Stanton noting that Cushing had referred to his own son's fate in conversation with a family after a particularly heartbreaking death in the operating room.[22]

∼

In tense surgical moments Cushing continued to be very hard on his assistants. During the Leonard Wood operation, Cairns wrote to his wife, 'The Chief began to blame everyone – but especially me. It seemed to me that the main cause of his behaviour was exhaustion ... I was not to blame. Today he spoke of "being tired," his "inhibitions going," "blaming me just as a golfer might blame his caddy."'

Cairns by then understood the rhythm. Before coming to Boston he had been warned that Cushing was a hard and selfish man. 'It is all true,' he told his wife in a long letter he wrote on New Year's Day 1927, four months into his service:

> He cursed me in front of everyone in the operating room the other day for doing something he had told me to do the previous day, and when I protested hotly with, I imagine, blazing eyes, he lied promptly and with perfect technique ... He seems to feel the need of fastening the blame for anything that goes wrong on someone else and he never hesitates to let his assistants down.
>
> The other day a patient we were operating on under local anesthesia had been placed in a very uncomfortable position on the operating table and felt and complained of considerable pain as the operation wore on. It had been partly my doing but not my fault as the Chief admitted afterwards. I got it hot for this from the Chief and then – for the patient heard it all – from the

patient himself ... The Chief realized he was behaving like a cad and more or less apologised to me afterwards – said he 'had made an ass of himself.'

He can be charming when he wants to be, and particularly in this contrite mood when it occurs ... Yet nothing comes of it for he as likely as not has soon behaved like a cad once more. He is positively Machiavellian in his attention to his reputation. It is almost incredible how detailed his little bluffings and plays are – and how universally applied. Even to his own family he presents the same face and it is all a gigantic bluff. One result of this is that all his permanent assistants are absolutely devoid of initiative: so much has he felt the need of being 'Il Prince' (or whoever Machiavelli's man was) that he has never encouraged them beyond a certain point, or given praise for good work, but has only blamed them and in a loud voice for their misdeeds. Behind their backs he belittles always the reputation of past assistants, and of his present assistants, including myself in all probability, though I haven't of course any evidence of this. It seems as though he cannot bear a rival or what he imagines to be a rival.[23]

Percival Bailey also remembered being belittled and blamed by Cushing, and being told in crises to 'act like a surgeon.' Cushing, Bailey remembered, was often discourteous and careless of other people's sensitivities: 'If he found he could hurt you, he took a malicious, sadistic pleasure in watching you squirm.' 'He's got that Jesus complex again,' a resident told Bailey one day in 1928 as Cushing was ordering one assistant after another out of the operating room for not being up to the job. Bailey himself lasted only half an hour that day before being told he would never be a surgeon and was sent out to find Gil Horrax.[24] Working with Jesus, a bearded man in a *New Yorker* cartoon says, is bound to create apostle issues.

Bailey and Cairns grew to become tough, egotistical, and eventually imperious surgeons, but as insecure apprentices they were especially sensitive to Cushing's slights. Bailey also had special problems. He was a product of a rural Illinois culture that made Walter Dandy's upbringing look like a model of elegance and privilege. In his autobiography, *Up from Little Egypt*, Bailey describes a sexual awakening that included experiences with animals and a prostitute in a graveyard, and also an orgy in France in which he was one of fourteen medics, in hospital garb, who ritually sodomized a Polish countess in a sewer. Not surprisingly, Bailey took offense when Cushing lectured him for groping a nurse at the Brigham. They disagreed often. Bailey walked out on Cushing on several occasions; and at the end of their relationship Cushing reiterated, correctly, that Bailey would never make a good brain surgeon. 'He never spoke ill of anyone,' Bailey summarized. 'He spoke ill to them.'[25]

But Cushing never held a grudge, Bailey conceded. He and Cairns and most assistants found that when the stress was over or when they stood up to Cushing and held their ground, he backed off. You had to learn 'how to handle the old boy,' W.P. Van Wagenen wrote. Thick-skinned disciples, such as Richard Light, thought Cushing's were normal reactions to the tremendous stress of the operating room and paid little attention to them. One particularly light-hearted Scots assistant would begin to chuckle when Cushing got angry. When Cushing glowered at him, he would break into laughter, and their standoff usually ended with Cushing going back to work.[26]

To some who had known Cushing in his Hopkins days, he seemed positively mellow in his later years at the Brigham – 'One of the best illustrations ... of a man whose heart becomes softer as his arteries hardened.' Even Cairns soon came to feel relatively comfortable in the operating room. One day when Cushing was scolding a second assistant for an unsteady hand, claiming he could tell the man was a smoker, Cairns dared to ask, 'Can you tell what brand he smokes?' The other oft-repeated story, told by Cushing himself, was the morning when he was in a bad temper and was chewing out Gus, his chauffeur, before they left for work. Gus silenced him by pointing out that he had breakfast egg on his face.[27]

Neurosurgery was a team game, but Cushing was the star – star player, star coach, and general manager, all in one. When new men arrived at the Brigham, Cushing welcomed them briefly, then ignored them for weeks, much as Kocher had ignored him in Berne years earlier.[28] Rook-

ies should know their place on teams, petty humiliation was part of the
initiation ritual, you were expected to prove yourself on the field. The
star was cold and concentrated and unapproachable. He taught by example and he overshadowed and smothered most of his teammates.
What basketball fans understand as the Michael Jordan syndrome was
for neurosurgeons the Harvey Cushing syndrome.

Cushing's attitude seemed to be 'Watch me and you'll see at least
one good way to do it,' Bronson S. Ray remembered. Cushing never
praised good performance by members of his team because he expected
it. 'Why should anyone need to be complimented for doing his job
well!' he exclaimed more or less good-humoredly when John E. Scarff,
later a distinguished professor of neurosurgery at Columbia, once dared
ask for approval.[29]

No mistake went unnoticed. Bandages that were too tight had to be
replaced. Bandages that were too loose had to be replaced. Patients
had to be put to bed. Patients had to be got out of bed. Residents were
responsible for their patients around the clock: 'Over histories & discharge letters Dr. Schreiber (principally) and Dr. Scarff had many plain
truths brought to their attention and were constantly adjured to "use
your beans,"' Madeline Stanton told her diary in 1928. 'It *was* needed
though at times a bit brusque.' A few weeks later she told Fulton, 'Dear
old Scarff got a frightful wigging ... yesterday – which was needed – He
is *so* vague & slow & almost *childish*.'[30]

If Osler's genius had been to teach students how to heal and cure,
Cushing was trying to teach his men, mostly by example, how to do
the impossible. This was not comfort doctoring to the folk in the
valley; it was high-alpine rescue work. The surgeons were on missions
where life and death hung in the balance, and no one could afford to
be soft or sloppy or make mistakes. Scarff wrote years later, 'It was
almost as though he regarded his young associates as an old maker of
Toledo plates regarded his metal, that one could only turn iron into
steel by constant hammering and polishing, and this hard philosophy
he never softened.'

It was hard because of days in the operating room like this one in the winter of 1930, recorded by Stanton in her diary. An operation on a Friday had not gone well:

> Saturday found the Friday woman doing badly, so the Chief started a re-elevation at 10. It was a bad task from the beginning and he kept on and on at the woman till she died on the table – He told L[ouise] E[isenhardt] this morning that the anesthetist who was new ... never told him the B[lood] P[ressure] was falling off, and that Scarff who was called to give a transfusion never told him he couldn't get into the vein & therefore failed to get any blood in the patient. The boys said when she died the Chief walked out of the room without a word. They stood around and waited and waited and finally Oldberg sewed up. Just as he was finishing the Chief walked in again & without a word proceeded to do a p.m. on the table. It was a tragic business, hard on everybody. Poor E[ric] O[ldberg] was terribly low this morning but he finally managed a smile this p.m. though he wasn't very cheery. The dear Chief – how does he stand it all! [31]

They wondered how Gil Horrax put up with the hammering year after year, never complaining, never striking out on his own, but also (according to Cairns) having no illusions about Cushing's game playing and pettiness. The answer, of course, is that Horrax was made of the kind of reinforcing steel that all teams built around a dominating tower must have. He had a passive, low-key personality and was perfectly content to play in the star's shadow, feed and assist, and get satisfaction from knowing he had been a player on one of the great surgical courts of all time. Not surprisingly, Cushing had more praise for Horrax's help – 'more than my crotchety manner would sometimes lead you to believe' – than for residents aiming at their own stardom. [32] When a man finally left the Brigham, he could almost always count on glowing references from the Chief; and Harvey faithfully wrote congratulatory notes to his students on their publications, always wishing them 'more power to your elbow.'

Every operation was like a championship game. The Chief's unvarying rituals were like an athlete's preparations, and visitors found it thrilling when he stepped onto the field, as it were, nattily dressed in his distinctive surgical grays. 'I remember well the electric charge which seemed to fill the air whenever he entered the operating room and then the calm which would eventually come once he was at work,' Scarff wrote. 'And then I remember the little swagger with which he would leave the operating room after a job well done. It was the swagger of a natural athlete, and I am sure that he walked off the baseball diamond in exactly the same jaunty fashion after he had made an exceptionally brilliant in-field put-out for Yale.' Other observers thought they had seen a great painter working at his easel, attended by valets.[33]

Cushing differed from some champion athletes and artists in staying around after each performance to supervise the winding-down and the preparation for the next day. His ward rounds were a kind of policing to make sure that everything had been done right. When he and Scarff once came upon a poor patient who had been left sitting uncomfortably on a bedpan, Scarff volunteered to go for the orderly. 'Scarff, you will what?' Cushing replied. 'Are you above taking care of this man yourself?'

> Whereupon he personally cleaned the patient and washed him, and then took the bedpan in his hands and walked down the center of the corridor of the private floor to the utility room where he washed out the bedpan and hung it over the drier. When this was done, he turned to me and said: 'Scarff, don't ever consider yourself too dignified to help a sick patient in distress.'

Another time Cushing and Scarff were doing operating rounds at 7:00 PM after a long day in the operating room and came across their patient lying in vomitus on a ward whose nurses were overwhelmed. 'Scarff, you and I will handle this matter':

> With that he went to the utility room, got a basin of warm water, some washclothes and towels, and some fresh linen and bedclothes for the patient. He then bathed the patient, dressed him in clean pyjamas and changed all of

the patient's bed linen, at the same time instructing me in how these things should properly be done.[34]

No one ever criticized Cushing for being callous towards a patient, though patients might have to wait long hours for a moment of his time. Burt Wolbach, the Brigham's pathologist, thought Cushing should be judged by his ability to win the absolute confidence and adoration of his patients. Of course, most successful physicians and surgeons receive head-swelling surfeits of patient gratitude, even when they fail, but some of the commendations to Cushing were unusually revealing. The touch of his hands was wonderfully gentle, even better than his brother Ned's, a cousin remembered. Another patient wrote of him in the operating room:

> When I came to the operating table you were not a very clear figure to me. I had been so busy with my own affairs that you were just a nice person I had met – kindly, more human than the god that the Peter Bent staff seemed to think you, and undoubtedly clever.
>
> But to the abnormally acute perceptions of the patient on the table you were very different. In fact there were three of you. There was the doctor talking to assistants or asking for things in a rather low assured voice that was not intelligible to the patient.
>
> There was a very worthy human who made me chuckle to myself when he showed that he did not 'suffer fools gladly' when a cold electrode was shoved under my chest.
>
> But the important you was the voice that at times spoke to me. It was most startlingly difficult from the casual you. It was so completely laden with sympathy and understanding that the memory thereof is ineffaceable, and this patient felt that if the time had come for his Fates to cut the thread it was very good to go with such a voice in ones ear.[35]

In Hugh Cairns's bitter, disillusioned letter about Cushing he eventually worked himself round to Horrax's view that Cushing was far and away the best operator among living brain surgeons. Most important:

He cannot bear to let a patient die and he would go on operating for 24 hours
without stop if he could by doing so save a patient. He is nearly 60 now and
is said to be sparing himself a little, but I have never seen his equal for
courage, determination and an entire absence of any regard for his own
personal comfort when that of a patient is concerned. Of course this is probably because he is anxious to publish good figures with low mortality rates,
in fact I am sure it is – but it is rather fine.

Bailey reached exactly the same conclusion: 'This lesson he taught me,
that no one has any right to undertake the care of any patient unless he
is willing to give that patient all of the time and thought that is necessary, and of which he is capable.' After Cairns had learned to stand up
to Cushing and was no longer under pressure, he became more toler-
ant, writing his wife: 'I do feel though that when the history of brain
surgery is written or perhaps when his life is written the smallness in him
will be considered as a very minor matter: and won't detract much if it
all from his reputation with posterity.'[36]

                                      ～

Cold and businesslike at the hospital, Cushing would unwind with his
young men when he invited them to Sunday dinner or to afternoon tea
at 305 Walnut. All of the Cushings, whose manners were superb, were
always gracious. 'Bailey & horrible McKenzie here for tea,' Mary told a
diary one day in 1927. 'I had 'em for hours before mum got home.' At
dinner the table talk was of family, dogs, rare books, medicine and
academia, but never 'shop' talk about patients in the hospital. Evenings ended early, when Dr Cushing retired to his study to work. 'It was
quite jolly up there tonight,' Hugh Cairns wrote to his wife in 1927, 'so
far as any American home can be jolly.'[37]

Sometimes in the afternoon there might be a friendly game of tennis
on the Cushing court or perhaps squash racquets at the hospital. The
Chief suddenly became a coiled spring again, relentless and ruthless in
his determination to win. He played tennis the way he operated, and

he operated the way he played tennis. He took every advantage he possibly could – opinions differed on whether he actually cheated – and when playing doubles he harrassed and chivvied his partners as though they were bumbling assistants.

One day on the Brigham court Loyal Davis watched the two chiefs of service, Cushing and Christian, play against their senior residents: 'Cushing gave orders to Henry Christian on every ball that came to him. Christian appeared not to hear him, or paid no attention to him.' Sometimes the residents, who wanted rest much more than exercise, just let the old man win. They told stories of how he practiced his baseball skills for weeks to be in shape for annual club games, and there was the probably apocryphal yarn of how he still refused to speak to a colleague who had once claimed that in a Harvard-Yale game in the 1880s he had tripped and fallen on his face and let in two runs.[38]

Davis, Cairns, and some of the other young men wondered how Cushing could carry on, fiercely determined to control his world, apparently almost friendless, respected by many, liked by a few, and loved, it seemed, by no one. The months or years which they spent working with Cushing were hellishly hard, exhausting, and humiliating. Cairns, who had been at Gallipoli and the battles of the Marne, told Fulton that they had not been as stressful as being Cushing's resident.[39]

Geoffrey Jefferson, a British neurosurgeon who got to know Cushing well but always had the perspective of distance, wrote perhaps the best evaluation:

That he was charming, tiresome, delightful, petty, and admirable all by turns is equally true. The real point is what was the dosage ... the great qualities very heavily outweighed the others. Some folk thought him almost sadistic in his treatment of them, but such a statement would puzzle others who never saw a trace of it ... The fact, no doubt, was that Cushing was a difficult man in competition ... A great creative artist is almost always a combative person ... Cushing pursued the scientific ideal with the utmost intensity and devotion. He sacrificed sometimes his friends to it. But of his honesty there is no doubt. He could be rough with his staff, he might nag interminably while operating,

but he sent them away at the end of their training better men than they would
have otherwise been; even if they had wounds to lick, they were proud of the
place where they had acquired them.

John Fulton, the closest of all observers, was on the spot when Cushing
himself had to lick the wound of losing Leonard Wood. Harvey spent
the day after Wood's death with his old books, rearranging them and
adding new acquisitions. One moment, noted Fulton, he was enthusing
over a 1545 Paré on gunshot wounds; the next, he was lamenting about
not being able to do the operation over again in two stages. Fulton
tried to suggest that Wood would have died no matter what had been
done and that the first operation had given him eighteen years of good
life: 'But Dr. C. wouldn't be consoled. However, he behaves in much
the same way over any of his patients who happen to die after an operation. It is always "bad surgical judgment" on his part.'[40]
   Fulton chronicled Cushing's gradual return to his old self. At dinner
one night that August he expressed great satisfaction that the laws of
Massachusetts had been upheld with the execution of the convicted
anarchist bombers, Sacco and Vanzetti. He also told many fine anecdotes from the old days in Baltimore, such as the story of the absent-
minded mathematician, Sylvester, 'who was asked to resign from the
Maryland Club because he had the misfortune in a darkened toilet to
urinate on a distinguished old Southern gentleman.' There was also the
tale of Sir Henry Halford, who had stolen the fourth cervical vertebra
of King Charles I from his tomb and showed it off at dinner parties in
London in the 1820s: 'It is extraordinary how at the Chief's one never
lacks for interesting topics of conversation.' Cushing had thrown himself into research as though he were starting out all over again, Fulton
noted, and was lamenting that Johns Hopkins medicine, once so full of
promise, was deteriorating from 'old foggydom.'[41]

∾

'I'm so darned fond of him I'd be miserable working for anyone else,'
Madeline Stanton told her diary about Cushing.[42] Miss Stanton's work

was the focus of her life, and it was all about keeping and furthering the Chief's agenda. She was a near-perfect secretary, who had mastered the technical language of neurosurgery as well as shorthand and typing, and could read Cushing's crabbed, semi–legible handwriting better than he could. She shared his passion for fine points of style – a raised eyebrow from Miss Stanton during dictation would cause Harvey to rethink a sentence. Boss and secretary would argue learnedly about hyphens and semicolons, then close ranks against the editorial eccentricities of American Medical Association journals and the journals' director, Morris Fishbein, known at the Brigham as 'Old Fishlegs.' Cushing put Miss Stanton in charge of his rare-book purchases; she came to know the dealers and the literature almost as well as he did, enjoyed the thrill of the hunt for hidden treasure, and probably had a better sense of prices. On any given day, Madeline could vamp a difficult acromegalic patient, persuade a grieving family to let Dr Cushing do a postmortem, clear a package of rare books through the Boston customs house, quietly suggest that important invitations and letters not go unanswered, and order flowers or a present for a member of the family.

When Cushing scolded her, she chalked up his bad temper to the stress of his life and tried harder to do better: 'Long acoustic case today and then the Chief cut brain for 2 hours, with the result that he was cross & tired at five. Poor dear, it made my heart ache to see how weary he was & how he limped. I wish he wouldn't push himself quite so far.' She often complained of the hours she had to work to keep up with him, but answered the bell for every extra round of typing or proofreading. He hardly ever commended her. Her feelings of inferiority and depression were sometimes almost overwhelming, but pride in doing her job, pride in and identification with Cushing's achievements, helped keep her going. 'Another long case today – Morrissey for the s'teenth time. The Chief thinks he got *all* the tumor this time & I hope to heaven he did.' 'What a man he is,' she would exclaim to her diary. 'Poor old dear – I'm *so* fond of him and yet can never let him know it in any way.'[43]

The young doctors who took the trouble to sit and chat with Miss Stanton and get to know her – often over lunch or tea – found that she knew everything about how the hospital and the Chief worked. Except in letters to Fulton and her harem friends, she was a model of discretion, but it did no harm to pass on tidbits of gossip and tips about how to get along:

> Dr Meagher paid me a visit in the afternoon – He is still not wholly happy – merely the 'caddy of the club' – I tried to cheer him on by telling him every one had to go through a period of seeming neglect by the Chief or being odd-job & handy man, that he was by no means the first & only one, and the best thing was to stick to his knitting and wait for things to work out themselves. He gave me the impression that the Chief was riding Dr. Oldberg rather unmercifully. Of course I think he deserves it, for I have never known anyone so utterly cocksure; but still, I hope he improves & the Chief lets up.[44]

She became friends with many of Cushing's assistants, including Oldberg, and despised others. Gil Horrax confided in her about his wife's depression. Elliott Cutler, 'the Cleveland whirlwind,' was astonishingly indiscreet and would tell everyone everything. John Fulton became her special confidant – their correspondence became massive, their friendship very close. Not so her relations with Percival Bailey, whose utter selfishness she despised: 'Of course the Chief & John are selfish too, the latter too much so for his years ... He will be much worse than the Chief as the years go by. But either of them do innumerable kind things, even so, when the mists of concentration which surround them nine tenths of the time clear away a bit, whereas P.B. never has any "remissions." '[45]

Miss Stanton longed to have an honorable relationship with a man or even a discreet affair, such as Louise Eisenhardt seems to have enjoyed with several doctors. Her joking references to Cushing's offices, below the operating rooms, as 'the nether regions' had Freudian connotations. But she abhorred the sexual predators in the hospital – on the one hand the treacly A.J. McLean, whom the harem nicknamed 'Liz,' and on the other a nurse who slept her way through much of the male hospital staff before suddenly marrying a doctor who happened to be a

Cabot. Miss Stanton used all her skill at hospital politics – the key was to work through Horrax – to have the 'unspeakable female' barred from contributing an article to the volume of essays that Cutler was editing in honor of Cushing's sixtieth birthday. Bailey, by these years, seems to have been settling down and did not bother anybody sexually.

Cushing noticed Madeline Stanton when his mists of concentration occasionally lifted. He sometimes gave her football tickets, sometimes invited her to a meal or a party at 305 Walnut, sometimes told her to take some time off. Miss Stanton was cultured and in her quiet way was sufficiently sociable and discreet to be invited occasionally to join the Cushing family circle. She had the trip of a lifetime when Cushing took her to Britain and the Continent in 1927 as a companion for daughter Betsey and to help with unfinished addresses and papers. She of course took the greatest personal interest in the Chief's family and their fortunes, which were only sometimes happy.

~

Kate may never have been the same after the death of her firstborn. The secretaries often remarked on how withdrawn and apathetic she seemed. Family friends had noticed a streak of reserve in her personality – that she could seem distracted, aloof, almost in a world of her own. Now it was as though she was tired, worn down from childraising, the war, compulsory medical entertaining, and being Mrs Harvey Cushing. The letter she wrote to Harvey in June 1927 about steeling themselves was also quietly resigned, as she tried to find a new balance:

> My theory is the same as yours – do the thing as well as you can while you are still in this world ... The problem is to keep soft & sweet inside while forming the hard outer shell which enables us to meet life ...
>
> I must set my house in order, and run it as well as possible, with as few people as possible, not for the sake of economy but for the sake of peace & a quiet life. I am old and tired. I have kept house summer & winter for 25 years. I am entitled to a little letting up of the strain of living & running a large

household ... I know you too are setting your house in order. Let us have a mutual tolerance and understanding.[46]

Kate had raised her daughters to have a sense of good taste and style and to appreciate beautiful things. She traveled a lot in these years, usually with one or more of the girls, sometimes with old friends, less than ever with Harvey. When he dropped in at Little Boars Head in the summer he slept in a separate cottage so that he could get as much rest as possible; but usually he stayed in Boston and worked. When Kate took the children to Ireland in the summer of 1929, he remarked to several friends how happy he was to be able to get down to work undisturbed and uninterrupted. The family knew that each spring he looked forward to their departure.[47]

Kate told the children that theirs was 'a family of individualists.' That the family often had an absentee father, even when he was at home, was well understood and sometimes regretted. 'The utter completeness of all of us being together is lacking without you,' Mary wrote her father while en route to Europe in 1929. Hugh Cairns, however, noticed that Cushing's presence in the family circle tended to 'subdue' everyone, and he told his wife that Kate and the girls were all 'just a little dull and lacking individuality.' They undoubtedly were subdued at Sunday dinners in the presence of the Victorian father and his guests. His dislike of being interrupted by ringing telephones, especially when the ringing was caused by young men asking to speak to his daughters, definitely put a damper on the girls' social life. Anyone who phoned for the Cushing girls after about 8.30 would be told they had gone to bed.[48]

Cairns changed his mind about Mary Cushing after he squired her to occasional concerts and dances, apparently as a favor to the family. Mary, who turned twenty-one in 1927, was working in a bookstore and dabbling at art; she seemed to have character and 'pep,' and knew her Jane Austen and Bernard Shaw. 'But it is perfectly dreadful that these young American girls – the "quite-quite" ones – should put stuff on their lips to make them look the colour of this red ink,' Cairns told his wife in red letters, betraying his own Victorian sensibility. A 1927 day-book of Mary's suggests that she had no particular interest in the married Australian, being much more attracted by such men as Barney Crile (George Crile's son) and Alger Hiss, who courted her and took her to the movies and the theatre. An intelligent young woman, perhaps the most intellectual of the children, Mary seemed to be biding her time until the right man came along.[49]

Younger sister Betsey followed Mary to Westover School, where her exuberant spirit could never quite be quelled by obnoxious teachers: 'Mlle says I'm dumb which is true and that I should be terribly bright as all my family are which is also true but still. Mlle is so rotten to everyone I can't stand her. We always have troubles with Mlle ... Another new girl is in the Infirmary and is trying to starve herself to death so that they'll let her go home.' Betsey was not a scholar and was not happy at Westover. A sprained back in an automobile accident in September 1926 became her official reason for dropping out of school, never to return or graduate. Family friends thought Betsey most resembled her father in her capacity to be engaging and single-minded.[50] No one in those days seems to have remarked on the oddity that the bright and personable Cushing girls apparently never considered attending university. Nowhere in his exhaustive correspondence does their father have a word to say about his expectations for his daughters.

On the other hand, there was never any doubt that Henry, like Bill before him, was bound for Yale. Henry thrived at Milton Academy, where he led his class, and he apparently profited, as his father had hoped, from summer on a western ranch with other Yale-bound boys in 1925. He entered Yale in September 1927, three months after his brother's death, to begin the long road to medicine.

He immediately got sidetracked by campus journalism and the competition for an editorial spot on the Yale *News*, among other temptations. He failed most of his first-year exams so badly that he was even denied the option of summer study. His father pulled every string he could to have the boy given a second chance. Thanks to what an administrator called 'ruthless executive action,' Henry was readmitted to Yale as a special student doing preliminary courses in the medical school.

Dean Milton Winternitz, clearly doing Harvey a personal favor, planned
to admit Henry directly into medicine in his second year. Henry came
down with jaundice, doubted that he really wanted to study medicine,
and spent all the money his father had given him; but he stuck it out at
Yale through 1928–9.[51]

Barbara, reported by her father to be 'growing like a weed and though
not a nervous child is highly keyed up all the time,' continued in the
family tradition of being seriously accident prone. In the spring of 1929
the thirteen-year-old ran her bicycle into an automobile, breaking her
tibia and receiving a mild concussion. Kate Cushing looked 'more than
weary' as she spent a night at the Brigham with Barbara, noted Madeline
Stanton: 'What next will the poor dear have to stand?'[52]

The 'next' for the whole family occurred that autumn when Harvey
decided he had to remove a tubercular growth from Barbara's neck
that was threatening to involve veins and nerves. The tradition that
doctors should not treat members of their families has often been
breached in minor situations or for emergency care. It has also been
breached by a few surgeons convinced of their superior competence.
Many years earlier W.H. Halsted had done a pioneering gallbladder
operation on his mother. Victor Horsley had operated on his son. In
1928 young Wilder Penfield in Montreal did not trust anyone else,
including Cushing, to attack a tumor in the brain of his sister and did
the operation himself. Cushing had taken out both Betsey's and Henry's
appendixes in circumstances that are not clear – perhaps as minor surgery, perhaps as an emergency procedure, most likely because of his
belief in his superior competence.

The sources contain no explanation of his decision to remove
Barbara's growth. Madeline Stanton captured the occasion, however,
in a remarkable diary entry, beginning with a comment that it had been
'one of the worst days I've lived through:'

> The family came in before nine & Barbara went up to get ready while the
> Chief tried to dictate to me ... but it was pretty difficult. He went up before
> ten and started in with his regular neurological team ... From then on till after

three the terrible ordeal went on – All was quiet except once around 12.30 when she evidently screamed terribly (I was at luncheon) and poor Mrs. C. & Betsey looked terribly frayed when I came back. I got them some hot broth & crackers but did not dream things would go on for so long.

It was utterly nerve-wracking for everyone. Upstairs the Chief looked like death & went on & on, fearing at one time he had injured the facial with the electrical current ... spending two hours trying to free the gland from the artery [actually the jugular vein]. And so on. Downstairs Mrs. C & Betsey playing canfield [solitaire] hour after hour, very meagre reports coming down infrequently via Dr. Sisson. When he told me sometime after one that the Chief was having quite a bit of bleeding, it seemed more horrible than ever. The family I don't believe could have had any active conception of the dangers, and I *hope* they didn't. Finally around 3 Miss Regan came down to say he was sewing up ... The Chief never came down at all but merely sent a note ... to Mrs. C. & word to me to have the bed in the examining room made up as he was spending the night. It all sounded too ominous.

I judge from what Dr. Oldberg told me today that when Barbara finally woke up & smiled *symmetrically* it was the greatest boon imaginable. She had none too good a night, but with morning was much better ... What it all portends I do not know. Anyway she's *alive* and that was so problematical all day yesterday.

Two weeks later Miss Stanton recorded that Cushing had achieved 'another of his usual perfect results' with the healing of Barbara's wound. There would be no scar.[53]

Two more weeks saw yet another family crisis when Henry dropped out of Yale, disappeared entirely for several days, and reappeared in murky circumstances involving press inquiries, the prospect of embarrassing though unspecified scandal, and consultations with a psychiatrist. 'It is tragic,' Madeline Stanton told her diary, 'the remaining son, so brilliant and promising and now in such a sorry plight.' Harvey got Henry off to the Maine woods to recover his health and then sent him west for another summer on a Montana ranch. He would never return to Yale.[54]

Harvey's first choice as an alternative would have been for Henry to go to Newfoundland to work as a volunteer in the Grenfell medical mission, whose rugged service delivering health care on one of North America's last frontiers Cushing greatly admired and financially supported. The world in general and Yale College in particular were becoming too soft, he told Wilfred Grenfell:

> These lads of the present generation, some of them who have perhaps been brought up too gently, are finding it difficult to adjust themselves to any sort of life that is in the end going to be worth while ... Such ability they possess, the present-day college does not seem to be adjusted to bring it out of them and I think it is due to the fact that the old rigours of the college pump and the 7.30 chapel and the curfew have all, one by one, been gradually withdrawn ... I wish that I had sent Henry to a smaller, old-old-time college like Williams or Dartmouth rather than to Yale which in my day was a country college but which now is engulphed in a growing city and, indeed, has been a sort of suburb of New York.[55]

Betsey became the first Cushing child to have a serious romance. She fell in love with a Harvard undergraduate, James Roosevelt, 'a tall, thin, lad with quite beautiful eyes, attractive manners, and on the whole seemingly very acceptable,' according to the ubiquitous Stanton.[56] Harvey did not really approve of twenty-year-olds becoming romantically entangled; nor, as a lifelong Republican, was he particularly impressed by the fact that young Roosevelt's father had succeeded Al Smith as the Democratic governor of New York. 'I should have known something of this kind would happen if we came here to Boston to live,' he wrote light-heartedly to the governor in January 1929, 'that one of my daughters would "take up" with a Harvard Democrat when there are so many desirable Yale Republicans in that part of the country where we really belong. The chief trouble with Jimmie is that he makes himself so agreeable, which is also one of Betsey's faults. So what can a man do?'

Despite their politics, the Roosevelts were highly spoken of, and the more Harvey learned about them the more impressed he became. He particularly respected Franklin D. Roosevelt's struggle with polio and the way he had beaten his handicap by dogged persistence. 'The Chief characterized him as a real hero,' Madeline Stanton wrote when Cushing told his staff of the young couple's engagement. 'I'm so glad he said all this, for I know he must disapprove of an undergraduate engagement, but he has never been able to manage his children.' Cushing told FDR that Kate favored letting the youngsters do as they liked: 'In the past when we have disagreed she has usually been in the right.'[57]

Betsey's impending engagement was the great item of family news at Harvey's sixtieth birthday celebrations in April 1929. His staff held a special birthday party at the hospital. Elliott Cutler presented him with a classic *Festschrift*, a 1,100–page volume of essays by his students, simultaneously published as a special issue of the *Archives of Surgery*. Cushing had accurately previewed the book two years earlier in trying to persuade Cutler not to bother: 'From what I know of festschrifts, they are merely cemeteries for a few good pieces of work and dumping grounds for a great many poor ones which otherwise would never have been written.'[58] Cutler and Cushing's students had gone ahead anyway.

Ken McKenzie made a surprise appearance from Toronto, bearing supplies of Canadian gin to lubricate birthday festivities in prohibition-bound Boston. Madeline Stanton noted that the gin was insipid but did take the polish off furniture when it was spilled. McKenzie also presented Cushing with a box of colorful ties and some doggeral verse about 'The Tie That Blinds.' After the party, select members of the group, Stanton among them, joined family and friends at 305 Walnut for a buffet supper, at which the well-stocked McKenzie produced champagne.

Madeline Stanton thought she saw flashes of the old Kate Cushing that day, but not many: 'On the whole she is terribly apathetic – almost alarmingly so ... She looks thin, wretched, effortless, and I was almost stunned at her reaction to certain situations. Poor dear, the Fates have buffeted her about cruelly these last few years, and with the Chief withdrawing more and more into his shell all the time, she must feel cruelly

at times the futility of playing a lone hand.'[59] The engagement was
formally announced a few weeks later at a tea attended by the governor and his wife, after which Kate took the family to Ireland while
Harvey rejoiced that they had left and he could get down to work.

'I've not always been over nice to you but I've always loved you,'
Harvey wrote Kate in a letter he appended to his will. 'You are the only
woman I've ever known I would have married and stayed by through
thick and thin. But for you we would all have blown up.' For all their
troubles, Kate and Harvey seem to have retained a kind of love for one
another, or at least a mutual respect. When the teenage girls complained to Kate about their father, she told them that they would always be proud of him, and added, 'I can never be bored with him.'[60]

As for Harvey, there was an occasion when he and his medical friends
got talking about their choice of partners: 'I married a nurse ... I married a nurse ... I married a nurse.'

'What about you, Harvey?' someone asked.

'I married a lady,' Cushing answered.

A lovely anecdote, made better by someone then commenting, 'Well,
Cush, you married above your class.'

Late in life, Betsey remembered one of the great good times between her two strong parents. They were playing tennis at Little Boars
Head and Harvey grumbled because Kate was not playing her usual
game. She snapped back that if he had to wear her skirt he would not
play so well either: 'The next day he came out in one of her skirts, and
fell down about four times.'[61] The resolution of the Cushing marital
match had usually been to play on separate courts – his was his profession and his writing, hers the household and the children. They played
together that way to the end of their lives.

Naturally, he grumbled about all the 'fuss and feathers' going into
the planning of Betsey's wedding. Maybe he would be too busy to attend; maybe Gus, the chauffeur, could give her away. To prepare for
marriage, Betsey took a housekeeping course that included cooking
lessons. 'That's all very well,' Harvey told Perry Harvey, 'but she tries it
out on us at home and if I have to eat any more of her buns or fried

puff-balls and things of that sort with a pleasant face, I shall succumb to chronic indigestion ... Please don't tell anybody about this as it sounds rather peevish.' The truly peevish relative in the Cushing-Roosevelt affair was Jimmy's grandmother, Sara Delano Roosevelt, who is said to have remarked to Betsey, 'I understand your father is a surgeon. Surgeons always remind me of my butcher.'[62] The Roosevelts were very much old American wealth, and while Eleanor and Franklin thought the Cushing family perfectly acceptable, Betsey would be marrying a bit above her class. Or so it seemed.

Harvey gave his daughter away to James Roosevelt in St Paul's Episcopal Church, Brookline, on June 4, 1930, two days after Jimmy's Harvard graduation. Groton School's Reverend Endicott Peabody conducted the ceremony. A reception for one thousand guests was held on the grounds at 305 Walnut. Harvey good-naturedly compared it to yet another circus, complete with tents and with parades of New York State motorcycle troopers guarding the governor. Everyone was agog about Mrs Al Smith having attended, Madeline Stanton noted. Had the former presidential candidate himself been there incognito?[63]

~

They were not in the Roosevelts' class financially, but money had never been a problem for the Cushings. Both Harvey and Kate had legacies from estates and trust funds that enabled them to live very comfortably by any standard. Through the 1920s the family received an annual income of about $20,000 from Harvey's father's estate alone, much of it from rents paid by the May Company, a great department store built partly on the Cushing properties in Cleveland. In 1931 Harvey's investment portfolio with Lee, Higginson & Company in Boston was still worth $840,000, despite two years of hard times. The Cushings' total income through the 1920s would have been about $50,000 a year – the equivalent of perhaps $750,000 in current purchasing power, but with lower taxes – more than enough to cover servants, private school fees, first-class travel, and all reasonable needs and luxuries.[64]

Harvey had conquered a passion for financial detail and now left their finances almost entirely in the hands of professional managers. He spent his time thinking medicine, not money. 'If I chose to make a large fortune out of my position and my specialty I could easily do so,' he wrote in 1924, 'but what I should do with it when made I do not know. I certainly wouldn't want my children to have it.'[65] A rather tough comment from a man who had built his own career on his father's and grandfather's generosity.

He was paid a remarkably unchanging $5,000 as chief surgeon of the Brigham and $3,500 as Moseley Professor at Harvard. In return for his salaries, he treated all the patients on the hospital's private wards without charge, taught medical students, and, under the geographic full-time system, did not practice outside the hospital. He also covered the wages of his personal staff, which in the early 1920s amounted to two or three times his salaried income.

Private patients who came to him at the Brigham were expected to pay a basic consulting fee, usually $25. If surgery was required, they were then asked about their means. Cushing's surgical fees ranged from about $500 for an exploratory craniotomy to $2,500 for a major tumor extirpation. For ganglionectomies he had charged $250. He waived his fees for physicians and their families, also often for teachers and servicemen. He thought people who could afford to should pay at least part of the costs of their care, but when in doubt or when patients balked, he erred on the side of generosity. His working rule for patients of moderate means was to suggest the equivalent of a month's income. He always felt guilty about sending a bill when he had failed to do all he had hoped for a patient, 'but at the same time, a doctor has more wear and tear when things do not go well than he does when they turn out fortunately.' So the bills were issued. H.L. Mencken once persuaded Cushing to waive a $1,000 fee charged to the widow of a literary critic only to find, to his chagrin, that his friend's estate was worth $100,000.[66]

'We are trying to conduct a hospital which considers the patient first and the business end of the affair only secondarily,' Harvey wrote to a doctor who inquired about his charges. To a worried patient he wrote,

'I am far more interested in getting people well of their maladies and in keeping track of them than in collecting bills for my services.' In 1920 he estimated that his professional income was about one-fifth of what it could be if he were in practice to maximize his wealth.[67]

Like Osler, but unlike many of his surgical colleagues, Cushing did not soak the very rich. There is no evidence in his papers of any unusually high charges for operating on the wealthy – or of any preferential treatment accorded to anyone, except perhaps friends, relatives of doctors, and Clevelanders. He was never asked to split a fee with a referring physician, a common but controversial practice on the fringes of the profession. His most cold-blooded comments on fees were in a letter advising Ken McKenzie, his Canadian former student, not to charge a rich patient all he could afford: 'Better under-charge than over-charge anybody any time. The reason why we have such a large clinic here is because the majority of the people are charged very little even on the private ward. They find it cheaper to come here and get a $250 dollar operation than to stay at home and pay a thousand for work possibly less well done. Moreover, another bit of advice to you: never pursue a patient with a collector, no matter how abused you may feel. You will be much happier, and your practice will grow in proportion.'[68]

Grateful patients sometimes insisted on paying more than Cushing billed. The grateful very rich were encouraged to donate to the hospital or to special funds to support Cushing's work. His most materially grateful patient was Mrs Philip H. Gray of Detroit, to whose tumor-ridden husband Cushing had given expert palliative care. From 1923 until his retirement, Cushing controlled the Philip H. Gray Fund for the Furtherance of Neurosurgery, to which Mrs Gray contributed $10,000 annually. He used it to pay Percival Bailey's and Louise Eisenhardt's salaries (previously funded from his own pocket), to bring visitors to the Brigham, and eventually to cover the wages of his harem, including the $2,000 he paid Madeline Stanton. The Gray money was also used to subsidize publications, to pay some patients' hospital bills, and on several occasions to pay families for agreeing to allow an autopsy. Cushing was always passionately ruthless in seeking consent for postmortems. 'I very often, as you know, pay out money to buy autopsies when they can only be gotten in this way,' he told the hospital superintendent in 1924; and, of course, his residents had many stories to tell of doing autopsies in very unfriendly circumstances. Cushing did not use consent forms either for operations or for autopsies.[69]

The Cushings donated regularly to charities. Their givings were on the order of $100 a year for the Red Cross and the Massachusetts Historical Society, $500 to the million-dollar campaign for a medical students' dormitory at Harvard, $10 to the Tennessee Evolution Case Defense Fund, and $250 to cover the hospital bills of an old family servant in Cleveland. Harvey felt that in-kind contributions by medical men to medical causes were worth more than money, but he often used his money to help patients pay bills, students to pay tuition, and residents to scrape by.

In the 1920s he formalized his subsidization of Brigham Hospital work by creating the Surgeon-in-Chief Fund to support house staff traveling abroad. When he retired in 1932, it was worth $32,000. In 1926 he gave $25,000 to Johns Hopkins to create a research fellowship at the Hunterian Laboratory. In 1928 he pledged $25,000 to the Yale endowment campaign to create the William Harvey Cushing Research Fellowship in surgery. In May 1929 he rushed to Cleveland to give moral support to George Crile in the aftermath of a terrible disaster at the Cleveland Clinic – an explosion and fire that caused 123 deaths, mostly from gas released in the combustion of nitrocellulose x-ray film. During the Depression of the 1930s, Cushing faithfully contributed to help down-and-out members of Yale '91 and veterans of Base Hospital No. 5, as well as his old mentor from Cleveland days, Newton Anderson.

~

Cushing had made his peace with the administration of the hospital after he returned from the war, and neither in his reports nor in his correspondence is there evidence of more than moderate crankiness through the 1920s. The lubricating effect of the Gray money and his own money and the general prosperity of the 1920s certainly helped – there was no more squabbling about paying for lunches. Having become conservative with age, Harvey no longer pressed expansion plans on the hospital. He now believed that medical bigness led to impersonality and bureaucracy. 'In medical science "smaller and better" would be the slogan after my own heart,' he wrote after visiting the New York Neurological Institute in 1929.[70] He thought the genius of the Brigham was its human scale, the staff's sense of itself as a family, and its reputation for patient care – for never losing sight of John and Mary while treating their maladies. He even had twinges of guilt about the way his clinic skewed Brigham surgery towards his own specialty. It was hard to keep the number of neurosurgical cases within bounds and was not healthy that the chief surgeon's interests should be narrowing while those of junior surgeons were expanding.[71]

The Harvard Medical School was a different kettle of fish. Under David Edsall, dean from 1918 to 1933, Harvard medicine raised its standards, continued to grow from a regional into a national institution, beefed up its research and scientific side, 'surpassed Johns Hopkins as the nation's archetypal medical school' (in historian Kenneth Ludmerer's judgment), and tried to reorient clinical training towards public health and prevention. Cushing sometimes praised Edsall's initiatives in recruiting, curriculum reform, and fundraising, but gradually decided that he profoundly disapproved of the school's direction and the dean's leadership.

He never quite got over the pricking of his belief that he was hired to be head of the surgery department of Harvard and chief surgeon at its primary teaching hospital. There continued to be no primary teaching hospital at Harvard and no head of the surgery department. The three teaching hospitals and their professors of surgery were all treated equally. As the authority of the dean of medicine increased – Edsall was the first full-time dean and the first dean with discretionary control of significant funds – all became equally subordinate. Cushing intensely disliked these developments. In letters, at faculty meetings, and occasionally in his annual reports, he complained constantly of budgetary and other slights to the Brigham and of increasing decanal autocracy. He lost faith in Harvard's willingness to allocate resources equitably among the young Brigham Hospital, the gigantic and venerable Massachusetts General Hospital, and the Boston City Hospital; and he began to advocate the creation of three separate and equally funded schools of clinical medicine in the hospitals, almost on a British model.[72]

He wanted to teach students his way in his hospital because he thought that Edsall and Harvard had bought into, or rather sold out to, a faddish Arrowsmith-like orthodoxy. The delicate balance of the art and science of medicine was becoming disrupted by excessive emphasis on science, the laboratory, bigness, and bricks and mortar. Too little attention was being paid to clinical medicine, doctor-patient relations, and the training of skilled healers. With considerable outspokenness, Cushing challenged the agendas of the Rockefeller Institute and the Rockefeller Foundation's General Education Board. These, he believed, were largely influenced by the Flexner brothers, who in turn had been overly influenced by a view of medicine that centered on bacteriology and the possibility of controlling or preventing infectious disease.

'They are chiefly interested in building up medical science and public health,' he wrote of the General Education Board in 1927. 'I am chiefly interested as a clinical teacher in improving the qualities of the medical practitioner.'[73] Edsall's main 'achievement' at Harvard had been to bring in Rockefeller millions to fund its new School of Public Health and other research-based chairs and activities. In doing this, Cushing thought, the medical faculty was going down the wrong road and losing its autonomy to boot. When Edsall agreed to sit on Rockefeller boards and committees, Cushing thought he was developing a clear conflict of interest.

It happened that Rockefeller money also found its way to Cushing's unit at the Brigham in the form of fellowships for visitors, such as Hugh Cairns, and travel grants to enable young neurosurgeons to study abroad. Cushing never directly solicited Rockefeller lucre, though, and prided himself on his independence: 'I have never had to go to anyone to beg for help in my work.'[74] The comment may have reflected old Cleveland medicine's disdain for the oil family that used to pay rent, a lingering bitterness about the full-time controversy, and recent memories of having virtually begged for support for a national neurological institute.

Issues of high principle have a way of becoming personalized to absurdity in academic cockpits. Dean Edsall had to grant that his son, who entered Harvard medical school in third year, had justly been failed in surgery for his ignorance of fractures, not having taken the second-year course. Could third-year surgical teaching be improved? the dean wondered. Not to the point where students could get away with skipping the second-year teaching on fractures, Cushing replied. Perhaps Harvard was admitting too many students on the basis of 'presumed scholarship,' he mused in a letter to the dean which he thought better of sending.[75]

To advance what seemed to be the modern approach to medicine, Edsall in 1929 arranged for the publication of a Rockefeller-funded Harvard Medical School introduction to the role of prevention in medicine. Even the dean's best friends admitted that the book, silly and slipshod in many chapters, was deeply embarrassing to the institution. Cushing was furious. When Edsall decided to require the departments to collaborate in reissuing a better version, Cushing, who was also angry about the dean's manipulation of appointments and his 'Wilsonian behavior' generally, led the resistance. In closed meetings in April 1930, he attacked Edsall's authoritarianism, his manipulation of money and dependence on the Rockefellers, and his foisting of a trite and questionable view of medicine on his colleagues.

It did become a matter of principle, a difference of opinion about the roles of doctors and the responsibilities of medical schools. Cushing published the gist of his views in the Brigham's annual report:

There is an old saying that money makes the mare go, and the emphasis in the School on preventive medicine – on keeping people well – is transparently due to the fact that large funds have been put at the disposal of this particular movement. It is a movement that deserves all praise, but there is no gainsay-

ing that however much we may prevent disease in the mass, just so many
more people will be kept alive some day to suffer accident or ill health
requiring the attention of a conscientious and experienced physician or
surgeon or both ...

Young surgeons need to have their manual dexterity with the tools of
their craft highly developed, to have the ritual of the operating room so
drilled into them that its observances come to be second nature, to have their
resourcefulness so developed that they instinctively know just what to do
when confronted by the fireman with a bad burn, by the comatose victim of
an automobile accident, by the child with a foreign body in its bronchus, by
the young wife with a ruptured tubal pregnancy, by persons with strangulation of the bowel, perforations of an ulcer, acute empyema and a host of
other emergencies – mostly preventable, of course, if one keeps away from
fires, avoids crossing the street, refrains from matrimony, and so on. These
and countless other emergencies that demand prompt surgical intervention
will continue to occur in spite of all precautions till the end of time, let
alone those far more numerous and equally unavoidable disorders with which
the path of life is strewn.[76]

Cushing probably hoped that his colleagues would force the dean's
resignation. They did not. Edsall always found Cushing's attacks trou-
bling – he reacted to them ponderously and clumsily, like an old bull to
a matador one of his friends observed – but he stayed in the ring and, as
administrators do, had a way of outlasting his opponents. He also
outlasted his first wife, divorcing her in Nevada at the height of the
controversy so that he could marry the medical school's secretary. The
newlyweds went off on a sabbatical year, intending on their return to
live in a decanal suite in the school's new student dormitory. The affair
outraged everyone, including the medical students, but there was a
feeling among the faculty that it would appear petty and improper to
try to overthrow the dean on a moral issue. Friends persuaded the Edsalls
not to live in the dorm. The dean and his bride carried on, running the
school together. 'What an amusing menagerie we have one way or another,' Madeline Stanton mused.[77]

By the late 1920s, Cushing seldom taught medical students, and when he examined in surgery he had a way of reducing candidates to terrified incompetence. He could be prickly, tactless, imperious, rude, and wrong in his assaults on Edsall and other Harvard colleagues with whom he disagreed – a paradigm of the surgeon as a tin-Jesus wanting to control the whole university or be left alone by it. There were times when he sounded like a hopeless reactionary railing against the priority of research and science in medical education, an old man turning his back on the sources of his own achievement. Often, though, he tore up his angriest letters, and sometimes he apologized for the ones he had sent.

More charitably, Cushing was advancing a traditional and important view of the responsibility of medical schools to produce real doctors, rather than clinically ignorant research scientists. He combined this with deep insight into the doctor's fundamental calling to treat disease and the need for educators to resist the allure of intellectual and philanthropic fashion. Preventive medicine and public health were as oversold in the 1920s as the system of full-time teaching – and mostly by the same people. The pendulum needed to swing back.

The medical career itself was becoming oversold in the 1920s, in the sense that the first-rank American medical schools found themselves for the first time with many more applicants than they could admit. Harvard's admissions committee tended increasingly to make decisions based purely on academic achievement (qualified by gender, for in Cushing's day there were no compelling proposals to admit women to Harvard medicine), and it resisted pressure to expand the size of incoming classes. Amiable doctors' sons who played football and coasted to C grades in prep school and college could no longer take it for granted that they would have access to the best medical schools. Cushing received many requests from friends and acquaintances for help getting Cleveland boys and Yale men into Harvard medicine. He usually replied that he would do what he could, and he did work hard to get more Elis admitted to Harvard; but typically, he warned his friends that the admissions committee had become 'pretty hard-boiled and apt to lay more stress on whether the candidates have done well in their pre-medical studies than upon whether they are likely to be good doctors, which is the thing you and I would both prefer to gamble on.'[78]

In 1929–30 Cushing 'brought all the pressure I could to bear' on the admissions committee to get a former captain of the Yale football team admitted to Harvard medicine. When the student failed his course in bacteriology, Cushing continued to plead for special treatment on the grounds of medical lineage. The young man's ninety-seven-year-old grandfather was still practicing medicine in Vermont and being honored as an ideal country doctor; the grandson would inherit the family practice. 'The qualities that people who employ doctors want first of all to see in them are honesty of purpose, a personality that wins confidence, unselfishness, an ambition to do good to his fellow men, and enough practical knowledge to know what are their own limitations,' Cushing argued, 'and on these grounds which we, alas, don't always take into consideration, I should place him in the first ten in his class.'[79]

Assuming that Harvard would be unbending, Cushing urged the dean of Boston's other medical school, Tufts, to take the young man:

> He was flunked in bacteriology and tells me that the theories of immunity were absolutely incomprehensible to him. As these same theories are incomprehensible also to me and as they are likely to be overthrown in a few years anyway, I had great sympathy with him. If I were looking for a man to be a good surgical house officer and one whom the patients would trust and adore, he is the kind of man I would pick out. Unfortunately the Medical School doesn't particularly favour that kind of man and that is why we have so few really bang-up surgeons.

Dean A.W. Stearns of Tufts agreed to stretch a point. The school was learning that some rejects from more academic medical schools, including one of Elliott Joslin's sons, did seem to have real clinical potential: 'Perhaps we had better be courageous rather than proud and take selected individuals whose personal qualifications are more important than their scholastic deficiencies.'[80]

Cushing told correspondents that he felt uneasy about intervening in Harvard's admissions process: 'But I think there are times when a certain amount of pressure has to be made if we wish to keep medicine the proper guild it is.'[81] It was a question of principle and priority in medicine, and it was a new chapter in the old contrast between the cultures of Harvard and Yale. When Harvard and Yale men could not find common ground, there was always Tufts.

THIRTEEN

Sprinting to the Tape

Had he seen the soul? What amazing experiences Harvey Cushing must have had as a brain surgeon! The man who drilled into people's heads, tapped their spirits, gazed on their minds, cut into their psyches, reconfigured their consciousness – what profound reflections the surgeon-artist-writer, who all his life had been interested in everything, might have had to share with the world! Did he have insight about the meaning of the mind – thoughts on the meaning of life? What would he say about the meaning of his own life – his achievement as the world's first brain surgeon – and about the modern miracles he wrought daily in his operating room? What was the spiritual, metaphysical, transcendent, existential significance of it all?

During his lifetime the press gradually lionized Cushing as the prototypical brain surgeon – which, of course, he was – and he was probably more in demand within the American medical world than any other figure.[1] He received scores of invitations to address medical meetings, speak to students, write textbook and journal articles, give interviews. His views were solicited on religion, the mind, psychoanalysis, leadership, and dozens of other topics. He could have commanded a very wide audience.

On most issues, other than the medical profession and medical education, he had little to say; and less as he aged. While some of his surgical contemporaries, notably George Crile and Alexis Carrel, felt moved to publish what appeared to be deep thoughts about the nature of man and the meaning of life, Cushing stuck to his shoemaker's last. He was a working surgeon and researcher, who would keep at it until the time came to retire. He politely declined most requests to speak or give interviews, variously citing busyness, uncertain health, the palpitations of his 'rabbit heart' when speaking in public, having nothing worth saying, and the physician's professional obligation to try to keep his name out of the newspapers. Privately, he thought that philosophic surgeons made fools of themselves.[2]

His aversion to the press was deep-seated. Journalists, he felt, should not be allowed to cover specialized medical events, such as professional meetings. Medicine was a difficult, hard-to-fathom subject, which was nearly always misunderstood by the laity and therefore best left to members of the guild. The romanticizing and popularizing of medicine made Cushing very uneasy, perhaps because there was so little that seemed very romantic about what he did from day to day. The adjective he most often applied to his surgical experiences was 'desperate.'

Cushing understood that times were changing and that there might be a case for a hospital carefully to court public favor, but personally he wanted no part of it. 'I have been brought up on an old-fashioned and rigid school,' he told an editor of the Boston *Globe* in 1926, 'one of whose tenets is that a doctor should keep his name out of the newspapers and remain unequivocably above any possible suggestion of lending himself to ... publicity. I know that times change and that many reputable doctors submit to interviews, but my brother, father, grandfather and great-grandfather would rest uneasy in their graves if they knew that times had so far changed that one of their tribe had voluntarily spoken in public in other than a medical journal.'[3] Cushing even objected to giving his picture to the press, pleading both familial and professional dislike of such vanities.

His nontechnical writing was for medical readers in the tradition of Osler, Oliver Wendell Holmes, and other medical essayists. Accordingly, he agreed to the 1928 publication of an anthology of his articles and speeches about medicine. Despite its unsnappy title, *Consecratio Medici and Other Papers*, the book was well received and had three printings in the winter of 1928-9. Its author turned down most other requests for more reflections because he was busy being a physician: 'I am engaged in the daily task of trying to save people's lives; and after six hours or so a day at the operating table, I am not very much good for composition.' To another correspondent he pleaded, 'If you knew what kind of a sixteen-hour-a-day life I lead, you would understand.'[4]

His views on the workings of the brain were not worth soliciting anyway, he explained: 'My knowledge of the brain is purely from the standpoint of an operator who exposes it and handles it and removes things from it.' To those who wanted help with life's mysteries, he had nothing to offer: 'The questions you ask are questions, I fear, for a philosopher or a psychologist, and I regret to say I am neither one nor the other, but merely a handicraftsman.'[5] He privately lamented the way psychiatry had divorced itself from organically based neurology and was succumbing to the harum-scarum chicanery of psychoanalysis. Psychiatry now stood to science, he thought, as astrology did to astronomy – 'but one can't very well say that in public.' Perhaps it was best just to ignore these questions: 'Happiness in this world consists in doing the best you can without puzzling too much over uncertainties.'[6]

Cushing certainly did not think that his handiwork was banal or uninteresting. 'Every surgical operation of course is a miracle,' he wrote in 1927. 'To take out a brain tumor with a patient under local anesthesia and talking to you for a period of eight hours while you are getting out a big meningioma is about as miraculous as anything one can record.' His record of his experiences would be in technical articles and monographs. These were wonderfully dramatic for those who could appreciate them but were largely inaccessible to the laity or the psychoanalytically inclined intelligentsia. Journalists were not encouraged to come to Cushing's operating room and observe and immortalize the miracles. Anyway, he said, it was just as miraculous when a surgeon removed an ingrown toenail without causing infection.[7]

He talked once in layman's terms about the excitement of medicine. In a commencement address to medical students at Dartmouth in 1928, he dwelt mostly on his admiration for the humdrum lives of hard-working general practitioners. Still able in that decade to claim with a straight face that the only rich doctors were those who married wealth, Cushing talked of the 'great game' of conquering disease and of the high adventure of the profession:

> Digging for buried treasure, climbing mountains, shooting big game, explor-ing unknown countries, are tame forms of sport in excitement and rewards compared to the sort of thing in which the doctor may engage ... It takes no less presence of mind, no less steadiness of hand, for a doctor in an emergency to tracheotomize a strangling and struggling child and to suck a diphtheritic membrane out of the wound into his own mouth; or, in these days when diphtheria has been conquered, to insert a tube into the trachea of a suffocat-ing child and remove a foreign body that has been inhaled.[8]

In 1929 they called back the dwarfs. After many months of fiddling, Harvey thought they had substances that contained the growth and sex hormones released by the pituitary's anterior lobe. 'Excitement about the pituitary body is on the up-grade again ...' Madeline Stanton re-corded. 'I suppose the pituitary body will be worked for all it is worth – I do hope that something exciting appears – comparable to insulin!'[9]

Cushing had entered into a joint venture with a major drug com-pany, Parke Davis, to develop his pituitary extract, and he knew that Herbert Evans was working with Eli Lilly and Company to the same end.[10] The kudos for winning the race to make effective growth hor-mone and/or sex hormone would be substantial, perhaps on the order of a Nobel Prize. Madeline Stanton provides glimpses of the work:

> Miss Edna Gordon, the pituitary dwarf, has arrived from Prince Edward Is-land and will come into the hospital next Monday to see what Mr. Teel can do for her in the way of growth. I don't feel very hopeful – the 'sex hormone'

– doesn't seem to have helped the young fat Jew from New York & maybe the
'growth hormone' is no more efficacious. However, their hope is high & it
would certainly be wonderful for the Chief to accomplish something so
evidently epoch-making, considering all the years of labour he has put on
the pituitary. But as in the case of insulin, it will probably be some newcomer
to the field who will have the final burst of glory.[11]

When Edna Gordon could not find lodging outside the hospital,
Cushing allowed her to spend a few weeks that July in his home at 305
Walnut – the family was away. He joked to his staff about the possibilities of filling the place with dwarfs, who did not take up much space.
Cushing lore held that he presided that summer over a house full of
munchkins. He did not, partly because it soon became apparent that
injections of the extracts in three patients had little or no effect. The
dwarfs went home, the researchers went back to their rats, and the
struggle to purify growth hormone continued. Eventually a colleague,
L.B. ('Laffy') Mendel, put a major damper on the research by showing
that with diet alone he could grow rats just as large as Cushing's injected ones.[12]

The Canadian ambassador to the United States and heir to a farm
implement fortune, Vincent Massey, was particularly disappointed by
the slow progress with growth hormone, for his son and heir Hart was of
very small stature and the family was becoming alarmed. Cushing eventually resorted to surgery on Hart Massey, but with little effect. After
Cushing's retirement, Vincent Massey helped subsidize J.B. Collip, one
of the discoverers of insulin, in the race to unlock the hormone that
might make his son grow. Nothing emerged in time to make a difference.[13]

❧

They still had a lot to learn about the use of the electric scalpel in
neurosurgery. Cushing told W.T. Bovie of the day he attempted a spinal cord incision, 'and the patient jumped like a frog and nearly went

off the table.' He gradually mastered the technique, and he worked with the manufacturers to improve the apparatus by using a foot switch and changing from clumsy pistol grip to penlike control. His enthusiasm caused other neurosurgeons to adopt the gizmo. Even Walter Dandy visited his operating room to see the electric loop. (He was 'the unspeakable Dandy,' in Miss Stanton's lexicon, but according to Bronson Ray he got on famously with Cushing that day. The only comparatively unwelcome, distrusted visitor, from whom research was hidden, was Wilder Penfield.) Cushing's confident predictions about the electric scalpel's adaptability for general surgery were also partly responsible for the innovation being overhyped and oversold. The American Congress of Surgeons made the mistake of endorsing a machine marketed by the Majestic Radio Corporation, which gave the congress two hundred free samples. Majestic soon went bankrupt, and Cushing had to warn against electrosurgery being performed by the wrong medical hands.[14]

In his hands, the instruments were particularly useful for excising encapsulated acoustic tumors and meningiomas. Operations became longer than ever, sometimes lasting eight to ten hours. Cushing increasingly relied on Gil Horrax to open and close for him in what he called 'relay' operations. These were fatiguing for everyone, and there were jokes about whether the tumors would recur before the operation ended, but Cushing was now able to accomplish in one exposure what had sometimes required several re-entries.

Another leap forward came when a visitor at the Brigham, Lawrence Kubie, showed the team how to identify tumors from smears of living cells. Now they could learn the histological nature of the enemy while they operated. This was particularly important now that they were attacking gliomas – tumors arising from the brain tissue itself, which were thought to be particularly malignant. Cushing was able to use his long series of results to show that certain gliomas, notably the astrocytomas, could be removed with a fair chance of nonrecurrence, even in children. If there was a chance of success, even in hitherto hopeless cases, it should be taken. 'He fights for the life of these unfortunate children with the ardor of a religious missionary,' John Fulton wrote in his diary, 'and seems never willing to admit that it is a losing game.'[15]

He was now attacking tumors everywhere in the brain, including those affecting the olfactory groove and the optic chiasm deep under the frontal lobes, as well as all the tumors of the cerebellum. His new tool for cutting tissue and cauterizing bleeding points gave him the option to be more aggressive, altering the risk-benefit trade-off in many subtle ways. Would he, for example, adopt the radical approaches of some of the younger surgeons, such as Dandy at Hopkins or Adson at the Mayo Clinic? They seemed increasingly willing to cut through and sometimes remove normal brain tissue to get at tumors.

Cushing usually remained more conservative. To attack tumors of the optic chiasm, for example, he favored surgical approaches that minimized dislocation of the brain and injury to its lobes. He did not support Walter Dandy's willingness to sacrifice an impaired optic nerve to get better access to a tumor, nor would he do a deliberate lobectomy.[16] On the other hand, animal studies seemed to support the view that the 'uncapping,' or removal, of an overlying shell of the cerebellum to get at acoustic tumors caused no permanent disability. In his major 1928 paper on the use of electrosurgery he foresaw the new problem:

> How far one may go with the adoption of this principle of removing the uninvolved shelf of brain that overlies a tumor rather than merely retracting it or incising through it down to the surface of the tumor with subsequent separation of the incised edges remains to be seen. The temptation will be great to extend the principle in regions where cortex registers no important function now that the excision of tissue is so greatly facilitated by electro-desiccation. And the same thing applies as well to lobectomies for the mass extirpation of gliomas – a principle which should of course not be carried too far. The mere prolongation of life unless it can be made better worth living is not an accomplishment for the surgeon to pride himself upon, as has often been emphasized.[17]

There could not be hard guidelines. No two operations were precisely the same. At best, brain surgery was complicated and hazardous. Words ultimately failed:

> When to take great risks; when to withdraw in the face of unexpected diffi-
> culties; whether to force an attempted nucleation of a pathologically
> favourable tumor to its completion with the prospect of an operative fatal-
> ity, or to abandon the procedure short of completeness with the certainty that
> after months or years even greater risks may have to be faced at a subsequent
> session – all this takes surgical judgment which is a matter of long experience
> and which can scarcely be transmitted by the written word.
>
> Surgical judgment, indeed, is a more or less inspirational quality which is
> variable and elusive, all surgeons being conscious of having it in hand on
> some occasions, of losing it on others. It is a good deal like a game which
> even the best and most consistent player foozles for some unaccountable
> reason at certain times. The surgery of brain tumors may be likened without
> being trivial to a form of major sport which is played against an invisible but
> utterly relentless antagonist quick to take advantage of every misplay and
> faulty move.[18]

Despite erratic health and occasional periods of depression, Cushing kept his team intact and his eyes on the ball. He sometimes used the metaphor of being in a marathon. In these years, he began sprinting for the finish. 'I do wish to heaven ... that he'd be sensible and take a decent vacation once in a while,' Madeline Stanton lamented in 1929.[19]

Wrapped in the rhythms of the desperate game, Cushing paid no attention to the stock market crash and the beginnings of hard times. 'I hear that the service has been steaming ahead with the safety valve tied down,' A.J. McLean told Eric Oldberg in the spring of 1930. 'It's great to look back on, but it's hell to participate in it.' Stanton found the days 'almost unbearably hectic.'[20] Cushing first noticed the economic downturn when fewer patients appeared at the Brigham later that year requiring his services. Not that he lacked business. He had many – too many – repeat customers, begging for more relief.

Multiple operations had always been fairly common. Sometimes it took two or three exposures to get at or find a tumor. Sometimes he had to go in again to clear up blod clots. Sometimes he never found a tumor and just bought his patients a little more time with repeated decompressions. The hardest cases were when tumors recurred. With the truly malignant ones, there was usually nothing to do but accept the inevitable. Not so with benign tumors, such as Leonard Wood's meningioma, which had recurred only because Cushing had somehow failed to make a complete removal. Often the huge meningiomas had worked their way deep into the brain and its ventricles, nerves, and vessels, and were impossible to extirpate totally. Then they grew back, fairly slowly over the years, becoming the kind of tumor that needed a second stab at fully excising, or a third ...

Wilder Penfield had operated on his sister's tumor in 1928, partly because of his belief that Cushing was too conservative about attempting total excision. Eighteen months later Cushing was asked to take the second stab at the recurring tumor, and he did. Less than twelve months later the woman died, apparently of another recurrence; because she was a Christian Scientist, there had been no consultation with a view to a third try.[21]

A more remarkable story of multiple operations had begun in 1919 when Cushing removed large paracentral meningeal tumors from the brains of a thirty-four-year-old Irish blacksmith, Timothy Donovan, and a twenty-two-year-old musician, Dorothy Russell. Both were difficult two-stage attacks on tumors that had burrowed deep into the brain, causing growing right-side paralysis and speech impediment, and Cushing was not sure how successful he had been. Within six months he had to remove recurrent tissue from Dorothy Russell's head, and he realized that in his first operations he had broken off an hourglass-shaped tumor at its neck, missing the more deeply embedded portion. By 1923 Donovan's symptoms had recurred so markedly that Cushing went in again and found much the same situation – substantial recurrent growth, which he painstakingly dissected and sucked out. In each case, the patient's symptoms dissipated and there was a return to normal life.

In each case they soon returned to the Brigham. Tim and Dorothy became familiar patients to a whole generation of workers on Cushing's service, 'whose respect and admiration they gained,' he wrote, 'while like a great tragedy there stalked before us the inevitable.' Cushing operated on Donovan eleven times between 1919 and 1930, taking out an estimated 1,350 grams of tumor, about the weight of a normal adult brain. Fairly early in the game, they 'knew that the battle was lost but not so Tim. Like many an Irish guardsman slogging back from the Menin Road, he would not admit defeat.'

Nor would Cushing admit defeat, despite some of his staff's belief that they should just let the poor man die. No matter how ultimately hopeless the struggle, no matter how steadily Donovan deteriorated or how many mishaps he suffered en route to the inevitable (including having to be reopened to retrieve a cotton pledget), the man wanted to live. 'To abandon him to his fate without a helping hand was un-thinkable; he would instinctively know why,' Cushing wrote of the situation in 1930. 'A death on the table would be preferable.'

He knew how easy it would be to make that happen but could not bring himself to do it. (In his later description of the ethical quandry, his normally clear prose becomes agonizingly muddled.) After the tenth operation in 1930, Donovan had an astonishing improvement in speech and body control. The eleventh followed soon after in an attempt to get out the last bit of tumor. Donovan lived on, in pain and struggle but with flashes of good cheer, for six more months, dying in July 1931.

Dorothy Russell had smaller recurrent tumors, an often baffling pat-tern of convulsions and emotional instability, and a fierce determina-tion to keep giving piano lessons to make her living and support her mother. Her bravery impressed everyone at the Brigham, which be-came a kind of second home, where she was welcome to come for rest, re-examination, and, if necessary, re-operation. Cushing's team oper-ated on her for the fifteenth time in January 1931: 'We were quite ready to acknowledge ourselves beaten; but not so this heroic young woman who hung on gamely.' The sixteenth operation was a negative re-exploration; on the seventeenth attempt, just a few weeks before he retired from surgery, Cushing removed eighty more grams of tumor.

Dorothy Russell was able to resume giving piano lessons for a few more months. For years, she had had to play mostly with her left hand. Always she had kept herself neat and tidy, wearing a wig to cover the ruin of her scalp. In November 1932 she stopped smiling and became immobilized by headaches. Her mother bought enough drugs to kill her; Dorothy found them and preferred to go back to the Brigham. She died there on Christmas Day 1932. She had given advance permission for a complete autopsy, and her brain was set aside for special study. For once in his career, Cushing did not bother. 'Even a pathologist surely might make allowances,' he wrote several years later, 'should a surgeon fail to show great enthusiasm over a lifeless brain he has handled a dozen or more times when pulsating and alive; learning meanwhile, both at and between sessions, things about its quondam possessor no microscope could ever disclose. One does not get the whole story from the autopsy.' These two cases, described in detail by Cushing in his 1938 monograph on the meningiomas (which would be read only by other neurosurgeons), were perhaps the closest he did come to seeing patients' souls.[22]

⌇

Louise Eisenhardt was his scorekeeper, keeping a little black book in which she cataloged and classified each case: yet another verified tumor, an unverified tumor, only a suspected tumor; if verified, a meningioma, a glioma, pituitary adenoma, et cetera. If the patient died while still in the hospital, from any cause, the death was attributed to the surgery. It was an easy matter to calculate the mortality rates – the final score, as it were. Cushing joked that he was like a golfer in needing an independent scorekeeper to keep him honest, but in fact he had himself established the rigid standards of recording. Few questioned Cushing's basic mortality figures. He did not pad his count of operations with trivial procedures, nor did he arrange early release from hospital to reduce the death count. The Brigham did not have a convenient con-valescent home for warehousing dying patients. Cushing often kept patients under observation for research purposes longer than was strictly necessary; his average tumor patient spent thirty-nine days in hospi-tal.[23]

Cushing always allowed that surgical statistics depended on so many variables as to be wildly imprecise. Over time, for example, he attempted increasingly difficult, riskier procedures, which ought to have driven his mortality rate up. It did rise slightly in the first year of electrosur-gery. On the other hand, the gradual medical and public acceptance of the possibility of a surgical approach to brain tumors, and Cushing's own fame, meant that over the years patients got to him earlier, when their tumors were smaller and easier to remove – though not necessar-ily easier to locate, except that locational techniques were also con-stantly improving.

Cushing's surgical technique had from the beginning defeated the threat of infection. He hardly ever lost a case to that complication – though in 1927 there was a sudden plague of streptococcal contamina-tion in the operating room, which was finally traced back to Cushing's own throat.[24] Postoperative care was also a major part of the effort to reduce mortality. At the Brigham, Cushing virtually invented the con-cept of intensive care in an age before the intensive care unit. Patients were observed on the operating table for hours after recovery, some-times in the operating room for days. Special nursing was supplied to charity patients out of a special fund, and in Cushing's final years spe-cial nurses were hired to oversee the whole neurosurgical ward. 'Un-questionably many lives have been saved in this way,' he wrote, 'for less experienced nurses or junior house officers can hardly be expected to appreciate the significance of symptoms which indicate that something is going wrong with a patient recently operated on for brain tumor.'[25]

Cushing's basic surgical 'score' for operations on verified tumors in the postwar years is provided in the following table. Over his whole career to 1929, working on more than twenty-four hundred men, women,

Operations for Verified Tumors Including New and Old Cases, 1922–1931

Successive May 1 to May 1	Number of patients	Patients operated on	Number of operations	Postoperative deaths	Case mortality (percent)	Operative mortality (percent)
1922–3	104	94	130	22	23.4	16.9
1922–4	156	140	190	26	18.6	13.7
1922–5	137	113	142	21	18.5	14.7
1922–6	155	133	172	25	18.8	14.5
1922–7	184	161	217	24	14.9	11.0
1922–8	185	149	183	28	18.7	15.3
1922–9	205	179	226	26	14.5	11.5
1922–30	178	147	191	24	18.3	12.5
1930–1	200	170	219	15	8.8	6.8
Total	1504	1286	1670	211	16.4	12.6

Source: Cushing, Intracranial Tumors

and children with verified and unverified tumors, he had lost 24.7 per-cent of his Hopkins patients and 16.2 percent of his Brigham cases.[26] He was extremely pleased that by 1930-1 he had driven his case-mor-tality rate below 10 percent. 'A neurosurgeon's responsibilities would be insufferable if he did not feel that his knowledge of an intricate subject was constantly growing – that his game was improving,' he had said in his Cameron lectures.[27]

It was difficult to enlarge upon the meaning of these figures for two reasons. First, rather like Babe Ruth's home run records in the 1920s, there was nothing to compare Cushing's scores with except his own earlier scores. No other neurosurgeon was in his league. When Eisenhardt surveyed the literature in 1929, all she could find was that Ernest Sachs had reported a mortality rate of 35.5 percent in 85 cases, Herbert Olivecrona in Sweden, a case mortality of 30 percent, and a German surgeon, Anton Eiselsberg, an operative mortality of 46 percent in 333 cases. Everyone used slightly different standards; most other clinics prob-ably received patients who were in a more desperate condition than the Americans referred to Cushing at the Brigham.[28]

Secondly, Cushing had come to emphasize that it would ultimately be more important to assess the quality of life afforded to the 90 percent of his patients who survived their operations. Amory Codman had been nearly fanatical on the need to measure the real end results of surgery. Cushing's elaborate record keeping, with obsessive follow-up inquiries, allowed for remarkable long-term study of his patients. He personally did no analysis of patient survival or quality of life – he saw too many problems establishing standards, let alone the issue of control cases – but in the 1930s he encouraged three of his former assistants to do some of the first studies of long-term surgical results. Both William P. Van Wagenen and Hugh Cairns traced the fortunes of the patients operated on in their year at the Brigham, while W.R. Henderson studied the results of 338 cases of pituitary adenomata.[29]

Everyone concluded that the end results varied hugely with the kind of tumor and could be measured in many different ways. Von Wagenen found that the 80 glioma cases who survived surgery in 1924-5 were given an average of two years of 'useful activity' (defined mainly as an ability to return to work) and 3.3 years of 'useful life'; patients with encapsulated tumors had 5 years of useful activity and 6.3 years of useful life. But some patients from his year were not evaluated because they were still living. Cairns was more interested in long-term survival, noting that 27.4 percent of the 135 patients who had survived operations in 1926-7 were still leading useful lives ten years later. Henderson thought the best measurement of results with pituitary tumors involved vision: in 176 of the 247 cases of chromophobe pituitary adenomata that he studied, the patients' vision had improved enough that they could return to work within six months of Cushing having operated. There was little difference in results between Cushing's transphenoidal and transfrontal approaches to the pituitary. Henderson found that radiation therapy appeared to have been more effective than Cushing had thought; Cairns's study tended to confirm the view that Cushing's cautious approach to acoustic tumors led to little improvement for the patient.

All the studies of Cushing's end results concluded with subjective comments about the excellence of his work, the lack of comparable data, and the fact that the results of operations once considered hopeless were now comparable to the results of tumor removal from other parts of the body. Cairns wondered how the gratitude of a family that had received eighteen months of the company of a healthy child could be quantified.

What about the hopeless cases? Cushing's policy had been to refrain as far as possible from operating on patients with obvious intracranial metastases. An early study by F.C. Grant of twenty-six cases of malignant metastases at the Brigham indicated that surgery had no effect on an average four-month life expectancy. 'This statement,' Cushing noted, 'however true in fact, failed to indicate that operations nevertheless may not infrequently afford a vast degree of symptomatic relief for which patients and their relatives are most grateful. Hence when the unfortunate victims of these disorders once come to be admitted to the hospital ward, it is difficult to refuse their appeals to give them at least the chance of temporary palliation of symptoms which a decompression may afford.' He privately chided Van Wagenen on his concept of 'useful life,' arguing that it was cruel to dismiss months of family happiness.[30] None of these discussions tried to weigh benefits against the financial cost of surgery. There were never any health economists looking over Cushing's shoulder, as there seldom are on medical frontiers.

⌁

Not only patients but also students and established surgeons continued to flock to the Brigham in Boston, the world's neurosurgical mecca. Madeline Stanton complained that there was 'a perfect swarm of foreigners under foot all the time.' Some came to work and study for a few weeks or months; others just to say that they had seen Cushing at work. By the late 1920s Cushing had trained or helped train the pioneering neurosurgeons of Canada and the United Kingdom and several countries on the Continent, as well as neurosurgeons in the United States. He had met practically everyone else in the field and had encouraged his own students to take a *wanderjahr* abroad and visit all the foreign neurosurgical stars, such as they were. A basic European list in the early

1930s might include Herbert Olivecrona in Stockholm, Clovis Vincent and Thierry de Martel in Paris, Ignaz Oljenick in Amsterdam, Otfrid Foerster in Breslau, and Geoffrey Jefferson, Norman Dott, and Hugh Cairns in the United Kingdom. Cushing had greatly influenced them all. 'I think often of you who represents for me the king of kings in chirurgy,' de Martel wrote to him as his retirement neared.[31]

Boston was particularly infested with medical guests when Harvard hosted the Thirteenth International Physiological Congress in July 1929. Almost every foreign visitor tried to get a ticket to visit Cushing's operating room. Russia's Ivan P. Pavlov, octogenarian father of the conditioned reflex and poster boy for Soviet science, was the meeting's guest of honor. He came, along with forty or fifty others, to see Cushing operate; afterwards he burned his name into a piece of beef with the electrosurgical knife. Cushing joked about eating the meat to improve his reflexes, hosted two hundred physiologists and neurosurgeons to lunch at the Brigham, and kept the Pavlov steak among his souvenirs.[32] After the congress he left town on what had become virtually an annual lecturing and book-buying trip to Europe.

In the winter of 1931 the old vascular problem in Cushing's legs flared up seriously. He tried to carry on. 'He fancies that no one notices he is limping and that half his shoe is cut away,' Fulton wrote. His left big toe was blue and very sore; gangrene and amputation loomed as possibilities.[33] Dr Cushing had to become, for the first time, a patient at the Brigham. After a week on the sidelines, he became a surgeon-patient. He rolled from his hospital bed to his offices and operating room in a wheelchair, tied a gown over his pyjamas, operated from a sitting position, and then returned to his room for another spell of 'lying doggo.' The experience became fodder for his annual report as Surgeon-in-Chief ('a man deprived of his pants gives up not only independence but identity – even hope'), and it marked the beginning of a terrible struggle to try and kick his cigarette habit, the only treatment other than rest for what was now diagnosed as Buerger's disease.[34]

Cushing was determined to keep operating, partly because his series

of verified tumors was approaching two thousand, an astonishing career total – reminiscent of Theodor Kocher's two thousand operations
for goiter – and an occasion for his last hurrah on the international
stage. The First International Neurological Congress was scheduled,
beautifully symbolically, to be held in Berne, Switzerland, in the summer of 1931. 'I feel a good deal like a Marathon runner who is in sight
of his goal but has gone lame and has made up his mind to stick it,
willy-nilly,' Cushing wrote in early March. 'Twenty-five more verified
tumours will make two thousand and then I shall quit.'[35]

Harvey's two thousandth tumor case was in the head of thirty-one-
year-old Ida Herskowitz, an acromegalic Jewish woman from New York,
who suffered from headaches and had lost half her field of vision in
both eyes. Relaying with Horrax, Cushing operated on her on April
15, 1931, easily removing a large, soft pituitary adenoma. After the
operation the staff presented Cushing in the operating room with a
silver cigarette case, said to contain two thousand cigarettes, and a
congratulatory telegram from Henry Ford. Then there was a party in
the lab with cake and all the fixings.[36] Part of the day's proceedings was
captured on film, a flawed but atmospheric visual record of the world's
first neurosurgeon at work.

Ida Herskowitz survived as well. The operation fully restored her
vision, but after a few months her headaches began to recur. In January
1932 Cushing lectured the patient on the need to be thankful for her
eyesight and ignore her headaches. 'She is a worthy soul,' he wrote to
her doctor, 'but has come to complain so much of her headaches that I
told her that if she ever mentioned the word to me again that I would
have nothing more to do with her and that she must make the best of it
because people with her malady often have bad headaches even when
the trouble is quiescent. I hope this may give her a psychotherapeutic
boost, if nothing else could.' Ms Herskowitz lived with her pains for
some years; then they went away, and almost thirty years after Cushing
had died she was reported to be headache-free and enjoying retirement
in Florida. The histological slides of her tumor have disappeared, however, possibly having been snitched as a historical souvenir.[37] (The slides

of Osler's brain that I reported missing in my biography of him have since been auctioned on eBay.)

Cushing warmed up for his European finale by giving a rich historical overview of American medicine, 'From Tallow Dip to Television,' at the hundred and fiftieth reunion of the Massachusetts Medical Society in June 1931. He noted how the torch of medical leadership had passed to America, 'where foreign medical graduates now flock as our ambitious and favored graduates once flocked abroad,' and he hoped that American medicine and American society would preserve the values that had worked in the past to lead to this greatness.[38]

None of the family went with Cushing to Europe in the late summer of 1931. His house and office staff assembled to see him off. John Fulton, the self-appointed Boswell, sailed with him on the SS *Deutschland*. Fulton recorded Cushing's interest in Charles Lindbergh's trip to Japan, his ability to work in his stateroom from 9:30 to 4:00 without moving from his desk, and his indulgence in a cocktail and caviar each night before dinner. Europe was now suffering from industrial stagnation, massive unemployment, and serious political unrest, but the world's leading neurologists and neurosurgeons gathered seven hundred strong in Berne to celebrate the coming of age of their disciplines. William Welch was on hand as American medicine's eldest statesman, and Pavlov again came from the Soviet Union. Sherrington was the star neurologist at the congress, Cushing the outstanding neurosurgeon. Both received honorary degrees at the opening session in Berne's municipal casino.

Cushing's paper to the congress was a report on his two thousand cases of verified tumors – an accounting of how he had spent the thirty years since that winter when he had worked in Berne with Kocher and Kronecker and had become committed to the nervous system. This would be his last statement on brain tumors as a whole, he said in this last bow. He paid tribute to his assistants and co-workers, and anticipated that they would better his score. He quoted Leonardo da Vinci: 'It's a mediocre pupil who does not excel his master.'

Fulton and most of Cushing's students felt more like weeping than joining in the thunderous applause for Cushing's paper. 'Old animosities were put aside,' Fulton wrote, 'and he was hailed by everyone as the supreme master of a great specialty. No one begrudged him his applause, and many observed with some astonishment his twenty-five pupils, most of whom had crossed the ocean primarily to hear him read his paper.' Welch remarked that Cushing had been the first American to found an international 'school' in medicine and said he had become 'the most influential man in the medical world today.'[39]

There were glittering, unforgettable dinners, one thrown by Cushing himself for the international neurosurgical establishment and his students. Towards the end of the congress, Cushing and Sherrington led a group of the delegates to the municipal cemetery where, in drenching rain, they laid wreaths on the graves of Kocher and Kronecker and the bacteriologist Edwin Klebs (whose son Arnold was present as one of Cushing's good friends and hosts). Welch gave a fifteen-minute extemporaneous speech; Cushing talked of medicine's most precious heritage lying in its noble traditions: 'What has been accomplished does not die.' The neurologists knew they were re-enacting the famous pilgrimage that Osler had led to the tomb of Pierre Louis in Paris in 1905.

After Berne and a visit to Klebs's alpine retreat, Cushing found himself eating oysters with Welch in Paris and – turning Boswell himself – taking down, in the haze of their cigarette and cigar smoke, the old man's reminiscences of Halsted and Mall and how the young New York surgeons had become addicted to spraying their noses with cocaine back in the 1880s. Popsy played a famous practical joke on Cushing when he spilled a bottle of red ink in his hotel room and declared that a murder had taken place. Harvey's last sightseeing in Europe that summer was to be driven around literary sights in Britain, accompanied by Hugh Cairns. They took in Keats's and Robert Louis Stevenson's house, and talked of books and plays.[40]

~

Cushing always intended to step down as Surgeon-in-Chief at the Brigham in 1932 when he reached sixty-three, the retirement age he and Christian had set many years earlier. He rejected a Brigham offer to extend his term by three years. Speculation on who would be appointed to fill Cushing's shoes centered on Elliott Cutler, Boston-born, a workaholic pioneer of cardiac surgery and also a Cushing protégé, a war comrade, and his friend for many years. In the mid-1920s Cushing had promoted Cutler's successful bid to become Crile's successor in the chief surgical job in Cleveland, and now he very much wanted to have Cutler brought back to Boston. He was a good surgeon, but Madeline Stanton's diaries make it clear that practically everyone who worked with Cushing disliked 'God Almightly Elliott,' considering him a shameless self-promoter and an indiscreet blowhard.[41]

The larger question was what would happen to Cushing. Automatic and pension-greased retirement to private life had not yet become the norm in North American academia. Cushing might take another position at the Brigham or Harvard, could go somewhere else, might well keep operating, sore feet and what he said was a tobacco tremor notwithstanding. His name alone made him a valuable commodity, a prize to any medical faculty, easily worth the cost of creating some kind of sinecure to let him do whatever he wanted.

Johns Hopkins had just such a sinecure in place, its chair in the history of medicine. Rockefeller money had endowed the chair in 1926 as a haven for seventy-seven-year-old William Welch, who was still lively, well-connected, and keen to buy books for the great Hopkins medical library which his friends were also promoting – and which later was named after him. As a historian of medicine, Welch was an easygoing dilettante compared with the Pulitzer Prize–winning Cushing, let alone some of the professional medical historians starting to be trained in Germany. Welch had told Cushing in 1926 that he intended to hold the chair for only a year or two 'for you to come and really develop the subject.' 'If you will hold it down until I am sixty,' Cushing had replied, 'I will be glad to try and follow on unless they can find somebody better, which ought not to be difficult.'[42]

Grumble though he did about the state of Johns Hopkins, Cushing deeply admired both the institution where he had done his most creative work and William Welch, the last of his mentors. His love of medical history and bibliography was also practically boundless – collecting, reading, and writing books would probably be his retirement hobby. He loved medical libraries, took a great interest in the plans for Hopkins' monument to Welch, and at that building's dedication gave one of the keynote addresses (a tedious one, John Fulton thought, but an important disquisition on the medical library as a professional unifier). Welch kept saying that he was only keeping his chair warm for Cushing and urged him to come home to Hopkins. In November 1930 Welch resigned his chair, and Hopkins instantly offered it to Cushing.[43]

The other university with at least as strong a hold on Cushing was his, and Welch's, alma mater, Yale. Everything had changed in the years since Yale's prewar attempts to bring Cushing home had floundered on its medical school's many inadequacies. In the 1920s both Yale and its School of Medicine had modernized spectacularly. A dynamic president, James R. Angell, supported by the magnificent Sterling and then Harkness bequests, had transformed Yale's old red-brick campus into an academic wonderland of neo-Gothic towers, quadrangles, and colleges. In 1920 Milton Winternitz, a Hopkins-trained pathologist and protégé of Welch, became dean of the moribund School of Medicine and worked demonically – Angell called him a 'steam engine in pants' – to create first-rate buildings, connections with a first-rate hospital, a first-class faculty, and an innovative, student-centered approach to medical education.

Cushing had been a mentor to 'Winter' back in Hopkins days, in fact had steered him into pathology. Through the 1920s he had been an enthusiastic booster of all the advances in Yale medicine. 'Nothing could be more ideal than a small, well conducted school in a college town,' he wrote to a friend in 1920. 'It ought to be like Heidelberg in the heyday of the school there. Winternitz has done superbly.' Cushing was one of many distinguished Yale alumni who had protested when Winternitz was refused election to the university's Graduate Club because he was Jewish. His own protégé, Sam Harvey, was recruited for Yale, and Cushing, taking greater interest in Yale medicine than even in Yale athletics, strongly supported Harvey's promotion to chief of surgery. In 1928 he encouraged Winternitz to give the chair of physiology to his newest protégé, John Fulton, telling him that Fulton would soon have the choice of any university in the country and 'has the qualities to make one of the most eminent physiologists we have ever had.' Fulton turned down Yale to return to Oxford as Sherrington's assistant. But Winternitz persisted, and in 1929 he renewed the offer on very generous terms. Cushing sent another archly Oslerian cable to Fulton: 'Do not procrastinate. Accept.' In the autumn of 1930 John Fulton became, at age thirty, the youngest of Yale's Sterling professors. Cushing was delighted.[44]

Winternitz was already courting the possibility of bringing Cushing to New Haven as one of Yale's oldest Sterling professors. In 1929 Cushing had protested that he just wanted to get on with his work in Boston. When Winternitz heard a year later that Hopkins was courting Cushing, he offered Cushing anything he would like – a sinecure if he wanted it; his own labs, research associates, residents, and nurses if he wanted to continue to be active; perhaps a starring role in Yale's new Institute of Human Relations, headed by the distinguished psychobiologist, Robert Yerkes.[45]

Cushing turned everyone down, pleading that he wanted to carry on at Harvard until his mid-1932 retirement. But he did not totally rule out going to either school when that time came, and both continued to woo him. Harvard chimed in belatedly and not very loudly. In the spring of 1931, Dean Edsall, who had many good reasons for hoping to see the last of Cushing, mentioned that he could stay on to give lectures in medical history in an honorary capacity.

Cushing continued to be noncommittal – in Fulton's view, 'the complete prima donna as far as his plans for the future are concerned.' Insider gossip was that Kate Cushing was firmly opposed to any return to Baltimore. To Hopkins friends she icily denied it, saying, 'There could be no happiness for any of us if HC should be unhappy.'[46] Fulton thought Kate might favor a move back to Cleveland, 'but the only intellectual stimulus he would have there would be in the communion with his

ancestors!' As for Cushing going to Hopkins, Fulton told Klebs, 'Can
you honestly envisage his remaining at peace in the same town with
Dandy whose personal hatred of H.C. knows no restraint? ... Can you
see him returning with Aequanimity to those haunts, now barren and
lifeless, where as a student he was inflamed by the divine spark of WO?'[47]

In the meantime, Harvard was considering who should succeed
Cushing as Moseley professor and the Brigham's chief surgeon. While
righteously abstaining from any formal role in the matter, Cushing lobbied hard for Cutler. Cutler's publication and research record was not
particularly strong, and the opposition, led by Edsall, would have preferred David Cheever. After much political maneuvering, a tense meeting of the full professors narrowly voted for Cutler. 'We can go about
making plans hand in hand,' Cushing happily – and naively – wrote to
Cutler at the end of 1931.[48]

So perhaps he would hang around Boston after retiring. President
Lowell now hinted about the possibility of his having a salaried chair in
the history of medicine and perhaps access to a few surgical beds at the
Brigham. Cushing had finally decided to rule out a return to Johns
Hopkins. Welch unwittingly laid the ground by inviting Henry E. Sigerist,
head of the University of Leipzig's Institute of the History of Medicine,
to give a series of historical lectures in Baltimore and other centers.
Sigerist had been trained in both medicine and history and was a dynamic, urbane lecturer, well received everywhere he went. He stayed
with the Cushings in Boston and impressed Harvey as a delightful house
guest and scholar. Harvey realized that Sigerist was an ideal candidate
to be a real professor of the history of medicine at Hopkins and decided
to forgo the option for himself and to support Sigerist instead.

'He has everything that I have not,' Cushing wrote to Lewis Weed,
'youth, training, linguistic abilities, a profound knowledge of history, a
wide acquaintance with historians, and a great career ahead of him ...
All said and done, it is a chair of medical history to be filled and not
merely a comfortable berth for the likes of me to enjoy for my declining
years.' Hopkins friends tried to suggest that Cushing stood for broad
medical humanism in the way that no narrow medical historian ever

could, but the surgeon was adamant. He had turned his back on the possibility reluctantly, he maintained, but in recognition of a better man. Johns Hopkins reluctantly offered its chair to Sigerist, who accepted. Cushing later said that if he had followed his heart and not his head, he would have chosen Hopkins.[49]

~

When he was asked what he was going to do, his simple, frustrating answer was, 'The day's work.'[50] He told President Lowell that he was like a marathoner in the last quarter-mile. He now tried to sprint even faster, not only in the operating room but in his surgical laboratories and at his desk. He hoped to complement his great brain tumor series with final research triumphs in his other great field of interest, the workings of the pituitary.

Clinically, the administration of pituitary extracts did not work during his lifetime. Effective human growth hormone would not come on the market for several more decades. Even so, laboratory research seemed to be enabling endocrinologists to continue to fill in the picture of pituitary functions and dysfunctions. In his final years at the Brigham, Cushing had many last words to say on the pituitary puzzle.

As the physiology of the gland continued to be elaborated in Cushing's and others' labs, mostly through cellular staining techniques, it became clear, for example, that pituitary tumors arising from the acidophilic cells of the anterior lobe (acidophilic adenomas) were the ones that stimulated the release of growth hormone, leading to acromegaly. Certain other anterior tumors – chromophobic ones – appeared to inhibit release of both the growth and the sexual hormones, leading to the syndrome first observed by Fröhlich of stunted sexual development and growth (infantilism, or dwarfism with sexual dystrophy). Could there be a third kind of tumor, Cushing wondered, arising from the anterior lobe's basophilic cells, which had a special impact in overstimulating the sexual hormone?[51]

Study of the secretions of the pituitary's posterior lobe was proving

even more baffling because of the complexities being revealed about
the relationship between the hypophysis (pituitary) and the hypothalamus, a portion of the diencephalon, or 'inner brain,' involving
the walls and floor of the third ventricle, above the pituitary, which
seemed also to have something to do with controlling the body's autonomic nervous system. In his first round of pituitary studies, twenty
years earlier, Cushing had ignored the hypothalamus entirely. By the
1930s it was realized that it played a role involving – reacting to,
controlling, or stimulating – the release of some pituitary secretions.
Cushing began to invest enormous amounts of energy and time working on this problem because of its relationship to his old belief that
there were direct secretions between the posterior lobe and the third
ventricle. He hoped to prove that pituitary posterior secretions acted
in the hypothalamic region to control many of the body's involuntary
responses.

Cushing and his researchers thought they could show that injections
of posterior pituitary extract (pituitrin) into the third ventricle caused
blood vessel dilation, sweating, tearing, and other visceral effects, thus
supporting the hypothesis of a vital role for the posterior lobe's secretion, almost as vital as the role of adrenalin. The effectiveness and
significance of the research was controversial even at the time. As friends
pointed out to him, the extracts Cushing used were probably contami-
nated by other stimulants; and the evidence from his injection experiments was much too vague to support the grand hypothesis which he
hoped to advance of pituitary control of the hypothalamus and the
autonomic nervous system through a parasympathetic center in the
hypothalamus. Generally, while there had been great advances since
Cushing's first foray into pituitary physiology before the war, investigators were still groping almost blindly to understand a hugely complex
relationship; it would be many years before the neuroendocrine functions of the hypothalamus would begin to be unraveled. Cushing would,
perhaps, have been struck by the irony that his working hypothesis – of
pituitary hormones controlling the hypothalamus – was almost the exact reverse of the true relationship.

As he grasped some of the difficulties in making his case, he fell back on having at least drawn attention to the intimate relation between hypophysis and hypothalamus. Some of his research students, who had been driven mercilessly to try to find supporting evidence for Cushing's hunches and hypotheses, never realized that this was no mean achievement, and they tended to be unduly critical of his scientific judgment. No one else in Cushing's lifetime made authoritative sense of these matters.[52]

His greatest strength as a researcher was rooted in clinical study. In 1931 he pulled together observations he had made in several patients to suggest that intracranial lesions, especially in the hypothalamic region, could lead to severe stomach ulcers. In a major paper, 'Peptic Ulcers and the Interbrain,' given as the Balfour Lecture at the University of Toronto, he argued for a re-emphasis on the old but generally discarded view of the possibility of neurogenesis of certain ulcers.

Unfortunately, Cushing then reasoned beyond his data to try to show that it supported the notion that high-strung persons, wracked by worry, anxiety, heavy responsibilities, and bad habits, were particularly susceptible to ulcers. He thought he had stumbled on the etiology of the majority of gastric ulcers and said so in his paper. Newspapers promptly played up his 'discovery': 'Cushing Lays Gastric Ulcer to Brain Storm ... Due to Mad Pace of Modern Life.' He was deluged with unwelcome publicity and letters and quickly backtracked, insisting that he knew nothing about ulcers. His paper was rejected for publication in the Canadian Medical Association's *Journal*.[53]

For several months he engaged in extensive correspondence trying to learn more about ulcers and to bolster his argument. Did the happy-go-lucky lifestyle of 'negroes' insulate them from ulcers? he wondered. His correspondents disagreed on the role of race in ulcers. Were cab drivers especially susceptible? What about smoking? 'The literature of ulcer is simply appalling and from it one could prove anything one wanted to,' he finally concluded. After a year's hesitation he toned down his paper, published it in *Surgery, Gynecology, and Obstetrics*, and had no more to say on the subject. While overstating his theories about the role of the hypothalamus, he had outlined an etiological basis for some ulcers.[54]

His most enduring contribution to clinical medicine developed out of background reading for his 1930 Lister Lecture on pituitary physiology. A 1924 paper from Czechoslovakia described a pituitary patient whose autopsy revealed a basophil adenoma. The photographs of the patient, Cushing noticed, showed a condition strikingly similar to that of one of the patients currently on his own wards. Surely they had the same disorder. This disorder, or 'syndrome,' involved a complex of ills, including the development of significant fat deposits, backache, weakness, fatigue, a weakening of the bones (about to be named osteoporosis), skin discoloration and streaking, exaggerated secondary sexual characteristics such as facial hair, high blood pressure, high blood sugar levels, and sexual dystrophy.

Cushing had noticed several patients like this over the years – including one mentioned in his 1912 study – and had labeled their disorder vaguely as 'polyglandular syndrome.' A few researchers had noticed that many of these symptoms accompanied tumors of the adrenal cortex, a gland which by the 1920s had been found to secrete a powerful hormonal cocktail, perhaps under control from the pituitary. Cushing scoured the clinical and pathological literature, studied his own patient records, and gradually pulled the puzzle together in the form of a long paper on the subject of pituitary basophilism.

He gave it in New York, Boston, New Haven, and finally in Baltimore in the early months of 1932, and had it published in the *Johns Hopkins Hospital Bulletin* under the title 'The Basophil Adenomas of the Pituitary Body and Their Clinical Manifestations (Pituitary Basophilism).'[55] His argument was that he had found a syndrome in the literature and in some of his patients that could be caused by basophilic pituitary tumors. Just as the more common acidophilic tumors caused hypersecretion of the growth hormone, these caused a hypersecretion of the sex hormone and perhaps other hormones through the medium of the adrenal cortex. Adrenocortical tumors themselves could cause the syndrome, though there was no evidence that they influenced the pituitary and they were not a necessary cause. In this first presentation, Cushing could cite only three cases where the syndrome had been shown to be associated with a basophilic pituitary adenoma. He concluded that more would be found.

He did not think his paper was particularly well received, commenting sourly that his Baltimore listeners had mainly discussed the pronunciation of 'syndrome' and that most in his New York 'ghetto' audience thought they suffered from it.[56] In fact, it was immediately realized in the medical world that Cushing had identified a distinct disease pattern. Other researchers had noticed parts of the picture – British clinicians had written about 'diabetes of bearded women' – but no one had put the puzzle together nearly as deftly and authoritatively. Medical journals immediately named it after him: 'Cushing's syndrome.' He was very pleased. 'Judging from the reactions I have received from all sides, it looks as though I may have made a ten-strike. I might have been more emphatic about it ... had I known what I have since learned. We now have three additional verified cases. In its milder forms it is apparently not an uncommon disorder.'[57]

Cushing's syndrome was and is the consequence of hypersecretion from the adrenal cortex, and could have multiple causes. The link to pituitary basophil adenomas as one significant cause of the hypersecretion was less obvious – a daring and controversial hypothesis on Cushing's part, based on only a few cases. There was considerable skepticism about this claim. Percival Bailey, for example, told Fulton that it was 'exceedingly far-fetched and founded on a very feeble basis,' and Hugh Cairns reported that London researchers were furiously cutting serial sections of the pituitary to prove Cushing wrong. The controversy began an immediate search, leaded by Cushing himself, for more evidence, and cases were very quickly uncovered where the link was clear.[58] Cushing himself found several basophilic adenomas on autopsy of his patients.

The old man's hunch had played out. After all those years of gathering information and misinformation about the pituitary, Cushing had correctly identified basophil pituitary adenomas as one significant cause of the hypersecretion from the adrenal cortex. In those cases, Cushing's syndrome becomes 'Cushing's disease,'[59] and both conditions are well known today in the field of endocrinology. Mild versions of Cushing's syndrome are often iatrogenic, or doctor induced, as a result of prescribing of the hormones of the adrenal cortex for inflammatory and other diseases.

⁓

Just as Harvey stood on the brink of retiring to live on his investments, the force of the depression finally hit the Cushing finances. In 1932 income from the family's Cleveland properties dried up entirely. Worse, Boston's venerable Lee Higginson & Company, which held most of the Cushing fortune, suspended operations. When Harvey looked into the state of his holdings with them he was appalled to find out that his nest egg had rotted. A portfolio worth $836,000 in July 1931 had shrunk to $365,000 by May 1932. Just one of many horror stories was the fate of $32,300 worth of the shares of International Match, suddenly revalued at $118.13.[60]

Cushing was staggered by the losses and not a little bitter. He joined the swollen ranks of Americans who took a dim view of financial manipulators. 'I had supposed that the trust fund that I had established for my family was as secure as anything could legally be,' he wrote to Yale's President Angell. 'I now learn that the people who had my affairs in hand have so manhandled them that I may have to start in afresh as a wage earner which is not so easy at my time of life.' How could he salvage the situation? In fact, he had many options, ranging from private practice in Boston to returning to Cleveland to succeed his successor by taking over Cutler's position. Far and away the most attractive possibility was Yale's open offer of one of its Sterling professorships at a salary of $10,000. In June 1932 Cushing agreed in principle to become Sterling Professor of Neurosurgery at Yale, effective in 1933. He could not yet see his way clear to setting the date for his move, and until he did the announcement would not be made.[61]

Cushing continued to operate through the spring and summer of 1932, but his business fell off drastically. Oddly, it sort of included Babe Ruth, who was given a neurological examination on Cushing's service at the Brigham after claiming to be paralyzed by a foul tip that hit his foot. The aging athlete's real need, it seemed, was rest.[62] So was Cushing's. Madeline Stanton found him so crotchety to work with at close quarters – 'Talk about temperamental! No female would have a show beside him' – that she wondered how anyone would be able to live with him when he had no surgery to take up his time.

The young neurosurgeons of the United States (absent Walter Dandy) paid him a remarkable tribute that spring in naming a new professional organization in his honor. The Harvey Cushing Society, a junior alternative to the more exclusive Society of Neurological Surgeons, held its first meeting in Boston in May. Cushing launched its proceedings by removing a third-ventricle tumor. 'I have never seen him operate with greater ease and sureness,' John Fulton observed.[63]

Cushing tried to tell Cutler how he should do his job after the transition: 'I would keep exceedingly quiet and out of the limelight; don't agitate for reforms even if they are needed; keep off from all committees for several years at least; get other and younger people to do the writing; resist all invitations to give occasional addresses ... don't give your opponents the chance to say that you are shallow and superficial, which they do say. I of course know better; but you have laid yourself open to this criticism. It is not my business, I fully realize, even to hint to you what you may best do when you come here ... a word to the wise should be sufficient.'

Cutler politely but firmly rebuffed him. Cushing realized he had to get out of his successor's way. At the last moment, he delayed sailing for Europe so that he could do one final operation on a comatose child on August 17, 1932. It was a futile exploration, but the patient, who probably had encephalitis, survived. Cushing caught a ship to Europe the next day. Before leaving, he had helped obtain a job for Gil Horrax at Boston's growing Lahey Clinic. He had also begun to clean out the paper, in his office, giving his vast files on the Osler biography, for example, to the Osler Library at McGill, and throwing out reams of material that Madeline Stanton promptly rescued for history from his wastebaskets. Apart from Horrax, he kept his harem in place, waiting and wondering what would happen to them on his return.[64]

Harvard gave him some honorary titles and a small pension, but there were no special ceremonies to mark his departure after twenty years as the university's and Boston's outstanding surgeon. John Fulton was amazed by Harvard's insouciance: 'I sometimes think that there has never been a more flagrant instance of a great university failing so completely to recognize the greatness of one of its members. By common consent in Europe he is regarded as the outstanding figure in American medicine of this or any previous epoch. In Harvard he is merely a troublesome member of the medical faculty ... tolerated in Cambridge only because he happened at one time to win the Pulitzer Prize and to become a member of the Saturday Club ... [an] attitude of patronizing stupidity.'[65]

Kate did not go with him on his retirement holiday. Harvey junketed about Italy with Arnold Klebs, looking at art, architecture, and medical history sites and buying books. He gave a paper at the International Physiological Congress in Rome, where he again hobnobbed with Pavlov and heard Mussolini open the proceedings. In Munich one night he dined at the next table to Winston Churchill. He flew in an airplane from Berne to Paris and then over the Channel to England, where he visited Sherrington and other old friends, and Hugh Cairns and other new friends.

Cushing planned to move to New Haven within months of his return. But Kate had problems house hunting, and Yale was starting to have problems guaranteeing the support it had promised for his research. Harvey decided to stay in Boston over the winter of 1932-3, hoping to polish off his pituitary research and, with Louise Eisenhardt, to finish the long-intended book on the meningiomas. Cutler gave him quarters in the hospital, and he had access to all his patient records,

with no responsibilities. Fulton thought that Cushing found it discon-
certing and hurtful to be so completely out of the loop, as it were,
though in fact there is no evidence that he was badly treated. Madeline
Stanton, the best barometer, thought he was very put out, as she certainly was, by Cutler's changes. Neurosurgical operations at the Brigham,
done by Robert M. Zollinger, suddenly went much more quickly – very
badly, Stanton thought – 'every move almost being against the Chief's
firmest & most fundamental beliefs.'[66]

Cushing was apparently invited to return to operating at the Brigham,
but refused. On November 5, 1932, Gil Horrax virtually forced him to
take over a difficult tumor removal on a physician's daughter. Harvey
did it, one last time. 'The Chief in harness again – and it was grand,'
Stanton exulted. 'But they didn't even have the courtesy to give him
his own room which I consider was past forgiveness ... Just another
evidence of utter gracelessness ... It's too rotten.'[67]

Cushing worked very hard all winter on his pituitary articles. That
gland was 'the Chief's first and only true love,' according to Stanton.
He continued to feel that his health was fragile and doubted that he
would ever operate again. He had already asked that Yale change his
presumptive title from Professor of Neurosurgery to Professor of Neurology, with the proviso that if he really lost it he could become Professor of the History of Medicine. He kept putting off the timing of his
move, even as he admitted that his procrastinating was intolerable,
especially for his Yale friends. 'This business of letting go is difficult, and
I suppose I ought to have the courage to say so frankly.' He was almost
certainly battling waves of depression, brought on by the stress of adjusting to his new situation and planning for the future.[68]

By the spring of 1933 even John Fulton had lost patience with
Cushing's indecision. He warned his idol in March that the Yale Corporation would not tolerate further postponements and that it was 'now
or never.' Cushing procrastinated further and finally told President Angell
that he was holding back because of fear of failing health:

> If this was merely a question of legs I might like Mr. Roosevelt resort to a
> wheel chair and a valet. But it is more than that, and I am conscious from

week to week of a relentless advance in the malady and a lessening of my
capacity for mental concentration.

My repeated hints that I might not be able to come up to the scratch have
not been due to any false modesty but to the realization of an increasing loss
in powers of sustained application.

I had hoped that this might be transitory and due to something other than
physical causes, but I am obliged to face the fact that this is not so.

I find that I can peg along here accomplishing some little now and then:
but I am increasingly doubtful about the advisability of this proposed transplantation which might finish me and prove a disappointment to you ... I
don't propose to shout my ill health from the house-tops and even my family
are probably unaware of the full measure of it.

The day after he wrote this letter, Madeline Stanton told Fulton that he
was 'unhappy, moody, unsettled and all else that you can imagine ... It
is so unhealthy.' Angell sympathized with Cushing but suggested that
he would feel better once he had made up his mind. Yale was happy to
take the risks associated with his health he said. Cushing finally agreed
to go. He told Simon Flexner, 'They are frank enough to say they don't
expect much and merely offer me the opportunity of living among
them. This was what led me to accept.'[69]

Cushing wrote to President Lowell of Harvard explaining that he
would have preferred to stay in Boston but could not in conscience
teach medical history after telling Hopkins that he was unqualified. He
had also realized, he said, that he had to leave Cutler alone at the
Brigham; Yale offered him the possibility of continuing to work in some
small way. At the Yale commencement that June there was tempestu-
ous applause when Angell announced that the most distinguished Yale
graduate in all of medicine would be coming home. 'Once an Eli always
an Eli,' Cushing told a friend.[70]

The Cushings rented a big frame house in New Haven – much like
their Boston home – at 691 Whitney Avenue. They arrived in October
1933 to begin their new life with, in Fulton's words, 'all their goods and
chattels, including Miss Stanton.'[71]

FOURTEEN

Regius Professor at Yale

Income was not a problem for the Cushings, because the family investments gradually recovered. Economically, it was not a bad time to have left the Peter Bent Brigham Hospital, which was strapped for funds for the rest of the 1930s, creating endless, demoralizing problems for Harvey's successor, Elliott Cutler, who did not have a happy tenure. While Yale, too, had to implement minor austerity measures, life for the Cushings in New Haven and wherever they summered was materially comfortable and intellectually rich.

Harvey's major concern was his health. When he reached New Haven in 1933, he collapsed like an exhausted runner, suffering from a gastric ulcer and the effects of Buerger's disease in his feet and legs. He never fully recovered, and periodically he was hospitalized or confined to a wheelchair and crutches. He never operated at Yale, never taught a course, produced no significant new research, and in those respects did not fulfill the role of a high-performing Sterling professor.

He often complained that the vascular degeneration was spreading to his brain – a fear that apparently haunted him for years – but his mind remained sharp. In six years at Yale he published several elegant essays and addresses, a 500-page edition of his war diaries, and, with Louise Eisenhardt, his monumental 800-page work on the meningiomas. He participated in the intellectual life of the university community and in some of the ongoing affairs of the neurosurgical and American medical worlds. He enjoyed companionship and care from the protégé who was virtually a surrogate son, John Fulton. Thanks to daughter Betsey's marriage, he found himself suddenly connected to the president of the United States. He had this temperamental affinity with FDR: Cushing, too, was never photographed in his wheelchair or on crutches.

A friend, undoubtedly thinking of Osler's final years at Oxford, had observed that Harvey would be 'a sort of Regius' at Yale.[1] He was. He added distinction to the university and its medical school just by living among them.

~

In the last months in Boston, Cushing had pushed himself as hard as he possibly could, working through the summer of 1933 without even a pretense of a holiday. He wanted to finish the book on meningeal tumors that he had been thinking about for twenty years and was now writing with Louise Eisenhardt. They thought they had to finish it before he left the Brigham and all his case records. At the same time he pushed for final research success, working with a young investigator, Kenneth W. Thompson. He hoped to nail down his claims about pituitary basophilism by inducing it experimentally in dogs. Then he hoped to show that basophilism extended to the posterior pituitary lobe and – consistent with his old hobbyhorse about it secreting directly into the cerebrospinal circulation – that it was probably the cause of essential hypertension.

Neither of these projects panned out. The research results could not support the hypotheses. When Cushing tried them out anyway in papers delivered on a quick trip to Europe immediately after his move to Yale, he was rebuffed and they were rejected for publication. He continued to support Thompson's work at Yale for several years, but both it and his own thinking gradually became bogged down in the swamp of confusion in the late 1930s about pituitary hormones and 'antihormones.' Expressing no regret, he gradually let go of the pituitary and of active involvement in research.[2]

He was more frustrated at being unable to complete the tumor book that summer, in part because what he first thought was hunger pains was soon diagnosed as an ulcer. A milk-based 'Sippy' diet got him through the transplant to Yale and the European trip, but when he returned to New Haven he had to spend much of the winter of 1933–4 in hospital. His mobility had also bothered him in his final Boston months – he could not walk more than a hundred yards at a time – and even as his ulcer healed, his feet and toes rebelled and became extremely painful. He sometimes thought that the stress of everything to do with his retirement had exacerbated his condition, perhaps even causing the ulcer as per the theory he had propounded in his Toronto paper on just that subject. It was almost comforting and certainly traditional to fall prey to a disease one had written about.[3] In fact, his condition may have been exacerbated from time to time by Raynaud's phenomenon, spasms of vascular constriction in the extremities related to both Buerger's disease and stress.

The pressure of pituitary research was his excuse for not going to Washington to attend the inauguration of Betsey's father-in-law, Franklin Delano Roosevelt, as president on March 4, 1933. Everyone else in the family went. Kate burst with pride to see Betsey and Jimmy Roosevelt in the presidential party – 'Our little Betsey, I murmured to Min – it seemed so wonderful' – and then found FDR's ringing speech, declaring that there was nothing to fear but fear itself, the greatest moment of all. Kate became an ardent FDR supporter. Harvey, who had voted for Herbert Hoover, joked that with the bank holiday Roosevelt had mandated, he wasn't sure how the family would get home.[4] The Roosevelts had spent a night at Little Boars Head while en route to Campobello Island in the summer of 1932 and had entertained the Cushings at Hyde Park that Christmas. In April 1933 Harvey visited the White House, where he found FDR bantering with British Prime Minister Ramsay MacDonald.[5]

Cushing was in Washington that spring to give a presidential address to the Fifteenth Congress of American Physicians and Surgeons. He used the glittering occasion – an audience of fifteen hundred colleagues

– to talk about 'Medicine at the Crossroads,' portraying a profession being seduced by the false gods of overspecialization and science, and falling prey to modern society's love of 'Babylonian' hospitals and laboratories. The next big public issue, already on the table, was a report of a Committee on the Costs of Medical Care, created by several charitable foundations, recommending that America move to some form of national health insurance. Harvey argued in his speech that the profession should have no interest in 'socialized' medicine. The best voluntary health insurance that citizens could take out would be to cut their tobacco usage, he claimed, speaking from painful experience. Medicine needed fewer commissions made up of well–intentioned philanthropists, sociologists, economists, and lawyers. It needed more humanists and historians to speak from and for its great traditions.[6]

He did not think that his connection with FDR would lead him into political adventures. He told correspondents that he certainly would not abuse his position by lobbying the White House. He could not resist, however, writing to FDR on several occasions on behalf of the Surgeon-General's Library, which wanted a new building. He also suggested to FDR that some kind of superbureau of public health should be created. Responding with polite evasiveness, FDR decided to make his own use of Cushing. In 1934 Secretary of Labor Frances Perkins asked him to sit on a medical advisory committee giving input on the health insurance issue to the administration's Committee on Economic Security. Harvey was reluctant to serve, but his son-in-law urged him to find the time.[7]

For about six months in 1934–5 Cushing found himself at the center of one of the first rounds of serious political infighting about health insurance for Americans. Uncharacteristically, he at first slipped into the role of a moderate centrist, bombarded on one hand with the statist views of the leaders of the Milbank charitable foundation and, on the other, with the American Medical Association's fierce opposition to any government role in health insurance. Cushing conscientiously canvassed friends at home and abroad, collecting thick packets of conflicting views. His middle-of-the-road conclusion was that some form of health insurance was bound to come, but local experimentation and much study were needed.

His bottom line was that nothing should be imposed on medicine without its consent. He was very uneasy, he admitted, at the thought of 'turning the management of our old profession, which has done pretty well for the world so far, over to an organization of social workers who may be very high-minded but who really don't know what the practice of medicine is all about or its difficulties.' If the state were to take over American medicine, bright young men would chose other professions.[8] When the Milbank-connected advocates, J.A. Kingsbury and Edgar Sydenstricker, seemed to be manipulating the advisory committee into endorsing health insurance – the maneuvering was byzantine even by New Deal standards – Cushing balked and wrote several letters, including one to FDR, making clear his dissent and determination not to be used as 'window-dressing.'[9]

The advisory committee fizzled – its final report never saw the light of day and had no influence. Almost everyone who had participated in the debate realized that American opinion on health insurance had not crystallized and that much more study and debate were needed. Neither the Committee on Economic Security nor the White House was prepared to go to bat for any scheme of national health insurance – it would be hard enough trying to pass Social Security – and the matter was dropped. The American Medical Association spanked the Milbank Fund by threatening to boycott the Borden's milk products that were the source of its money. Through 1933–4 Cushing had been promoted by some of his friends as a possible president of the AMA. He urged them to drop the idea as he could not possibly stand up to the 'barnstorming' it would entail.[10] The state of his health suggests that he was sincere. If he had ever had medical-political aspirations, the time had long since passed. He told Edgar Sydenstricker how alarmed he was at committee meetings to observe Sydenstricker's chain-smoking and apparent development of a gastric ulcer similar to his own. The health reformer died from a coronary within two years.[11]

~

Betsey Roosevelt also smoked heavily, and she wore herself out helping with the presidential campaign in 1932. The secretaries and medics in Cushing's circle often remarked on how thin she was and wondered about her health. She had evidently been unsure of the role she wanted to play in life, earlier telling her mother about a friend who had suggested that she might take a law degree. Kate revealed much about her own conservatism in chiding her daughter:

> Why yes Betsey I always thought you would make a good lawyer. Why not start right in summer school & let the little house go to pot. Intellect's the thing, the legal mind & all that. Never mind about keeping the house neat & planning J's meals. Anybody can do that ha ha & when he makes speeches don't grin admiringly in the back ground but tell him how much better you could do it. It all goes to make a happy lawyer's home.
>
> You have the priceless asset of a natural dignity, good taste and sound common sense – & a sense of humor.[12]

Betsey settled down to be a housekeeper and mother, first in Boston, where Jimmy went into the insurance business, then, soon after FDR's election, in Washington. Harvey's first two grandchildren, Sara, born in 1933, and Kate, in 1936, remembered their Cushing grandfather, whom they called 'No-papa,' only as a dim figure who must not be disturbed. Both Betsey and Jimmy were soon drawn to the flame of FDR's power. In 1936 Jimmy became his father's principal secretary. She was his favorite daughter-in-law – smart, spontaneous, funny, and loyal – and often filled in as White House hostess when Eleanor Roosevelt was away.

The politician and the brain surgeon were cordial though not close. In June 1934 the presidential yacht dropped in at New Haven harbor long enough for FDR to get an honorary degree from Yale. John Fulton was chagrined that because of his wife's violent anti–New Deal views, the Cushings did not invite them to meet the man she hated. Cushing himself was a little miffed when he dropped in at the White House over

Easter 1935, apparently unannounced, and found the welcome a bit chilly.[13] On the other hand, after Barbara graduated from Westover School (at the top of her class, much to her father's pleasure), Betsey threw a coming-out party for her at the White House. Babe Cushing began her public life in American society at the top.

Babe's entrance on the social scene was particularly welcome to the family because some months earlier she had been a badly hurt passenger in an automobile accident following a party on Long Island – another liquor-driven crack-up – and had to have major reconstructive surgery on her teeth and face. Franklin D. Roosevelt Jr had been at the same party and in the next car. He was also on the scene with Babe in early 1936 when she was photographed, looking glamorous and unscarred, in a New York night club. Harvey did not approve of either nightclubs or society photographers. His postscript on an otherwise bantering note to the president had an obvious bite: 'You might tell son Franklin that the next time he takes Barbara to a nightclub, whether or not he allows photographs of the face to be taken, all will be over between us.' The wordly president asked the puritanical surgeon, 'When will you ever become old enough to realize that the new generation goes to a Night Club instead of Sunday School and that being photographed there is the modern parallel of the pretty colored card you and I used to get for good behavior and perfect attendance?'[14]

Cushing warmed politically to FDR. As the 1936 presidential campaign developed, he decided that he preferred Betsey's father-in-law to the hapless Republican candidate, Alf Landon. Cushing believed that the medical profession ought to feel indebted to Roosevelt for having helped sidetrack health insurance, and he was one of those rentiers who thought the New Deal protected his pocketbook: 'So many people in those days of rugged individualism forever ended by the crash in 1929 found like myself that they had been deluded in their trust of supposedly reputable bankers that they strongly sympathize with the President in having laws passed that now make it possible for them to leave their money in banks with safety and to make investments with reasonable security.'[15]

The Cushings agreed to host a luncheon at their New Haven home on October 22 for the campaigning president, his entourage, the mayor of New Haven, the governor of Connecticut, and other guests. FDR enjoyed a large meal and several cocktails in Cushing's study, leaning casually against the doctor's priceless editions of Vesalius while chatting with selected Yale students. The crippled president seemed fresher and more exuberant than anyone else in his campaign team. The Yale Faculty Club's catering manager reported to John Fulton that she was 'quite taken aback by two things, the utter charm and resilience of Mr. Roosevelt, and the complete stupidity and bourgeoisie of all the henchmen who accompanied him.' After lunch, FDR briefly addressed a crowd of thirty to fifty thousand people on the New Haven Green. 'The Hospital did a rushing business collecting people who had fallen out of windows, off fire escapes and out of the stately elms,' Fulton noted. Two days after FDR's landslide re-election, the Cushings motored to Hyde Park for the christening of granddaughter Kate.[16]

~

Cushing expressed no regret at leaving the operating room and showed no hankering to return to it. If he was not visibly unhappy at giving up the job of taking out tumors, he did become distressed at having given up all the tumors he had taken out over many years. When he moved to Yale, he left all his specimens and patient records in Boston. He thought he had an agreement that they would be retained at Harvard or the Brigham as the crux of a national brain tumor 'registry,' a center for the study and classification of tumors, old and new. The impetus for creating the Cushing Tumor Registry came from some of his students, who thought they could profit from access to such material, but it was also inspired by the example that Amory Codman had set some years earlier in creating a Bone Sarcoma Registry. Louise Eisenhardt was to tend the collection in Boston as its curator, and Harvard had more or less committed itself to providing some space and a little money to launch the project.[17]

Immediately after Cushing's exit from Boston there were problems allocating space and finding money. Everything, of course, was a matter of priorities, and nurturing Cushing's tumor collection was not high on anyone else's list of priorities. Louise Eisenhardt, a scholarly faithful servant, lacked the leadership skills to advance the cause. As tumor registry correspondence between New Haven and Boston descended into predictable acrimony, both parties realized that the best solution would be for Cushing to reclaim his specimens and their nanny. In 1935 Eisenhardt and approximately eight hundred jars of brains and tumors moved to New Haven. Cushing also decided to have all of his Brigham patient records, some 50,000 pages of them, photographed at his expense. The cost was $3,500, the equivalent of more than $100,000 today. With Eisenhardt, his specimens, and his records all at hand at Yale, Harvey could think about going back to work on the meningioma book.[18]

First he gave the best of his war diaries to the world. While working on *Consecratio Medici* he had told his editor, Edward Weeks of Little, Brown and Company, that his war journals were full of rich material but could not be published until after his death. Weeks called Cushing at intervals to tease him about being so healthy, and, as the Boston establishment was about to close, finally was given access. Weeks arranged to have four long excerpts published in *Atlantic Monthly* in 1934. They generated a flood of mostly favorable letters to Cushing (though, not surprisingly, the Boston Common Society was offended by his lighthearted account of 'The Battle of Boston Common') and brought in 1,900 new subscriptions to *Atlantic* from the medically connected. Weeks immediately began to pester Cushing to agree to a book. In 1936 Little, Brown published *From A Surgeon's Journal*, a 510-page edition of the diaries. Harvey dedicated it to Kate, 'for her sympathy and understanding through all this.'

He had deleted excess detail, toned down some of his disdain for certain individuals and allies, and eliminated potentially libelous passages. Little of the spirit and tone of the originals was lost, and many maps and illustrations complemented a handsome design. To modern readers the book seems excessively detailed, as are most of Cushing's writings. Most reviewers in 1936 found *From A Surgeon's Journal* a fascinating and harrowing read. The *New York Times* critic said that Cushing was 'one of the most alert-minded observers ever to report on a war.' His former colleague and doctor, Sidney Schwab, told him, 'You have gotten into your book the atmosphere of war, its rush, resiliency, its strangeness, its foolishness, stupidities, its heroism and its wastefulness.' Cushing himself and some of his reviewers thought the volume's effect should be to further the peace movement. So did Mark Van Doren, writing in the *Nation* of his horror at what he thought were Cushing's appalling passages about enjoying the war and comparing it to a football game. The only serious fuss by anyone actually mentioned in the book issued from the British firm of Burberry and Company, makers of raingear, who threatened legal action if the British edition repeated a comment that one of the two greatest failures of the war had been the Burberry raincoat. The phrase was changed to 'waterproof raincoat.' There was no complaint from the institution Cushing named as the other great failure, the Church of England.[19]

In his memoirs Edward Weeks rated Cushing the most exacting author he had ever dealt with. He had never seen the likes of Cushing's fastidiousness and attention to minute detail – almost matched, he added, by Madeline Stanton's. Stanton faithfully served in New Haven as Harvey's secretary and jack-of-all-manuscripts. Unfortunately, she had stopped keeping a diary. The editing of *Surgeon's Journal* included arcane and lengthy discussions of the use of dots versus dashes, the need to use en-dashes instead of em-dashes, and who should pay the large cost of all the changes Cushing insisted upon in the galley proofs. Surgical and literary persnicketiness had a common root.[20]

Harvey had almost had enough. He had neither the appetite nor the energy to write another book-length biography – certainly not an autobiography, and not the biography of William Welch, which many urged him to undertake (it was eventually written by Simon Flexner and son). He had no interest in rewriting his Osler biography, say, to make it shorter and more readable, but he did attend to detail, issuing a four-page 'Corrigenda and Addenda' for future printings.

~

'Writing comes after reading.'[21] Cushing's collection of medical volumes, most of them beautifully bound in vellum and calf, had lined the locked glass bookcases in his office at the Brigham. For years, Harvey had lived a triple life – not only an obsessed surgeon and a driven author but also a hopeless bibliomaniac. He scoured dealers' catalogues, firing off orders, haggling over prices, tearing open the packages from England, Italy, Austria, and France which Madeline Stanton brought up from the customs house. His favorite relaxation while traveling was visiting second-hand book shops. He spent relatively lavishly – far more freely than Osler had – and by the 1920s the European book dealers, like the European neurosurgeons, began coming to him.

Beginning with Vesalius, he had broadened out into collecting practically anything to do with the history of anatomy. Cushing wanted any book with bones in it, the dealers liked to say. E.P. Goldschmidt, antiquarian bookseller of London, had been impressed when Cushing bought a rare treatise on anatomy from him at a high price 'without wincing.' According to Stanton, Cushing paid $1,500 for a single book in 1929, whereas $1,000 had previously seemed embarrassingly high. Osler, on the market a generation earlier and a bit less affluent, had never paid more than about $250. Today, many of the books they bought are worth hundreds of thousands of dollars. Goldschmidt selected a rare octavo of Paré's *Dix livres* to take on his 1929 visit to Cushing in Boston. He was humbled to find that Cushing's shelves contained two slightly differing copies of that work, plus a dozen more scarce Parés.[22]

Cushing was connected with most of the principals in Anglo-American medical bibliophilia and with all the leading book dealers, medical librarians, and medical bibliographers on two continents. He was a close friend of the great builders of the U.S. Surgeon-General's Library (now the National Library of Medicine), John Shaw Billings and Fielding Garrison. He was thoroughly disliked by an Osler protégé and librarian at the New York Academy of Medicine, Archie Malloch, who believed that Harvey had purloined Lister letters that belonged to Malloch's

father (Cushing denied the insinuation, saying that his only Malloch-
Lister letter had come from Osler).[23] He had been a crucial patron of
Osler's hapless nephew, William W. Francis, who had cataloged Osler's
books at Oxford while Harvey was working on the biography and had
then moved to McGill as curator of the Osler Library, built to house
Osler's gift of his magnificent collection. Cushing spoke at the opening
of the Osler Library in 1929, just as he spoke at the opening of the
Welch Library at Hopkins, the opening of the Allen Medical Library in
Cleveland, and innumerable other bibliocentric events.

On these occasions he reflected wittily on the breeding habits of
books (their tendency to multiply faster than rabbits), their diseases
('they have worms; they wear out their clothing, break their backs,
dislocate their joints, and require the constant care of a
bibliotherapeutist'), the importance of libraries to the medical profession, and the need to inoculate medical students with the library habit
(more important than familiarity with the kymograph or the laboratory, but not easy to instill 'in these days when reading as a fine art is
about gone'). His favorite book anecdote was of a physician coming up
to his display of Vesaliana at a conference and asking for a sample,
thinking he would be given vaseline. Seriously and personally, Cushing
spoke of books as a doctor's 'greatest source of relaxation, his greatest
solace in times of trouble.' Both Madeline Stanton and John Fulton
noticed how books comforted him while he was mourning death in his
operating room and in the family. 'He cuddled old books and hugged
them close' was said of Cushing, as it had been of Oliver Wendell
Holmes.[24]

Unlike some book collectors, Cushing read and thought about his
books – not only absorbing their contents but learning all he could
about their authors, designers, printers, binders, illustrators, and imita-
tors. Geoffrey Jefferson wrote that Cushing was one of the few men who
was a hero to his booksellers, respected not just for his pocketbook but
for his love of the product. 'Here was one of the greatest surgeons of the
epoch,' Goldschmidt wrote, 'the acknowledged master of all the intri-
cacies of the convolutions of the human brain, who would question me

on a problem of early printing with the modesty and eagerness of a fourth-form schoolboy.' When the subject changed to Vesalius, Goldschmidt added, Cushing spoke with the authority of an expert.[25]

His bibliographic friends included Geoffrey Keynes in England, the workaholic surgeon brother of John Maynard Keynes, and the eccentric and hard-drinking *New York Times* book antiquarian, Leonard L. Mackall. John Fulton represented the next generation, spending his wife's money to collect all the classic works in physiology. Fulton was even more enthusiastic about medical books and medical biography than Cushing. In the 1920s Cushing had introduced Fulton to many of his bookish friends, most importantly to Arnold Klebs, an acquaintance since Hopkins days.

Klebs was the physician son of Edwin Klebs, co-discoverer of the diphtheria bacillus. Arnold moved to America with his father in the 1890s, and he met Cushing and other members of the Johns Hopkins group during the years he was practicing medicine. He became an ardent Osler worshipper. After the war, he retired to his native Switzerland to live with his second wife and his medical books in a villa on the shores of Lake Geneva. Klebs had once hoped to teach medical history at Johns Hopkins. He began collecting the earliest printed medical books – the incunabula, published before 1500 – and kept up a long-distance correspondence and friendship with Cushing that ripened over the years. On his European trips in the late 1920s and early 1930s, Cushing spent much of his time with Klebs, much of it discussing the fine points of very rare books. He came to consider Klebs – who was writing what everyone thought would be the definitive guide to the medical incunabula – his bibliographic mentor.[26]

Harvey insisted that Klebs be their house guest on his American trips – to the disgruntlement of Kate Cushing and Madeline Stanton. To Stanton, he was 'the unspeakable Klebs,' a Hunnish Teuton who was rumored to have mistreated his wives and whose presence gave her the shivers: 'How the Chief can stomach him I don't see – except as a bibliophile.'[27] Kate told Harvey that Klebs was a kind of 'bibliophilic octopus' who had him in his tentacles. She almost certainly resented

the large amounts of money that her husband, who for years had lectured her on the need for frugality, was pouring into incunabula and
other rare books, often on Klebs's advice. Cushing, who appears to
have tried to hide his extravagances from his wife, rationalized to a
friend that they were 'a better investment I believe than bonds – certainly better than mining stock which is the usual way in which doctors
impoverish their families.'[28] Kate seems to have spent her discretionary
money on antiques, another form of collecting.

What would he do with his investment? When he left Boston, he
gave away his runs of journals and recent medical texts. It was unlikely
that any of his children would want his books, and his first assumption
was that his executors would sell them. As he began setting his affairs in
order, the idea grew on him that perhaps he should will his library to
Yale, the institution to which he owed so much. In September 1934 he
and Fulton went to Canada for the opening of Wilder Penfield's Montreal
Neurological Institute. Harvey gave the keynote address, one final plea
for psychiatrists, neurosurgeons, and other mind-workers to unite under the banner of neurology. He again visited the beautiful Osler Library at McGill. On the train home, he told Fulton that he was going to
leave his books to Yale and suggested that his young friend might do
the same with his collection. Fulton was thrilled at the idea of such a
posthumous collaboration. A few days later, Cushing woke up in the
night with the idea that Klebs might be persuaded to do likewise, 'so
that the three could go down to bibliographic posterity hand in hand.'

Cushing put the idea to Klebs, who announced that he was 'heart
and soul' in favor of the plan. The trio began revising their wills and
adjusting their purchases to avoid overlapping, and Cushing began to
consult Yale friends about the kind of building that might eventually
house the great trinitarian collection. Both Fulton and Klebs worried
from time to time that their friend was still an easy mark in the business: 'He has no guile or cunning when it comes to dealing with these
high-powered Hebraic booksellers,' Fulton wrote in 1936, 'and I shudder to think how much they have extracted from him during the past
year.'[29]

Cushing intended that his personal papers, including his diaries, would go with his books. He had saved practically everything – and Madeline Stanton had salvaged material he tried not to save – and he spent many hours in his Yale years arranging his massive correspondence files, often writing important autobiographical and biographical notes. Cushing was always comfortable looking back, comfortable analysing history and tradition and exploring the circumstances that influence character. He had the nostalgist's inclination to label each period of his past – boyhood, Yale, Hopkins – as the best years of his life. Friends of a lifetime were dropping away now – Perry Harvey died in 1932, W.T. Councilman in 1933, William Welch in 1934 – thereby inspiring him to write elegant obituary essays stressing the roots of achievement in American life and values. His personal sense of history inclined him to celebrate the culture of the Puritans of New England and their descendants who had journeyed over the mountains to settle western Massachusetts and upstate New York and the Western Reserve, and had built the towns, cities, colleges, libraries, and medical schools of the American heartland.

~

While Cushing did not like the passing of the old order in America, he did not identify with the conservative dinosaurs satirized in two of the popular novels of the 1930s: John P. Marquand's *The Late George Apley* and George Santayana's *The Last Puritan*. He had known those types in Boston – inbred, hidebound, narrow-minded descendants of old families, who set their faces against all kinds of change. Cushing enjoyed seeing them mocked in fiction. Of course, he knew he was a puritan – some of his friends teased him that he was the true last Puritan – but his achievement in life was nothing if not progressive.

Cushing had worked unremittingly hard, eschewed vanities and pleasures, respected family values and traditions, and been a great innovator in American and world medicine. Following the trails of his ancestors, following a trail partly blazed for him by the brilliant drug-debilitated Halsted, Cushing had been the puritan as perfectionist surgeon – no germs, no bleeding, no sloppiness, no shortcuts. In applying these conservative methods in a previously rough-and-ready, blood-drenched surgical milieu, he had, Cromwell-like, wrought a revolution. He had created modern neurosurgery. If he was the product of a culture and region aptly characterized as 'the last distinct footprint of Puritanism,' then his surgical achievement, neurosurgery as he created it, might be characterized as the last distinct handiwork of Puritanism.

One flaw in this generalization is that puritanism's handiwork is by no means over in American medicine or in American life. Many, perhaps most, of the most important innovations are still made by neopuritanical practitioners of many religious backgrounds and of non-religious backgrounds. Even in Cushing's day, no one had to be of New England Puritan descent to become a driven, high-achieving neurosurgeon. A strong argument can be made that the Jewish American experience of the twentieth century brought to neurosurgery and many other fields of American life intensity, discipline, and creativity – also egotism and competitive fire – that were similar to the fuel of Cushing's ambition. Cushing never blindly idolized the past or sweepingly condemned the present. The rebuilt, modernized, and progressive Yale University to which he returned the 1930s, for example, seemed to him to represent a fulfillment, not the shortcomings of its founders' values. It was Eden updated. Putting his sons' experiences behind him, he made a point of celebrating the high quality of campus life and the improved educational experience that Yale gave its men.

There were two problems with Cushing's version of applied, secularized Puritanism. The conservative side of it, reinforced by age, did have a bias against innovation, both cultural innovations in the 1920s and Walter Dandy's invention of ventriculography in neurosurgery. Hesitancy to opt for the new and the unproven is often sound practice and usually was for Cushing. Sometimes, usually in nonprofessional areas of life, Cushing seemed to resist change for no good reason. 'His first impulse is always no,' Kate once told daughter Barbara after she had had an argument with her father. The Cushing women must have found it particularly exasperating to be lectured about the evils of cigarette smoking by a father who had been a heavy smoker for forty years. More seriously, Cushing was also suspicious of most other changes in women's roles. He had not seen the need for women to vote, go to college, or go into medicine. He did not like makeup or fashionable clothes – which once caused Barbara to satirize his taste by visiting him in full Puritan plainness of dress and meekness of spirit.[30]

A second problem was Cushing's addictive personality. Addicted to tobacco, addicted to work. A driven man, lacking a sense of balance in life, perhaps knowing that he lacked it. Harvey Cushing the American Puritan was a different type from William Osler the British Anglican, who taught that the most important qualities in life were balance, proportion, moderation. Cushing interpreted Osler literally but incorrectly, I think, in believing that the 'master word' in both medicine and life was 'work.' He worked too much and too hard. He tried to be too many things – surgeon, researcher, teacher, author, administrator. His family, among others, paid a price. Later generations of neurosurgeons may also have paid a price for believing that their specialty required the stamina and genius of macho supermen, that they had to work like Cushing and other overachievers, relaxing differently perhaps but usually not relaxing at all. There has been a similar dynamic in other fields of surgery and medicine. Does workaholism necessarily go with the job?

Could there have been the achievement without the work? Harvey Cushing achieved more than William Osler in advancing a medical specialty – indeed, he was the principal figure in an epic medical and American drama. William Osler, more peripatetic, less driven, and more cosmopolitan, may have had a better life. Certainly he was much easier to live with. Both great physicians served their patients wonderfully well. Both had discarded faith in the supernatural for a commitment to medicine as a divine calling, a total commitment to the well-being of patients, to serving suffering humanity: *Consecratio medici*.

Neither physician advocated socialized medicine, and in this sense both were individualists, Cushing the more pronounced. Both deeply believed that the state should promote public health. Both saw the medical profession, the old guild itself, as the defining social component of their lives and thought. Collectively, medicine was the sum of the strivings of every medical student, every family practitioner, every specialist and researcher, every nurse, and every orderly. The striving was not for money, not for fame in the secular (nonmedical) world. It was for human betterment, and its overall effect seemed to be overwhelmingly positive. In Osler's and Cushing's lifetimes, medicine was a profession on the frontier of the best kind of social change: the saving, improving, and prolonging of human life.

In the United States it was a profession that was forced to be especially conscious of the needs of its patients because the patients were so especially demanding. In the democratic, egalitarian America in which the Cushing doctors practiced medicine, physicians could not so easily disdain patients, could not unaccountably hurt patients, could not dismiss patients' demands for treatment. In rich America, physicians such as Cushing, who were idealistically unconcerned about making money in medicine – though it helped to live off the rent paid by the May Company in downtown Cleveland or to get grants from Rockefeller oil money – were free to take the treatment of patients, generals, and housemaids alike to stunningly high levels of complexity and excellence. The rise of American medicine in general and neurosurgery in particular was a product of American puritanism, American democracy, and American wealth.

∼

In 1938 a Jewish reader of *From A Surgeon's Journal* wrote to Cushing wondering what in the world he meant by describing a wind at sea as 'a veritable "white squall" which only lacks the scratching Jew to larboard.' His correspondent was fairly certain that this was a racial slur, and she sarcastically asked if Dr Cushing noticed any difference when he opened the brain of a 'scratching Jew' and that of a New England Yankee.

Cushing replied immediately and apologetically. The phrase, he said, was an unfortunate one; and had I known it was going to cause confusion or distress on the part of some of my Jewish friends, I would not have permitted it to be printed. It happens to be taken from a poem called 'The White Squall' written by William M. Thackeray once on a time when crossing the Eastern Mediterranean in a small boat crowded with seasick passengers.

You have a very natural and entirely praiseworthy pride of race; and during the War the body louse, which was shown to be a carrier of trench fever, showed no respect either for Jew or Gentile.[31]

On another occasion, a Boston medical librarian, Zoltàn Haraszti, was thrilled to be invited to dinner at the Cushing home to meet Henry Sigerist. He became deeply embarrassed, though, when the postprandial conversation turned to Jewish jokes, and he realized that no one in the company knew he was Jewish. 'I chiefly blame myself for the initial mistake which I made ...' he wrote Cushing the next day. 'I do not mind Jewish jokes if it is clearly understood that I am a Jew – so that I am in a position to laugh or to reply in kind. Further, I too have a sense of humor and know that Jewish jokes can be an excellent pastime, almost indispensable, especially when for some reason or other the Irish ones are barred.' He was writing to Cushing, he said, out of respect for the surgeon and for his own self-respect. Cushing replied briefly, thanking him for the letter and stating, 'I take people for what they are, not for their color, or race, or religion.'[32]

Cushing lived most of his life in a society that traded continually and unself-consciously in ethnic stereotypes, some harmless, some ugly. His correspondence files, both incoming and outgoing, are speckled with references to 'Hebrews,' Irish, 'darkies,' 'niggers,' and 'coons.' Cushing and most of his friends believed that there were distinct ethnic and racial traits. Sometimes they made fun of them – when citing the folk wisdom of uneducated old darkies – or, as Cushing did, in becoming fans of the popular black-face radio show 'Amos and Andy.' Sometimes in their professional correspondence they commented on whether or not a person's ethnicity would cause problems. What we now see as the racist overtones of such language came naturally and almost innocently. There is no evidence that it directly affected Cushing's surgical practice. He was not a bigot. He appears to have operated indiscriminately on black and white patients, gentiles and Jews. Open the skull, and a brain is a brain is a brain. There is no evidence that Cushing ever gave a moment's credence to crude views that race significantly affected brain structure.

(The one qualification may be the notion he – and others – tried out in the 1930s that blacks, being happy-go-lucky, might be less prone to gastric ulcer. When the evidence seemed inconclusive, he dropped the idea. Similarly, writing about pituitary basophilism, but with evident self-doubt, he told a friend, 'I have never heard of one of these cases in a negro; in fact, negroes seem far less prone to endocrinological disorders than white people – particularly Hebrews, if Hebrews are white people. Perhaps it is because I have gotten out of touch with darkies since I came north.')[33]

He accepted the structure of black-white relations in the United States and in the medical world as he found it. Throughout his lifetime, there was formal and informal segregation everywhere in the country, including in many hospitals and doctors' offices. Cushing accepted the status quo wherever he worked. The Harvard Medical School, for example, did admit a few black students. In 1916 one of them asked Cushing's advice about whether he should apply for a hospital position in Boston: 'I gave him a very frank opinion, doubtless tinged by my experiences in the South, as to the utter impossibility of it so far as the Brigham was concerned. He, however, is a very worthy young fellow, and did excellent work in the School, and I think would be a perfectly satisfactory person to send abroad, where there is less racial feeling, – in fact no racial feeling.'[34]

In 1929 Cleveland's director of public health and welfare asked his opinion about having colored nurses and interns at the municipal hospital. Cushing's answer was a clear statement of his views and very representative of his time:

> My opinion in this particular matter is not worth much and is perhaps colored by my long experience in Baltimore where white and colored folks are

necessarily separated in the Hospital. We have much to learn from the South in these matters. They handle the negro problem with far greater understanding, appreciation and, I may add, respect for the colored race than we show in the North.

We occasionally have a colored medical student in our school. They sometimes have done well and have come up for our hospital examinations. I have always frankly told these young men that I thought they would do far better for their race if they would take their hospital appointments in an institution that was devoted to colored people; that this would save them embarrassment as well as ourselves. We have a good many Southern women who are patients here, and that they should be given a physical examination by a negro, however well educated, is simply unthinkable. This, I am sure, you can understand.

I think it would be far better for the City of Cleveland, if the colored population has reached that stage, to establish a hospital for negros in which they can prove their worth. The time may come when we will perhaps have to take a different attitude in these matters, but I don't think the time is here yet. If you should put colored nurses and colored internes in the City Hospital to-day, you would have to put them in the Lakeside to-morrow as pressure would promptly be brought upon you to do so. I am sure that colored women would often make excellent trained nurses as they have shown themselves to be excellent nursery maids. But this will mean that colored men who are their friends and visitors will have to appear at the nurses' parties and receptions and this would be absolutely disastrous to the whole social status of your training school.

These are not things that I like to say, but I am quite sure the more intelligent of the colored people in any community would feel that they are true.[35]

The treatment of members of America's Jewish population had to be more subtle. In Cushing's youth, the 1880s, descendants of the early Jewish Americans, most of whom had immigrated from Germany and were assimilated into the German or American culture, or both, were beginning to enter medicine and other professions in significant numbers. At the same time, a major new wave of poor Jewish immigrants from Eastern Europe was beginning to pour into the United States. They were forced to start at the bottom of American society, but they aimed for the top. By the 1920s and 1930s, their children were rising very fast and were the harbingers of what would become one of the most spectacular ethnic immigrant achievements in American history.

As the Jews rose, they had to cope with the stereotype, grounded in some measure of forced reality, of their people as money-hungry, pushy, and culturally crude. William Osler seems never to have held such views. But Harvey Cushing and almost all of his friends – certainly such members of his circle as Cutler, Fulton, and Stanton, and Britishers such as Geoffrey Jefferson – took the image for granted and measured the Jews they met against it. Was a young Jewish man a 'typical' Hebrew? – in which case he was not very attractive or welcome. Or was he untypical, in being, say, well mannered, sophisticated, and professional, and thus perfectly acceptable? Simple ability was not sufficient. 'I just now seem to be surrounded by Hebrews of unquestioned ability but they simply don't get along with anybody,' Cushing wrote to W.G. MacCallum at Johns Hopkins in 1925. 'Since writing Osler's biography, I have rather come to conclude that personality is the most important thing in the world. It almost always goes with ability, of course, but ability without personality falls like a seed on the desert.' MacCallum concurred and said that his department, pathology, was 'going to be like the proverbial eye of a needle for all the sons of Israel – even tho I have about four or five of them now.'[36]

Letters of recommendation often included comments on how well a Jew would fit in. There was seldom a problem and hardly ever a comment about it with completely assimilated German Jews such as the Flexner brothers, Milton Winternitz at Yale, and Ernest Sachs in neurosurgery. Cushing had no hesitation about urging Harvard to invite Charles Singer, 'a very erudite Hebrew,' to give lectures. He was pleased to support the application to Phillips Exeter Academy of a patient's son named Cohen, 'an especially attractive and fine looking youngster with, so far as I can see, little of the Jew about him except his name.'[37] In 1928 Cushing worked hard to find a job for his former resident Leo

Davidoff, 'a very un-Hebraic Hebrew ... escaped the effects of the ghetto ... a Hebrew but a most attractive lad ... You will have to have a Hebrew or two on your staff, and he is about as good a one and as unhebraic as anyone you could find.'[38] Similarly, in recommending a Harvard graduate for a Jersey City hospital job, Cushing commented, 'Although he has some negro blood in his veins he comes nearer to being a white man than a good many white men I know.'[39]

There were so many bright Jews that hospitals and medical schools decided to restrict their access, usually by applying quotas. These could be informal. Cushing in 1925 decided that he did not want three Jews on his small Brigham staff at the same time. 'I have no objection to Hebrews but I do not like too many of them all at once.' But he would not tell young Weinberg that this was the reason for his rejection – and he did recommend that Sam Harvey hire him at Yale. Cushing never expressed concern about the Yale Medical School's formal quota on Jewish students, which Winternitz himself had been instrumental in imposing. When asked in 1939 for advice on getting a Jewish lad into medicine, Cushing said that he knew about the quota situation: 'Some schools, I am aware, feel obliged to limit the percentage of Jewish applicants for the reason that so many of them have better undergraduate records and are more able than other students that on that basis an unduly large percentage of students would be Jewish. But on what basis the selections are made I do not know.'[40] Yale's admissions committee based its selections roughly on Winternitz's formula: 'Never admit more than five Jews, take only two Italian Catholics, and take no blacks at all.'

'I wish things looked better in Europe,' Cushing wrote to Klebs in April 1933. 'This jew-baiting in Germany sounds bad but it may be news talk.' A former student wrote him that it was indeed bad, and soon there were appeals from German Jews and American Jews about the need to help their people relocate from Nazi Germany. Cushing's first response was to urge restraint, arguing that the good sense of the German people would put limits on 'the mad career of Hitler' and that the Jewish community's essential contributions to German life would not be suppressed.[41] He soon realized that he was wrong, and found himself doing what he could on behalf of former students and acquaintances who were trying to escape from Nazi oppression. He wanted to keep his activities private, but he agreed to Ernest Sachs's request that he serve on the New York–based Emergency Committee in Aid of Foreign Displaced Physicians, and to have his name on the letterhead.[42]

Cushing's correspondence files indicate that he tried to help or give advice to two or three dozen German and Austrian physicians or researchers, including his old friend Alfred Fröhlich, who did escape to America, and a distinguished former student, the Viennese neuro-anatomist Benno Schlesinger, about whom he corresponded extensively with Leo Davidoff. The main problem was to find jobs in American institutions, which had few vacancies and ongoing prejudices. Yale itself hired no Jewish refugee scientists in the 1930s, though Milton Winternitz personally managed to bring out at least one fellow Jew.[43]

The volume of appeals increased as the decade wore on, reaching a crescendo after the German takeover of Austria in 1938. In April that year, Cushing wrote a sentence in a letter to an old friend that would be horrifying if it were not read in context:

> What sticks in my craw is the Nazi treatment of the Jews. It would be almost better, it seems to me, to exterminate them as the Turks attempted to exterminate the Armenians. Can you imagine the terror of these poor intellectual people now trapped in Austria, trying to find some way to extricate themselves! Naturally they all wish to come over here, and places are being found for a good many of them. But even so, they may not be allowed to leave Austria; and should they finally be, they are stripped of their worldly possessions before being let loose. The whole world seems to me more or less mad, and I sometimes feel I won't be sorry to leave it.[44]

Two weeks after writing this letter, Cushing tried to confront his feelings honestly to his friend Klebs, who was showing little sympathy for bleeding hearts on the 'Jew question.' Klebs observed that persecutions happened periodically throughout history and the Jews themselves were partly responsible. Maybe, Cushing replied, but 'I can't help from sympathizing with them from afar even though I am aware that I might be irritated by them and inclined to dodge them if they were able to land here all at once; indeed my conscience smites me about a man whom Winternitz in the kindness of his heart has taken on ... He happens to be a bibliophile ... I know of course that this has been going on for centuries, but nevertheless it seems to me it might have been avoided or at least made less cruel.' In July 1939 he agreed to be one of the representatives from Connecticut on the National Committee for the Resettlement of Foreign Physicians, formed under the chairmanship of David Edsall. By the end of his life, Cushing had learned not to take the old prejudices completely for granted.[45]

❧

The vascular problems in his lower legs incapacitated him for much of the winter of 1934–5 and again in the autumn of 1936. Several toes became ulcerous and gangrenous and excruciatingly painful. In December 1935 various colleagues who examined him in the New Haven hospital – John Homans, Gil Horrax, and George Heuer – all thought it would be necessary to amputate toes or a foot, or perhaps sever the sciatic nerve. Harvey briefly became dependent on barbiturates and was deeply depressed.

The nerves from one toe were cut, and in January 1936 most of the toe had to be removed. Cushing also managed to break his heavy cigarette habit. Noticing an immediate improvement in his condition, he instantly became a convert to 'nicotine teetotalism': 'I'm really making surprising progress. Why? Three weeks without tobacco. I'm going on the road when I recover completely to lecture on the cigarette habit. Every consultant who came to see me "reached" for a cigarette before he looked at my foot. They all advised amputation of leg. None of them advised omission of tobacco. I was better in three days ... I am nasty now to people who smoke in my room.'[46]

His toe problems recurred and so did his smoking. He tried using denicotinized tobacco and corncob pipes. Fulton urged him to smoke less and drink more (Harvey had always been a very moderate drinker, with a low tolerance for alcohol). He was unable to attend his son Henry's wedding in Boston in June 1936 and was probably in his wheel-chair during the FDR luncheon that October. He was hospitalized again a few weeks later, and more toe was removed. This time, his circulation improved markedly as did his mobility. He seems to have stopped smoking more or less permanently. Even before these years, he had realized that smoking aggravated his disease and he had warned others not to be addicted.

Could things have been different? What about the option of smoking moderately? In a 1939 letter, at a time when smoking was still glamorous and years away from being medically condemned, he forgot about Osler's moderate tobacco use and addressed the issue:

> There is of course no such thing as a moderate smoker. Tomorrow under some stress or trouble such a one quickly becomes an excessive smoker and damages himself just at the time he should be taking good care of his health. There is no question whatever but that tobacco is extremely damaging to the neuro-vascular system.
>
> It is unfortunate that the victims of the habit are often doctors and still more often highly-strung surgeons who are loath to acknowledge to other lay-habitués the damaging effect of tobacco ... There seems to be at present no possible legislation to prevent the radio advertising of tobacco as a source of 'chemical consolation.' It would be just as sensible to allow the smoking of opium to be advertised in similar fashion for the same reasons.[47]

❧

Cushing saw a few patients in New Haven when his health permitted, mostly his old cases reporting in, but also a few new ones whom he referred to colleagues for neurological or neurosurgical treatment. Under Yale's mandatory retirement rule he had to retire a second time, in 1937 at age sixty-eight. Yale gave him the honorific title of Director of

Studies in Medical History. He neither directed nor formally studied medical history but was a living legend for the medical history he had made. Honors had kept coming his way, most notably a fellowship in the enormously prestigious Royal Society, a unique distinction for an American surgeon. He was nominated for the Nobel Prize in Physiology or Medicine on several occasions between 1934 and 1936 – possibly in other years as well – both for his achievements in neurosurgery and for the delineation of pituitary basophilism. He knew about the nominations, one of which, probably counterproductively, enlisted support from the White House. He expressed no regret when the prizes went to others. 'Fame lies in the silence – not in the song,' he told Klebs. Fulton observed, though, that he accepted his second retirement 'philosophically but just a little ungraciously.'[48]

In the summer of 1938 Cushing found the energy for his first trip to England and the Continent in five years, sailing on the *Queen Mary*. The main occasion was to receive an honorary Doctor of Science degree from Oxford. His physician nephew, Pat Cushing, and his surrogate son, John Fulton, accompanied him on what became a kind of grand rounds with old friends. In London he stayed at his and Osler's favorite hotel, Brown's, he toured the new facilities at the Royal College of Surgeons, lunched with C.S. Sherrington, (now an octogenarian Nobel laureate), talked books with Geoffrey Keynes, took in a meeting of the Osler Club, and spent an evening with old Sir Almroth Wright. Perhaps he even dropped in at the Cheshire Cheese.

At Oxford he was proudly hosted by Hugh Cairns, who had managed to break through the constraints of the British neurological establishment to become the university's first Nuffield Professor of Surgery. Cairns arranged a glittering luncheon at Balliol College for Cushing and thirty of his students, colleagues, and friends. At the presentation of his degree in the Sheldonian Theatre, he was cited for having navigated surgery's Northwest Passage, served in war, and written Osler's biography. The next day he gave a bedside clinic, his first in five years, at the Radcliffe Infirmary.

Back in London there was a great book sale at Sotheby's that attracted Maggs, Quaritch, Goldschmidt, and all the other prominent London dealers. Queen Mary opened a new wing at the Queen Square National Hospital for Nervous Diseases. Then the Americans flew to Paris and then to Geneva to spend time at Klebs's villa. Coming home on the *Queen Mary*, Cushing heard more horror stories about suicides by Jewish academics in Vienna. He urged Cairns to help relocate one of their mutual friends.[49]

Meningiomas: Their Classification, Regional Behaviour, Life History, and Surgical End Results, by Harvey Cushing with the collaboration of Louise Eisenhardt, was released in the autumn of 1938 by Charles C Thomas, America's leading medical publisher. In thirty-two chapters, comprising 741 pages of text, with hundreds of photographs, sketches, and tables, the authors told the complete history of Cushing's thirty-year assault on the class of tumors which had most interested him and which he had named. Narrative case histories of Leonard Wood, Tim Donovan, and Dorothy Russell were presented by name. Cushing dedicated the book to his collaborators and to his patients.

Meningiomas was hailed by reviewers as a masterpiece, a classic, an epic of neurosurgery, and proof of Cushing's stature 'as one of the great surgeons of all time.' Geoffrey Jefferson observed that it contained a whole philosophy of surgery and of the doctor-patient relationship.[50] The stories of Donovan and Russell still make harrowing reading.

The book was Cushing's last published word as a neurosurgeon. He ended it Hippocratically by remarking that new methods would make his survival percentages appear to be 'amateurish and the work of tyros – *Truly the Art is long.*' In retirement he was the grand old man of a specialty whose largest professional organization, the Harvey Cushing Society, bore his name but whose art was still short. Most American and European neurosurgeons were indebted to him for their basic operative techniques, for many of their specific procedures, and for much of their knowledge of tumors. The Cushing Brain Tumor Registry, he hoped, would become an international center for tumor studies. When it soon became clear that this was not happening, he began to wonder if the registry and its curator, Louise Eisenhardt, should be relocated to a place where some of his younger disciples, such as Oldberg and Bailey in Chicago, could keep it going after his death.[51]

Cushing had nothing to say about a major trend in neurosurgery in the 1930s. The radical young surgeons, led by Dandy at Johns Hopkins and Penfield in Montreal, were much less hesitant about sacrificing healthy brain tissue than he had been. The justification, of course, was to get at tumors and the source of epileptic seizures. Evidence from lobectomies performed by Dandy on some of his patients, and in John Fulton's laboratory on primates, seemed to show that quite a bit of brain tissue could be removed or disconnected, especially in the frontal lobes, without destroying basic intelligence or motor skill. By 1936 some neurosurgeons were beginning to do prefrontal lobotomies to try and ease the sufferings of certain patients who exhibited extreme mental illness but no identifiable organic disorder.

In Cushing's prime, his principle of respect for tissue, his surgical conservatism, and his insistence on locating real lesions would have made what came to be called 'psychosurgery' seem like a recrudescence of crude surgical aggression. I have not found any Cushing comments for or against lobotomy, a procedure that would be performed thousands of times in the 1940s and then discarded in the 1950s for want of evidence of effectiveness as the age of psychopharmaceuticals dawned. Cushing's conservative instincts and surgical conscience would almost certainly have cautioned him against doing lobotomies. In any case, the paternity of the procedure, and responsibility for it at the bar of history – a verdict not yet in – rested more with Dandy, Fulton, and others of the radical school.[52]

There is one intriguing exchange of letters in 1937 between Cushing and Dr Richard Brickner, who had written an influential book about a case of Dandy's that, more than any other, seemed to suggest that lobectomies did not harm basic intelligence. Cushing could not understand from Brickner's account exactly why Dandy had undertaken such a radical operation. He let the matter drop, though, telling Brickner, 'If enquiries were made from Dandy, he would think he was being criticized and to this he does not take kindly ... Probably no one else will

ever raise any question as to the nature of the tumor or the propriety of
the procedure.'[53]

A session on lobotomy captured the most attention at the April
1939 meeting of the Harvey Cushing Society in New Haven, timed to
celebrate the patriarch's seventieth birthday. Harvey himself gave a
talk on the end results of surgery for pituitary adenomas. The Cushings
and the Fultons lavishly entertained about one hundred neurosurgeons
and spouses, Arnold Klebs made a surprise appearance, FDR sent best
wishes, and Harvey's old operating-room orderly, Adolf Watzka, came
out of retirement to mop speakers' brows at the birthday dinner on
April 8, just as he had so many times in the past. Fulton and Eisenhardt
had arranged for the publication of a bibliography of Cushing's writings, and a group of Scandinavian disciples presented him with a special *Festschrift*. Harvey paid tribute to his co-workers and to the emergence of neurosurgery as 'perhaps the most arduous and responsible of
the many surgical specialties. We can have the great satisfaction of
knowing that only men of a certain type will venture to make it their
life work.'

Cushing closed this last speech to his colleagues with a quotation
from the Talmud: 'The day is short and work is great. The reward is also
great and the Master praises. It is not incumbent on thee to complete
the work but thou must not therefore cease from it.'[54] His new work
would be on a bio-bibliography of Vesalius and a new anthology of his
historical and biographical essays.

~

The family had gathered for his birthday, and Arnold Klebs, a house
guest, had a warm memory of overhearing Kate and Harvey giggling
together as they rehashed the party.[55] Otherwise, Fulton noted that
Cushing was often alone in these years, and thought he was lonely.
Kate spent much of her time with the girls, summering in rented homes
on Long Island. Harvey and Kate had not traveled together for years.
Son Henry was making his way more or less independently in the in-

vestment business in Boston. Fulton, Cushing's closest friend at Yale, was constantly traveling and was beginning to suffer from the effects of prodigious work – and, on too many occasions, prodigious intake of alcohol. Except for a fine dinner in Philadelphia in 1937 with the old Hopkins crowd to honor Max Brödel, and his trip to England the next year, Harvey stopped attending conferences, reunions, and other such occasions. He was the most prominent missing person at both the Peter Bent Brigham Hospital's twenty-fifth anniversary celebration and the Johns Hopkins's fiftieth.

All but one of his siblings had been dead for many years. The survivor, older brother George, had disappeared in the 1880s and turned up again more than thirty years later as a man whose only vocation or interest was in the Boy Scout movement. George's occasional visits to the Cushings in the 1930s were a semi-comedy of uneasy fraternizing, especially on occasions when he and his charges all arrived in their short pants. Harvey and his cousins pooled resources to give George a decent income in the 1930s. George suffered from the same circulatory problems as Harvey, who advised him to stop smoking. George Cushing died on April 7, 1939, in his seventy-fifth year. Harvey paid the cost of having George buried in his and Kate's family plot in Cleveland.[56]

Harvey participated when he could in Yale social and intellectual events, notably the meetings of the undergraduates' Elizabethan Club, Thursday dinners at Trumbull College, gatherings of the Beaumont Medical Club, and meetings of an exclusive club named The Club. He occasionally gave talks to medical students, getting along with them much better, Fulton noticed, than in the years when he had been so fiery and intimidating. He was visited by former students, colleagues, and classmates (he persuaded Star Childs to give several millions to Yale to support cancer research), and by such interesting figures as his literary bête noir, Sinclair Lewis. The Cushings liked dining out in New Haven, but Kate had the habit of becoming visibly indignant at criticism of FDR, of which there was much.[57]

Other than reading, Cushing's only recreation in his Yale years was croquet, which he played with his old competitive zeal. He brought a croquet team to play at Fulton's home in hundred-degree heat in July 1934. The 'hot lunatics,' Fulton noted, kept at it by the light of automobile headlights until nearly midnight. 'Father insists on croquet which is the most boring game in the world and I mean boring,' Babs wrote to sister Betsey in 1938. 'He plays it like chess and plots and plans every play for ten minutes while his partner oozes cold sweat.' The ever-gracious Kate noted that Harvey's croquet friends were 'a strange & unattractive group ... He is mad for his game & I sit and give tea to the left overs, some of them half-witted.'[58]

He was not happy about the lives his daughters were beginning to lead. Mary, or 'Minnie,' perhaps the most independent-minded of the girls, had been introduced to the fabulously rich Vincent Astor, either through Betsey and the White House or through Richard Meagher, a Cushing trainee who became Astor's doctor. From about 1936, Mary had an intimate relationship with Astor, who was openly estranged from his wife. A devoted family servant, Maud Herlihy, remembered how indignant Cushing became when Astor and his chauffeur brought Mary home one weekend. He apparently insisted that Kate go and find out Astor's intentions.[59]

In the meantime, Barbara, who wanted to have a career in New York City and floated continually in a cloud of beaux, decided that she would move to Manhattan and live with Mary. In September 1938 she broached the subject to her father: 'I have talked to father about NY – everything was no NO NO – well Va give me reasons *please* – New York is no place for young girls – especially pleasure loving y.g.'s. There was a great deal of talk about Minnie and I felt 12 yrs old.' Babe went off anyway, and Harvey told Kate that they should get a smaller house.[60]

The White House took its toll on Betsey and Jimmy Roosevelt in several ways. Neither FDR's mother nor his wife made life easy for Betsey, whose chosen-daughter status with the president they resented. Jimmy came down with an ulcer, which everyone thought had been caused by the stress of politics. He went to the Mayo Clinic for surgery. Betsey went too. Doctors there advised her father that she smoked too much and was too thin (many people commented in these years on the thinness of all three Cushing girls). Whatever Jimmy Roosevelt felt about Betsey, he found a nurse at the Mayo Clinic whom he liked better. After his discharge, he and the nurse ran off to California, where he planned to enter the film business. When Harvey heard that Betsey and Jimmy were considering divorce, he commented that there had never been a divorce in the Cushing family.[61]

In September 1939 war broke out again in Europe. Once again the United States stayed neutral. Despite his Midwestern origins, Cushing had always been an internationalist. He believed that Hitler had to be stopped, and he hoped the United States would take a stand. He urged congressmen to support all possible aid to Britain, and he gave his Canadian friends, again at war from the beginning, advice on how to organize a neurosurgical service.[62]

When he was not glued to the radio to hear war news, Cushing fiddled with his books, corresponded with old friends such as Elliott Joslin, and kept on writing. In September 1939 he published an obituary essay for his two surgical friends, Will and Charlie Mayo, who had both died that summer. He compared the Mayos to Wilbur and Orville Wright as men who in their youth had imbibed 'the flavor of the old Northwest Territory where the offspring of the early settlers were reared to think more highly of serving mankind than of helping themselves.' He agreed to write a foreword to an edition of a W.S. Halsted article on the use of silk in surgery, and he was called on to arrange for the shipment of the body of Thomas McRae's widow, a niece of Osler's, who was found dead on a train. He took in a Yale-Harvard baseball game that month and complained that Harvard had brought in a bunch of semiprofessionals. Perhaps the universities should compete at croquet instead.[63]

On October 2, Cushing sent $100 in response to a special appeal to help a down-and-out member of the class of '91. He also wrote a letter on behalf of a Jewish doctor who was trying to immigrate to the United States.[64] He had been having occasional chest pains all summer but apparently just thought his ulcer was acting up. He had tea at the Fultons on October 3. That night he was lifting a heavy edition of Vesalius when he felt serious, continuing pain. Servants called an ambulance the next morning. At the New Haven hospital he was diagnosed as suffering from a heart attack. He survived long enough in hospital to compliment his nephew Pat on having the touch of a good doctor, to complain about the view from his oxygen tent, and to hear that Yale was about to proceed with the library that would house his books.

Harvey Cushing died from the effects of a myocardial infarction at 2:30 AM on October 7, 1939. Thinking he would make it through the night, none of his family was with him when he died.[65] His life span, the psalmist's three score and ten, had been only two weeks longer than that of his mentor and friend, William Osler.

Inheritance and Memory

Postmortem examination of Harvey Cushing's body confirmed the cause of death. He had suffered from general arteriosclerosis and atherosclerosis, which had caused the blockage of major coronary arteries that killed him. His lungs had been damaged by smoking and were also scarred from an old bout with tuberculosis. His brain had more or less normal vascular damage and a small cyst. It was a medically and historically unremarkable autopsy. Unlike Osler in an earlier era, Cushing knew there was nothing to be learned from further study of his brain, so it was not preserved. The funeral at Center Congregational Church in New Haven was attended by 500 people inside the building and 2,000 outside on the Green. The body was cremated and the ashes taken to Cleveland for burial in the family plot in Lakeview Cemetery.

Cushing's estate was worth about $650,000 (but the complexity of trust funds makes all figures unreliable) and passed mostly to his family. He willed small sums to some of the servants and left $5,000 each to Madeline Stanton, Julia Shepley, Louise Eisenhardt, and Gil Horrax. He gave Yale his books, papers, and literary properties, and a further $100,000. A special $5,000 bequest was to cover the cost of cataloging the books, and there was a further $5,000 to underwrite the costs of publishing his biography, should someone choose to write one.[1]

John Fulton had arranged for the instant publication of obituary
notices and the funeral service. Julia Shepley came out of retirement to
help Madeline Stanton acknowledge some 1,100 expressions of sympathy that were sent to the family. Kate was calm and serene throughout the death ritual, only remarking to Barbara that none of them had
realized how much their lives had revolved around him: 'We're a tail
without a kite.' Within a week of the funeral, Kate asked Fulton to
write Harvey's biography. She then did not take much interest in the
project, except to express the hope that it would say little about their
private life.[2] It was said that when Kate was one day shown the sixteen
volumes of Harvey's published articles, she ran her hand over them,
remarked, 'What industry!' and then turned away.[3]

Harvey closed his farewell letter to Kate with a reference to Bill and
a lighthearted order: 'Don't mourn for us too much or we will be unhappy while waiting for you.'[4] Within a few months of her husband's
death, Kate was fully occupied by her daughters' marital events: Mary's
wedding to Vincent Astor, Barbara's wedding to Stanley Mortimer, and
Betsey's divorce from Jimmy Roosevelt. Eventually Betsey remarried,
to John Hay Whitney, and both Mary and Barbara also divorced and
remarried. Kate died in 1949 at the age of seventy-nine. Of the children, Betsey lived the longest, dying in 1998 at the age of eighty-nine.
There are many surviving grandchildren and great-grandchildren.

The lives of the 'fabulous Cushing sisters,' as they were known in
New York society in the 1940s and 1950s, became the stuff of journalists' columns and society gossip, much of it collected in a 1990 book,
The Sisters, by society journalist David Grafton. Retailing bitchy hear-
say, Grafton contended that Kate Cushing had raised the girls to be
gold diggers, their only ambition in life being to marry money. Not a
scrap of paper anywhere in the Cushing Papers or the Cushing-Whitney
Archive supports this view. Like Harvey, Kate had hoped the girls would
find happiness and fulfillment in good marriages and in lives characterized by the exercise of good taste and service. Money was not a factor,
if only because the Cushings and Crowells were more than comfortable, even in the 1930s. The girls did become famous for their exquis-

ite taste in clothes, decor, art, and entertaining, though not in husbands. They were very close to one another and to their mother. Mary Astor Fosburgh tended to be the most retiring. Betsey Roosevelt Whitney's second marriage was a warm and enduring success. Babe Mortimer Paley had a glittering career in fashion, becoming America's perennial best-dressed woman, and then was highly visible as the wife of William Paley, a broadcasting mogul with an enormous appetite for life.

Such an odd transformation in gender history – In the body and personality of Babe Cushing, her brain-surgeon father's lean, austere, almost classical physique and character became a model of feminine beauty at the highest levels of American society. Barbara possessed her father's form and features, his intensity and nervous energy, his hunger for nicotine. While Harvey Cushing found a kind of fulfillment in making a great contribution to medicine and humanity, Barbara's life in Manhattan was less obviously creative. It is not clear that she found contentment – she had an unfulfilled interest in sculpting, for example – and she died at age sixty-three of the ravages of lung cancer.[5]

Both of her parents were responsible for the way in which Barbara and, to a degree, her sisters spent their lives as helpmate wives, offering gracious hospitality in their homes and taking a serious interest in the arts. It was a woman's sphere that still made sense to puritans leaving their last footprint on American life in the nineteenth century, but it steadily became challenged by shifting female choices and societal values in the twentieth century. With different parental guidance, the talented Cushing sisters could have gone to university or at least tried to embark on professional careers. One or more of them, especially Barbara, might have kept faith with the family vocation by going into medicine, even surgery. The Cushing sisters did maintain a family interest in health care as well as their mother's independence of spirit. All three were tough enough to get out of bad first marriages. It is not clear, though, that in their traditional and privileged social circles the Cushing women fully realized their potential. Theirs was a way of life now disappearing throughout North America and Europe. In a sense, they were part of what Fitzgerald in *Tender Is the Night*, referring to the Divers, characterized as 'the exact furthermost evolution of a class.'

Louise Eisenhardt, MD, was the first woman to specialize in neuropathology and in 1944 became the first editor of the *Journal of Neurosurgery*. She was the leading pillar of the Harvey Cushing Society and continued to keep track of some of Cushing's patients as head of the Cushing Brain Tumor Registry. As the autopsy on her chief was being concluded in 1939, she had come into the room and cut a lock of Cushing's hair.[6]

Madeline Stanton, BA, became chief curator of the books in Yale's Medical Historical Library, which inhabits a wing of the Grosvenor Atterbury–designed medical library that was opened in 1941 and is now known as the Harvey Cushing/John Hay Whitney Medical Library. The Historical Library, centering on a kind of gothic great hall, received first the Cushing, then the Klebs, and finally the Fulton collections of rare anatomical books, incunabula, and physiological works. Miss Stanton was initially the library's secretary, working under John Fulton's direction. Fulton appears to have seduced her in the late 1930s, and for a time she was also his mistress, making pointed comments about having joined a new harem. In 1939-40 Fulton did initial work gathering material for the Cushing biography while also arranging for publication of a collection of Cushing's later essays, *The Medical Career*, and of the Vesalius bio-bibliography. But then he turned to war service in Washington.

When Fulton returned to the biography in 1945, he was on the brink of disintegrating from too many years of hard work and high living. Julia Shepley did virtually all of the work of sorting, reading, and annotating Cushing's letters. In a kind of alcoholic haze, Fulton then assembled the material into a 714-page volume, *Harvey Cushing: A Biography*, which was published jointly by the Historical Library and Charles C Thomas in 1946.[7] The book was reasonably well received but was thought to be dense and long, modeled too closely on Cushing's *Osler*. Fulton cutely avoided making any reference to himself. He was so close to self-destruction that the surprise is to find that (as with F. Scott

Fitzgerald's later writing) many passages were tolerably good. Elizabeth Thomson's 1950 book, *Harvey Cushing: Surgeon, Author, Artist*, stressed both the attractiveness of Cushing's personality and the toll he imposed on his family. Many, including the family, thought she had presented a more rounded and readable portrait of Harvey.[8]

John Fulton, who had become diabetic as well as alcoholic, had to relinquish his Sterling Professorship of Physiology in 1951, and was put out to pasture as chairman of the Department of the History of Medicine. For the rest of his life he was a sorry figurehead, often pathetically ill, who was shielded by the women at the library and by his rich wife. When Fulton died in 1960, Madeline Stanton formally became what she had been for many years, the head of the Medical Historical Library at Yale, curator of one of the world's priceless collections of medical books. Until her retirement in 1968 and for several years afterwards, she was a model to Yale medical students of gracious New England manners, book-loving scholarship, conscientious attention to duty, and perfectionist attention to detail.[9]

After Cushing's death, Walter Dandy at Johns Hopkins was probably the most prominent neurosurgeon in America. His life was cut short in 1946 by a heart attack. Debate still rages in neurosurgical circles, especially at Johns Hopkins, about the relative merits and contributions of Cushing and Dandy, but it is not much of a contest. An old Hopkins hand concluded that Dandy may have been a more brilliant operator, but otherwise there was no comparison: 'Dandy couldn't begin to approach Cushing in breadth of learning, interest, culture, general stature. Dandy was a one-man surgeon. Cushing was a one-man army.'[10]

If Cushing's brain did not survive, his collection of brains did. The Cushing Brain Tumor Registry has outlived all of the principals in this biography and the patients. For many years after Louise Eisenhardt's retirement, the jars of preserved brain tissue and tumors, the patient records and photographs, gathered dust on shelves in the basement of Yale's medical student residence. After a night at Mory's, medical whiffenpoofs would venture into the 'brain room' in the dead of night,

leaving graffiti behind. In the 1990s the collection was officially redis-
covered, its amazing collection of photographic plates rescued, and
plans developed for its long-term preservation as a unique contribution to medical Americana.[11]

There are no more medical Cushings in Cleveland. No spirits watch
over the modest family headstones in the little plots near the big
Rockefeller monument. The Harvey Cushing Society continued to grow
as the leading professional organization of neurosurgeons in the United
States. In 1965 it changed its name to the American Association of
Neurological Surgeons, and with some seven thousand members at the
beginning of the twenty-first century it is the leader in its field. Around
the world, which now comes to North America to learn advanced medicine and surgery, the members of the AANS and other neurosurgeons
recognize and remember Harvey Cushing as the founder of their specialty.

They now work with the assistance of amazing imaging devices, elec-
tronic navigation aids, and operating microscopes and endoscopes that
hugely enlarge their field of vision. They repair aneurysms, treat hydrocephalus and epilepsy, and shrink and extract tumors with success rates
that were barely conceivable in Cushing's era. Some neurosurgeons
think theirs has become a surgical trade like any other. The main issue
in some operating rooms is whether the music will be rock or bluegrass.
Others still see neurosurgery as a high-tension, high-skill frontier, an
Everest of medicine, requiring Cushingesque, priestly, or simply obsessive levels of work and dedication.

For all their technology, the neurosurgeons open and close the human cranium with drills, saws, scalpels, clips, and clamps much as Harvey
Cushing mastered and then taught the technique a hundred years ago.
They can no more afford to make slips and errors in their handiwork,
their science, and their art than he could. One way or another, most of
them acknowledge that they are Harvey Cushing's spiritual descendants – his surgical sons and, as the world evolves, his surgical daughters. This is memory at its best. As Cushing said in homage to his predecessors, 'What has been accomplished does not die.'

Notes and Sources

This book is based on extensive study of the Harvey Williams Cushing Papers (CP) at Yale University. The Cushing Papers are housed partly in the Manuscripts and Archives division of the Sterling Library and partly in the Historical Library of the Harvey Cushing/John Hay Whitney Medical Library. The whole Cushing collection, amounting to about 121 linear feet in bulk, has been carefully microfilmed onto 159 reels containing about 200,000 exposures. Scholars are required to use the microfilm, which is unusually reader-friendly and is also purchasable. The finding aid to the Cushing Papers is available online.

Even more than Osler, Cushing was a natural saver and collector, instincts that were further honed when he became Osler's biographer. His own 'Boswells,' John Fulton and Madeline Stanton, hovered anxiously over Cushing's files while he was alive and added to them after his death by soliciting donations of letters. The Cushing Papers are wonderfully rich, perhaps uniquely so in the medical world. While other libraries do have small collections sometimes labeled Cushing Papers, Yale's is far and away the mother lode. It contains, for example, copies of all of Cushing's patient records from his years in Boston, as well as many files from his Hopkins years. The only other significant collection of Cushing Papers (CPOL) is a number of important files relating to the Osler biography, which he gave to the Osler Library at McGill University in the early 1930s.

Kate Cushing's personal papers, containing many letters to and from Harvey and the children, passed to her daughter Betsey (Roosevelt) Whitney and were made available to me, without restriction, as the Whitney-Cushing Archive (WCA), which will eventually be accessible through a university repository.

Much of the revealing correspondence generated before, during, and after the publication of John Fulton's *Harvey Cushing: A Biography* (1946) is now available in the major collection of John Farquhar Fulton Papers, held at Yale's Sterling Library. Fulton's diaries are available at the Medical Historical Library. The Medical Historical Library has a small collection of Madeline Stanton Papers, but a much larger and more important collection, including her diaries, is held at the Sterling. The Sterling's collection of the papers of Elizabeth H. Thomson, author of *Harvey Cushing: Surgeon, Author, Artist* (1950), is less revealing than the Thomson Scrapbook held in the Archive of the American Association of Neurological Surgeons (AANS). Yale's Medical Historical Library also holds important Cushing-Klebs correspondence. The Department of Neurosurgery in the Yale Faculty of Medicine controls access to the Cushing Brain Tumor Registry.

Minor but sometimes important collections of Cushing-related material are held at the Countway Medical Library in Boston, the Dittrick collections in the Allen Memorial Medical Library in Cleveland, the Western Reserve Historical Society in Cleveland, the Archive of the American Association of Neurological Surgeons in Chicago, Flinders University in Australia, and the Chesney Archives of the Johns Hopkins Medical Institutions in Baltimore. While working on my earlier biography of Osler, I consulted at the Chesney Archives and the Osler Library many collections relating to Osler, Halsted, Welch, and others of Cushing's era, and that research also became background for this volume. The Walter E. Dandy Papers at the Chesney Archives contain important correspondence, notably that between Dandy and his parents. With additions, most of these letters have been privately distributed in usable format by the Dandy family.

The most accessible guide to and sampling of Cushing's surgical publications is *Harvey Cushing: Selected Papers on Neurosurgery*, edited by Donald D. Matson et al. (New Haven & London: Yale University Press, 1969), which contains an amended reprint of the 1939 *Bibliography of the Writings of Harvey Cushing*. I found it both convenient and important (because of his insertions and comments) to work from Cushing's own volumes of his reprints, as microfilmed from his papers.

A very large number of other primary and secondary sources have been consulted and, where useful, are cited appropriately in the notes. Altogether, the research base for this book was about five times as voluminous as the sources used in my Osler biography. Still, I complete this project with a sense that many more gems of Cushing and perhaps Osler material are waiting to be discovered in archives and private homes and attics.

ABBREVIATIONS

AANS	American Association of Neurological Surgeons
BMC	Betsey Maria Cushing (mother)
CAJHMI	Chesney Archives, Johns Hopkins Medical Institutions
Career	Harvey Cushing, *The Medical Career and Other Papers* (Boston: Little, Brown, 1940)
Consecratio	Harvey Cushing, *Consecratio Medici and Other Papers* (Boston: Little Brown, 1928)
CP	Harvey Williams Cushing Papers, Yale University
CPOL	Cushing Papers, Osler Library, McGill University, Montreal
FD	Fulton Diaries, [Medical] Historical Library, Yale University

FP	John Farquhar Fulton Papers, Yale University
Fulton	John F. Fulton, *Harvey Cushing: A Biography* (Springfield, Ill.: Charles C Thomas, 1946)
GRO	Grace Revere Osler
HC	Harvey Cushing
HistNeurosurg	Samuel H. Greenblatt, ed., *A History of Neurosurgery, in Its Scientific and Professional Contexts* (Washington: American Association of Neurological Surgeons, 1997)
HKC	Henry Kirke Cushing (father)
Intracranial Tumours	Harvey Cushing, *Intracranial Tumours: Notes upon a Series of Two Thousand Verified Cases with Surgical-Mortality Percentages Pertaining Thereto* (Springfield, Ill.: Charles C Thomas, 1931)
KC	Kate Crowell Cushing (wife)
JAMA	*Journal of the American Medical Association*
JF	John Fulton
JHH	John Hopkins Hospital
Meningiomas	Harvey Cushing, with Louise Eisenhardt, *Meningiomas: Their Classification, Regional Behaviour, Life History, and Surgical End Results* (Springfield, Ill.: Charles C Thomas, 1938)
MGH	Massachusetts General Hospital
MHLY	[Medical] Historical Library, Harvey Cushing/John Hay Whitney Medical Library, Yale University
MS	Madeline Stanton
Pituitary Body	Harvey Cushing, *The Pituitary Body and Its Disorders* (Philadelphia & London: Lippincott, 1912)
Selected Papers	*Harvey Cushing: Selected Papers on Neurosurgery*, ed. Donald D. Matson et al. (New Haven & London: Yale University Press, 1969)
SJ	Harvey Cushing, *From A Surgeon's Journal, 1915–1918* (Boston: Little, Brown, 1936)
SP	Madeline Stanton Papers, Yale University
Thomson	Elizabeth H. Thomson, *Harvey Cushing: Surgeon, Author, Artist* (New York: Schuman, 1950)
WCA	Whitney-Cushing Archive, privately held
WD	Walter E. Dandy
WO	William Osler

NOTES

The sources of all direct quotations and other significant facts and incidents are noted. The annotation is often summary, a single note identifying several quotations. Articles whose authorship is not given are by Cushing. For manuscript sources, enough detail is provided to locate material with the help of standard finding aids and my index of abbreviations. References to the Cushing Papers at Yale (CP) are usually followed by a microfilm reel and page number, e.g., CP 156/987. Readers with queries about any notes or sources should contact the author at the University of Toronto or refer to the master manuscripts of this book deposited at the Historical Library in the Harvey Cushing/John Hay Whitney Medical Library at Yale.

Opening: The Surgeon and the General

1 Hermann Hagedown, *Leonard Wood: A Biography* (New York: Harper & Bros., 1931), 1: 210.
2 Leonard wood File, CP 125.
3 Harvey Cushing (HC) to Kate Crowell Cushing (KC), July 14, 1909, CP 18/352.
4 Geoffrey Jefferson, 'Harvey Cushing,' in *Sir Geoffrey Jefferson: Selected Papers* (New York: Pitman, 1960).
5 HC operative notes and later comments, Leonard Wood File, CP 125; slightly differing accounts are in HC (with L. Eisenhardt), *Meningiomas: Their Classification, Regional Behaviour, Life History, and Surgical End Results* (Springfield, Ill.: Charles C. Thomas, 1938), 409–12, and Samuel James Crowe, *Halsted of Johns Hopkins: The Man and His Men* (Springfield, Ill.: Charles C. Thomas, 1957), 76–7.
6 HC note, CP 125/2.

1: Western Reserve

1 Notes on family background, CP 154/80; genealogy and ancestral tables files, 154/53ff; William E. Cushing notes on conversations with Erastus Cushing, CP 155/744ff.
2 Erastus Cushing, 'Thesis,' Berkshire Medical School, 1824, CP 155/662ff.
3 Erastus Cushing to Cornelia Cushing, Aug. 31, 1855, CP 154/1257.
4 Cornelia Briggs Cushing, correspondence, photographs, and memorabilia, 1835–56, CP 154/858ff; the white cat story is in William E. Cushing's notes on conversations with Erastus Cushing in 1876, 155/751.
5 HC, 'The Western Reserve and its Medical Traditions,' in *Consecratio Medici* (Boston: Little Brown, 1928) (hereafter *Consecratio*), 208.
6 William Williams, 'Autobiographical Fragment' (1887–8), CP 158/470.
7 William E. Cushing notes in 1876, CP 155/751.
8 William Williams, 'Autobiographical Fragment,' CP 158/563; Lucien Price, 'Olympians in Homespun,' *Atlantic Monthly*, Apr. 1926.
9 Mary Cushing to [mother], Apr. 7, 1836, CP 154/869.
10 HC memo, Sept. 22, 1910, CP 155/735; William E. Cushing notes in 1876, 155/751.
11 Howard Dittrick, 'Dr. Erastus Cushing,' *Bulletin of the Academy of Medicine, Cleveland* [1930], CP 154/874; drug store, 154/885.

12 Erastus Cushing ledgers, Cushing family account books, [Medical] Historical Library, Yale (MHLY); HC, 'Western Reserve,' in *Consecratio*, 216.

13 Cornelia Platt to Mary Cushing, Dec. 25, 1845, CP 154/909; Henry Kirke Cushing (HKC) to Charlotte Platt, Feb. 10, 1838, 154/888; Erastus Cushing to Geo. P. Briggs, Nov. 25, 1856, 155/364.

14 Cushing-Briggs letters, 1856, CP 154/1279–89.

15 HKC entry, 'Erastus Cushing, Mary Ann Platt, and Their Forebears,' CP 154/701ff; Erastus Cushing to HKC, Oct. 13, Dec. 13, 1850, 157/78, 97.

16 HKC entry, 'Erastus Cushing, Mary Ann Platt, and Their Forebears,' CP l54/701ff; Mary Cushing Diary, Apr. 1851, 154/1078.

17 Laura Fitch Williams to William Williams, Nov. 21, 1838, CP 154/601–2; Mary Cushing letter, Feb. 5, 1848, 154/990; notes by Charles Tudor Williams, Mar. 1910, CP 154/793ff.

18 Betsey Maria Cushing (BMC) to HKC, May 26, July 9 and 26, 1861, CP 155/1068, 1124, and 156/20.

19 BMC to HKC, June 2 and 11, 1861, CP 155/1077, 1085.

20 HKC to BMC, May 18, July 4 and 18, 1861, CP 154/360, 403, 428.

21 F.T. Brown to Rev. W.H. Goodrich, Aug. 12, 1861, CP 157/178.

22 HKC to BMC, Aug. 26, 1861, CP 154/454.

23 'Recollections of HKC begun by William Edward Cushing,' Feb. 22, 1910, CP 157/11.

24 HC to KC, Oct. 24, 1903, CP 17/1212.

25 HKC note and Certificate of Enlistment of Substitute, CP 157/205.

26 Cushing ledgers and account books, MHLY.

27 HC, 'Something of BMC by her Youngest Son' (HC memoir), June 1934, CP 154/807ff; Will Cushing to BMC, Mar. 17, [187?], 154/456.

28 Notes by Charles Tudor Williams, Mar. 1910, CP 154/793ff.

29 HC to Loyal Davis, Nov. 23, 1931, CP 20/851; HC to Lucien Price, Jan. 12, 1937, 43/1235; HC to Mrs. Louise Price Parker, May 23, 1936.

30 HC memoir, CP 154/807ff; Julia Parson to John Fulton (JF), Sept. 30, 1940, Fulton Papers, Yale (FP) 215/321; Elizabeth H. Thomson, *Harvey Cushing: Surgeon, Author, Artist* (New York: Schuman, 1950), 12.

31 HC memoir; HC to Will Cushing, approx. 1877, CP 19/261.

32 Notes by Charles Tudor Williams, Mar. 1910, CP 154/793ff; HC, 'Perry Williams Harvey,' in HC, *The Medical Career and Other Papers* (Boston: Little, Brown, 1940) (hereafter *Career*), 258; HC to KC, June 3, 1894, CP 17/241.

33 HC draft recollections, CP 154/771.

34 HC, *Career,* 256; HC memoir, CP 154/807ff; A.F. Harvey to JF, Nov. 27, 1939, FP 214/308.

35 Laura Baldwin to JF, Nov 28, 1939, FP 213/296; Robert S. Carroll to JF, Sept. 24, 1943, FP 213/299.

36 Obit. of Henry Platt Cushing, *Science*, June 3, 1921, CP 158/751.

37 Helen M. Smith to JF, May 2, 1940, FP 213/326; Katrina S. Firlik and Andrew

Firlik, 'Harvey Cushing, MD: A Clevelander,' *Neurosurgery* 37 (Dec. 1995), 1178–86.

38 Obit. of George Briggs Cushing, CP 154/91; John F. Fulton, *Harvey Cushing: A Biography* (Springfield, Ill.: Charles C. Thomas, 1946), (Hereafter Fulton), 22–5.

39 Firlik and Firlik, 'Harvey Cushing ... Clevelander'; HC memoir, CP 154/807ff; HC to Arnold Klebs, July 21, 1936, Arnold Klebs correspondence, MHLY.

40 J. Milton Dyer to JF, Mar. 23, 1940, FP 213/302.

41 Graduation program, FP 216/335; J.J. Thomas to JF, Nov. 16, 1939, FP 216/329.

42 J.J. Thomas to JF, Nov. 16, 1939, FP 216/329.

43 HC bio. for Yale Reunion Class Book, CP 55/160; BMC to HC, May 22, 1888, 14/175.

2: Making a Yale Man

1 HKC to HC, May 7, 1888, CP 16/78.

2 HC to BMC, Sept. 18, 1887, CP 16/3; HC to HKC, Sept. 18, 1887, 14/22; HC to BMC, Sept. 25, 1887, 14/24.

3 For background on Yale, see Brooks Mather Kelley, *Yale: A History* (New Haven and London: Yale University Press, 1974); Owen Johnson, *Stover at Yale* (1912; Yale Bookstore reprint, 1997), 325.

4 HC to HKC, Feb. 19, 1888, CP 16/42; HKC to HC, Feb. 23, 1888, 16/44.

5 HC to BMC, Nov. 20, 1887, CP 14/46.

6 HC to BMC, Nov. 27, 1887, CP 14/50; Richard M. Hurd, 'A History of American College Athletics,' *Outing Magazine*, Feb. 1889, CP 105/301.

7 HC to HKC, Dec. 4, 1887, CP 16/19.

8 HKC to HC, Jan. 7, 1888, CP 16/28.

9 BMC to HC, Jan. 11, 1888, CP 14/64; HC to BMC, Jan. 14, 1888, 14/64; BMC to HC, Jan. 24, 1888, 14/74.

10 HC to BMC, Feb. 5, 1888, CP 14/84; BMC to HC, Feb. 8, 1888, 14/86.

11 HC to HKC, Apr. 8, 1888, CP 16/61; HKC to HC, Apr. 10, 1888, 16/65.

12 HC to BMC, Mar. 4, 1888, CP 14/111; HC to BMC, Apr. 15, 1888, 14/147.

13 See various clippings in HC Yale Scrapbook, CP 105/949ff.

14 BMC to HC, Feb. 14, 1888, CP 14/93; BMC to HC, Apr. 24, 1888, 14/155; HKC to HC, May 1, 1888, 16/73; HC Yale Scrapbook, 105/949.

15 HC to BMC, Mar. 10, Apr. 8, 1888, CP 14/115, 141; HC to HKC Apr. 29, May 4 and 13, 1888, 16/69, 83, 88.

16 HKC to HC, May 7, 1888, CP 16/78; BMC to HC, May 8, 1888, 14/163.

17 HC Yale Scrapbook, CP 105/972, 977; HC to BMC, May 27, 1888, 14/179.

18 BMC to HC, May 29, 1888, CP 14/181; HC to BMC, June 3, 1888, 14/184.

19 HC to HKC, Mar. 10, 1888; CP 16/51; HC to BMC, Apr. 22, 1888, 14/153; HC to BMC, Mar. 25, 1888, 14/130.

20 HC to BMC, May 20, 1888, CP 14/173.

21 Ibid.; Egerton Swartout to JF, Feb. 28, 1940, FP 215/328; HC, Yale Scrapbook, July 7, 1888, CP 105/1019.

22 Scholarship record of HC, FP 213/302.

23 HC Yale Scrapbook, CP 105/949; HC to HKC, Mar. 27, 1889, 16/131; Kelley, *Yale*, 303 (a 1903 report).

24 HC to HKC, Dec. 9, 1888, CP 16/121; HC to BMC, Nov. 11, 1888, 14/208; HC to BMC, Feb. 10, 1889, 14/225.

25 HC to HKC, Nov. 10, 1889, June 6, 1890, CP 16/152, 171; HC to BMC, Oct. 5, 1890, 14/332.

26 HC to HKC, May 19, June 2, 1889, CP 16/144, 146; HC to HKC, Sept. 3, 1889, 16/150.

27 HC to BMC, Oct. 5 and 12, 1890, CP 14/332; HC to HKC, Oct. 10, 1890, 16/189.

28 HC to Ludwig Kast, Nov. 14, 1935, CP 31/1311; HC to BMC, Feb. 9, 1890, 14/282.

29 HC to HKC, Feb. 1, 1891, CP 16/204; HC to HKC, Nov. 2, 1890, 16/191; HC Notebook from Physiological Chemistry, 1890–1, 125/360.

30 HC Yale Scrapbook, CP 105/372, 440; HC to BMC, Apr. 13, 1890, 14/302; (Washington) HC to HKC, Apr. 28, 1889, 16/135; Fulton, 195.

31 HC Yale Scrapbook, CP 105/634, 647, 624.

32 Program of the Thanksgiving Jubilee of Delta Kappa Epsilon, Nov. 26, 1889, HC Yale Scrapbook, CP 105/482.

33 HC to HKC, Mar. 27, 1889, CP 16/131; HC to HKC, Feb. 2, 1890, 16/161; HC to BMC, May 25, 1890, 14/314.

34 HC Yale Scrapbook, CP 105/372; HC to BMC, Feb. 24, 1889, 14/229; HC to BMC, Oct. 5, 1890, 14/332; also Kelley, *Yale*, 307.

35 Notes by Grace MacBride Crile, FP 213/300; Fulton, 144.

36 HC to HKC, Sept. 21, 1890, CP 16/183; HC to BMC, Sept. 28, 1890, 14/330.

37 HC to BMC, Jan. 25, 1891, CP 14/359.

38 HC to HKC, Nov. 29, 1890, CP 16/193.

39 HC to HKC, Mar. 1, 1891, CP 16/206; HC to D. Bryson Delavan, Feb. 11, 1937, 20/1230.

40 HC to BMC, June 14 and 21, 1891, CP 16/413, 425; HC Yale Scrapbook, 105/677, 699, 700, 831; damages: W.H. St John to HC, July 10, 1891, 47/831.

3: Making a Harvard Doctor

1 HC to HKC, Sept. 28, 1891, CP 16/219; HC to BMC, Oct. 4, 1891, 14/421.

2 HKC to HC, Oct. 3, 1891, CP 16/225; HC to BMC, Sept. 20, 1892, 14/502.

3 HC to Lewis Bremar, Sept. 12, 1927, CP 6/87.

4 C.R.L. Putnam to JF, undated (c. 1940), FP 215/322.

5 HC to HKC, Nov. 1, 1891, CP 16/234; M.H. Richardson to Edward F. Cushing, Nov. 17, 1891, 15/227.

6 HC to Edward F. Cushing, n.d., CP 15/231.

7 HC to HKC, Feb. 27, 1892, CP 16/242.

8 Perry Harvey to HC, Dec. 14, 1892, CP 28/980.

9 Will Cushing to HKC and BMC, Mar. 17 [1877 or 1878], CP 154/456–7.

10 Caroline Crowell to HC, Sept. 30, 1891, CP 11/151; HC to BMC, Mar. 6, 1892, 14/456.

11 HC to HKC, Mar. 6, Apr. 3, 1892, CP 16/246, 248; Perry Harvey to HC, Apr. 10, 1892, 28/951.

12 HC grades at Harvard Medical School, FP 213/301; William J. Mallon, *Ernest Amory Codman: The End Result of a Life in Medicine* (Philadelphia: Saunders, 2000).

13 KC to HC, Sept. 1, 1892, CP 17/156; HC to KC, Sept. 12, 1892, 17/168.

14 HC to KC, Sept. 22, 1892, CP 17/173; HC to BMC, Oct. 9, 1892, 14/504.

15 HC to KC, Oct. 15, 1892, CP 17/177.

16 HC to BMC, Oct. 23, 1892, CP 14/506; HC to BMC, Nov. 13, 1892, 14/514.

17 HC to BMC, Nov. 6 and 27, Dec. 11, 1892, CP 14/512, 518, 522.

18 HC to BMC, Nov. 6, 1892, CP 14/512.

19 HC to BMC, Jan. 1, 1893, CP 14/533; HC to HKC, Jan. 3, 1893, 16/287.

20 HC to BMC, Dec. 25, 1892, CP 14/526.

21 HC to HKC, Jan. 1, 1893, CP 16/285.

22 Fred G. Barker, II, 'The Massachusetts General Hospital: Early History and Neurosurgery to 1939,' *Journal of Neurosurgery* 79 (1993), 948–59; 'The Personality of a Hospital,' *Consecratio*, 131.

23 HC Diary, 1892–3, CP 67/1155ff; HC to Dr Washburn, Feb. 10, 1920, 53/912–14; Frank Lynam to JF, 1944, FP 214/314.

24 HC to BMC, Jan. 15, 1893, CP 14/540; HC Diary, 67/1164; Frank Lynam to JF, 1944, FP 214/314 (autopsy incident misattributed to Lynam in Fulton, 69n).

25 'The Personality of a Hospital,' in *Consecratio*, 125; HC Diary, CP 67/1168.

26 HC Diary, Jan. 30, 1893, CP 67/1158; HC to HKC, Feb. 25, 1893, 16/291.

27 HC to HKC, Apr. 3, 1893, CP 16/294; HC notes and text, Anthrax, 1892, 114/1162; HC Diary, Apr. 21 and 19, 1893, 67/1167–9.

28 HC Diary, May 4 and 2, 1893, CP 67/1171.

29 HC to KC, July 2, 1893, CP 17/195; HC Diary, May 24, 1893, 67/1174; C.R.L. Putnam to JF, c. 1940, FP 215/322.

30 HC to BMC, June 4 and 11, 1893, CP 14/586, 588; HC to HKC, June 19, 1893, 16/304; HC Diary, 67/1177.

31 HC to HKC, June 19, 1893, CP 16/304; HC Diary, 67/1179; J. Bissell Speer to HC, Mar. 19, 1937, 113/1139.

32 HC to HKC, July 6, 1893, CP 16/316.

33 HC to BMC, July 23, 1893, CP 14/604.

34 HC Diary, Aug. 12 and 24, Sept. 25, 1893, CP 67/1185, 1188, 1193.

35 HC Columbian Exposition Diary, 1893, MHLY; HC to KC, Sept. 25, 1893, CP 17/205.

36 HC to HKC, June 11, 1894, CP 16/345; HC to HKC, Nov. 26, 1893, 16/332.

37 HC to G. Atterbury, Jan. 13, 1894, CP 4/1125; HC, 'Neurological Surgeons: With the Report of One Case' (1923), in *Selected Papers*, 595–6; HC Diary, Dec. 3, 1893, 67/1202; HC to KC, Dec. 6, 1893, 17/220.

38 HKC to HC, Oct. 21, 1893, CP 16/329; HC Diary, Nov. 1, Oct. 9, 1893, 67/1198, 1195; HC to HKC, Nov. 16, 1893, 16/332.

39 HC to BMC, Feb. 11, 1894, CP 14/367; HC Diary, Dec. 22, 1893, 67/1205; HC to BMC, Jan. 21, Feb. 20, 1894, 14/631, 640, 642; Fulton, 84.

40 HC Diary of a trip to Havana, 1894, CP 106/9ff; HC to KC, Mar. 10, 1894, 17/228; HC to KC, Mar. 31, 1894, 17/234.

41 HC to G. Atterbury, Jan. 13, 1894, CP 4/1125.

42 HC to HKC, Apr. 8, 1894, CP 16/341. There is no record of the advice HC received from his family and no supporting evidence relating to HC's note thirty years later (CP 114/673ff, notes on Halsted) of having applied to work with Osler.

43 HC to HKC, June 11, 1894, CP 16/345; HC to BMC, May 13, 1894, 14/658.

44 HC to HKC, undated, CP 16/349.

45 HC Diary of a trip to London and the Derbyshire 'Peak Country,' 1894, CP 106/100ff; HC letters to parents and KC, July 16–31, 1894, passim.

46 HC to KC, Aug. 22, 1894, CP 17/255.

47 HC to KC, Oct. 29, 1894, CP 17/261; HC to Dr Walter P. Bowers, Mar. 23, 1916, 75/965.

48 HC Bermuda Diary, 1895, MHLY; John Fulton Diary (FD), Mar. 25–31, 1928, 88.

49 HC to KC, Mar. 2, 1894, CP 17/226; HC to BMC, May 5, 1895, 14/735. An elusive reference in HC to E.A. Codman, July 25, 1894, Codman Papers, Countway Library, Boston, suggests that he may have renewed acquaintance with Kate, 'the only girl I ever loved,' on his trip to England in 1894.

50 HC to F.A. Washburn, Feb. 10, 1920, CP 127/367; correspondence and charts also in a bound volume compiled by HC, *Anesthesia Charts of 1895 with Explanatory Notes*, Countway Library, Boston; Mallon, *Ernest Amory Codman*, ch. 2; also HC, 'On the Avoidance of Shock in Major Amputations by Cocainization of Large Nerve-Trunks Preliminary to Their Division: With Observations on Blood-Pressure Changes in Surgical Cases,' *Annals of Surgery* 35 (Sept. 1902), 321–45.

51 HC to BMC, June 16, 1895, CP 14/739; HC to HKC, July 13, 1895, 16/387.

4: Making an American Surgeon

1 HC to BMC, July 28, 1895, CP 14/747.

2 F.G. Barker II, 'The Massachusetts General Hospital: Early History and Neurosurgery to 1919,' *Journal of Neuosurgery* 79 (1993), 948–59; *also* Edward D. Churchill, ed., *To Work in the Vineyard of Surgery: The Reminiscences of J. Collins Warren (1842–1927)* (Cambridge, Mass: Harvard University Press, 1958).

3 Edward Cushing to HC, July 6, 1895, CP 15/243.

4 HC to HKC, Aug. 1895, CP 16/389; HC to BMC, Sept. 9, 1895, 14/753; HC to BMC, May 10, 1896, 14/784.

5 HC to HKC, June 18, 1896, CP 16/412; also HC notes on Halsted, 1925, 114/673ff, and HC to BMC, Jan. 31, 1897, 14/823.

6 Edward Wyllys Taylor, 'Two Cases of Tumor of the Brain, with Autopsy,' *Boston Medical and Surgical Journal*, Jan. 16, 1896, 57–60; 3rd patient, Henry R. Viets to JF, July 18, 1945, FP 216/331; also Fulton, 259–60.

7 Henry R. Viets to Charles McDonald, Apr. 2, 1942, in Viets to JF, Apr. 16, 1942, FP 216/331; also HC, 'Neurological Surgeons: With the Report of One Case' (1923), in *Selected Papers*.

8 HC to HKC, Feb. 23, 1896, CP 16/404.

9 HC to BMC, Feb. 15, 1896, CP 14/772.

10 HC to BMC, May 10, 1896, CP 14/784; Samuel James Crowe, *Halsted of Johns Hopkins: The Man and His Men* (Springfield, Ill.: Charles C. Thomas, 1957), 65. The evidence does not support a claim that HC took the first x-rays at the MGH.

11 F.S. Newell to JF, Apr. 6, 1942, FP 215/319.

12 Frank H. Linnehan to HC, June 4, 1930, CP 55/1187; Henry Viets to JF, Apr. 7, 1942, FP 216/337; H.W. Linnehan to JF, Oct. 30, 1939, 214/314.

13 HC, 'The Personality of a Hospital,' in *Consecratio*, 137; HC to Edward Cushing, Apr. 12, 1896, CP 15/252.

14 HC to HKC, Oct. 30, Nov. 17, 1895, CP 16/395, 397; HC notes on Halsted, 1925, 114/673ff.

15 W.S. Halsted to HC, Dec. 7, 1895, CP 27/921; HC notes on Halsted, 114/673ff; HC to BMC, Mar. 22, 1896, 14/777.

16 Halsted to HC, Apr. 15, 1896, CP 114/684; HC to HKC, Apr. 30, 1896, 16/409; HC to BMC, May 10, 1896, 14/784; HC to HKC, July 17, 1896, 16/414.

17 Travel diary, quoted in Fulton, 113; HC to HKC, Aug. 16 and 23, 1896, CP 16/420, 424.

18 C.A. Porter to HC, summer 1896, quoted in Fulton, 116.

19 HC to BMC, Oct 4, 1896, CP 14/791.

20 HC to 'Alice,' Oct. 4, 1896, CP 11/266; HC to KC, Oct. 11, 1896, 17/274; HC to BMC, Oct. 17, 1896, 14/793; HC to HKC, Oct. 15, 1896, 16/426.

21 HC to HKC, Oct. 15, 1896, CP 16/426; HC notes on Halsted, 1925, 114/673; for the embellished version, see J.H. Pratt, interview notes with HC, June 1939, FP 216/238.

22 HC notes on Halsted, 1925, CP 114/673ff.

23 HC Diary, Nov. 2, 1900, CP 107/2; also J.M.T. Finney, *A Surgeon's Life* (New York: Putnam's, 1940), 89; Hugh Young, *A Surgeon's Autobiography* (New York: Harcourt Brace, 1940), 58–9; W.G. MacCallum, *William Stewart Halsted, Surgeon* (Baltimore: Johns Hopkins University Press, 1930), 96–7; S.J Crowe, *Halsted of Johns Hopkins: The Man and His Men* (Springfield, Ill.: Charles C. Thomas, 1957), 50.

24 HKC to HC, Oct. 18, 1896, CP 16/427; Edward Cushing to HC, autumn 1896, 15/309.

25 HC to BMC, Oct. 17, Nov. 1, 1896, CP 14/793, 797; HC notes on Halsted, 1925, 114/673; HC to HKC, Nov. 30, 1896, 16/431.

26 HC to BMC, Nov. 1 and 21, 1896, CP 14/797, 803.

27 HC to KC, Dec. 31, 1896, CP 17/276.

28 HC to HKC, Feb. 7, 1897, CP 16/437; HC to HKC, Apr. 5, 1897, 16/445.

29 MacCallum, *Halsted*, 245.

30 Ibid., 92.

31 Young, *A Surgeon's Autobiography*, 62.

32 Geoffrey Jefferson, 'Harvey Cushing,' in *Selected Papers of Geoffrey Jefferson* (London: Pitman, 1960); more florid version, Fulton, 121–2.

33 Ibid.

34 'Haematomyelia from Gunshot Wounds of the Spine,' *American Journal of the Medical Sciences* 115 (June 1898), 654–83, CP 127/394ff; Young, *A Surgeon's Autobiography*, 73; HC to William A. Evans, Aug. 7, 1933, CP 21/877.

35 'Observations upon the Origin of Gall-Bladder Infections and upon the Experimental Formation of Gall-Stones,' *JHH Bulletin* 10 (Aug.–Sept. 1899); 'A Comparative Study of Some Members of a Pathogenic Group of Bacilli of the Hog Cholera ...' *JHH Bulletin* 11 (July–Aug. 1900); HC to HKC, Sept. 24, 1899, CP 16/602; Young, *A Surgeon's Autobiography*, 73.

36 HC and Louis E. Livingood, 'Experimental and Surgical Notes upon the Bacteriology of the Upper Portion of the Alimentary Canal ...' *JHH Report* 9 (1900), 543–91, CP 127/614ff.

37 Halsted to HC, Aug. 4, 1897, CP 114/703; Halsted to HC, July 2, 1897, 114/696.

38 J.F. Mitchell, 'Memories of Dr. Halsted,' *Surgery* 32 (1952), 451–60; Finney, *A Surgeon's Life*, 97; HC to HKC, May 1897, CP 16/449.

39 Henry Hurd to HC, Aug. 11, 1898, CP 31/579; HC Diary, Nov. 6, 1900, 107/13.

40 Ida M. Cameron to HC, Dec. 16, 1933, CP 10/388 (re nurses); Margaret B. Hoyt to JF, Dec. 10, 1939, FP, folder 309. The incident echoes in HC, 'The Medical Career,' in *Career*, 31.

41 HKC to HC, Oct. 1, 1897, CP 16/470; MacCallum, *Halsted*, 134; HC to S.C. Harvey, Oct. 2, 1934, 28/1233; HC to Charles Camac, Sept. 27, 1897, 11/624; HC to KC, Oct. 6, 1897, 17/294.

42 HC to HKC, Oct. 1897, CP 16/478; Fulton, 130–1, for HC's notes on the case; HC to A. Jentzer, July 26, 1937, 87/519.

43 HC to KC, Mar. 15, 1898, CP 17/343; HC to HKC, Sept. 25, 1898, 16/552; FD, Aug. 18, 1929.

44 'Operative Wounds of the Thoracic Duct: Report of a Case with Suture of the Duct,' *Annals of Surgery* 27 (June 1898), 719–28.

45 'Remarks upon a Case of Jejunal Fistula,' *JHH Bulletin* 10 (July 1899), 136–7. In the early nineteenth century, William Beaumont published pioneering studies of digestion as a result of his observations of St Martin, who had a permanent opening in his stomach.

46 HC to KC, Apr. 20, 1899, CP 17/726; HC to KC, Sept. 21, 1898, 17/562; HC to HKC, Nov. 15, 1898, 16/564; Fulton, 139, ignores Cushing's doubts about a cure in

HC 'Two Cases of Splenectomy for Splenic Anemia: A Clinical Lecture, Jan. 21, 1920 ...' *Archives of Surgery, Chicago* 1 (July 1920), 1–20; WO to Edward Cushing, Feb. 9, 1899, CP 89/700.

47 Halsted to HC, July 2, 1897, CP 114/696; HC notes on Halsted, 1925, 114/673ff.

48 'Cocaine Anesthesia in the Treatment of Certain Cases of Hernia and in Operations for Thyroid Tumors,' *JHH Bulletin* 9 (Aug. 1898), 192–3, CP 127/427ff; HC notes on Halsted, 1925, 114/673ff.

49 WO, 'On Perforation and Perforative Peritonitis in Typhoid Fever,' *Philadelphia Medical Journal*, Jan. 1901.

50 HC to KC, Aug. 14, 1898, CP 14/472.

51 'Laparotomy for Intestinal Perforation in Typhoid Fever: A Report of Four Cases ...' *JHH Bulletin* 9 (Nov. 1898), 257–69.

52 Ibid.; also 'Concerning Prompt Surgical Intervention for Intestinal Perforation in Typhoid Fever: With the Relation of a Case,' *Annals of Surgery* 33 (May 1901), 544–57.

53 C.A. Porter to HC, Aug. 21, 1899, CP 127/466.

54 HC undated and unindexed review of Crile, CP 127/508; Peter C. English, *Shock, Physiological Surgery, and George Washington Crile: Medical Innovation in the Progressive Era* (Westport, Conn.: Greenwood Press, 1980).

55 HC to KC, Aug. 21, 1898, CP 17/495.

56 HC to KC, Oct. 7, 1897, CP 14/851.

57 HC to KC, Nov. 19, 1897, CP 17/300; HC to KC, Nov. 24, 1897, 17/303.

58 KC to HC, 'Tuesday,' 1898, Whitney-Cushing Archive (hereafter WCA); HC to KC, Nov. 27, 1900, CP 17/898.

59 Caroline Crowell to HC, Mar. 10, 1898, CP 17/340; HC to KC, Mar. 15, 1898, 17/343.

60 KC to HC, 'Thursday no Friday,' 1898; 'Sunday,' 1898; 'Tuesday,' 1898, WCA.

61 HC to KC, Jan. 1, 1898, CP 17/317.

62 HC to KC, Jan. 7, 1898, CP 17/321.

63 HC to BMC, Feb. 20, 1898, CP 15/03; HC notes on Halsted, 1925, 114/673ff ; HC to KC, Nov. 15, 1898, 17/630.

64 Halsted notes to HC, CP 114/715–37; HC to Lyman Richards, Nov. 2, 1929, 96/1095; 'William Stewart Halsted,' in *Career*, 225.

65 See Michael Bliss, *William Osler: A Life in Medicine* (Toronto: University of Toronto Press, 1999), chs. 5, 6.

66 Halsted to HC, undated, in HC to KC, Apr. 29, 1899, CP 17/728; HC to KC, Apr. 28, 1898, 17/383.

67 HC to KC, July 7, 1898, CP 17/416; HC notes on Halsted, 1925, 114/673ff; Halsted to HC, July 23, 1898, 114/710; HC to KC, July 10, 1898, 17/429.

68 HC to KC, Aug. 12, 24, and 28, 1898, CP 17/457, 499, 510.

69 HC to KC, Mar. 18, 1899, CP 17/705.

70 HC to KC, Oct. 25, 1898, CP 17/605.

71 HC to BMC, July 19, 1899, CP 15/53; HC to KC, Apr. 14, 1898, 17/381.

72 HC to KC, Sept. 21, 1898, CP 17/562; HC to KC, Sept. 26, 1898, 17/566; HC to KC, Aug. 28, 1898, 17/510.

73 HC to KC, Oct. 22, 1898, CP 17/601; HC to KC, Sept. 16, 1898, 554/17.

74 HC to KC, Nov. 25, 1898, CP 17/636.

75 HC to KC, June 22, 1899, CP 17/752.

76 HC to KC, Dec. 20, 1900, CP 17/909.

77 Thomas McCrea to HC, Aug. 18, 1899, CP 36/797; HC to KC, Dec. 23, 1899, 17/795; BMC to HC, Feb. 17, 1900, 15/70; HKC to HC, Feb. 20, 1900, 16/621.

78 HC to HKC, May 10, 1900, CP 16/635; KC to HC, 'Friday,' apparently misdated 1901, WCA.

79 John B. Townsend to JF, Apr. 18, 1940, FP 216/330.

80 Unless otherwise noted, details are from HC, 'A Method of Total Extirpation of the Gasserian Ganglion for Trigmental Neuralgia ...' JAMA 34 (1900), 1035, reprinted in *Selected Papers*; and 'The Surgical Aspects of Major Neuralgia of the Trigeminal Nerve: A Report of Twenty Cases ...' JAMA 44 (Mar. 11, 18 and 25, Apr. 1 and 8, 1905), 773–8, 860–5, 920–9, 1002–8, 1088–93.

81 Jefferson, 'Harvey Cushing.'

82 Walker Evans to HC, Dec. 18, 1907 (misdated 1902), CP 127/1541.

83 HC, 'The Surgical Aspects of ... Major Neuralgia.'

84 Undated *Journal American* clipping, CP 127/582; Newcomb clipping, Apr. 25, 1900, in HC Baltimore scrapbook, 106/28; HC notes on Newcomb, in Fulton, 263–5 ('He did not remain permanently well'); HC to KC, June 20, 1900, 17/830.

5: A Window on the Brain

1 HC travel diary (hereafter Diary), June 23, 1900, CP 106/772; HC to KC, June 24, 1900, 17/831.

2 HC to BMC, June 29, July 2, 1900, CP 15/83, 85.

3 HC to BMC, July 17, 1900, CP 15/87; Diary, July 19, 1900, 106.

4 Diary, July 5, 1900, CP 106/733; HC to HKC, July 7, 1900, 16/640; HC to KC, July 10, 1900, 17/838.

5 Diary, July 19 and 24, 1900, CP 106/750, 781.

6 HC to BMC, July 22, 1900, CP 15/89; Diary, July 22, 1900, 106/754.

7 HC to HKC, Aug. 3, 1900, CP 16/649; HC to KC, Aug. 6, 1900, 17/846; HC to BMC, Aug. 6, 1900, 15/96.

8 HC, 'The Society of Clinical Surgery in Retrospect,' unpublished 1921 ms, CP 49/74.

9 Diary, July 17 and 27, 1900, CP 106/796; HC to HKC, July 7, 1900, 16/640.

10 Diary, July 4, 1900, CP 106/731; HC to Ernest Sachs, Aug. 8, 1933, 47/624. See Fulton, 163, for an embellished description of the ganglionectomy.

11 HC to Edward Cushing, Sept. 6, 1900, CP 15/261; HC to HKC, Sept. 15, 1900, 16/666; Diary, Aug. 18, 1900, 106/890.

12 J.M.T. Finney, *A Surgeon's Life* (New York: Putnam's, 1940), 126–7; also John Harley Warner, *Against the Spirit of System: The French Impulse in Nineteenth-Century American Medicine* (Princeton: Princeton University Press, 1998), 257–60, 304–5.

13 Diary, Oct. 12, 1900, CP 17/878; HC to KC, Oct. 21, 1900, 17/880.

14 Diary, Oct. 14, 15 and 17, 1900, CP 106/945–7, 960.

15 Diary, Oct. 22, 1900, CP 106/976; HC to BMC, Oct. 26, 1900, 15/113; Diary, Oct. 25, 1900, 106/987.

16 Diary, Oct. 26 and 30, 1900, CP 106/991, 996–8.

17 Diary. Oct. 30, 1900, CP 106/996.

18 Diary, Nov. 1 and 4, 1900, CP 107/2, 10.

19 Diary, Nov. 6, 1900, CP 107/13.

20 HC to KC, Nov. 15, 1900, CP 17/896; also HC to BMC, Nov. 16, 1900, 15/121.

21 Diary, Nov. 18 and 24, 1900, CP 107/20–1.

22 HC to KC, Nov. 27, 1900, CP 17/898; HC to HKC, Dec. 9, 1900, 16/687.

23 HC to KC, May 21, 1901, CP 17/941; HC to Jeanne Michaud, Jan. 2 and 5, Apr. 1, Dec. 14, 1901, 38/897–8, 904, 913.

24 Diary, Mar. 31, 1901, CP 107/207; HC to HKC, Jan. 13, 1901, 16/695.

25 Diary, Apr. 5, 1901, CP 107/237.

26 HC, beginning of notebook of observations in Kocher's Laboratory at Berne, CP 107/696, 705, 792.

27 'Concerning a Definite Regulatory Mechanism of the Vaso-Motor Center Which Controls Blood Pressure during Cerebral Compression,' *JHH Bulletin* 12 (Sept. 1901), 290–2, CP 127/811.

28 Francis M. Forster to JF, Nov. 5, 1946, FP 317/239; reply, Nov. 7.

29 Diary, June 5, 1901, CP 107/395. Fulton, 191–2, confuses his K's.

30 Peter C. English, *Shock, Physiological Surgery, and George Washington Crile: Medical Innovation in the Progressive Era* (Westport, Conn.: Greenwood Press, 1980); on 'Cushing's law,' see E.A. Archibald, 'Retrospect of Current Literature,' *Montreal Medical Journal*, Feb. 1905, CP 127/913; Fulton, 192. For an overview that emphasizes the importance of HC's early work on intracranial pressure, see Samuel H. Greenblatt, 'Cushing's Paradigmatic Contributions to Neusorugery,' *Bulletin of the History of Medicine* 77 (2003), 789–822.

31 Diary, Feb. 5, 1901, CP 107/112; Fulton, 186 (referring to Turin notes which cannot now be located); Diary, May 5, 1901, 107/356; HC to HKC, May 12, 1901, 16/712.

32 Diary, May 21, 1901, CP 107/380; Albert Kocher to HC, Mar. 2, 1902, 107/446.

33 HC to HKC, June 10, 1901, CP 16/719; W.S. Halsted to HC, May 25, 1901, 114/740–1; HC to KC, May 21, 1901, 17/941.

34 HC Special Diary, 'A visit to "Le Plus Pittoresque Endroit du Monde,"' CP 107/597; HC to HKC, Aug. 29, 1900, 16/659.

35 HC to HKC, undated postcard, CP 107/314; HC to HKC, May 12, 1901, 16/712.

36 Fulton, 188; HC to HKC, Apr. 14, 1901, CP 16/709; Diary, Apr. 6, 1901, 107/237.

37 HC to KC, Apr. 18, 1901, CP 17/931.

38 AC, 'Haller and His Native Town: A Letter from Berne,' *American Medicine*, Oct. 5–12, 1901, in *Career*, 266–84.

39 HC to BMC, July 3, 1901, CP 15/158.

40 HC to KC, July 7, 1901, CP 17/948.

41 HC to Edward Cushing, July 7, 1901, CP 15/263; HC to Walter B. Cannon, Oct. 11, 1927, 11/752.

42 Diary, July 12, 1901, CP 107/498.

43 HC to HKC, July 14, 1901, CP 16/729.

44 Diary, July 21, 1901, CP 107/503.

45 Diary, notes from Scotland, CP 107/563; HC to A.N. Richard, Feb. 8, 1936, 51/1271.

46 T. McCrae to HC, Feb. 4, 1901, CP 36/819.

47 WO to HC, Apr. 12, 1901, CP 107/307; T. McRae to HC, June 11, 1901, 36/284; WO to HC, 'Saturday' [July 1901], 107/523; H. Hurd to HC, July 8, 1901, 123/18.

48 KC to HC, Apr. 1, apparently 1901, WCA; HC to HKC, Sept. 29, 1901, CP, 16/737.

49 HC to KC, Oct. 3, 1901, CP 17/977; HC, 'Neurological Surgeons: Report of One Case' (1923), *Selected Papers*.

50 KC to HC, undated letters, 1901, WCA.

51 HC to KC, Oct. 9, 1901, CP 17/981.

52 HC to HKC, Oct. 13, 1901, CP 16/743; also HC, 'The Story of the Old Hunterian,' Jan. 24, 1920, 126/640; HC notes, 1913, 1915, 123/3–16.

53 'The Surgical Aspects of Major Neuralgia of the Trigeminal Nerve: A Report of Twenty Cases ...' *JAMA* 44 (Mar. 11, 18 and 25, Apr. 1 and 8, 1905), 773–8, 860–5, 920–9, 1002–8, 1088–93.

54 HC to KC, Nov. 28, 1901, CP 17/1011; 'Some Experimental and Clinical Observations concerning States of Increased Intracranial Tension,' *American Journal of the Medical Sciences* 124 (Sept. 1902), 375–400; HC to HKC, Dec. 4, 1901, 16/755.

55 HC to KC, Nov. 4, 1901, CP 17/998; HC to KC, Jan. 13, 1902, 17/1039.

56 L.F. Barker to HC, Feb. 24, 1902, WCA; W.T. Councilman to HC, Feb. 22, 1902, CP 123/19; Charles W. Eliot to HC, Mar. 11, 1902, 21/1153.

57 N. Bowditch Potter and George Crile to KC, Engagement File, WCA; KC to BMC, undated, 1902, WCA; Amory Codman to HC, undated, Engagement File, WCA; HC to KC, Mar. 15, 1902, CP 17/1061.

58 HC to KC, Jan 20, 1902, CP 17/1049.

59 WO to HC, Mar. 3, 1902, also undated, CP 89/709–11.

60 'The Surgical Aspects of Major Neuralgia of the Trigeminal Nerve: A Report of Twenty Cases ...'

61 Abe [Garfield?] to HC, undated, 1902, Engagement File, WCA; KC to HC, 'Wednesday evening,' 1902, WCA.

62 KC to HC, 'Sunday night,' 1902, WCA; KC to HC, Mar. 28, 1902, WCA; HC to KC, Mar. 22, 1902, CP 17/1067; HC to KC May 3, 1902, CP 17/1122.

63 'The Blood-Pressure Reaction of Acute Cerebral Compression: Illustrated by Cases of

Intracranial Hemorrhage,' *American Journal of the Medical Sciences* 125 (June 1903), CP 127/1125.

64 Case 1 in 'Sexual Infantilism with Optic Atrophy in Cases of tumor Affecting the Hypophysis Cerebri,' *Journal of Nervous and Mental Disease* 33 (Nov. 1906), CP 128/207; identified in *Intracranial Tumours*, 2, as first tumor experience; HC to KC, Apr. 28, 1902, 17/1117.

65 'The Surgical Treatment of Facial Paralysis by Nerve Anastomosis: With the Report of a Successful Case,' *Annals of Surgery* 37 (May 1903), 641–59; HC to KC, May 13, 1902, CP 17/1131; HC to HKC, May 26, 1902, 16/775.

66 HC to HKC, May 18, 1902, CP 16/773; KC account book, 1902, WCA; *Cleveland Plain Dealer*, June 11, 1902; notes from HC/KC honeymoon diary, enclosed in Phyllis A. Horan to Kate Whitney, Oct. 27, 1989, WCA.

6: Opening the Closed Box

1 HC to HKC, Feb. 26, 1902, CP 16/766; HC to KC, July 2, 1908, 18/225.

2 KC to HC, Sept. 2, 5 and 8, 1902, WCA.

3 KC to HC, Sept. 1 and 18, 1902, WCA.

4 HC to HKC, Nov. 15, 1903, CP 16/901.

5 Fulton, 699.

6 Unless otherwise noted, this discussion rests on the rich anthology of articles edited by Samuel H. Greenblatt, *A History of Neurosurgery, in Its Scientific and Professional Contexts* (Washington: American Association of Neurological Surgeons, 1997) (hereafter *HistNeurosurg*), particularly Greenblatt's own contributions; also John E. Scarff, 'Fifty Years of Neurosurgery, 1905–1955,' *International Abstracts of Surgery* 101 (Nov. 1955), 417–513; A. Earl Walker, *A History of Neurological Surgery* (New York: Williams & Wilkins, 1951; reprint Hafner, 1967); Ernest Sachs, *The History and Development of Neurological Surgery* (New York: Harper Brothers and Yale University School of Medicine, 1952); Gilbert Horrax, *Neurosurgery: An Historical Sketch* (Springfield, Ill: Charles C. Thomas, 1952).

7 Robert H. Wilkins, 'Treatment of Craniocerebral Infection and Other Common Neurosurgical Operations at the Time of Lister and Macewen,' *HistNeurosurg*, 90.

8 Ibid.; also S.H. Greenblatt, 'Cerebral Localization: From Theory to Practice. Paul Broca and Hughlings Jackson to David Ferrier and William Macewen,' *HistNeurosurg*.

9 Arthur E. Lyons, 'The Crucible Years, 1880 to 1900: Macewen to Cushing,' *HistNeurosurg*; A. Hughes Bennett and Rickman J. Godlee, 'Case of Cerebral Tumor,' *Medico-Chirurgical Transactions, London* 68 (1885), 243–75, reprinted in Robert H. Wilkins, ed., *Neurosurgical Classics* (New York & London: Johnson Reprint Corp., 1965), 361–71.

10 Perpetuated in Fulton, 256, by his complete misreading of the Cushing and Eisenhardt paper that he cites, which shows that the Durante operation came after Godlee-Bennett.

11 HC, *Intracranial Tumours: Notes upon a Series of Two Thousand Verified Cases with Surgical-Mortality Percentages Pertaining Thereto* (Springfield, Ill.: Charles C. Thomas, 1921) (hereafter *Intracranial Tumours*), 1.

12 'On Routine Determination of Arterial Tension in Operating Room and Clinic,' *Boston Medical Surgical Journal*, Mar. 5, 1903, 250–6, in *Selected Papers*, 94–103; Jerome P. Webster to JF, Nov. 1, 1939, FP 216/332; Greenblatt, 'Cushing's Paradigmatic Contributions to Neusorugery,' *Bulletin of the History of Medicine*, 77 (2003), n. 57.

13 Fulton, 212–14, drawing on HC ms, 'The Society of Clinical Surgery in Retrospect,' 1921, CP 49/74ff; Division of Surgery of the Medical School of Harvard University, Bulletin no. 11, *Report of Research Work, 1903–* (Mar. 1904); HC, 'On the Avoidance of Shock in Major Amputations by Cocainization of Large Nerve-Trunks Preliminary to their Division ...' *Annals of Surgery* 36 (Sept. 1902), 321–45; 'Treatment by the Tourniquet to Counteract the Vasomotor Spasm of Raynaud's Disease,' *Journal of Nervous and Mental Disease* 29 (Nov. 1902), 657–63.

14 HC, 'The Society of Clinical Surgery in Retrospect,' 1921, CP 49/74ff; James Mumford to HC, June 1, 8, 1903, 39/189, 193; Grace Crile, ed., *George Crile: An Autobiography* (Philadelphia: Lippincott, 1947), 1: 140–3.

15 HC to HKC, Apr. 5, 1904, CP 16/947.

16 'The Special Field of Neurological Surgery,' *Cleveland Medical Journal* 4 (Jan. 1905), 1–25, and *JHH Bulletin* 16 (Mar. 1905), 77–87, CP 127/1528ff.

17 'Pneumatic Tourniquets: With Especial Reference to Their Use in Craniotomies,' *Medical News*, Mar. 26, 1904, 577–80, CP 127/1453.

18 'The Blood-Pressure Reaction of Acute Cerebral Compression, Illustrated by Cases of Intracranial Hemorrhage,' *American Journal of the Medical Sciences* 125 (June 1903), 1017–44, CP 127/1125.

19 'Concerning Surgical Intervention for the Intracranial Hemorrhages of the Newborn,' *American Journal of the Medical Sciences* 130 (Oct. 1905), with handwritten notes, CP 128/13; 'Surgery of the Head,' in W.W. Keen, ed., *Surgery: Its Principles and Practice* (Philadelphia: Saunders, 1908), 3: 215, 233; HC to HKC, Aug. 13, 1906, 16/1075; Thomson, 136.

20 'Consequences of Cranial Injuries: A Discussion Based on three clinical Histories Which Illustrate the Extradural, Subcortical, and Intermeningeal Types of Intra-Cranial Haemorrhage,' *New York Medical Journal*, Jan. 19 and 26, Feb. 2, 1907, CP 128/266; 'Surgery of the Head,' in Keen, *Surgery*, 251.

21 'Intradural Tumor of the Cervical Meninges: With Early Restoration of Function in the Cord after Removal of the Tumor,' *Annals of Surgery* 39 (June 1904), 934–55, CP 127/1463; HC to HKC, Nov. 23, 1903, 16/904.

22 'The Establishment of Cerebral Hernia as a Decompressive Measure for Inaccessible Brain Tumors: With the Description of Intermuscular Methods of Making the Bone Defect in Temporal and Occipital Regions,' *Surgery, Gynecology and Obstetrics* 1, (Oct. 1905), 297–314, in *Selected Papers*, 106–23, CP 128/41; 'Exhibition of Cases:

Decompressive Craniectomy for Brain Tumor,' *JHH Bulletin* 18 (Apr. 1907), 142–5, CP 128/260.

23 'Technical Methods of Performing Certain Cranial Operations,' *Surgery, Gynecology and Obstetrics* 6 (Mar. 1908), 227–46, CP 128/538.

24 'Consequences of Cranial Injuries. A Discussion Based on Three Clinical Histories Which Illustrate the Extradural, Subcortical, and Intermeningeal Types of Intra-Cranial Haemorrhage,' *New York Medical Journal*, Jan 19 and 26, Feb. 2, 1907, 97ff, CP 128/266.

25 'The Surgical Aspects of Major Neuralgia of the Trigeminal Nerve: A Report of Twenty Cases ...' *JAMA* 44 (Mar. 11, 18 and 25, Apr. 1 and 8, 1905), 773–8, 860–5, 920–9, 1002–8, 1088–93, CP 127/1571; KC to HKC, Feb. 11, 1904, 156/188.

26 'The Sensory Distribution of the Fifth Cranial Nerve' *JHH Bulletin* 15, (July-Aug. 1904), 213–32, CP 127/1481; 'The Taste Fibers and Their Independence of the N. Trigeminus: Deductions from Thirteen Cases of Gasserian Ganglion Extirpation,' *JHH Bulletin* 14 Mar.–Apr. 1903, 71–8, CP 127/1022; 'On Preservation of the Nerve Supply to the Brow, in the Operative Approach to the Gasserian Ganglion,' *Annals of Surgery* 43 (Jan. 1906), 128/075; 'Exhibition of Cases,' *JHH Bulletin* 18 (Apr. 1907), 142–5, 128/260.

27 William G. Spiller and Charles H. Frazier, 'The Division of the Sensory Root of the Trigeminus for the Relief of Tic Douloureux ...' *Philadelphia Medical Journal* 8 (1901), 1039–49, reprinted in Robert H. Wilkins, ed., *Neurosurgical Classics* (New York & London: Johnson Reprint Corp., 1965); HC, previous citations, plus 'Remarks on Some Further Modifications in the Gasserian Ganglion Operation for Trigmental Neuralgia (Sensory Root Evulsion),' Southern Surgical and Gynecological Association *Transactions* 19 (1907), 128/307; 'Remarks on the Surgical Treatment of Facial Paralysis and of Trigeminal Neuralgia ...' American Surgical Association *Transactions* 25 (1907), 128/314.

28 'Perineal Zoster: With Notes upon Cutaneous Segmentation Postaxial to the Lower Limb,' *American Journal of the Med. Sciences* 127 (Mar. 1904), 375–91, CP 127/1430; Brödel sketch, 127/1446.

29 HC to HKC, May 31, 1903, CP 16/841; KC to HKC, Aug. 18, 1905, 156/197.

30 Gerald A. Birks, 'A Layman's Tribute to Harvey Cushing,' FP 213/297; HC to KC, June 21 and 24, 1904, CP 17/1245, 1251; Birks obit. clipping, 127/1609.

31 HC to KC, Dec. 16, 1902, WCA.

32 GRO to KC, received Aug. 15, 1903, CP 157; HKC to HC, apparrently Dec. 4, 1903, 16/908; Michael Bliss, *William Osler: A Life in Medicine* (Toronto: University of Toronto Press, 1999), 240.

33 HKC to HC, Apr. 26, 1903, CP 16/836; BMC to HC, Apr. 27, 1903, 15/175.

34 HKC to HC, Aug. 3, 1903, CP 16/882; Edward Cushing to HC, Aug. 17, 1903, 15/268.

35 HC to KC, Oct. 22 and 24, 1903, CP 17/1210–12.

36 Caroline Cushing to KC, Oct. 29, 1903, CP 157/727; HC to KC, Dec. 30, 1901, 17/1026.

37 The 'pushing' issue is raised in George C. Ebers, 'Osler and Neurology,' and Dee James Canale, 'William Osler and "the Special Field of Neurological Surgery,"' both in Jeremiah Barondess and Charles G. Roland, eds., *The Persisting Osler*, 2: (201–26).

38 HC to HKC, May 31, 1903, CP 16/841.

39 Ibid.

40 KC to HC, Oct. 20, 1903, and 'Wednesday,' apparently 1903, WCA.

41 HC to KC, numerous letters, June–July, 1904, CP 17/1226ff.

42 HC to KC, July 16 and 19, 1904, CP 17/1287–92.

43 HC to KC, July 24 (misdated July 21), 1904, CP 17/1293.

44 HC Diary, July 28, 1904, and passim, CP 107/906ff.

45 GRO to KC, Aug. 17, 1904, CP 157; HC to KC, Aug. 2, 1904, 17/1309.

46 HC to KC, 'Tuesday,' c. Sept. 29, 1904, CP 17/1349; HC to KC, Oct. 2, 1904, 17/1358.

47 HC to HKC, Apr. 29, 1905, CP 16/1005; GRO to KC, May 22, 1905, 157; HC to KC, July 2, 1905, 18/49.

48 KC to HKC, Aug. 18, Oct. 27, 1905, CP 156/197, 203.

49 C.M. Faris et al., intro. by HC, 'Comparative Surgery: With Illustrative Cases,' *JHH Bulletin* 16 (May 1905), 170, CP 127/1656; HC, 'Instruction in Operative Medicine: With the Description of a Course Given in the Hunterian Laboratory of Experimental Medicine,' *JHH Bulletin* 17 (May 1906), 182, CP 128/138; Miley B. Wesson to JF, Mar. 25, 1940, FP 216/332; Carl W. Rand, 'Harvey Cushing: Scientist, Teacher, Friend,' Los Angeles County Medical Association *Bulletin*, July 20, 1961.

50 Conrad Jacobson essay on HC, FP 214/310; student thanks, Apr. 28, 1903, CP 106/297; also KC to HKC, Jan. 5, 1906, 156/207.

51 HC to HKC, Oct. 15, 1905, CP 16/1024; HC to Jay McLean, Jan. 24, 1920, 78/35; HC, 'Realignments in Greater Medicine,' in *Consecratio*, 60.

52 HC to HKC, Oct. 15, 1905, CP 16/1024; CP 56 passim, esp. 56/72, HC to W.B. Cannon, Jan. 8, 1909.

53 HC to KC, Sept. 29, 1904, CP 17/1351; HC to HKC, Apr. 2, 1908, 16/1163; Theodor Kocher to HC, Sept. 22, 1907, 32/801.

54 Appointment files, CP 123; KC to HKC, Mar. 14, 1906, 156/211.

55 Baltimore Scrapbook, 112c, CP 106/518; KC to HKC, Dec. 11, 1906, 156/211.

56 HKC to HC, Mar. 10, 1907, CP 16/1109 ff.

57 HC to KC, May 26 (misdated May 27), 1907, CP 18/65; HC to KC, June 11, 1907, 18/88.

58 H.M. Thomas and HC, 'Removal of a Subcortical Cystic Tumor at a Second-Stage Operation without Anesthesia,' *JAMA*, Mar. 14, 1908, 847–56, CP 128/555.

59 James Bordley Jr and HC, 'Observations on Choked Disc: With Especial Reference to Decompressive Cranial Operations,' *JAMA*, Jan. 30, 1909, 353–60, CP 128/630; HC and James Bordley Jr, 'Observations on Experimentally Induced Choked Disc,' *JHH Bulletin* 20 (Apr. 1909), 95–101, CP 128/670; HC, 'Some Aspects of the Pathological Physiology of Intracranial Tumours,' *Boston Medical and Surgical Journal*, 161, July 15, 1909, 71–80, CP 128/743.

60 'Recent Observations on Tumours of the Brain and Their Surgical Treatment,' *Lancet*, Jan. 8, 1910, 90–4, CP 128/843.
61 'The Special Field of Neurological Surgery: Five Years Later,' *JHH Bulletin* 21 (Nov. 1910), 325–39, CP 129/113.
62 Ibid.; 'Recent Observations on Tumours of the Brain and Their Surgical Treatment,' *Lancet*, Jan. 8, 1910, 90–4, CP 128/843.

7: The Bottom of the Box

1 John Homans to JF, Nov. 29, 1939, FP 214/309.
2 HC to HKC, Apr. 11, 1909, CP 16/1243; G.W. Crile to HC, June 14, 1909, 13/407; HC to HKC, June 16, 1909, 16/1255.
3 'Sexual Infantilism with Optic Atrophy in Cases of Tumor Affecting the Hypophysis Cerebri,' *Journal of Nervous and Mental Disease* 33 (Nov. 1906), 704–16, CP 128/207; HC handwritten note on original.
4 Fulton, 276, incorrectly states that E.A. Schäfer's lectures on the pituitary at Hopkins in Apr. 1908 probably stimulated Cushing's interest; Schäfer (CP 106/592) said that to lecture on the pituitary at Hopkins was like carrying coals to Newcastle.
5 Cited in Ock-Joo Kim, 'The Integration of Science with the Healing Art: Harvey Cushing's Development of Neurosurgery, 1896–1912' (PhD thesis, University of Minnesota, 1998), 193.
6 John Homans to JF, Nov. 29, 1939, FP 214/309; S.J. Crowe, *Halsted of Johns Hopkins: The Man and His Men* (Springfield, Ill.: Charles C Thomas, 1957), 74; HC, 'The Hypophysis Cerebri: Clinical Aspects of Hyperpituitarism and of Hypopituitarism,' *JAMA*, July 24, 1909, 249–55, CP 128/773; HC handwritten note on original. HC later learned that Otto Marburg had suggested the same terms, but without experimental evidence.
7 HC to HKC, Apr. 11, 1909, CP 16/1243; Hemens is discussed in 'The Hypophysis Cerebri: Clinical Aspects of Hyperpituitarism and of Hypopituitarism'; 'Partial Hypophysectomy for Acromegaly: With Remarks on the Function of the Hypophysis,' *Annals of Surgery* 50 (Dec. 1909), 1002–17, CP 128/828; HC, *The Pituitary Body and Its Disorders* (Philadelphia & London: Lippincott, 1912) (hereafter *Pituitary Body*), 140–3, 293–4; and correspondence CP 126/506ff.
8 *Pituitary Body*, 256.
9 Ibid., 294.
10 Ibid., 320.
11 *New York Herald*, Mar. 26, 1912, CP 126/879 ff; case follow-up in HC, 'Psychic Disturbances Associated with Disorders of the Ductless Glands,' *American Journal of Insanity* 69, no. 5 (1913), 965–90.
12 *Pituitary Body*, 300–2.
13 Ibid., 97.
14 Correspondence re case XX, in CP 126/449ff.

15 *Pituitary Body,* 167; S.J. Crowe to JF, Aug. 4 and 10, 1945, FP 213/300; Fulton, 303. For similar HC autopsy stories, see William Sharpe, *Brain Surgeon: The Autobiogrpahy of William Sharpe* (New York: Viking, 1952), ch. 6.

16 S.J. Crowe to JF, Aug. 10, 1945, FP 213/300; Charles D. Humberd, 'A Twenty-Five-Year-Old Error in Measuring a Giant,' *JAMA,* May 16, 1936, 1713–15, CP 99/331ff; but also E.L. Crosby to JF, Apr. 22, 1940, FP 214/310, stating that Hopkins's studies showed Turner had been 7 ft. 9 in.

17 Leon Asher to HC, July 29, 1912, CP 126/92; M. Allen Starr to HC, Sept. 14 [1912], 126/150; anon. review in *Maryland Medical Journal,* Sept. 1912, 126/157; DM review in *Cleveland Medical Journal,* 126/154.

18 Other letters and reviews, CP 126/150ff; *Pituitary Body,* 171; HC to F.C. Shattuck, apparently 1912, B Ms c 4.2, Countway Library, Harvard Medical School.

19 'The Control of Bleeding in Operations for Brain Tumors: With the Description of Silver "Clips" for the Occlusion of Vessels Inaccessible to the Ligature,' *Annals of Surgery* 54 (July 1911), 389–410; reprinted variously.

20 Conrad Jacobson profile of HC, FP 214/310.

21 Helen F. Adams to JF, Nov. 16, 25 and 28, 1939, FP 213/295; Miley B. Wesson to JF, Nov. 21, 1946, FP 217/340; Wesson to JF, Mar. 25, 1940, 216/332.

22 Jacobson profile of HC, FP 214/310; Crowe, *Halsted,* 75.

23 Adams, to JF, Nov. 16, 1939, FP 213/295; Sharpe, *Brain Surgeon,* 54.

24 Roy McClure to JF, Dec. 22, 1939, FP 214/315; John Homans to JF, Nov. 29, 1939, 214/309.

25 Jacobson profile; R. Eustace Semmes, 'Memories of Doctor Cushing,' ms in possession of Dr D.J. Canale; also quoted in Henry L. Heyl, 'A Selection of Harvey Cushing Anecdotes,' *Journal of Neurosurgery* 30 (Apr. 1969), 369.

26 Jacobson, profile; Crowe, *Halsted,* 75–6; Francis Grant to WD, Feb. 15, 1934, Dandy Papers, CAJHMI.

27 Roy McClure to JF, Dec. 22, 1939, FP 214/315; HC, 'Experiences with the Cerebellar Astrocytomas: A Critical Review of Seventy-Six Cases,' *Surgery, Gynecology and Obstetrics* 52 (Feb. 1931), 129–204, CP 133/567.

28 Crowe, *Halsted,* 78.

29 Cary B. Gamble to JF, Mar. 8, 1940, FP 213/306; Crowe, *Halsted,* 77–8; Helen Adams to JF, Nov. 16, 1939, 213/295; Roy McClure to JF, Dec. 22, 1939, 214/315.

30 Bertram M. Bernheim to JF, June 14, 1947, FP 217/339.

31 HC to KC, June 23, 1909, and undated 1909, CP 18/325, 312; KC to Mother, misdated Aug. 11, 1909, WCA.

32 KC to Mother, Aug. 13, 18 and 20, 1909, WCA.

33 KC to Mother, Aug. 31, 1909, WCA: HC to HKC, Sept. 12, 1909, CP 16/1279.

34 HC to HKC, Oct. 3, 1909, CP 16/1285; KC to HKC, Oct. 28 [1908], 156/221.

35 HC to HKC, Jan. 21, 1910, CP 16/1300; HC notes on appointments, 123/3–16.

36 Nurse's notes on HKC illness, Feb. 8–11, 1910, CP 157/289; WO to HC, Feb. 25, 1910, reel 89.

37 A. Lawrence Lowell to HC, Mar. 29, 1910, CP 123/178; HC notes on appointments, 123/3–16; Robert Brookings to HC, May 7, 1910, 123/257; Edward Cushing to HC, Apr. 6, 1910, 15/300. For the state of the Harvard Medical School see Saul Benison, A. Clifford Barger, and Elin L. Wolfe, *Walter B. Cannon: The Life and Times of a Young Scientist* (Cambridge: Harvard University Press, 1987).

38 J.C. Warren to HC, Apr. 14, 1910, CP 123/193; Joseph Pratt to HC, June 30, 1910, 123/412; Robert M. Yerkes to HC, May 9, 1910, 123/269; W.B. Cannon to HC, May 13, 1910, 123/274; Cannon to HC, c. May 20, 1910, 94/103; E.A. Codman to HC, undated, 123/186.

39 WO to HC, Apr. 20, 1910, CP 123/234; GRO to KC, June 11, 1910, 89/792; HC 1910 diary, 123/250ff; HC notes on appointments, 123/3–16.

40 HC to Simon Flexner, May 20, 1910, CP 23/395; HC notes on appointments, 123/3–16; Robert M. Brookings to HC, May 23, 1910, 123/318.

41 KC to HC, undated, refiled in 1910 series, CWA.

42 HC to KC, 'Wednesday,' CP 18/454.

43 Fulton, 313; George and Grace Crile accounts of 1910 trip, Crile Papers, folder 56, Western Reserve Historical Society, Cleveland; WO to HC, July 10, 1910, CP 89/798.

44 HC to J.G. Mumford, Mar. 19 [1909?], Countway Library, Boston;

45 Ernest Jones, *Free Associations: Memoirs of a Psycho-Analyst* (New York: Basic Books, 1959), 190.

46 HC to KC, July 1, 1911, CP 18/399.

47 HC memorandum, Mar. 22, 1911, CP 155/334.

48 E.A. Codman to HC, Apr. 15, 1911, CP 12/477; WO to James Mumford, Countway Library, Boston, undated; James Mumford to HC, May 31, June 15, July 19, 1911, CP 39/262–6.

49 *Correspondence of Walter E. Dandy and His Parents John and Rachel Dandy, 1907–1914*, ed. Kitty Dandy Gladstone (Wellesley, Mass.: n.p., 1997), John Dandy to WD, Oct. 27, 1908. See also William Lloyd Fox, *Dandy of Johns Hopkins* (Baltimore and London: Williams & Wilkins, 1984); Fox, 'The Cushing-Dandy Controversy,' *Surgical Neurology* 3 (1975), 61–6; Eugene S. Flamm, 'New Observations on the Dandy-Cushing Controversy,' *Neurosurgery* 35 (Oct. 1994), 737–40.

50 *Correspondence of Walter E. Dandy*, WD to Mother and Father, May 4, 1914; John Dandy to WD, Mar. 16, Dec. 20, 1909, June 13, 1912.

51 Ibid., Rachel Dandy to WD, May 8, 1909.

52 Ibid., WD to Mother and Father, Oct. 28, 1910; Rachel Dandy to WD, Oct. 31, 1910.

53 Ibid., WD to Mother and Father, Nov. 3, 1910.

54 Ibid., WD to Mother and Father, Nov. 3, Dec. 3, 1910.

55 Lewis H. Weed and Paul Wegefarth, 'Studies on the Cerebro-Spinal Fluid and Its Pathway,' Introduction by HC, *Journal of Medical Research* 21, no. 1 (1914), 1–176, CP 129/521ff.

56 *Correspondence of Walter E. Dandy*, Rachel Dandy to WD, Nov. 6, 1911.

57 Dandy to JF, Nov. 26, 1945, FP 42/627; Crowe, *Halsted*, 86; Jacobson profile of HC, FP 214/310.
58 Roy McClure to JF, Dec. 22, 1939, FP 214/315; *Correspondence of Walter E. Dandy*, WD to Mother and Father, Mar. 16, 1912, Jacobson profile of HC, FP 214/310; HC, 'The Third Circulation and its Channels,' in *Studies in Intracranial Physiology and Surgery* (Oxford: Oxford University Press, 1926); HC to KC, 'Saturday,' 1911, CP 18/498.
59 *Correspondence of Walter E. Dandy*, John Dandy to WD, Nov. 30, 1911; Rachel Dandy to WD, c. Jan. 10, 1912.
60 Ibid., Rachel Dandy to WD, c. spring 1912; John Dandy to WD, June 7, 1912.
61 Ibid., WD to Mother and Father, Mar. 6, 1912; John Dandy to WD, Mar. 18, 1912; WD to Mother and Father, Mar. 16, 1912.
62 Ibid., WD to Mother and Father, Apr. 6, 1912.
63 Ibid., WD to Mother and Father, Mar. 16, 1912.
64 HC to KC, Aug. 26, 1912, CP 18/591; *Correspondence of Walter E. Dandy* WD to Mother and Father, Dec. 29, 1913; WD to JF, Nov. 26, 1945, FP 42/627.
65 HC to KC, Aug. 26, 1912, CP 18/591.

8: Adieu the Simple Life

1 HC to KC, June 4, Aug. 3 and 7, 1912, CP 18/509, 571, 576.
2 KC to Mother, Aug. 5, 1913, WCA.
3 KC to Mother, Aug. 11, 1913, WCA.
4 For the vision of the Brigham, see Morris J. Vogel, *The Invention of the Modern Hospital, Boston, 1870–1930*, (Chicago: University of Chicago Press, 1980), ch. 4; also, Edward D. Churchill, ed., *To Work in the Vineyard of Surgery: The Reminiscences of J. Collins Warren, 1842–1927* (Cambridge: Harvard University Press, 1958); Henry K. Beecher and Mark D. Altschule, *Medicine at Harvard: The First Three Hundred Years* (Hanover, N.H.: University Press of New England, 1977); David McCord, *The Fabrick of Man: Fifty Years of the Peter Bent Brigham* (Boston: Peter Bent Brigham Hospital, 1963); Lowell quote in Jerome D. Green to HC, Oct. 28, 1910, CP 25/534.
5 HC to H.B. Howard, undated, 1911, CP 97/109ff; also H.A. Christian to HC, Feb. 15, 1911, 96/443; HC to Fielding Garrison, Apr. 7, 1913, 25/777; Churchill, *Vineyard*, 249. Much of the Christian-Cushing correspondence is also found in the Henry Christian Papers at the Countway Medical Library, Boston.
6 HC to Alexander Cochrane, draft, c. Apr. 15, 1910, CP 123/220, published in Fulton, 345; HC to C.F. Hoover, Aug. 3, 1923, 123/455.
7 HC to Alexander Cochrane, Dec. 18, 1911, CP 96/483; HC to Christian, Jan. 25, 1912, 96/498; Christian to HC, Jan. 27, 1912, 96/500.
8 HC to Christian, Mar. 4, 1912, CP 96/510; Christian to JF, Dec. 9, 1913, FP 213/299; John Morton to JF, Jan. 25, 1946, FP 215/318.

9 Christian to HC, Nov. 3, 1911, CP 96/452.

10 HC to Lowell, Apr. 22, 1910, CP 123/235; Francis B. Harrington to HC, May 1, 1910, cited in Joseph C. Aub and Ruth K. Hapgood, *Pioneer in Modern Medicine: David Linn Edsall of Harvard* (Cambridge: Harvard Medical Alumni Association, 1970), 229; John Homans to JF, Dec. 11, 1939, FP 214/308; Christian to JF, Oct. 3, 1947, and reply, FP 217/339.

11 HC to Christian, Jan. 25, 1912, CP 96/498.

12 Brookline property file, CP 103, esp. John P. Reynolds to HC, May 10, 1912, 103/316; Mrs Albert Bigelow, 'Memoir of a Friend and Neighbor' (1939), FP 213/297.

13 HC to KC, July 30, 1912, CP 18/562.

14 Helen Clapesattle, *The Doctors Mayo* (Minneapolis: University of Minnesota Press, 1941).

15 HC to KC, June 7, 1904, CP 17/1220; HC to HKC, Oct. 15, 1905, 16/1024.

16 Grace Crile, ed., *George Crile: An Autobiography*, 2 vols. (Philadelphia and New York: Lippincott, 1947), chs. 1, 18 and 19.

17 HC, 'The Society of Clinical Surgery in Retrospect,' Nov. 16, 1921, CP 49/74ff; Cushing-Carrel correspondence, 11/862ff; Ira M. Rutkow, 'The Letters of William Halsted and Alexis Carrel,' *Surgery Gynecology, and Obstetrics* 151 (Nov. 1980), 676–88; S. McKellar, 'Innovations in Modern Surgery: Alexis Carrel (1873–1944),' in Darwin H. Stapleton, ed., *Creating a Tradition of Biomedical Research: The Rockefeller University* (New York: Rockefeller University Press, 2003).

18 R.D. McClure, 'Hydrocephalus Treated by Drainage into a Vein of the Neck,' *JHH Bulletin* 20 (Apr. 1909), 217, CP 128/697; Carrel to HC, July 9, 1908, 11/898; Carrel to HC, May 1, 1912, 11/906; *George Crile: An Autobiography*, 162; W.T. Councilman to HC, Mar. 7, 1907, 123/92.

19 James Mumford to HC, Dec. 27, 1912, CP 39/315.

20 HC to KC, June 30, 1912, CP 18/547.

21 Ibid.; HC Diary, July 2, 1912, 108/449.

22 *George Crile: An Autobiography*, 240; Grace Crile Diary, Crile Papers, folder 56, Western Reserve Historical Society, Cleveland.

23 Ira Rutkow, *American Surgery: An Illustrated History* (Philadelphia: Lippincott-Raven, 1998), 248.

24 L.W. Jeffries to HC, Aug. 25, 1911, CP 30/1258; David Cheever to HC, May 30, 1912, CP 11/1248.

25 Fulton, 355.

26 *First Annual Report of the Peter Bent Brigham Hospital, for the Years 1913 and 1914* (Cambridge: The University Press, 1915), 41, CP 129/832.

27 'Report of the Surgeon-in-Chief' (1919), in Peter McL. Black, et al., eds., *Harvey Cushing at the Brigham* (Park Ridge, Ill.: American Association of Neurological Surgeons, 1993); *Correspondence of Walter E. Dandy and His Parents*, ed. Kitty Dandy Gladstone (Wellesley, Mass., 1997), WD to Mother and Father, Feb. 2, 1913.

28 HC note on full-time issue, 1932, CP 114/2–3; C. Jacobson profile of HC, FP 214/310.

29 HC to KC, Sept. 1 or Aug. 6, 1912 [*sic*], CP 18/573.

30 Lewis H. Weed, Harvey Cushing, and Conrad Jacobson, 'Further Studies on the Role of the Hypophysis in the Metablism of Carbohydrates: The Autonomic Control of the Pituitary Gland.' *JHH Bulletin* 24 (Feb. 1913), 40–52, CP 129/357; HC, 'Concerning the Symptomatic Differentiation between Disorders of the Two Lobes of the Pituitary Body ...' *American Journal of the Medical Sciences* 145 (Mar. 1913), 313–28.

31 HC and Emil Goetsch, 'Hibernation and the Pituitary Body,' *Journal of Experimental Medicine*, July 1, 1915, 25–47, CP 129/756; Hibernation file, CP 77.

32 'Psychic Disturbances Associated with Disorders of the Ductless Glands,' *American Journal of Insanity* 69, no. 5 (1913), 965–90, CP 129/499.

33 HC to Simon Flexner, Mar. 8, 1915, CP 23/402; HC 'Surgical Experiences with Pituitary Disorders, JAMA, Oct. 31, 1914, 1515–25.

34 Lewis H. Weed and Paul Wegefarth, 'Studies on the Cerebro-Spinal Fluid and its Pathway,' Introduction by HC, *Journal of Medical Research* 21, no. 1 (1914), 1–176; *Correspondence of Walter E. Dandy*, WD to Mother and Father, May 25, 1913.

35 HC to WD, June 4, 1913, Dandy Papers, CAJHMI; *Correspondence of Walter E. Dandy*, WD to Mother and Father, June 22, 1913, Dec. 16, 1912.

36 Ibid., Dec 8 and 29, 1913, Jan. 4, 1914; KC and HC diary, Jan. 1, 1914, WCA; HC to WD, Jan. 20, 1914, Dandy Papers, CAJHMI.

37 Walter E. Dandy and Kenneth D. Blackfan, 'An Experimental and Clinical Study of Internal Hydrocephalus,' JAMA, Dec. 20, 1913, 2216–17; 'Internal Hydrocephalus: An Experimental, Clinical and Pathological Study,' *American Journal of Diseases of Children* 8 (1914), 406–82, reprinted in Robert H. Wilkins, ed., *Neurosurgical Classics* (New York: Johnson Reprint Corp., 1965), 71–118; Weed and Wegefarth, 'Studies on the Cerebrospinal Fluid and Its Pathway.'

38 *Correspondence of Walter E. Dandy*, WD to Mother and Father, Jan. 4, 1914, Mar. 15, 1914.

39 Ibid., Aug. 16, Feb. 22, June 27, 1914.

40 HC remarks at Peter Bent Brigham Hospital, Boston, Founder's Day, Nov. 12, 1914, CP 129/686.

41 James Ford Rhodes to HC, Jan. 31, Feb. 14, 1914, CP 44/1284–5; John T. Morse to HC, Feb. 13, 1914, 39/25; Fulton, 356–60; HC to Dr Frederick P. Gay, Nov. 23, 1934, 25/950.

42 Fulton, 356, modified by Henry A. Christian to JF, Dec. 12, 1946, FP 217/339; KC to Mother, Feb. 17, 1913, WCA.

43 Mrs Albert Bigelow, 'Memoir of a Friend and Neighbor,' FP 213/297; KC to Mother, Mar. 3, 1913, Apr. 13 and 29, 1914, WCA.

44 William J. Mallon, *Ernest Amory Codman: The End Result of a Life in Medicine* (Philadelphia: Saunders, 2000).

45 'Concerning the Results of Operations for Brain Tumor,' JAMA, Jan. 16, 1915, 189–95, CP 129/675.

46 Memo on Harvard situation (possibly by HC) enclosed in A. Flexner to HC, Oct. 1,

1913, CP 114/38. For the origins of the full-time debate, see Michael Bliss, *William Osler: A Life in Medicine* (Toronto: University of Toronto Press, 1999), 379–90, 399–400.

47 Saul Benison, A. Clifford Barger, and Elin L. Wolfe, *Walter B. Cannon: The Life and Times of a Young Scientist* (Cambridge: Harvard University Press, 1987), 339–47.

48 HC notes, CP 114/49; HC correspondence with Lowell, spring 1914, 114/61–6.

49 Walter Cannon to HC, Mar. 6, 1915, CP 114/85: Cannon's biographers note that Christian and Edsall were almost as intransigent.

50 HC to A. Lawrence Lowell, Mar. 7, 1915, CP 114/94; Alexander Cochrane to Lowell, Apr. 15, 1915, 114/97; Cochrane to HC, May 14, 1915, 114/101.

9: Adieu America

1 HC to Rutherford Morison, Feb. 24, 1938, CP 36/219.

2 HC to Prof. Hermann Küttner, Oct. 8, 1914, CP 31/1251; Henry Head to HC, Sept. 8, 1914, 29/109; Max Brödel to HC, Nov. 2, 1914, 9/659.

3 HC to J. Lorthoir, Nov. 2, 1914, CP 35/159; HC to Henry Head, Dec. 7, 1914, 29/100.

4 'The American Hospital of Paris: Section for the Wounded,' brochure, Sept. 1914, CP 109/897; Grace Crile, ed., *George Crile: An Autobiography* (Philadelphia: Lippincott, 1947), 247–8; G.W. Crile to HC, Dec. 21, 1914, 109/1156; also American Ambulance file, CP 56.

5 HC to Joseph Blake, Jan. 26, 1915, CP 56/48; G.W. Crile to HC, Jan. 15, 1915, 109/1166.

6 HC to Dr Théodore Tuffier, Mar. 8, 1915, CP 56/092; Crile to HC, Mar. 11, 1915, 109/1178.

7 HC to Simon Flexner, Mar. 8, 1915, CP 23/402; HC to Will. Cushing, Mar. 12, 1915, 56/98; HC to Crile, Mar. 6, 1915, 56/089; Crile to HC, Mar. 11, 1915, 109/1178.

8 HC war diary (hereafter War Diary), Mar. 18–27, 1915 (citations are by date, occasionally by page number, by preference to the published version, HC, *From A Surgeon's Journal* [Boston: Little, Brown: 1936], hereafter *SJ*, but where necessary for accuracy or completeness to the original war diary, CP reels 109–13; often the differences between the unpublished and published diary are slight).

9 War Diary, Mar. 28–31, 1915.

10 *SJ*, Apr. 1, 2, 1915.

11 HC to KC, Apr. 4, 1915, CP 18/641; HC, 'The Harvard Unit at the American Ambulance in Neuilly, Paris,' *Boston Medical and Surgical Journal*, May 27, 1915, 801–3, 129/178.

12 War Diary, Apr. 11, 1915.

13 Ibid., Apr. 14, 1915.

14 Ibid., Apr. 21, 1915.

15 Ibid., Apr. 29, 1915; also HC, 'Concerning Operations for the Cranio-Cerebral

Wounds of Modern Warfare,' *Military Surgeon*, June–July 1916, CP 130/06. For other views of the impression Cushing left at Neuilly, see the 1915 Diary of Robert B. Osgood, Countway Library, Boston; and E.C. Cutler, *A Journal of the Harvard Medical School Unit to the American Ambulance Hospital in Paris: Spring of 1915* (privately printed, 1915).

16 War Diary, Apr. 23, 1915.

17 'Concerning Operations for the Cranio-Cerebral Wounds of Modern Warfare.'

18 War Diary, Apr. 26, 1915; HC to KC, Apr. 16, 1915, CP 18/651.

19 War Diary, Apr. 24, 1915.

20 Ibid., Apr. 28, 1915.

21 Ibid., May 2, 1915.

22 SJ, May 3, 1915.

23 HC to KC, Apr. 20, 1915, CP 18/656; SJ, May 6, 1915.

24 War Diary, May 7, 1915; HC to Robert B. Greenough, June 5, 1915, CP 56/129.

25 War Diary, May 8 and 9, 1915.

26 John Finney to HC, Oct. 19, 1915, CP 65/571.

27 HC to Crile, May 21, 1915, CP 56/118; HC to KC, Apr. 29, 1915, 18/662; HC to Crile, July 29, 1915, 56/139.

28 HC to Robert B. Greenough, June 16, 1915, CP 56/135; HC to WO, Sept. 13, 1915, 42/136.

29 *Report of the Surgeon-in-Chief of the Peter Bent Brigham Hospital, 1916*, CP 130/100; HC to Elsie Hopper, Sept. 17, 1915, 30/152.

30 HC to G.W. Crile, Aug, 18, 1916, CP 13/427; HC and Christian statement for trustees, Mar. 26, 1917, 94/280ff; HC to Fred T. Murphy, Jan. 3, 1917, 96/617.

31 Saul Benison, A. Clifford Barger, and Elin L. Wolfe, *Walter B. Cannon: The Life and Times of a Young Scientist* (Cambridge: Harvard University Press, 1987), 333ff; also W.T. Councilman to A. Lawrence Lowell, May 4, 1916, CP 67/957.

32 HC to Geo. W. Crile, Feb. 11, 1916, CP 56/476; HC to W.G. MacCallum, Mar. 22, 1917, 36/515; War Diary, Mar. 22, 1916.

33 HC, *Tumors of the Nervus Acusticus and the Syndrome of the Cerebellopontile Angle* (Philadelphia and London: Saunders, 1917), 14.

34 Ibid., 177.

35 Ibid., 246, 18.

36 Ibid., 244.

37 Ibid., 274.

38 Ibid., 278.

39 Ibid., 265; 'Proceedings of Societies ... Exhibition of Cases.' *JHH Bulletin* 28 (1917), 96.

40 *Report of the Surgeon-in-Chief of the Peter Bent Brigham Hospital, 1916*, CP 130/100; SJ, 79–83; HC, 'The Boston Tins,' in *Consecratio*, 174–85.

41 United States Surgeon General's Office, *The Medical Department of the United States Army in the World War* (Washington: Government Printing Office, 1923), vol. 1, ch.

2; *The Story of U.S. Army Base Hospital No. 5*, By a Member of the Unit [HC] (Cambridge, Mass.: University Press, 1919); *George Crile: An Autobiography*, CP 110/09ff.

42 *Base Hospital No. 5*, 16; *Consecratio*, 177.

43 *SJ*, 89, 83; *Base Hospital No. 5*.

44 *SJ*, 85–6; Seth M. Fitchet to HC, Jan. 21, 1937, CP 113/1130.

45 War Diary, Apr. 9–18, 1917; HC to Leonard Wood, Apr. 27, 1917, CP 110/740.

46 War Diary, Apr. 28, 1917; *Base Hospital No. 5*, 27.

47 *The Medical Department of the United States Army in the World War*, 2: 19–20; *Base Hospital No. 5*, 28; clipping, *New York Sun*, CP 110/811.

48 HC to M.W. Ireland, Nov. 10, 1919, CP 113/367; War Diary, Apr. 28–30, 1917.

49 HC exchanges with A. Lawrence Lowell, Apr. 30, 1917 et seq., CP 110/791ff; *SJ*, May 11, 1917.

50 *SJ*, May 6, 1917.

51 Clippings and notes, CP 110/881ff; KC to Mother, May 2, 1917, et seq., WCA; War Diary, May 6, 1917.

52 Benison, Barger, and Wolfe, *Walter B. Cannon*, 392; *SJ*, May 11, 1917.

10: An American Surgeon at Passchendaele

1 *SJ*, June 7 and 8, 1917, 123, 124.

2 Grace Crile, ed., *George Crile: An Autobiography* (Philadelphia: Lippincott, 1947), 285. Bowlby may have realized this on his own.

3 War Diary, May 19–21, 1917.

4 Ibid., May 24, 1917; HC to KC, May 27, 1917, CP 18/687.

5 War Diary; *The Story of Base Hospital No. 5* [by HC] (Cambridge, Mass.: University Press, 1919); HC to KC, May 31, 1917, CP 18/683.

6 HC to KC, July 1, 1917, CP 18/711; HC to Col. Jacob C.R. Peabody, June 4, 1917, 110/1365.

7 HC to KC, June 16, 1917, CP 18/701; *SJ*, June 13, 1917, 137–8.

8 War Diary, July 1, 1917; HC to KC, July 1, 1917, CP 18/711.

9 War Diary, July 4, 1917.

10 HC to KC, July 6, 1917, CP 18/713; War Diary, July 8, 1917.

11 HC to KC, July 10, 1917, CP 18/717; War Diary, July 11, 1917.

12 A.T. Sloggett memorandum, Aug. 4, 1917, attached to Knutsford to Derby, July 30, 1917, Wellcome Library, Archives and Manuscripts, RAMC, 4462/20. Thanks to Dr Ann Crichton-Harris for bringing this to my attention.

13 1917 Diary of Robert B. Osgood, June 22, July 3 and 12, Countway Library, Boston.

14 *SJ*, 165–6, 219.

15 *SJ*, July 24, 1917, 168.

16 *SJ*, July 27, 1917, 172.

17 See n. 12 above; War Diary, Aug. 3, 1917.

18 *SJ*, Aug. 24, 1917, 184.
19 HC to KC, Aug. 13, 1917, CP 18/736; *SJ*, Aug. 17, 1917, 187.
20 *SJ*, Aug. 17, 187.
21 War Diary, Aug. 21, 1917.
22 Ibid., Aug. 23, 1917.
23 GRO to HC, Aug. 19, 1917, CPOL, 52.
24 *SJ*, Aug. 30, 1917, 197–8; HC to Susan [Chapin], Aug. 30, 1917, CP 18/743; HC to KC, Oct. 6, 1917, 18/764; unpublished memoirs of George Brewer, courtesy Norman H. Horwitz.
25 *SJ*, Sept. 4, 1917, 119; KC to HC, Sept. 7, 1917, CP 18/75.
26 War Diary, Sept. 19, 1917.
27 *SJ*, 213, 215, 217.
28 'Notes on Penetrating Wounds of the Brain,' *British Medical Journal*, Feb. 23, 1918, 221–6; HC to KC, Sept. 23, 1917, CP 18/757.
29 *SJ*, 241; HC to KC, Oct. 28, 1917, CP 18/774.
30 *SJ*, Oct. 31, 1917.
31 KC to HC, Sept. 15, 1917, WCA.
32 Ibid., May 15, June 11 and 25, 1917, WCA.
33 Ibid., July 21, 1917 and, 'Monday evening,' summer 1917, WCA.
34 Ibid., Aug 21 and, 28, 1917, Mar. 20, 1918, WCA.
35 Ibid., Feb. 8, 1918, Nov. 10 and 14, 1917, Dec. 8, 1917, WCA.
36 Ibid., Oct. 20, 1917, Jan. 27, 1918, WCA.
37 Henry L. Higginson to HC, Mar. 7, 1918, CP 111/1167.
38 KC to HC, Sept 2, 1917, WCA.
39 War Diary, Dec. 13, 1917.
40 HC to KC, Oct. 28, 1917, CP 18/774; Betsey Cushing to HC, Aug. 16, 1917, Feb. 16, 1918, Oct. 31, 1918, WCA; KC to HC, Sept. 28, 1917, WCA.
41 HC to KC, Nov. 21/17, CP 18/784; HC to KC, Dec. 2, 1917, 18/789; War Diary, Dec. 2, 1917, Feb. 9, 1918; HC to KC, Oct. 19, 1918, 18/1071.
42 *SJ*, Jan. 6 and 28, 1918, 274, 280.
43 *SJ*, 274; HC to KC, Dec. 31, 1917, Jan. 7, 1918, CP 18/817, 829.
44 War Diary, Jan. 1 and 10, 1918.
45 *SJ*, Feb. 9, 1918, 287.
46 'A Study of a Series of Wounds Involving the Brain and Its Enveloping Structures,' *British Journal of Surgery*, Apr. 1918, 558–684; note on British use of the article in CP 130/176; United States Surgeon General's Office, *The Medical Department of the United States Army in the World War*, vol. 11: *Surgery* (Washington: Government Printing Office, 1923), sec. 3, ch. 3.
47 *SJ*, Jan. 30, 1918, 285.
48 War Diary, Jan. 16, 1918.
49 Ibid., Mar. 4, 1918.
50 *SJ*, Mar. 10, 1918, 297–8.

51 War Diary, Mar. 18, 1918.
52 *SJ*, Mar. 27, 1918, 316.
53 'Bob' to HC, Apr. 21, 1936, CP 113/764 (banana peel); *SJ*, Apr. 10, 1918, 326.
54 *SJ*, Apr. 19, 1918, 358–9; HC to KC, Apr. 21, 1918, CP 18/910.
55 War Diary, Apr. 24 to May 3, 1918.
56 KC to HC, May 20, 1918, WCA.
57 War Diary, May 9–18, 1918, HC to KC, May 17, 1918, CP 18/930; J.M.T. Finney, *A Surgeon's Life* (New York: Putnam's, 1940), 198–9; M.W. Ireland to JF, Jan. 14, 1946, FP 214/310; Hugh Bayne to HC, July 14, 1918, CP 112/408.
58 *SJ*, June 10, 1918, 378.
59 HC to KC, June 30, 1918, CP 18/993; KC to HC, June 10, 1918, WCA.
60 *SJ*, July 22, 1918, 406; HC to KC, July 22 and 28, 1918, CP 18/1002, 1005.
61 War Diary, Sept. 10, 15, 1918.
62 HC to KC, Sept. 28, 1918, CP 18/1046.
63 *SJ*, Oct. 4, 1918, 466.
64 Carl W. Rand, 'Harvey Cushing: Scientist, Teacher, Friend,' Los Angeles County Medical Society *Bulletin*, July 20, 1961; HC to William Welch (57 varieties), Mar. 1, 1919, CP 40/461; Stephen G. Reich, 'Harvey Cushing's Guillain-Barré Syndrome: An Historical Diagnosis,' *Neurosurgery* 21, 2, (1987), 135–41.
65 *SJ*, Oct. 31, 1918, 490.
66 HC to KC, Oct. 19, 1918, CP 18/1071; Sidney I. Schwab to JF, Nov. 7, 1939, Dec. 20, 1945, FP 215/325.
67 KC to HC, Oct. 20 and 31, Sept. 4, 1918, WCA.
68 Ibid., Sept. 9 and 21, 1918.
69 HC to KC, Nov. 30, 1918, CP 18/1097; Pearce Bailey to HC, Dec. 6, 1918, 112/1078; *Senior Consultant in Neurological Surgery Report to Chief Surgeon, AEF*, Dec. 2, 1918, CP 112/1000; War Diary, Dec. 6, 1918.
70 War Diary, Jan. 2–10, 1919.
71 HC to KC, Jan 19, 1919, CP 19/3.
72 HC to Benedict Crowell, Apr. 9, 1919, 13/651; KC Diary, 1919, WCA. In *SJ*, 511, HC incorrectly dates both his arrival at Hoboken and his discharge.
73 HC to Warwick Deeping, Dec. 1, 1936, CP 20/24.

11: Fathers and Sons

1 Betsey Cushing notes to father, enclosed in Betsey to KC, Feb. 5, 1919, WCA.
2 KC Diary, Feb. 14, 1919, WCA; KC to HC, Dec. 18, 1918, WCA.
3 KC to HC, July 13, 1920, CP 19/20.
4 KC to HC, July 8, 1920, CP 19/123; KC to HC, July 13, 1920, 19/20.
5 HC correspondence re the institute is at CP 40/457ff. Published pleas are 'Concerning the Establishment of a National Institute of Neurology,' *American Journal of Insanity* 76 (Oct. 1919), 167–83, CP 130/301; 'Some Neurological Aspects of Reconstruction,'

Archives of Neurology and Psychiatry 2 (Nov. 1919), 493–504; on Flexner, see Fulton Diaries (FD),1: 109, Apr. 30, 1928.

6 HC to Joseph M. Flint, Mar. 1, 1919, CP 23/544; HC to Richard B. Dillchunt, May 3, 1920, 20/211; David Cheever to HC, Feb. 5, 1918, 111/1104; Cheever to HC, 1918, 112/474; also, re Jacobson, CP 31/384ff.

7 HC to George W. Coy, July 30, 1919, CP 31/603; reply, Aug. 2, 61/604.

8 HC to Sidney I. Schwab, Apr. 7, 1919, CP 40/505; FD, Jan. 15, 1928; Percival Bailey, 'Pepper Pot,' in Paul C. Bucy, ed., *Neurosurgical Giants: Feet of Clay and Iron* (New York: Elsevier, 1985), 86.

9 Jacobson memoir of HC, FP 214/310; *Report of the Surgeon-in-Chief of the Peter Bent Brigham Hospital, 1920*, 125, CP 130; Fulton, 454.

10 HC to Myra Warner, Apr. 4, 1919, 52/1034.

11 HC to L.F. Barker, Nov 6. 1919, CP 7/314; HC to A.W. Adson, Dec. 16, 1919, 1/976; HC to J. Chalmers Da Costa, Dec. 6, 1919, 20/496; HC to Wilfred Harris, Oct. 13, 1932, 28/529.

12 HC to Elliott Cutler, July 19, 1919, CP 19/652; Ernest Sachs to HC, Jan. 6, 1920, 49/140.

13 'Notes on a Series of Intracranial Tumors and Conditions Simulating Them: Tumor Suspects; Tumors Unverified; Tumors Verified,' *Archives of Neurology and Psychiatry* 10 (Dec. 1923), 605–68, CP 131/436.

14 HC to H.B. Jacobs, Apr. 23, May 26, 1919, CP 31/258–9.

15 HC to Archie Malloch, Dec. 29, 1919, CP 37/415; *Consecratio,* 97.

16 GRO to KC, Feb. 9, 1920, CP, 157; David Edsall to HC, Feb. 19, 1920, 73/251; reply, Mar. 10, 73/253.

17 GRO to HC, quoted in Fulton, 458.

18 HC to Norman Gwyn, Mar. 20, 1920, CP 81/538; HC to GRO, Mar. 13, 1920, 83/577; HC to Lewis Perry, Sept. 11, 1925, 83/581

19 HC to L.F. Barker, Mar. 13, 1920, CP 79; GRO to Archie Malloch, Apr. 7, 1920, Malloch Papers, Osler Library, 573/6/33.

20 HC to Prof G. Bastianelli, Sept. 24, 1923, CP 79.

21 HC to KC, July 9 and 15, 1920, CP 19/16–27.

22 HC to F.J. Shepherd, Apr. 3, 1920, CP 84/598; GRO to Archie Malloch, Aug. 20, 1920, Malloch Papers, Osler Library, 573/6/61.

23 HC to Norman Gwyn, Jan. 14, 1921, CP 81/539; GRO to Archie Malloch, Apr. 4, 1920, Malloch Papers, Osler Library; HC to Archie Malloch, Jan. 28, 1929, Muirhead and Lady Osler Papers, Osler Club of London archive, Royal College of Physicians.

24 HC to Thomas McRae, Dec. 1, 1923, CP 82/567; Jeannette Osler to HC, Sept. 12, 1921, and reply Oct. 12, 42/113–15.

25 HC to Fielding Garrison, July 10, 1922, CP 25/816; KC to Mother, June 2, 1922, WCA; HC to G. Crile, July 27, 1922, CP 13/436.

26 HC to KC, July 25, 1917, CP 18/725; HC to KC, Oct. 26, 1918, 18/1084; HC to A.M. Stearns, Feb. 11, 1920, and reply Feb. 12, 19/338.

27 HC to W.L.W. Field, July 23, 1919, CP 22/980; HC to Bill, Oct. 26, 1920, 19/379.

28 HC to Bill, July 22, 1922, CP 19/483; HC to KC, Aug. 9, 1922, 19/48.

29 HC to Frank O'Brien [English teacher], undated, CP 19/490; HC to Fred Walcott, Oct. 26, 1922, 53/679; HC to R.W. Angier, Yale, June 9, 1923, 19/497.

30 HC to S.W. Childs, Apr. 9, 1924, CP 12/55; HC to W.G. Harrison, Dec. 4, 1925, 26/1226.

31 WD, 'Ventriculography Following the Injection of Air into the Cerebral Ventricles,' *Annals of Surgery* 68 (1918), 5–11.

32 WD, 'Röntgenography of the Brain after the Injection of Air into the Spinal Canal,' *Annals of Surgery* 70 (1919), 397–403.

33 HC to WD, May 21, 1919, CP 20/561.

34 WD, 'Presentation of Two Cases of Epilepsy Apparently Cured ...' *JHH Bulletin* 31 (1920), 137–8; 'The Diagnosis and Treatment of Hydrocephalus Resulting from Strictures of the Aqueduct of Sylvius,' *Surgery, Gynecology, and Obstetrics* 31 (1920), 340–58; 'Prechiasmal Intracranial Tumors of the Optic Nerves,' *American Journal Opthalmology* 5 (Mar. 1922), 169–88.

35 HC to George J. Heuer, Nov. 10, 1920, CP 29/659

36 'The Special Field of Neurological Surgery after Another Interval,' *Archives of Neurology and Psychiatry* 4 (Dec. 1920), 603–37.

37 HC to George J. Heuer, Dec. 2, 1920, CP 29/661; WD to HC, June 30, 1921, 20/566; William Lloyd Fox, *Dandy of Johns Hopkins* (Baltimore: Williams and Wilkins, 1984), 67–8.

38 HC to George E. Brewer, Jan. 23, 1917, CP 9/571; William Sharpe, *Brain Surgeon: The Autobiography of William Sharpe* (New York: Viking, 1952).

39 Abraham Flexner to Simon Flexner, Jan. 30, 1919, cited in Fox, *Dandy*, 54; W.S. Halsted to W.W. Keen, Apr. 1919, cited in S.J. Crowe, *Halsted of Johns Hopkins*, (Springfield, Ill. Thomas, 1957), 107; Halsted to Dandy, June 21, 1919, Halsted Papers, CAJHMI; Loyal Davis, *A Surgeon's Odyssey* (New York: Doubleday, 1973), 128.

40 WD, 'The Treatment of Brain Tumors,' *JAMA*, Dec. 10, 1921, 1853–9.

41 WD exchange with Caroline McGill, Jan. 1922, Dandy Papers, CAJHMI.

42 HC to Ernest Sachs, Dec. 12, 1921, CP 47/585; Sachs to HC, Dec. 13, 1921, 95/182; HC reply, Dec. 16, 95/183; W.P. Bowers to HC, Dec. 19, 1921, reply Dec. 20, 8/459–60; HC to George J. Heuer, Dec. 22, 1921, 29/664.

43 Wilder Penfield, *No Man Alone: A Neurosurgeon's Life* (Boston: Little Brown, 1977), 67–8; Minutes of the Fifth Meeting of the Society of Neurological Surgeons, Apr. 28–9, 1922, CP 49/220.

44 'American Neurological Association Transactions,' *Archives of Neurology and Psychiatry* 8 (1922), 570–5; HC to WD, May 12, 1922, CP 20/569; WD to Israel Strauss, May 15, June 7, 1922, Dandy Papers, CAJHMI; WD to JF, Nov. 26, 1945, FP 42/627.

45 WD, 'An Operation for the Total Extirpation of Tumors in the Cerebello-Pontine Angle: A Preliminary Report,' *JHH Bulletin* 33 (1922), 344–5.

46 HC to WD, draft, Sept. 13, 1922, CP 20/570; HC to W.G. MacCallum, Sept. 18, 1922, 36/525.

47 HC to Will Mayo, Sept. 8, 1922, and reply, Sept. 26, CP 38/154–5; HC to Alfred W. Adson, Oct. 11, 1922, 1/982.

48 HC to Winford H. Smith, Sept. 25, 1922, CP 48/894 (two drafts), also 20/571 with HC handwritten note to WD; WD to HC, Sept. 29, 1922, 20/573.

49 WD to HC, Oct. 20, 1922, and reply Oct. 23, CP 20/577–8.

50 HC to E.R. Carpenter, Jan. 8, 1924, CP 11/850; HC to Francis C. Grant, Nov. 14, 1924, 26/404.

51 WD to C.L. Bradford, Nov. 25, 1921, Dandy Papers, CAJHMI; WD to HC, Jan. 22, 1923; WD to HC, Nov. 23, 1932.

52 See especially the portrait of Dandy in Davis, *A Surgeon's Odyssey*, 125, 128–9.

53 WD to Israel Strauss, Oct. 31, 1927, Dandy Papers, CAJHMI; Francis Grant to WD, Dec. 23, 1927, June 1, 1933; Fred L. Reichert to WD, Dec. 30, 1936.

54 HC to Elliott Cutler, Aug. 21, 1925, CP 19/708; HC to Lewis H. Weed, Sept. 22, 1922, 53/1063.

55 'William Stewart Halsted,' in *Career*, 232.

56 F.M. Pottenger to HC, May 5, 1920, CP 4/513; HC to Milo P. Ridge, Sept. 30, 1920, 44/561; Madeline Stanton (MS) to Eric Oldberg, Feb. 8, 1932, Oldberg Papers, Yale.

57 'Disorders of the Pituitary Gland: Retrospective and Prophetic,' JAMA, June 18, 1921, 1721–6, CP 130/900.

58 HC to Paul D. White, Jan. 18, 1922, CP 2/1058; HC to J.J.R. Macleod, July 29, 1922, 37/168.

59 HC to W.W. Keen, Nov. 2, 1921, et seq., CP 2/334ff; 'Surgical End-Results in General: With a Case of Cavernous Haemangioma of the Skull in Particular,' *Surgery, Gynecology and Obstetrics* 36 (Mar. 1923), 303–8, 131/257.

60 HC to S.J. Crowe, Jan. 1, 1923, CP 13/573; also HC to W.S. Thayer, Dec. 13, 1922, 50/896.

61 W.J. Mayo to HC, Dec. 18, 1922, CP 123/447; GRO to HC, Dec. 26, 1922, 123/442.

62 Fulton, 456.

63 *Report of the Surgeon-in-Chief of the Peter Bent Brigham Hospital. Reprinted from the Fourteenth Annual Report, 1927*, CP 132/642.

64 *Report of the Surgeon-in-Chief ... Seventh Annual Report, 1921*, CP 130/840.

65 HC to J.B. Howland, July 31, 1923, CP 97/432; Thomas P. Morley, *Kenneth George McKenzie and the Founding of Neurosurgery in Canada* (Toronto: Fitzhenry and Whiteside, 2004).

66 Geoffrey Jefferson, letter to *Lancet*, Dec. 20, 1924, CP 131/677; 'Report of the Eighth Meeting of the Society of Neurological Surgeons, Boston,' Dec. 7–8, 1923, 49/262; Loyal E. Davis and HC, 'Experiences with Blood Replacement during or after Major Intracranial Operations,' *Surgery, Gynecology, and Obstetrics* 40 (Mar. 1925), 310–22, 131/676.

67 HC to I.W. Voorhees, July 27, 1923, CP 52/264; HC to W.W. Keen, Mar. 5, 1924, 32/192.

68 'The Meningiomas (Dural Endotheliomas): Their Source, and Favoured Seats of Origin,' *Brain* 45 (Oct.1922), 282–316, CP 131/144.

69 'Notes on a Series of Intracranial Tumors and Conditions Simulating Them: Tumor Suspects; Tumors Unverified; Tumors Verified,' *Archives of Neurology and Psychiatry* 10 (Dec. 1923), 605–68, CP 131/436.

70 HC to W.G. MacCallum, Dec. 7, 1927, CP 36/559.

71 HC to Corbet Locke, Nov. 28, 1925, CP 82/557; Fielding Garrison to HC, Mar. 29, 1920, 81/535; HC to C.L. Starr, Aug. 20, 1925, CP 97/1140. We do not know whether Dr Herbert Bruce's feelings were hurt by Cushing's biography; his son's feelings were greatly hurt by my less disguised retelling of the story seventy-five years later.

72 GRO to Archie Malloch, Aug. 11, 1924. Malloch Papers, Osler Library, 573/10/35; HC to Irman J. Ridgeway, Dec. 2, 1925, CP 44/535.

73 HC to Florence Keen, Mar. 3. 1938, CP 32/65.

74 HC to Leonard Mackall, Jan. 22, 1924, CP 82/568; W.M. McIntosh (OUP) to HC, undated, Cushing Papers, Osler Library, folder 57; Julia Shepley to MS, July 2, 1924, Madeline Stanton Papers (SP).

75 GRO to Archie Malloch, May 25, 1924, Malloch Papers, Osler Library, 573/10/23; Julia Shepley to MS, Dec. 13, 1924, SP.

76 Julia Shepley to MS, Oct. 7, 1924, SP; Archie Malloch to JF, Dec. 19, 1945, FP 1236/316; HC to W.G. MacCallum, Dec. 22, 1925, CP 72/610.

77 'Laboratories: Then and Now,' *Canadian Medical Association Journal* 13 (Jan. 1923), CP 131/206.

78 'The Clinical Teacher and the Medical Curriculum,' in *Consecratio*, 187.

79 'Experimentum Periculosum: Judicium Difficile,' in *Consecratio*, 247.

80 'The Clinical Teacher and the Medical Curriculum,' in *Consecratio*, 196–7.

81 HC to Mrs William Hooper, June 16, 1925, CP 30/204.

82 'The Western Reserve and Its Medical Traditions,' in *Consecratio*, 201–2.

83 'Experimentum Periculosum; Judicium Difficile,' in *Consecratio*, 239; also *Report of the Surgeon-in-Chief ... Ninth Annual Report, 1922*, 131/229.

84 HC to Editor, *Brookline Chronicle,* Apr. 10, 1923, CP 6/208; Fulton, 516, 520; HC to KC, Oct. 4, 1925, WCA.

85 HC to Joe Collins, Apr. 29, 1925, CP 80/515; Zinsser review, *New Republic*, Dec. 22, 1925, CP 121/124.

86 Mencken review, *American Mercury*, Aug 25, 1925.

87 Arthur Keith to HC, May 4, 1922, CP 81/552; FD, Aug. 2, 1929. According to Fulton, Cushing was hurt, however, that none of Osler's family had responded to him in any way about the book.

88 HC to Dr M. Allen Starr, July 3, 1925, CP 84/595; HC to G. Grey Turner, July 23, 1925, 84/603; H.C. to William M. McIntosh, July 2, 1925, 83/579.

89 Percival Bailey and HC, *A Classification of the Tumors of the Glioma Group on a Histogenic Basis with a Correlated Study of Prognosis* (Philadelphia: Lippincott, 1926); E.E. Manuelidis, 'A Neuropathologist's Perspective on the Celebration of the 2000th Operation of Harvey Cushing,' *Journal Neurosurgery* 50 (Jan. 1979), 13–16.

90 *Studies in Intracranial Physiology and Surgery: The Third Circulation; the hypophysis; the gliomas* (Oxford: Oxford University Press, 1926); 'Ductless Glands: Discussion by Dr. Harvey Cushing,' Congress of American Physicians and Surgeons *Transactions* 13 (1925), 61–4.

91 *Studies in Intracranial Physiology and Surgery.*

92 Lewis H. Weed to HC, Jan. 26, 1925, CP 53/1079, 131/607.

93 HC to Edgar H. Wells, May 12, 1926, CP, 83/608; 'Consecratio Medici,' in *Consecratio*, 13.

94 HC to Bill, undated, 'Thursday,' WCA; Bill Cushing to 'Va,' May 19, 1924, CP 19/595.

95 HC to Bill, Dec. 16, 1925, CP 19/622; HC to Bill, Feb. 15, 1926, 19/623.

96 The account of the disaster is based on coverage in the *New Haven Register* and *New Haven Courier*, June 12–16, 1926, plus clippings from unidentified newspapers in the A.C. Klebs correspondence, item 82, MHLY. There is no mention of the accident in any Yale publications. Fulton, 534, mentions the accident without detail, except for the story about telling the operating-room team. The patient, Mrs Lillian Murphy, wrote to KC about the event after HC's death in October 1939, WCA. Betsey Cushing many years later told her daughters that Bill had quarreled with his father at their last meeting and they had not been reconciled at the time of his death. Her memory was erroneous about factual detail, though, and the story cannot be corroborated.

12: Johnson and Boswells

1 Elliott Cutler to MS, June 1926, SP 2/15; Leo Davidoff, 'Harvey Cushing as We Knew Him,' *Bulletin of New York Academy of Medicine* 30 (Nov. 1954), 903.

2 KC to HC, June 5, 1927, WCA; HC to KC, 'Friday Eve' [1927], WCA, and HC to KC, Aug. 15, 1934, in Estate Papers box, Will file, WCA; pages of automatic writing and notes from a seance, Estate Papers box, Will file; Edward Weeks, *In Friendly Candor* (Boston: Little, Brown, 1959), 105.

3 HC to Codman and Shurtleff, Aug. 27, 1925, CP 94/421; HC to V. Mueller, Jan. 31, 1933, 94/769; also 10/903ff, 94/377ff.

4 *Intracranial Tumours*, 32. His best discussion of radiotherapeutics is in 'Experiences with the Cerebellar Astrocytomas ...' *Surgery, Gynecology, and Obstetrics* 52 (Feb. 1931), 129–204, reprinted in *Selected Papers*, 184.

5 'The Meningiomas Arising from the Olfactory Groove and Their Removal by the Aid of Electro-Surgery,' Macewen Memorial Lecture, June 22, 1927 (Glasgow, 1927) reprinted in *Selected Papers*, 246; also 'Electro-Surgery as an Aid to the Removal of Intracranial Tumors,' *Surgery, Gynecology, and Obstetrics* 47 (Dec. 1928), 751–84, CP

132/747; E.R. Berry, Howard Kelley files, Dandy Papers, CAJHMI; HC operative note, quoted in Fulton, 537.

6 HC to Cecil Drinker, Apr. 20, 1927, CP 21/377; HC to Francis C. Grant, Apr. 20, 49/356.

7 HC to Curtis F. Burnam, Apr. 4, 1927, CP 68/582.

8 '"Dyspituitarism": Twenty Years Later,' *Archives of Internal Medicine* 51 (Apr. 1933), 487–557), reprinted in *Selected Papers*, 544; HC to Francis Benedict, Sept. 1, 1926, CP 7/883; HC to David Edsall, Oct. 11, 1927, 73/629; also HC to Herbert M. Evans and reply, Jan. 17, 1928, 22/183.

9 'Acromegaly from a Surgical Standpoint,' *British Medical Journal*, July 2 and 9, 1927, 1–9, 48–55, reprinted in *Selected Papers*, 357; HC and Leo. M. Davidoff, 'The Pathological Findings in Four Autopsied Cases of Acromegaly with a Discussion of Their Significance' (New York: Rockefeller Institute for Medical Research, Monograph no. 22, 1927); *Time*, May 2, 1927, in *Selected Papers*, 393.

10 'Experiences with Orbito-Ethmoidal Osteomata Having Intracranial Complications: With the Report of Four Cases,' *Surgery, Gynecology, and Obstetrics* 44 (June 1927), 721–42, CP 132/386; James Mitchell to HC, May 20, 1927, 132/398.

11 HC to Alexander Lambert, Oct. 24, 1919, et seq., CP 103/814ff.

12 HC to Leonard Wood, May 24, 1927, CP 54/1146. Details of the operation from the Wood file, CP 125/263ff, including HC's operative notes. The operation is also described in *Meningiomas*, 409–13; and in HC to Arnold C. Klebs, Sept. 8, 1927, 119/127, and HC to Gen. Hugh Scott, June 7, 1928, 46/310.

13 *Meningiomas*, 413.

14 Hugh Cairns to Barbara Cairns, Aug. 7, 1927, Cairns Papers, Flinders University, Australia.

15 HC memo, Sept. 1, 1927, CP 125/2.

16 FD, Aug. 28, 1927, MHLY.

17 J. Shepley to MS, Nov. 29, 1924, SP.

18 MS Diary, Sept. 27, 1926, SP; Hugh Cairns to Barbara Cairns, Sept. 28, 1926, Cairns Papers, Flinders University. See also G.J. Fraenkel, *Hugh Cairns: First Nuffield Professor of Surgery, University of Oxford* (Oxford: Oxford University Press, 1991).

19 Julia Shepley to MS, Feb. 6, 1925, SP; Lycurgus Davey, 'Obituary: John Farquhar Fulton,' *Journal of Neurosurgery* 17 (1960), 1119–26; Arnold Muirhead, 'John Fulton: Book Collector, Humanist, and Friend,' *Journal of the History of Medicine* 17 (Jan. 1962), 2–15.

20 HC to Worth Hale, Nov. 24, 1924, CP 24/21; FD, 1: 56.

21 For published biographical appreciations of MS by Elizabeth Thomson and others, see *Journal of the History of Medicine*, 1981, 129–67.

22 MS Diary, June 29, 1928, SP.

23 Hugh Cairns to Barbara Cairns, Aug. 7, 1927, Cairns Papers, Flinders University; the original letter of Jan. 1, 1927, could not be located in the Cairns Papers but is published in Fraenkel, *Hugh Cairns*, 52–3.

24 P. Bailey, 'Pepper Pot,' in Paul C. Bucy, ed., *Neurosurgical Giants: Feet of Clay and Iron* (New York: Elsevier, 1985), 74–89; a possibly less embellished version is in Bailey to JF, Sept. 4, 1945, FP 213/296.

25 Percival Bailey, *Up from Little Egypt* (Chicago: Buckskin Press, 1969), 30–1, 41, 112, 211; (groping) Bailey, 'Pepper Pot.'

26 W.P. Van Wagenen to A.J. McLean, May 23, 1932, *Notes on the History of the Founding of the Harvey Cushing Society*, AANS Archive; Henry L. Heyl, 'A Selection of Harvey Cushing Anecdotes,' *Journal of Neurosurgery* 30 (Apr. 1969), 370; also H.P. Sawyer to JF, Nov. 20, 1946, FP 217/340.

27 Hugh H. Trout to JF, Mar. 30, 1940, FP 216/330; Cairns anecdote in Edgar A. Kahn, *Journal of a Neurosurgeon* (Springfield, Ill.: Thomas, 1972), 186; MS Diary, July 25–9, 1929, SP.

28 Frederic Schreiber reminiscences, FP 215/325.

29 Ray and Scarff reminiscences, in 'Harvey Cushing as We Knew Him,' *Bulletin of New York Academy* (Nov. 1954), 902, 908.

30 MS Diary, Nov. 13, 1928, SP; MS to JF, Feb. 4 and 5, 1929, FP 2329.

31 Scarff in 'Cushing as We Knew Him,' 909; MS Diary, 31 Jan. to 3 Feb., 1930, SP.

32 HC to Gil Horrax, Apr. 12, 1929, CP 30/420.

33 Scarff in 'Cushing as We Knew Him,' 909; Loyal Davis, *A Surgeon's Odyssey* (New York: Doubleday, 1973), 139; also Richard A. Davis, 'The Brigham Diary of Loyal Davis: A Portrait of Harvey Cushing and a Neurosurgical Acolyte,' unpublished ms, 1993, AANS Archive.

34 Scarff in 'Cushing as We Knew Him,' 908.

35 Burt Wolbach to JF, Nov. 8, 1946, FP 217/340; Laura Baldwin to JF, Nov. 9, 1939, FP 213/296; Max Roesler to HC, Dec. 4, 1928, CP 44/701.

36 Fraenkel, *Hugh Cairns*, 53–4; Bailey, *Up from Little Egypt*, 210; Hugh Cairns to Barbara Cairns, May 5, 1927, Cairns Papers, Flinders University; Fraenkel, *Hugh Cairns*, 57.

37 Mary Cushing Diary, Mar. 28, 1927, WCA; Hugh Cairns to Barbara Cairns, Jan. 17, 1926, Cairns Papers, Flinders University.

38 Davis, *A Surgeon's Odyssey*, 185–6; Jacobson, 'Dr. Cushing,' FP 214/310; also Bailey, 'Pepper Pot.'

39 Fulton, 539.

40 Ibid.; Sir Geoffrey Jefferson, 'Harvey Cushing, 1869–1939,' in Bucy, *Neurosurgical Giants*, 52–67, and in *Selected Papers of Sir Geoffrey Jefferson* (London, 1960); also Jefferson notes on observing Cushing, 1924, 1937, AANS Archives; JF to parents, Aug. 14, 1927, CP 125/318.

41 JD, Aug 28, Sept. 5, Oct. 9, 1927.

42 MS Diary, June 27, 1928, SP.

43 Ibid., July 2, Oct. 30, 1928, Jan. 12, 1929, Aug. 14, 1928.

44 Ibid., Dec. 2, 1929.

45 Ibid., Mar. 2, 1929.

46 Mrs Albert Bigelow, 'Memoir of a Friend and Neighbor,' FP 213/297; KC to HC, June 5, 1927, WCA.

47 MS to JF, July 2, 1929, FP 2329; HC to H.R. Burgess, July 6, 1929, CP 6/397; Betsey Whitney, 'Draft of Information regarding Barbara Paley,' WCA.

48 Mary Cushing to HC, June 23, 1929, CP 19/184; Hugh Cairns to Barbara Cairns, May 5, 1927, Cairns Papers, Flinders University; Betsey Whitney, 'Draft of Information Regarding Barbara Paley,' WCA.

49 Hugh Cairns to Barbara Cairns, Jan 21, 1927, Cairns Papers, Flinders University; Mary Cushing Diary, 1927, WCA; also Mrs. Albert Bigelow, 'Memoir of a Friend and Neighbor,' FP 213/297.

50 Betsey Cushing to Kate Cushing, 'Sunday,' 1925, WCA; HC to Mary R. Hillard, Oct. 4, 1926, CP 27/412; Mrs Bigelow 'Memoir of a Friend and Neighbor.'

51 HC correspondence re Henry and Yale, CP 52/904–15; with Winternitz, 54/928ff; also HC to SC Harvey, July 6, Oct. 6, 1928, 28/1187–9.

52 HC to Warren R. Sisson, Feb. 9, 1928, CP 48/766; MS Diary, Mar. 24, 1929, SP.

53 MS Diary, Nov 25–9, SP; HC's appendectomies, Thomson, 226; William B. Spaulding, 'Should You Operate on Your Own Mother?' *Pharos of Alpha Omega Alpha* 55 (Summer 1992), 23–6; HC account of the operation is in HC to T.B. Futcher, Jan. 2, 1930, CP 25/26; MS to JF, Dec. 11, 1929, FP 2329.

54 MS Diary, Jan. 27 to Feb. 3, 1930, SP; HC to Wilfred Grenfell, Feb. 15, 1930, CP 26/725; HC to Arthur R. Ruggles, Feb. 15, 1930, 44/933; HC to Fred C. Walcott, Mar. 22, 1930, 53/698.

55 HC to Wilfred Grenfell, June 22, 1930, CP 26/739.

56 Diary, Apr. 4–9, 1929, SP.

57 MS Diary, Apr. 4–9, 22–4, 1929, SP; also HC to Milton Winternitz, Apr. 23, 1929, CP 54/953; HC to FDR, Jan. 26, Mar. 16, 1929, cited in Richard L. Rovit and William T. Couldwell, 'No Ordinary Time, No Ordinary Men: The Relationship between Harvey Cushing and Franklin D. Roosevelt, 1928–1939,' *Journal of Neurosurgery* 95 (Aug. 2001), 354–68.

58 HC to Elliott Cutler, May 23, 1927, CP 19/750.

59 MS Diary, Apr. 3 and 5–9, 1929, SP.

60 HC to KC, apparently Aug. 4, 1934, Estate Papers box, Will file, WCA; Mary C. Astor to Elizabeth Thomson, undated, ET Scrapbook, AANS Archives; also, Betsey Whitney, 'Draft of Information regarding Barbara Paley,' WCA.

61 Betsey Whitney, 'Draft of Information regarding Barbara Paley,' WCA.

62 HC to Perry Harvey, Jan. 8, 1930, CP 28/1074; David Grafton, *The Sisters* (New York: Villard Books, 1992), 8.

63 HC to Lucien Price, May 15, 1930, CP 43/1109; HC to Arnold C. Klebs, June 4, 1930, 32/667; HC to George Gorham Peters, June 11, 1930, 95/810; MS Diary, June 2–11, 1930, SP.

64 CP 10/20ff; also HC to Ed Bushnell, Apr. 16, 1927, 9/1288.

65 HC to C.F. Hoover, Aug. 3, 1923, CP 123/455.

66 Patient accounts files, CP 90–2 passim; HC to John Roodin, Mar. 4, 1926, 93/1008; H.L. Mencken to JF, Mar. 6, 1940, FP 1236/317.

67 HC to Lyman G. Richards, Feb. 27, 1926, CP 96/871; HC to Herman Plaut, Jan. 6, 1928, 93/955; HC to Richard M. Pearce, Apr. 23, 1920, 70/10.

68 HC to K. McKenzie, May 25, 1924, CP 37/9.

69 Gray Fund correspondence, CP 70/668ff; HC to J.B. Howland, Feb. 2, 1924, 97/450; Bronson S. Ray, *As I Remember It: An Autobiography* (New York: privately published, 1990), 106, 110; JF to Hugh Cairns Sept. 30, 1927, FP 13.

70 HC to B. Brouwer, Dec. 4, 1929, CP 9/944.

71 FD, Apr. 26, 1928; *Fourteenth Report of the Surgeon-in-Chief of the Peter Bent Brigham Hospital, 1927*, CP 132/640; *Eighteenth Report of the Surgeon-in-Chief … 1931*, 133/1038; Ray, *As I Remember It*, 98.

72 Kenneth M. Ludmerer, *Time to Heal: American Medical Education from the Turn of the Century to the Era of Managed Care* (New York: Oxford University Press, 1999), 56; HC, annual reports, passim; HC to A. Lawrence Lowell, Mar. 13, 1925, CP 76/190. See also Joseph C. Aub and Ruth K. Hapgood, *Pioneer in Modern Medicine: David Linn Edsall of Harvard* (Cambridge: Harvard Medical Alumni Association, 1970).

73 HC to Emile Holman, Feb. 15, 1927, CP 29/1287.

74 HC to Adolf Hanson, Mar. 26, 1935, CP 28/106; also 45/233ff for Rockefeller Foundation correspondence.

75 HC to David Edsall, May 25, 1927, CP 73/619; HC to Edsall, Apr. 8, Nov. 27, 1929, 73/749, 794; HC to Edsall, Sept. 5, 1927, unsent, 73/625.

76 Kenelm Winslow to HC, Mar. 5, 1930, CP 77/08; MS Diary, Mar. 17–18, 1930, SP; HC notes, 77/31ff; *Sixteenth Report of the Surgeon-in-Chief of the Peter Bent Brigham Hospital, 1929*, 133/315.

77 Edward D. Churchill, *Wanderjahr: The Education of a Surgeon* (Boston: Countway Library, 1990), 27; HC to Elliott Cutler, Apr. 5, 1930, CP 77/21; MS to JF, May 19, 1930, FP 2330; Aub and Hapgood, *Pioneer in Modern Medicine*, ch. 22.

78 HC to Arthur W. Elting, Apr. 10, 1929, CP 75/646.

79 HC to. S.B. Wolbach, Harvard Medical School, June 11, 1931, CP 54/1001.

80 HC to A. Warren Stearns, June 13, 1931, CP 47/36; Stearns to HC, June 12, 75/703.

81 HC to Philip Bard, Apr. 27, 1932, CP 75/723.

13: Sprinting to the Tape

1 Samuel H. Greenblatt, 'The Image of the "Brain Surgeon" in American Culture: The Influence of Harvey Cushing,' *Journal of Neurosurgery* 75 (1991), 808–11; David Riesman to HC, Sept. 27, 1926, CP 45/86.

2 HC to Arnold Klebs, Feb. 19, 1936. Klebs correspondence, MHLY.

3 HC to W.D. Sullivan, Dec. 24, 1926, CP 5/1052.

4 HC to E.G. Conklin, Sept. 16, 1927, CP 10/1086; HC to Wilbur Cross, Oct. 7, 1930, 13/516.

5 HC to Lieut. H.B. Sterling, Jan. 25, 1926, CP 47/72.

6 HC letter, Feb. 23, 1933, CP 13/357; HC to Charles S. Corey, Jan. 30, 1922, 10/1236.

7 HC to Hilbert F. Day, May 7, 1927, CP 20/1054.

8 *Career*, 30–1.

9 MS to JF, Jan. 21, 1929, FP 2329.

10 HC to L.G. Rowntree, July 5, 1928, CP 45/805; HC to Geo. W. Corner, Apr. 26, 1929, 7/13; also 76/984ff.

11 MS Diary, Apr. 16 and 17, 1929, SP.

12 '"Dyspituitarism": Twenty Years Later,' *Archives of Internal Medicine*, 51 (Apr. 1933), 487–557, *Selected Papers*, 531.

13 Vincent Massey to HC, Apr. 30, 1929, CP 35/905; HC to J.B. Collip, Feb. 25, 1933, 10/989.

14 HC to W.T. Bovie, May 19, 1928, CP 68/679; WD to HC, Dec. 7, 1927, CP 20/590; MS Diary, Apr. 29, 1929, SP; MS to JF, Apr. 29, 1929, FP 2329; Bronson S. Ray, *As I Remember It: An Autobiography* (New York: privately published, 1990), 99, 113; HC correspondence with G.H. Leibel, CP 68/567ff.

15 'Experiences with the Cerebellar Medulloblastomas: A Critical Review,' *Acta Pathologica et Microbiologica Scandinavica*, 7 (1930), 1–2, CP 133/346; Louise Eisenhardt and HC, 'Diagnosis of Intracranial Tumors by Supravital Technique,' *American Journal of Pathology* 6 (Sept. 1930), 133/555; *Report of the Surgeon-in-Chief of the Peter Bent Brigham Hospital*, 1929, 133/315; FD, Apr. 1–29, 1928.

16 HC and Louise Eisenhardt, 'Meningiomas Arising from the Tuberculum Sellae with the Syndrome of Primary Optic Atrophy and Bitemporal Field Defects Combined with a Normal Sella Turcica in a Middle-Aged Person,' *Archives of Opthalmology* (Jan. 1929), 1–41, and (Feb. 1929), 168–205; *Intracranial Tumours*, 74; Ray, *As I Remember It*, 104.

17 'Experiences with the Cerebellar Astrocytomas,' *Surgery, Gynecology, and Obstetrics* 52 (Feb. 1931), 129–204, reprinted in *Selected Papers*, 184–245; also *Intracranial Tumours*, 89–90; 'Electro-Surgery as an Aid to the Removal of Intracranial Tumors,' *Surgery, Gynecology, and Obstetrics* 47 (Dec. 1928), 751–84, CP 132/747.

18 'Cerebellar Astrocytomas,' in *Selected Papers*, 185.

19 HC to M.P. Smithwick, June 30, 1932, CP 46/840; MS to JF, Lincoln's birthday, 1929, FP 2329.

20 McLean to Oldberg, Mar. 15, 1930, Oldberg Papers, Yale; MS Diary, Apr. 21–3, 1930, SP.

21 Jefferson Lewis, *Something Hidden: A Biography of Wilder Penfield* (Toronto and New York: Doubleday, 1981), 118–25; HC to JF, July 21, 1931, CP 24/623.

22 *Meningiomas*, ch. 21.

23 *Intracranial Tumours*, 140–1.

24 HC to JB Howland, Oct. 22, 1927, CP 97/618; Fulton, 555.

25 *Intracranial Tumours*, 147.

26 Louise Eisenhardt, 'The Operative Mortality in a Series of Intracranial Tumors,' *Archives of Surgery* 18, part 2 (Apr.-June 1929; Cushing birthday volume), 1927–35.

27 HC, *Studies in Intracranial Physiology and Surgery* (Oxford: Oxford University Press, 1926), 121.

28 Eisenhardt, 'Operative Mortality.'

29 *Intracranial Tumours,* vii–viii, 4; William P. van Wagenen, 'Verified Brain Tumors: End Results of One Hundred and Forty-Nine Cases Eight Years after Operation,' *JAMA,* May 5, 1934, 1454–8; Hugh Cairns, 'The Ultimate Results of Operations for Intracranial Tumors: A Study of a Series of Cases after a Nine-Year Interval,' *Yale Journal of Biology and Medicine,* 8 (May 1936); W.R. Henderson, 'The Pituitary Adenomata: A Follow-Up Study of the Surgical Results in 338 Cases (Dr. Harvey Cushing's Series),' *British Journal of Surgery* 26 (1939), 811–921.

30 *Intracranial Tumours,* 105; HC to William P. Van Wagenen, Dec. 16, 1932, Feb. 25, 1933, CP 52/416, 419.

31 MS to JF, May 19, 1930, FP 2330; T. de Martel to HC, May 14, 1932, CP 37/998.

32 Richard F. O'Neill to JF, Apr. 11, 1942, FP 1236/320; HC, Aug. 22, 1929, Note on the Physiological Congress, in Fulton Memorabilia, Physiological Congress, Boston, 1929, MHLY; Fulton, 577–9.

33 JF to Arnold Klebs, Feb. 5, 1931, FP 100/1383; MS Diary, Oct. 18, 1931, SP.

34 HC letter, Mar. 18, 1931, CP 46/341; *Report of the Surgeon-in-Chief of the Peter Bent Brigham Hospital, 1930,* 133/628; Richard D. Light, 'Remembering Harvey Cushing: The Closing Years,' *Surgical Neurology* 37 (1992), 147–57. In several letters HC refers to his case of 'Berger's disease.'

35 HC to Arnold Klebs, Mar. 5, 1931, Klebs Papers, MHLY.

36 MS Diary, Oct. 18, 1931, SP; HC to W.G. MacCallum, Apr. 16, 1931, CP 36/583; Fulton, 604.

37 Elias E. Manuelidis, 'A Neuropathologist's Perspective on the Celebration of the 2000th Operation of Harvey Cushing,' *Journal of Neurosurgery* 50 (Jan. 1979), 13–16.

38 *Career,* 37–67.

39 FD, Aug. 20, 1931, et seq.; Fulton, 606–9; *Intracranial Tumours,* 147; HC note, CP 124/450–1; Light, 'Remembering Harvey Cushing: The Closing Years.'

40 HC, remarks at tomb, WCA; HC notes on Welch in Paris, CP 124/477–8; G.J. Fraenkel, *Hugh Cairns* (Oxford: Oxford University Press, 1991), 79.

41 HC to M.P. Smithwick, June 30, 1932, CP 46/840; MS Diary, Oct. 16, 1929, Dec. 2, 1929, SP; MS to JF, Nov. 10, 1928, FP 162/2328.

42 Simon Flexner and James Thomas Flexner, *William Henry Welch and the Heroic Age of American Medicine* (Baltimore: Johns Hopkins University Press, 1941), 419; Welch to HC, Apr. 12, 1926, HC to Welch, Apr. 13, CP 54/64.

43 William Welch to Elliott Cutler, May 2, 1929, CP 105/245; Joseph Ames to HC, Dec. 1, 1930, Cushing Papers, Correspondence about file, CAJHMI.

44 HC to John Howland, Nov. 27, 1920, CP 27/737; HC to Admission Committee,

Graduate Club, Yale University, Nov. 23, 1920, 26/348; HC to M.C. Winternitz, Feb. 11, 1928, 24/69; FD, May 6–9, 1929; HC to JF, May 8, 1929, 24/304-7; on Yale medicine generally, see Gerard N. Burrow, *A History of Yale's School of Medicine: Passing Torches to Others* (New Haven: Yale University Press, 2001).

45 M.C. Winternitz to HC, Nov. 20, 1930, CP 123/462; Robert M. Yerkes to James R. Angell, Dec. 22, 1930, 123/476.

46 David L. Edsall to HC, Apr. 27, 1931, CP 123/488; FD, May 26, 1931; KC to W.G. MacCallum, June 20, 1931, MacCallum Papers, CAJHMI.

47 JF to Arnold Klebs, Dec. 7, 1930, Klebs Papers, MHLY.

48 MS Diary, Oct. 18, Nov. 2–9, 1931, SP; Cushing-Cutler correspondence, CP 19/848ff; HC to Elliott Cutler, Dec. 15, 1931, 19/863.

49 A. Lawrence Lowell to HC, Nov. 12, 1931, CP 123/501; HC to Lewis Weed, Nov. 23, Dec. 3, 1931, et seq., 123/500–5; HC note on Welch, 123/582.

50 MS Diary, Nov. 5–7, 1931, SP; HC to A. Lawrence Lowell, June 29, 1932, CP 75/908.

51 Percival Bailey and Harvey Cushing, 'Studies in Acromegaly. 7: The Microscopical Structure of the Adenomas in Acromegalic Dyspituitarism (Fugitive Acromegaly),' *American Journal of Pathology* 4 (Nov. 1928), CP 132/692.

52 In her good doctoral thesis, 'The Integration of Science with the Healing Art: Harvey Cushing's Development of Neurosurgery, 1896–1912' (University of Minnesota, 1998), Ock-Joo Kim marshalls impressive evidence from the 1980s and 1990s to show that Cushing's early observations were substantially correct (212–36). Cushing's later work on the posterior pituitary hormone and the parasympathetic nervous system was published as six papers in the *Proceedings of the National Academy of Science* 17 (April and May 1931), 163–80, 239–64; his papers contain vast amounts of correspondence with J.J. Abel and Walter Cannon, among others, on the relevant physiological and research issues.

53 CP 70/340ff; HC to John Beattie, Apr. 25, 1932, 7/722

54 HC to Davie Marine, Mar. 12, 1932, CP 70/181; 'Peptic Ulcers and the Interbrain,' *Surgery, Gynecology, and Obstetrics* 55 (July 1932), 1–34. See also Gerald N. Grob, 'The Rise of the Peptic Ulcer, 1900–1950,' *Perspectives in Biology and Medicine* 46 (Autumn 2003), 550–66.

55 *JHH Bulletin* 50 (Mar. 1932), 137–95.

56 HC to JF, Mar. 4, Jan. 6, 1932, CP 24/725, 686.

57 HC to John Beattie, Apr. 25, 1932, CP 7/722; also HC to Leon Asher, Apr. 25, 4/368.

58 Percival Bailey to JF, Apr. 4, 1932, et seq., FP 13; Hugh Cairns to MS, June 2, 1932, SP; Parkes Webber to HC, May 25, 1932, CP 133/869; HC to W.G. MacCallum, Mar. 10, May 5, 1933, MacCallum Papers, CAJHMI; 'Further Notes on Pituitary Basophilism,' *JAMA* 99 (July 1932), 281–4; HC to Pierre Pusch, Feb. 11, 1935, CP 42/1143.

59 'A New Pituitary Syndrome,' editorial, *New England Journal of Medicine*, Mar. 24, 1932; 'A New Pituitary Syndrome,' editorial, *Lancet*, May 21, 1932; 'Basophil Adenoma of the Pituitary,' *British Medical Journal*, Aug. 20, 1932, 358, CP 133/879ff.

60 HC to Malcolm C. Ware, Lee Higginson Trust Company, May 4, 1932, et. seq., CP 34/293.

61 HC to James R. Angell, May 31, 1932, CP 4/110; HC to A. Lawrence Lowell, June 29, 1932, 75/908; James Angell to HC, June 12, 1932, et seq., 123/517.

62 Bronson S. Ray, *As I Remember It: An Autobiography* (New York: privately published, 1990), 109.

63 For the founding of the Harvey Cushing Society, see the two volumes of *Notes on the History of the Founding of the Harvey Cushing Society* in the AANS Archives; MS to JF, Apr. 26, June 9, 1932, FP 2331; FD, May 6, 1932.

64 HC to Elliott Cutler, Feb. 6, 1932, reply Feb. 12, CP 19/879; HC to M.P. Smithwick, June 30, 1932, 46/840; Ray, *As I Remember It*, 114; MS to JF, July 13, 1931, FP 2331.

65 FD, Jan. 19, 1932.

66 MS Diary, Oct 2–9, Nov. 8, 1932, SP.

67 Ibid., Nov. 5, 1932.

68 MS to Eric Oldberg, Jan. 11, 1933, SP, 7/100; HC to M.C. Winternitz, Oct. 22, 1932, CP 24/812; HC to S.C. Harvey, Dec. 31, 1932, 28/1223.

69 JF to HC, Mar. 9, 1933, CP 24/877; HC to James R. Angell, June 13, 1933, 123/547; MS to JF, June 14, 1933, FP 2332; Angell to HC, June 15, 1933, CP 123/549; HC to Simon Flexner, July 11, 1933, 23/459.

70 HC to A. Lawrence Lowell, [June 1933], CP 123/551, 75/910; James R. Angell to HC, June 23, 1933, 4/116; HC to O.R. Lanman, July 11, 1933, 33/251.

71 FD, Oct. 12, 1933.

14: Regius Professor at Yale

1 G.R.L. Putnam to HC, July 16, 1933, CP 134/178.

2 Fulton, 638; the paper was published as 'Hyperactivation of the Neurohypophysis as the Pathological Basis of Eclampsia and Other Hypertensive States,' *American Journal of Pathology* 10 (Mar. 1934), 145–75; also HC and K.W. Thompson, 'Experimental Pituitary Basophilism,' *Proceedings of the Royal Society* 115 B (May 1934), 88–100.

3 HC to C.S. Sherrington, Feb. 18, 1934, CP 48/623; HC to J. Irving, July 21, 1933, 30/922; HC to W.G. MacCallum, Jan. 29, 1934, 36/610; HC to L. Minor Blackford, Sept. 25, 1933, 5/832.

4 KC to Betsey Roosevelt, Mar. 10, 1933, WCA; MS to JF, Mar. 6, 1933, FP 2332.

5 FD, May 16, 1933.

6 *Career*, 68–102.

7 HC to H.H. Kerr, May 18, 1933, CP 32/462; Richard L. Rovit and William T. Couldwell, 'No Ordinary Time, No Ordinary Men: The Relationship between Harvey Cushing and Franklin D. Roosevelt, 1928–1939,' *Journal of Neurosurgery* 95 (2001), 354–68. On health insurance, see the extensive correspondence at CP 66/146ff, also Daniel S. Hirshfield, *The Last Reform: The Campaign for Compulsory Health Insurance in the United States, 1932–1945* (Cambridge: Harvard University Press, 1970).

8 HC to Ronald Brown, Dec. 26, 1934, CP 6/265; HC to Alan Gregg, Jan. 11, 1935, 66/371.

9 HC to FDR, Feb. 1, 1935, CP 66/505; HC to Edwin E. Witte, Feb. 4, 1935, 66/507.

10 HC to Reginald Fitz, Apr. 18, 1934, CP 13/174.

11 HC to Edgar Sydenstricker, Sept. 27, 1935, CP 66/827.

12 KC to Betsey, May 4, 1931, WCA.

13 FD, June 20, 1934; Fulton, 660, citing log of Richard U. Light.

14 Maud Herlihy memo for Betsey Whitney, Sept 4, 1986, WCA; Sally Bedell Smith, *In All His Glory: The Life of William S. Paley* (New York: Simon and Schuster, 1990), 247; HC to FDR, undated; FDR to HC, Feb. 24, 1936, cited in Rovit and Couldwell, 'No Ordinary time, No Ordinary men.'

15 HC to Marjorie R. Nesbit, Sept. 9, 1936, CP 39/539; HC to Glen Wright, Sept. 1, 1936, 54/1214.

16 FD, Oct. 22, 1936; JF to Arnold Klebs, Oct. 23, 1936, FP.

17 Correspondence in the tumor registry file, CP 52/395ff, and the Codman file, 12/485ff; also Christopher John Wahl, 'The Harvey Cushing Brain Tumor Registry,' (DM thesis, Yale University School of Medicine, 1996).

18 Tumor registry file; HC to JB Conant, June 12 and 27, 1934, CP 65/351–2.

19 Robert Van Gelder, *New York Times*, May 5, 1936, CP 113/816; Sidney I. Schwab to HC, Apr. 25, 1936, 113/800; Mark Van Doren, *Nation*, June 3, 1936, 113/912; HC to John W. Cummin, Sept. 27, 1937, 13/894; *SJ*, 373.

20 Edward Weeks, *In Friendly Candor* (Boston: Little, Brown, 1959), 98–116.

21 'The Doctor and His Books,' in *Consecratio*, 286.

22 E.P. Goldschmidt, 'Recollection of Harvey Cushing and His Book-Collecting,' *Journal of the History Medicine and Allied Sciences* 1, no. 2 (1945), 229.

23 Archie Malloch to HC, Mar. 15, 1938, et seq., CP 37/827ff.

24 'The Doctor and His Books,' in *Consecratio*, 270; also 'The Binding Influence of a Library on a Subdividing Profession,' in *Career*, 153–71; Geoffrey Jefferson, 'Harvey Cushing and His Books,' *Journal of the History of Medicine and Allied Sciences* 1, no. 2 (1945), 250.

25 Jefferson, 'Harvey Cushing and His Books,' 252; Goldschmidt, 'Recollections of Harvey Cushing,' 229; also Madeline Stanton, 'Harvey Cushing: Book Collector,' *JAMA*, Apr. 12, 1965, 149–52.

26 HC to Arnold Klebs, June 25, 1930, Klebs Papers, MHLY

27 MS Diary, Jan. 10–11, 1929, SP; MS to JF, Mar. 5, 1929, FP 2329; MS to JF, Jan. 19, 1929, FP 2329.

28 KC to HC, Jan. 28, 1927, WCA; HC to Dr Cullen, July 10, 1928, CP 103/209.

29 Fulton, 646–8; FD, Sept. 28, 1934; HC to Arnold Klebs, Oct. 4, 1934, reply Oct. 14, Klebs Papers, MHLY; JF to Arnold Klebs, Mar. 18, 1936, FP.

30 Barbara Cushing to Betsey Roosevelt, Sept. 13, 1938, WCA; Fulton, 640.

31 Jill Schulman to HC, Jan. 19, 1938, CP 46/549, reply Jan. 24, 46/555.

32 Zoltàn Haraszti to HC, Dec. 3, 1931, and reply Dec. 4, CP 28/470–1.

33 HC to Rudolph Matas, Apr. 4, 1932, et seq., CP 70/230–68; HC to James Bordley III, Dec. 12, 1936, 8/377.
34 HC to Francis W. Peabody, Aug. 3, 1916, CP 43/222.
35 HC to Dudley S. Blossom, Dec. 19, 1929, CP 5/905.
36 HC to W.G. MacCallum, Dec. 22, 1925, and undated reply, CP 72/610–11.
37 HC to A. Lawrence Lowell, Mar. 15, 1920, CP 35/230; HC to Joseph S. Ford, Dec. 2, 1922, 21/893.
38 HC to Emil Goetsch, May 8, 1928, CP 26/108; HC to G.J. Heuer, Mar. 19, 1931, 20/751; HC to Foster Kennedy, Dec. 10, 1928, 20/724; HC to Heuer, Mar. 25, 1931, 29/724.
39 HC to George O'Hanlon, Sept. 14, 1926, CP 75/522.
40 HC to Dr Robert T. Miller Jr, July 22, 1925, CP 76/658; HC to Sam. Harvey, Aug. 20, 1925, 28/1167; HC to Harry H. Barthman, Apr. 4, 1939, 5/353; Winternitz quoted in Edward C. Halperin, 'The Jewish Problem in United States Medical Education 1920–1955,' *Journal of the History of Medicine* 56, no. 2 (2001), 140–67.
41 HC to Arnold Klebs, Apr. 1, 1933, Klebs Papers, MHLY; HC to Franz Boas, Apr. 27, 1933, CP 12/737; C.F. List to HC, Mar. 21, 1933, and reply Mar. 30, 34/1046–8.
42 HC to C.F. List, Dec. 29, 1933, CP 34/1060; correspondence re the Emergency Committee, CP 69.
43 Brooks Mather Kelley, *Yale: A History* (New Haven: Yale University Press, 1974), 416; HC to Arnold Klebs, May 10, 1938, Klebs Papers, MHLY.
44 HC to Elsie Hooper, Apr. 29, 1938, CP 30/339.
45 HC to Arnold Klebs, May 10, 1938, Klebs Papers, MHLY; *Bulletin of the National Committee for the Resettlement of Foreign Physicians*, July 1939, CP 69/531.
46 HC to Dick Meagher, Jan. 10, 1936, CP 38/309; HC to Norman Dott, Feb. 2, 1936, 21/286.
47 Fulton, 697–700; HC to George W. Gray, Sept. 16, 1939, CP 25/488.
48 HC to Arnold Klebs, June 4, 1935, Klebs Papers, MHLY; FD, Dec. 10, 1936.
49 Fulton, 697–700; HC to Hugh Cairns, Aug. 11, 1938, CP 11/619.
50 Reviews at CP 87/01ff, especially *Archives of Neurology and Psychiatry*, Mar. 1939; Geoffrey Jefferson to HC, Dec 7, 1938, 87/93.
51 HC to Eric Oldberg, Mar. 29, 1938, et seq., CP 65/554ff.
52 Jack D. Pressman *Last Resort: Psychosurgery and the Limits of Medicine* (Cambridge: Cambridge University Press, 1998); Elliot S. Valenstein, *Great and Desperate Cures: The Rise and Decline of Psychosurgery and Other Radical Treatments for Mental Illness* (New York: Basic Books, 1986).
53 HC to Richard W. Brickner, July 20, 1937, and reply July 30, CP 87/198–9.
54 Fulton, 708.
55 Arnold Klebs to JF, May 7, 1939, FP.
56 HC to Rev. and Mrs. Peterson, Dec. 27. 1935, CP 42/690; HC correspondence with George Cushing, 15/551ff.
57 JF to Arnold Klebs, Mar. 1, 1935, FP; FD, Mar. 1–7, 1937.

58 FD, July 4–7, 1934; Barbara Cushing to Betsey Roosevelt, Sept. 13, 1938, WCA; KC to Betsey Roosevelt, Sept. 17, 1938.

59 Maud Herlihy memorandum, Sept. 4, 1986, WCA.

60 Barbara Cushing to Betsey Roosevelt, Sept. 13, 1938, WCA; KC to Betsey Roosevelt, Sept. 17, 1938.

61 Maude Herlihy letter, Feb. 21, 1992, WCA; Jimmy Roosevelt to 'Dr. Cush,' Dec. 19, 1938, WCA.

62 HC to Sen. Francis T. Maloney, Sept. 23, 1939, CP 35/762; HC to K.W. McKenzie, Sept. 14, 1939, 37/82.

63 HC, 'The Mayo Brothers and Their Clinic,' in *Career*, 301; HC to Malcolm Farmer, Sept. 15, 1939, CP 22/274.

64 HC to William H. St John, Oct. 2, 1939, CP 47/860; HC to Whom It May Concern, Oct. 2, 1939, 44/809.

65 Fulton, 712–13; JF to Arnold Klebs, Oct. 5 and 7, 1939, FP.

Closing: Inheritance and Memory

1 Autopsy: H.M. Zimmerman to John Fulton, May 24, 1940, FP, 216/334; Cushing Estate file, FP 219/351; earlier version in WCA.

2 Barbara Cushing to Watson Webb, 'Friday,' WCA; KC to JF, c. Sept. 29, 1943, FP 301.

3 Percival Bailey, 'Pepper Pot,' in Paul C. Bucy, ed., *Neurosurgical Giants: Feet of Clay and Iron* (New York: Elsevier, 1985), 88.

4 HC to KC, Aug. 15, 1934, Kate and Harvey Cushing Estate Papers, Will file, WCA.

5 David Grafton, *The Sisters: Babe Mortimer Paley, Betsey Roosevelt Whitney, Minnie Astor Fosburgh. The Lives and Times of the Fabulous Cushing Sisters* (New York: Villard, 1992); Sally Bedell Smith, *In All His Glory: The Life of William S. Paley* (New York: Simon and Schuster, 1990).

6 Lycurgus M. Davey, 'Louise Eisenhardt, MD: First Editor of the *Journal of Neusorugery* (1944–1965),' *Journal Neurosurgery* 80 (Feb. 1994), 342–6.

7 MS to Paul D. MacLean, Mar. 12, 1963, SP 7/93; 'Between the Lines,' ms on the writing of the Cushing biography, Fulton shelves, Cushing Room, MHLY.

8 Elizabeth H. Thomson, *Harvey Cushing: Surgeon, Author, Artist* (New York: Schuman, 1950); reaction from Betsey, Mary, and Barbara is in the Thomson scrapbook, AANS Archives.

9 'In Memory of Madeline Earle Stanton,' tributes and reminiscences, *Journal of the History of Medicine* 36 (April 1981), 129–50.

10 Bertram M. Bernheim to JF, June 14, 1947, FP 217/339.

11 Christopher John Wahl, 'The Harvey Cushing Brain Tumor Registry: Changing Scientific and Philosophic Paradigms and the Study and Preservation of Archives' (DM thesis, Yale University School of Medicine, 1996).

Acknowledgments

The warm and wise patience with which Elizabeth Bliss has lived with my research and writing was never more in evidence than during this project, and I am deeply grateful. Our lives are not like Harvey's and Kate's were, but I suspect Liz can sometimes see parallels.

The University of Toronto, where I have spent my academic career, made it possible for me to do this book by providing me with both time and research support as a consequence of my attaining our special rank of University Professor. I am particularly grateful to the Faculty of Medicine and the History of Medicine Program for providing me with a wonderful on-campus home and to Professor Edward Shorter and our administrator, Andrea Clark, for the best kind of professional companionship. In the company of Master John Fraser and other Fellows of Massey College, I was able during the course of the work to pause, take refreshment, and resume. Amanda Rogers did valuable spot library research, while Erica Charters made a side trip to the United Kingdom unnecessary. Susan Lamb lashed me into Power Point literacy, and Terry Dagradi handled picture research at Yale.

While this was not in any way an official or sanctioned biography, I received only enthusiastic help from the several members of the Cushing family I approached. I am particularly indebted to Harvey Cushing's (and FDR's) granddaughters, Kate Whitney and Sara Wilford, for making available to me the Cushing-Whitney Archive and for sharing memories. Kate Whitney offered insightful comment on early drafts of some of the chapters. Harvey Cushing's other line of descendants – neurosurgeons – also enthusiastically supported this project. I am particularly indebted to Dr Mark Bernstein in Toronto and Dr Dennis Spencer at Yale for allowing me to come into their operating rooms to observe some of the miracles of modern neurosurgery and patiently explaining how their procedures relate to the Cushing era. I saw Mark take out a meningioma and Dennis operate for epilepsy, and in Toronto I was also privileged to observe Drs Mike Tymianski and John Rutka remove an acoustic neuroma. All other neurosurgeons with whom I discussed Cushing were helpful and enthusiastic: special thanks to Dr Sam Greenblatt for early encouragement, Dr Ed Laws for reading the manuscript and making available to me his Geoffrey Jefferson documents, Dr Henry Brem at Johns Hopkins, and Dr Peter Maclaren Black at Harvard and at the Peter Bent Brigham Hospital.

Of the many librarians and archivists who helped provide me with access to material, Toby Appel of the Medical Historical Library at Yale bore by far the heaviest burden and always handled it easily. My special thanks also go to the staff in Manuscripts and Archives at Yale's Sterling Library, to Nancy McCall and her staff at the Chesney Archives at Johns Hopkins, to Jim Edmonson at the Dittrick Medical Museum in the Allen Medical Library in Cleveland, to Chris Phillips at the American Association of Neurological Surgeons, to Gillian Doolley at the Flinders University Library in Adelaide, and to those who helped at the Countway Medical Library, the Osler Library, the Western Reserve Historical Society, and the other institutions I approached.

I am indebted to Len Husband at the University of Toronto Press and Jeff House and Susan Ferber at Oxford for shepherding me from proposal to publication. Susan's editorial comments on the manuscript were particularly helpful, as were those of the anonymous readers used by the publishers. The manuscript was also read critically and helpfully by Dr Martin Edelstein, Dr Ed Laws, and Elizabeth Bliss. Jack Granatstein caught several errors in the chapters on the war, and Dr Bob MacBeth helped with an early draft of the first technical chapters. Carlotta Lemieux again did a wonderful copy edit. All remaining errors of fact and interpretation are my responsibility.

This project was a long and often solitary communion with Cushing and his times. For bits of help and encouragement and support along the way I am grateful to Dr Jeremiah A. Barondess, Dr John Carson, William Cushing, Dr John Dirks, Dr Earl Nation, Dr William Gibson, Kitty Dandy Gladstone, Drs Arthur Gryfe and the other members of the Toronto Medical Historical Club, Dr Norman H. Horwitz, Richard Landon, Shelley McKellar, Dr David Naylor, Ron Pruessen, Dr William Seidelmann, Eric and Lois Sinclair, Dr Ron Tasker, and Janice E. Mellian and Caren Nelson Schubart of the Cushing cottages at Little Boars Head, New Hampshire. Thanks and apologies to those whom I have inadvertently neglected to mention.

Illustration Credits

Alan Mason Chesney Medical Archives of the Johns Hopkins Medical Institutions: Johns Hopkins Hospital.

American Association of Neurological Surgeons: Victor Horsley; Cushing and Walter Dandy; Percival Bailey; Cushing at sixty; Welch, Klebs, Cushing; book collector; croquet player; last picture.

Max Brödel Archives, Department of Art as Applied to Medicine, Johns Hopkins University School of Medicine: Transphenoidal approach to the pituitary.

Countway Library of the History of Medicine, Harvard University: Harvard Medical School; Massachusetts General Hospital.

Cushing, Harvey. *The Pituitary Body and Its Disorders* (Philadelphia: Lippincott, 1912): Crowe and giant, p. 163.

Cushing, Harvey. *From a Surgeon's Journal* (Boston: Little, Brown, and Company, 1936): No. 46 Casualty Clearing Station.

Cushing (Brain Tumor) Collection, Yale University: Leonard Wood's tumor; dwarf patient; Timothy Donovan composite.

Cushing-Whitney Archive, privately held: The latch-keyers; Kate Crowell, 1894; the Cushing sisters.

Cushing-Whitney Medical Library, Yale University: Erastus Cushing; Henry Kirke Cushing; Betsey Williams Cushing; Harvey, aged two; Cleveland cousins; Cushing at Yale; the Yale Nine; Harvey Cushing, Yale '91; Cushing sketches; all-star surgeons; Harvey Cushing, 1900; Harvey Cushing, moustache; Harvey wooing Kate; Cushing's sketch of the brain; Theodor Kocher; Brödel sketch of sacral nerve; Research pose; Peter Bent Brigham Hospital; 305 Walnut Street; Alexis Carrel; reunited family; Fulton; Horrax; the 'harem'; Madeline Stanton; Cushing at bedside; Cushing and Foerster; Cushing, 1928; 2000th tumor; Kate Cushing.

Dittrick Medical History Center – Case Western Reserve University: Ned Cushing; G.W. Crile.

Mayo Foundation for Medical Education and Research: William & Charles Mayo.

National Library of Medicine, Bethesda, Md.: Henry Christian; E.A. Codman; Wm. T. Councilman.

National Portrait Gallery, Smithsonian Institution: Leonard Wood, by John Singer Sargent, 1903, oil on canvas, 76.5 cm x 63.8 cm.

Sterling Library, Yale University: New Haven *Evening Register*, 1926.

***U.S.S. Sequoia, Presidential Yacht*, Picture Gallery:** Surgeon and president.

William Paley Collection: Kate Cushing raising children.

Yale Museum of Art: Harvey Cushing by John Singer Sargent, 1916, charcoal (frontispiece).

Index

Also by Michael Bliss

Medical History

William Osler! A Life in Medicine
The Discovery of Insulin
Banting: A Biography
Plague: A Story of Smallpox in Montreal

Canadian History

Right Honourable Men: The Descent of Canadian Politics
from Macdonald to Chrétien
Northern Enterprise: Five Centuries of Canadian Business
A Canadian Millionaire: The Life and Business Times
of Sir Joseph Flavelle.
A Living Profit: Studies in the Social History
of Canadian Business, 1883–1911